Community Health
and Wellness 5
Primary Health Care in Practice

Anne McMurray

Jill Clendon

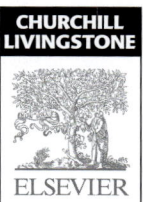

CHURCHILL
LIVINGSTONE

ELSEVIER

Sydney   Edinburgh   London   New York   Philadelphia   St Louis
Toronto

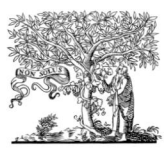

Churchill Livingstone
is an imprint of Elsevier

Elsevier Australia. ACN 001 002 357
(a division of Reed International Books Australia Pty Ltd)
Tower 1, 475 Victoria Avenue, Chatswood, NSW 2067

National Library of Australia Cataloguing-in-Publication Data

National Library of Australia Cataloguing-in-Publication entry

McMurray, Anne, author.

Community health and wellness: primary health care in practice/Anne McMurray, Jill Clendon.

5th edition.

9780729541756 (paperback)

Public health—Social aspects—Australia.

Health promotion—Social aspects—Australia.

Social medicine—Australia.

Clendon, Jill, author.

362.120994

Senior Content Strategist: Libby Houston
Content Development Specialist: Martina Vascotto
Project Manager: Anitha Rajarathnam and Srividhya Shankar
Edited by Laura Davies
Proofread by Shaukia Mir
Cover and internal design by Georgette Hall
Index by Robert Swanson
Typeset by Toppan Best-set
Printed in China by China Translation and Printing Services

Dedication

This book is dedicated to all those who care for communities.

Anne McMurray, Jill Clendon September 2014

Contents

Foreword

Dr **Rosemary Bryant AO, FACN**
Commonwealth Chief Nurse and Midwifery Officer

I am delighted to have been asked to write the foreword to this pertinent and valuable resource.

Primary health care, and the role of the nurse within this sector, is a very important topic for the nursing community and the health care system more broadly.

It is particularly timely given that we are rapidly moving from a demographic structure that was once characterised as an 'age pyramid' to one that is increasingly becoming dominated by the very elderly.

It is paramount that, as a first-class health system, we are able to offer excellence in nursing care to our ageing population in their homes, and in their communities.

As well as providing information about healthy ageing, this resource also offers a detailed section on sustainable health for families and individuals, emphasising the significance of healthy families and healthy children.

It is my strong opinion that health must be viewed on an age continuum, and the early acknowledgement of the importance of maternal, child and adolescent health, and healthy lifestyles, cannot be underestimated.

I firmly believe that inclusiveness and cultural sensitivity of our Indigenous population must always remain one of nursing's key goals. As the authors acknowledge in Chapter 13, a lack of cultural inclusive has an enormous impact on Indigenous health and wellbeing. As a population already experiencing disparate health outcomes, inclusiveness must remain at the core of nursing and midwifery care.

In Chapter 15, the authors acknowledge the variability of effective, efficient and appropriate care. With our fast-paced lives—both personal and professional—and our often changing workplaces, it is imperative that nurses are adaptive, and abreast of new evidence-based practice. The implementation of evidence-based practice is, in my opinion, the skill of the future.

In order for nurses to deliver high-quality care they also need access to the necessary resources that can empower them to deliver the right care and access to support mechanisms to encourage them to continue on their chosen path of delivering care for their communities. I believe this publication is one such resource.

I commend the authors on taking the initiative to write this well-informed publication, and I thoroughly recommend it to all nurses employed within the primary health care sector.

Rosemary Bryant
Chief Nurse and Midwifery Officer

Preface

This book is intended to guide the way nurses and other health professionals work with people to try to maintain health and wellbeing in the context of living their normal lives, connected to their families, communities and social worlds. Life is lived in a wide range of communities, some defined by socio-cultural factors such as ethnicity or Indigenous status, some defined by geography or 'place', others by affiliation or interest, and some by relational networks such as social media. Because most people live within multiple communities it is important to understand how their lives are affected by the combination of circumstances that promote or compromise their health and wellbeing. Knowing a person's age, stage, family and cultural affiliations, employment, education, health history, and recreational and health preferences has an enormous effect on the way we, as health professionals, interact with them. Likewise, our guidance and support are heavily influenced by the environments of their lives: the physical, social and virtual environments that contribute to the multilayered aspects of people's lives. Knowing how, why and where people live, work, play, worship, shop, socialise, and seek health care, and understanding their needs in these different contexts, underpins our ability to develop strong partnerships with people and communities to work together as full participants, in vibrant, equitable circumstances to achieve and enable *community health and wellness.*

This edition of the text represents contemporary thinking in community health and wellness from the local, trans-Tasman and global communities. We have added two new chapters, one on community assessment and another on working with groups. *Primary health care* (PHC) continues to be an integral approach to promoting health and wellness throughout the world and we apply the principles of PHC to our practices in this part of the world. These principles are outlined in Chapter 1 and elaborated throughout the text. A PHC approach revolves around considering the *social determinants of health* (SDH) in working in partnership with individuals, families and communities. The text examines the inter-relatedness of the SDH throughout the various chapters, to examine where such things as biological factors, employment, education, family issues and other social factors influence health and the way we approach our role in health promotion and illness

prevention. As partners our role is to act as enablers and facilitators of community health, encouraging community participation in all aspects of community life. Another foundational element that guides our consideration of community health is the notion that health is a *socio-ecological* construct. As social creatures we are all influenced by others and by our *environments,* sometimes with significant health outcomes. The relationship between *health* and *place* is therefore crucial to the opportunities people have to create and maintain health. Interactions between people and their environments are also *reciprocal*; that is, when people interact with their environments, the environments themselves are energised, revitalised, and often changed. Analysing these relationships is therefore integral to the processes of assessing community strengths and needs as a basis for health promotion planning, as we outline in the chapters of Section 1.

Our knowledge base for helping communities become and stay healthy is based on understanding the structural and social determinants of health that operate in both the global and local contexts. We also know with some certainty that what occurs in early life can set the stage for whether or not a person will become a healthy adult and experience good health during the pathways to ageing. Along a person's life pathway it is helpful to know the points of critical development and age-appropriate interventions, particularly in light of intergenerational influences on health and wellbeing. We outline some of these influences and risks in Section 2 of the book, which addresses healthy families, healthy children, adolescents, adults and older persons. After nearly a quarter of a century, the *Ottawa Charter* is still acknowledged by health promotion experts as the most useful guide for strategic health promotion planning with each of these groups. We use the symbol of the Ottawa Charter in each chapter in Section 2, to signal that the discussion is moving toward the challenges and solutions in assisting people to work towards the five elements of the Charter: healthy public policies, creating supportive environments, strengthening community action, developing personal skills and reorienting health services.

Maintaining an attitude of *inclusiveness* is the main focus of Section 3. Within the chapters of this section we suggest approaches that promote cultural safety and sensitivity in helping Indigenous people and others disadvantaged or discriminated against to develop their capacity for change. To enable capacity development we need to use knowledge wisely, which means that we need evidence and innovation for all of our activities. Clearly, our professional expertise rests on becoming research literate and developing leadership skills for both personal and community capacities to reach toward greater levels of health, vibrancy and sustainability for the future. Section 3 also addresses the policy and research interface, to consolidate some of the research information we provide throughout the book, and to emphasise the importance of evidence-based and evidence-informed practice to develop policies that promote and sustain health and wellbeing.

As you read through the chapters you will encounter the Mason family in Australia and the Smiths in New Zealand, both fly-in fly-out (FIFO) families. Their home lives revolve around their respective communities, but both families also deal with the challenges of male partners who work away from home in a Pilbara mining community. Throughout the chapters you will see how they deal with their lifestyle challenges and opportunities as they experience child care, adult health issues, and some of the characteristics of their communities that could potentially compromise their health and wellbeing. We hope you enjoy working with them and develop a deeper sense of their family and community development and how nurses can help enable health and wellness. At various stages of the chapters we outline important research studies that are helping to advance the knowledge base and a number of prompts to help refresh the main topics of our conversation with you and stimulate your thoughts on community health. We also urge you to be thinking of the 'big issues', which will be outlined in the reflective section at the end of each chapter.

Throughout the text we have added a series of reminders and practice strategies to connect each chapter with the foundational principles presented in the early chapters. We have also included some group exercises that can be used in practice or tutorial groups to help add depth to your considerations of how best to achieve community health and wellness.

About the Authors

Anne McMurray is a registered nurse, a Fellow of the Royal College of Nursing Australia and Member, Order of Australia (AM). She is Emeritus Professor, School of Nursing and Midwifery, Griffith University, Queensland, Emeritus Professor, School of Nursing, Murdoch University, Perth and Adjunct Professor, School of Nursing and Midwifery, University of the Sunshine Coast. Anne has practised in a range of nursing and community health settings in Canada and Australia, and is actively involved in research and research supervision, publishing and mentoring. She is an Expert Advisor on Primary Health Care to the International Council of Nurses. Anne was made a Member of the Order of Australia in the 2006 Queen's Birthday honours list for services to nursing, particularly in the development of nurse education and community health practices, and as a contributor to professional publications.

Jill Clendon is a registered nurse, member of the College of Nurses, Aotearoa, and is currently working as a nursing policy advisor and researcher for the New Zealand Nurses Organisation. She is also an Adjunct Professor at Victoria University, Wellington. Jill spent the 12 years previous to her current position in nursing education, teaching at both undergraduate and post graduate levels with a specific interest in primary health care and child and family health. Jill's research has examined the efficacy of community-based nurse-led clinics, and the historical and contemporary context of community-based well child care in New Zealand. Jill holds a PhD in Nursing and a Masters of Philosophy in Nursing from Massey University and a Bachelor of Arts in Political Studies from Auckland University. She is Chairperson of Victory Community Health in Nelson, and member of the Nelson Bays Primary Health Care Nurse Advisory Group. Jill has a background in public health nursing and, in her spare time, runs a volunteer, after-hours nurse-led clinic in Nelson.

Acknowledgements

We would like to acknowledge those who helped shape our thinking during the contemplation and writing of this book: students, colleagues and friends, who continue to provide stimulating ideas. Our thanks go to all of those who shared their stories and their photos with us to make the text come alive in the hearts and minds of community practitioners. We are grateful to our reviewers who helped strengthen the book, and the team at Elsevier who provided invaluable assistance in producing this work. Bringing a trans-Tasman perspective to the book has been both challenging and rewarding. Being able to bounce ideas off one another and melding together the various perspectives we bring has been both inspirational and enjoyable. We hope that communities on both sides of the Tasman will benefit from the insights that working together has brought. We would also like to thank our families for their support and patience.

Reviewers

Sharon Laver
RN; Master Arts (Social Ecology); Grad Dip Adult Education and Training, and Grad Dip. Health Management
Member, Australian College of Nursing (MACN)

Ailsa Munns
RN RM CHN BachAppSc (Nursing); Master Nursing
Lecturer, Course Coordinator Child and Adolescent Health Programs
Coordinator Community Mothers Program (WA)
School of Nursing and Midwifery
Curtin University

Louise O'Brien
BA RN PhD
Conjoint Professor of Nursing, University of Newcastle, Australia

Naumai Smith
RGON, BA(Ed), MHSc
Associate Dean (South Campus)
Faculty Equity and Diversity Portfolio Holder
Auckland University of Technology, New Zealand

Jane Taylor
PhD, MHlthProm, GCIntHlth, BEd
Lecturer in Public Health, School of Health and Sport Sciences, University of the Sunshine Coast, QLD, Australia

Judy Yarwood
RN, MA (Hons), Dip Tchg (Tertiary), FCNA (NZ)
Nursing lecturer, Department of Nursing and Human Services
Christchurch Polytechnic Institute of Technology, Christchurch

SECTION 1
Working with Communities

Introduction to the Section

The six chapters that introduce this text provide a foundation to help frame what we understand about communities in contemporary society, and how community health and wellness is achieved and maintained. Chapter 1 defines 'community' and the principles and foundations for creating and maintaining community health. The overall goal for those working with communities is to nurture health within a primary health care (PHC) philosophy; that is, providing care for the community and its people in a way that is socially just. This overarching goal is guided by an understanding of the social determinants of health (SDH). The SDH outlined in Chapter 1 explain that health is a product of social and environmental factors, which underlines the importance of *place* in health. In Chapter 2 we address communities of place, beginning with the global community and examining features of urban and rural communities in Australia and New Zealand. We take an in-depth look at FIFO communities, and some of the circumstances of these communities which influence the lifestyles of the Mason and Smith families. The chapter then examines relational communities of people bound together virtually through electronic and social media, and communities of affiliation, which create a bond based on occupation, religious or cultural characteristics.

As we outline in Chapter 3, working with communities requires comprehensive knowledge of their circumstances. A number of models of assessment are outlined to illustrate unique features of each as well as common elements that provide the foundations for planning. We track the development of these assessment models, and provide some critique of their usefulness in the current context where assessment strategies should be informed by knowledge of the social determinants of health (SDH). We introduce a new model, the *SDH Assessment Circle*, as a unique approach to including the SDH in community assessment, and provide some examples of its appropriateness in assessing families such as the Smith and Mason families within the context of their communities.

Community assessment provides a guideline for health promotion, as we explain in Chapter 4. The PHC principles situate people's aspirations for health within an ethos of *social justice*. The challenge of PHC lies in promoting *inclusive* conditions that would provide *equity* and *access* to supports, care and services for all members of a community or a population. The strategies for achieving these goals are embedded within the roadmap of the Ottawa Charter, based on community partnerships for empowerment, intersectoral collaboration, appropriate use of technology and cultural sensitivity. These strategies reflect the focus on health promotion in the settings of people's lives; healthy neighbourhoods, healthy schools, healthy workplaces and places of worship, healthy villages, cities and communities. Two critical, inter-related concepts are fundamental to helping communities: *empowerment* and *health literacy*. Community empowerment is possible when members of a community have genuine opportunities and support for health decision-making. Such decisions are informed by adequate, appropriate and useful knowledge; that is, health literacy. A health literate community is one where people are not only aware of the things that keep them healthy, but they feel confident making choices that influence their health, and they are comfortable working with health professionals to improve their health and the health of their community.

Health literacy and community empowerment are revisited throughout the text as central themes in health promotion. As current researchers argue, if people have a functional understanding of the reasons they are being urged to create a smoke-free environment, grow healthy foods for consumption, and lobby their local government for space to engage in a physically and socially vibrant lifestyle, they are more likely to participate in these aspects of healthy lifestyles. If they are able to access appropriate and accurate information on the internet to help alleviate any health problems, this can also be helpful. And when they are in the process of recovery from illness or rehabilitation, health literacy can help allay fears and anxieties by providing greater predictability in their pathway to better health. Importantly, members of health literate communities can become a resource for others who may need a greater understanding of the structural and social determinants of health as a basis for making appropriate choices for good health.

Chapter 5 extends our discussion of health promotion strategies to a wide range of nursing roles and the many ways in which we can enable community capacity. Nurses and other health professionals assist communities using a *comprehensive primary health care* approach, which supports all aspects of community life, helping to conserve what is special and helpful, and assisting them in countering what is not. Other activities are aimed at *selective primary health care*, which is a more targeted approach, where specific groups or issues are given priority attention. Because PHC has become integral to professional practice in both Australia and New Zealand we examine the PHC roles in the context of various

models of practice and the situations that guide role development, including rural and remote nursing, child, school and occupational health nursing, community mental health and the more generic roles of practice nurses and nurse practitioners. In today's health care environments nurses undertake a range of these traditional roles and some that have evolved in response to contemporary lifestyles. We describe some of these new roles and examine their effectiveness in a range of health service contexts.

In this era of instant communication, nurses and other health professionals are using accessible technologies to help people change. Chapter 6 outlines some of these strategies and explores their viability for working with groups. As nurses, we can become fully engaged with our community some of the time, and sit as a 'guide on the side' at other times, but always using our expertise and our evidence as resources to their efforts. The chapter therefore deals not only with the dynamics of group work, but leadership in helping people change and achieve their goals.

CHAPTER 1

Creating and maintaining a healthy community

Introduction

For most people, 'community' is a friendly term, conjuring up a sense of place, a sense of belonging. Healthy communities are those places where belonging is valued, where the connections between individuals, families and the environments of their lives are as important as the life forces within. This is essentially an ecological relationship. *Ecology* embodies the idea that everything is connected to everything else. Health is both a social and ecological phenomenon, in that it is created and maintained in the context of community life. Although as individuals we can experience relative states of health or ill health because of our biological make-up, these are manifest within the social ecology of a community. Health is therefore dynamic, changing as a function of the myriad interactions between biology and our genetic predispositions, and the psychological, social, cultural, spiritual and physical environments that surround us.

As health professionals our role in working with communities is quite different to working within a health care institution. Whereas institutional care is focused on an episode of illness, the community role ranges from preventing illness to protecting people from harm or worsening health once they have experienced illness, to recovery and rehabilitation. To undertake this type of role requires extensive knowledge of people in the many contexts of their lives. Community practice also revolves around caring for the community itself. It is *multilayered* in that it can include protecting communities from harm or stagnation, helping its citizens to enhance their existing capacity for future development by fostering *health literacy* (that is, knowledge that contributes to health and wellbeing), working in partnership with them to become *empowered* to make decisions that will maintain the community's viability and capability to cope with any future challenges.

Working with communities to promote health and wellness requires a combination of foundational knowledge about health, including the role of social and environmental factors, having the intellectual curiosity to seek out and, in some cases, generate research evidence for interventions, and commitment to social engagement with the community. Specifically, there is a need for thorough assessment skills, ongoing surveillance and monitoring, intervention and evaluation strategies, and political advocacy to lobby for family and community resources and supports.

The philosophical foundation for this type of practice is entrenched in the World Health Organization's (WHO) definition of health, where health is not seen as one half of a dichotomy of health and illness, but 'a state of complete physical, mental and social wellbeing and not merely the absence of disease or infirmity' (WHO 1974:1). The WHO definition of health also reflects the importance of the social determinants of health (SDH). What this means is that health is determined within the social world that circumscribes people's lives. Researchers have found that the SDH are even more influential on the health of the population than medical care, with studies showing the greatest health gains in the population over the past two centuries are from changes in broad economic and social conditions (CSDH 2008). Based on this knowledge that it is the real world conditions of people's lives that make them healthy, our health care agenda is not one of providing endless services, but a carefully considered primary health care (PHC) approach to helping people create and maintain health.

> **WHAT IS ... HEALTH?**
>
> A multilayered social and ecological phenomenon created in the context of community life.

> **WHAT DO YOU THINK?**
>
> The World Health Organization defines health as 'a state of complete physical, mental and social wellbeing and not merely the absence of disease'.
>
> How is this definition congruent with the idea of health as a social and ecological phenomenon?

OBJECTIVES

By the end of this chapter you will be able to:

1   explain health, wellness and community health as socio-ecological concepts

2   identify the social determinants and structures of health and wellness

3   analyse the principles of primary health care and their usefulness in promoting individual and community health

4   examine the factors that influence community sustainability

5   explain the concept of social capital and its contribution to community health

6   explain the importance of health literacy in empowering people to enhance community health capacity

7   investigate the role of research and evidence-based practice in promoting community health.

Healthy communities are dynamic, constantly changing as people respond to the circumstances of their life and their environments and as they make decisions that help enhance their community's health capacity. Positive interactions change environments, conserving what is precious, rejecting influences that could be destructive. In a perfect world, there would be no need for health professionals to meddle in these interactions, but we all live in situations that could be improved. As health professionals we can help inform community members about the political, economic and cultural conditions which have an impact on their health and the health of their community. In this respect, we are a resource to the community, using our scientific knowledge and access to information to help promote and preserve health and treat illness.

This chapter examines the various social and ecological determinants of health, and some of the ways they influence the health of the local and global communities and the people who live there. With this knowledge we can develop strategies for using the principles of PHC to help people make decisions for personal and community health and wellbeing. We provide several examples of research studies to provoke your thinking about the rationale for various practice strategies, and how research findings can be used to optimise health. The case study for this chapter also introduces the Masons and the Smiths, both fly-in fly-out (FIFO) families, the Masons from Maddington in Western Australia, and the Smiths from Papakura in South Auckland. We hope you enjoy working with the families and find their lives interesting in terms of their challenges and potential for community health and wellness.

THE ECOLOGICAL, MULTILAYERED PERSPECTIVE OF COMMUNITY HEALTH

What is health?

As mentioned previously, health is a product of reciprocal interactions between individuals and their environments. Each of us brings to our environmental interactions a number of factors unique to us alone. These include the following:

*   a personal history
*   our biology as it has been established by heredity and moulded by early environments
*   previous events that have affected our health, including past illnesses or injuries
*   our nutritional status as it is currently, and its adequacy in early infancy
*   stressors; both good and bad events in our lives that may have caused us to respond in various ways.

REMINDER: Health is ecological

Biological factors provide the foundation for an individual to develop into a healthy person, but these are shaped by the environments or conditions of their lives.

Clearly, health is multifaceted. Becoming and staying healthy 'depends on our ability to understand and manage the interaction between human activities and the physical and biological environment' (WHO 1992: 409). Biological factors provide the foundation for an individual to develop

5

as a relatively healthy person, which is an adaptive process. Personal development occurs when an individual is engaged in progressively complex, regular reciprocal interactions with their environment (Bronfenbrenner 1979). Reciprocal exchanges between people and their environments therefore build the capacity for individual and community health. This process begins with the individual. From birth, individuals are programmed to develop certain biologically preset behaviours at critical and sensitive developmental periods. This is called 'biological embedding', and it influences how people interact with the genetic, social and economic contexts of their lives (Best et al. 2003). However, the environments or conditions of a person's life shape biological factors and the way individuals respond to the world around them (Hertzman 2001; Hertzman & Power 2006). These include both physical and social environments that include family and community characteristics and aspects of the wider society that create opportunities or threats to health.

spaces they inhabit and the resources they use. There are almost as many definitions of community as there are communities. When people are asked to articulate what community health means to them, the answers vary from different beliefs, to various ways of becoming healthy, to determinants of health in their community. Researchers often define community in terms of the context, and this can be geographical or social. For example, when members of a self-help community were asked to define what community meant to them, they came up with a consensus view that it was:

> *A group of people with diverse characteristics who are linked by social ties, share common perspectives, and engage in joint action in geographical locations or settings. (MacQueen et al. 2001:1929)*

Implicit in this definition of 'community' is the notion that a community is goal directed; that is, the community is a context for action.

BUILDING THE FOUNDATIONS FOR HEALTH

Ecological: everything is connected to everything else

Dynamic and socially determined: health is situated in the multilayered, real-world, social contexts of community life

Reciprocal: health is created in the exchanges between people and their environments

Health literacy: adequate knowledge to inform health decisions

Empowerment: knowledge and opportunity to have control over one's life and health decisions

---

WHAT IS ... COMMUNITY?

- A place we share with others?
- A network of like-minded people?
- A group who live, work and play together?
- An interdependent group of people inhabiting a common space?
- A context for action?

What do we mean by community?

In the most basic terms, the word community simply means that which is common. We often think of a community as the physical or geographical place we share with others, or the place from which care is delivered (Crooks & Andrews 2009). However, the ecological view focuses on the community as an interdependent group of plants and animals inhabiting a common space; that is, a natural ecosystem (Hancock 2011). People depending on one another, interacting with each another and with aspects of their environment, distinguish a living community from a collection of inanimate objects. Communities are thus dynamic entities that pulsate with the actions and interactions of people, the

GROUP EXERCISE: The impact of social and physical environments on health

Throughout the text we have included shaded boxes like this one to introduce group exercises. These exercises are designed to encourage students to work together on a topic and may require ongoing work throughout a chapter.

Working in small groups, make a list of the types of social and/or physical environments that may impact on health. You may want to make two lists—environments that impact on health positively, and those that impact negatively.

As you work through the chapter, keep adding to your lists.

What is community health?

When people are asked to define community health, their responses usually reflect a philosophical view of community, or *how* health is achieved in the community rather than what constitutes community health. For example, Baisch (2009:2472) defines community health as 'grounded in philosophical beliefs of social justice and empowerment. It is achieved through participatory, community development processes based on ecological models that address broad determinants of health' (Baisch 2009:2472). Healthy communities are the *synthesis* or product of people interacting with their environments when they work collaboratively to shape and develop the community in a way that will help them achieve positive health outcomes.

Our definition of community health is as follows:

Community health is characterised by the presence of strong social capital, engaged and empowered community members, a dynamic and healthy physical, social and spiritual environment, accessible, affordable and equitable services and resources, and a system of governance that is inclusive and responsive to community members in addressing the SDH.

This and other definitions of community health embody an ideal where all community members strive towards a common state of health. Of course, in real life, communities and societies are neither consistent nor stable, which reflects the variability among individuals and the dynamic changes that occur in people's social lives. Social conditions are particularly important to community health, because social environments provide the context for interactions in all other environments. When the social environment is supportive, creating a climate of trust and mutual respect, people are more likely to be *empowered,* in control of their life, and therefore their health (Wiggins 2011). We call this *social inclusion.* On the other hand, if their social situation is plagued by civil strife, an oppressive political regime, crime, poverty, unemployment, violence, discrimination, food insecurity, diseases or a lack of access to health and social support services they may be *disempowered,* leaving them less likely to become healthy or recover from illness when it occurs. As Wallerstein (2002:73) explains, empowerment is 'a social action process by which individuals, communities and organisations gain mastery over their lives in the context of changing their social and political environment to improve equity and quality of life'. When people live in situations of disadvantage or disempowerment they are unable to access the same resources for health as those who live in more privileged situations and their lives and potential for the future are compromised. This is called *social exclusion.*

WHAT IS ... EMPOWERMENT?

Empowerment is a key construct in health promotion wherein people are enabled to feel in control of their lives.

The issues that arise from power imbalances and unfair societal structures create inequalities in health across the community and society itself (Edwards & MacLean Davison 2008; Marmot 2006). To redress the inequalities and create a more just, equal and inclusive society requires community empowerment, where individuals become motivated to bring about community change through advocacy (Wiggins 2011). Advocacy involves promoting or 'championing' the needs of the community in such a way as to help people participate fully in decisions that affect their lives, their health and their communities. This type of 'people power' or community activism, supported by health professionals and other community advocates, can equalise power relationships, resulting in improvements to health, reduction in community risk factors and rearrangement of the structural conditions that support health and wellness.

BUILDING THE FOUNDATIONS FOR A HEALTHY COMMUNITY

Community: a shared place, a network, an interdependent group, a dynamic entity, a context for action

Community health: a product of

- participatory community development
- collaborative interaction with the environment to create and maintain health
- social inclusion
- empowered citizens
- healthy physical, social and spiritual environment
- accessible, affordable, equitable, responsive services and resources.

The role of health professionals in community health:

- promoting health and providing care where people live, work and play
- advocating for the community, its people and its physical, social, spiritual environments

- promoting equity, access, social inclusion and adequate resources by assessing community needs and disadvantage and then lobbying for change where required
- encouraging empowerment and health literacy to promote citizen participation in decisions for health and wellbeing
- generating the evidence base relative to community health needs.

COMMUNITY HEALTH AND WELLNESS

Healthy people's lives are characterised by balance and potential. In a balanced state of health there is harmony between the physical, emotional, social and spiritual. When they are part of a healthy community there are opportunities for them to reach and maintain high levels of health or wellness. Wellness, in this context, means the dynamic relationship between people and their environment that arises when individuals use that environment to maintain balance and purposeful direction (Dunn 1959). This socio-ecological connectivity between people and their environments embodies community health and wellness in that people feel supported and able to develop health capacity. For example, they may feel they have lifestyle choices, and if they choose, they will be able to exercise or relax in safe spaces. They have access to nutritious foods; students balance study with recreation; young families immunise their children and have time out from work to socialise. Older people are valued for their contribution to the community, inclusive policies promote opportunities for all citizens to participate fully in the community and lead a high-quality, happy life.

WHAT IS ... WELLNESS

A state of harmony between the physical, emotional, social and spiritual health of the individual and their environment.

What does happiness have to do with it?

The importance of happiness has been acknowledged by many researchers, who recognise that happiness, quality of life and our interactions with the environment are all instrumental in creating health and wellbeing in any given community (Helliwell et al. 2012; Rossouw &

Pacheco 2012; Tafarodi et al. 2012). Although most of us enjoy having something to strive for, consumer goods and possessions offer hollow outcomes compared to meaningful interactions in our social world. The importance of these interactions also extends to the global community. In 1972, the King of Bhutan made the world take notice of that small country by taking a leadership role in arguing that nations should be concerned with the ultimate purpose in life, which is happiness. He proposed a gross national happiness (GNH) index comprised of psychological wellbeing, the use of time, community vitality, cultural diversity and resilience, health, education, environmental diversity, living standard and governance, rather than focusing on economic indicators of success such as gross domestic product (GDP) (GNH. Online. Available: www.grossnationalhappiness.com [accessed 11 January 2013]). Since that time, many initiatives have been developed to try to bring this balanced and socially responsive perspective of health and happiness into mainstream thinking. The Happy Planet Index, developed in the UK, refocused wellbeing on the criteria of average life expectancy, life satisfaction and the ecological footprint. The Canadian Index of Wellbeing has also adopted this approach, computing measures of quality of life into social, economic and environmental trends in Canadian cities (Hancock 2009). Australia and New Zealand have also developed a number of happiness indicators, some of which tend to survey satisfaction with life while others ask people to rank their level of happiness. Importantly, both countries report that most of the population is highly satisfied with their lives and/or very happy (UMR. Online. Available: http://umr.co.nz/updates/how-happy-are-new-zealanders, http://www.abs.gov.au/ausstats/abs@.nsf/mediareleasesbytopic/C4BC45C467B5B87 [accessed 11 January 2013]).

Our self-happiness ratings have been reinforced by comparisons with other nations in the annual World Happiness Report, where New Zealanders and Australians are considered among the top ten happiest nations (8 and 9 respectively) (Helliwell et al. 2012). Because researchers have used a variety of conceptual approaches to methodologies and measurement, cross-country comparisons (see Box 1.1) are somewhat imprecise, but there is no disputing the fact that being happy with one's life and opportunities is a good thing. However, with the privilege of happiness comes the responsibility to take our place as global citizens and participate in creating an equitable, inclusive and viable global community.

BOX 1.1 'Happy' research

An interesting study at the University of Toronto explored whether there are distinctive culturally determined aspects of happiness. The researchers asked university students from Canada, China, India and Japan what they held to be most important for assessing the worth of their lives. In other words, they were asked 'what makes your life worth living? What is or should your life be about? If you were at the end of your life what would you point to as evidence that you had led a worthy or good life?'

Interestingly, the most frequently occurring responses showed common, rather than culturally unique, values. These included the following:

1 having close and enduring friendships
2 happy and healthy family
3 positive impact on others
4 loving marriage or romantic partnership
5 good wealth or assets
6 successful career
7 achievement of great things
8 a moral life
9 wisdom.

So what does this tell us?

Although there were some minor cultural differences among the responses, the researchers were led to conclude that in today's globalised society there are more shared, common elements in our values, meanings and commitments than there are differences. This is interesting in relation to our understanding of what constitutes 'culture' (Tafarodi et al. 2012).

HEALTH, HAPPINESS AND SUSTAINABLE DEVELOPMENT

WHAT DO YOU THINK?

Would happiness and sustainability provide a better basis for a world economy than the current financial system?

The World Happiness Report, which is produced by the Earth Institute at Columbia University in the US links happiness and health to sustainable development, arguing that human wellbeing, social inclusion and environmental sustainability are inextricably linked (Earth Institute. Online. Available: www.earth.columbia.edu/worldhappinessreport [accessed 11 January 2013]). Like other measures of a good life, the Earth Institute addresses health from a socio-ecological perspective, on the basis that happiness and wellbeing increase longevity and make immune systems more robust (Helliwell et al. 2012, Layard 2005). As one of the key Earth Institute researchers laments, the great contradiction in our world is that many of us enjoy sophisticated technologies and unprecedented wealth, while one billion people go without enough to eat each day (Sachs 2012). Yet the paradox of modern life, called 'Modernity's Paradox', is that in achieving affluence and progress in our developed nations we succumb to new crises of obesity, smoking, diabetes, depression and other ills (Li et al. 2008). Many of these illnesses are 'disorders of development', and they are accompanied by the loss of community, the decline of social trust, and rising anxieties about the global economy and unemployment (Sachs 2012). Clearly, economic issues and consumerism are limited in terms of creating health and happiness. Although most of us enjoy having something to strive for, consumer goods offer hollow outcomes. Instead, we may find higher levels of wellness in communities that allow people to live in a stable, democratic society, to enjoy the company of family and friends, to have rewarding work that yields sufficient income, to feel personal happiness with the ability to address any mental health problems, to set goals related to common values, and to have some means of attaining guidance, purpose and meaning (Diener & Seligman 2004). To help the global community achieve similar levels of health and wellbeing requires commitment to global sustainability.

SUSTAINABILITY

The ability of communities to function effectively with available services for the foreseeable future by mobilising resources.

In today's society we hear much discussion about sustainability, particularly in relation to global warming, climate change and a plethora of environmental factors that have far-reaching effects around the globe. For example, we know that systemic inequities interfere with our ability to protect all people from the effects of climate change (Bowen et al. 2012). It is therefore important that policymakers and those making decisions for the

> **BOX 1.2 Five principles of sustainable development**
>
> 1   Living within environmental limits
> 2   Ensuring a strong, healthy and just society
> 3   Achieving a sustainable economy
> 4   Using sound science responsibly
> 5   Promoting good governance
>
> (Source: Sustainable Development Commission in Porritt 2012 S24).

good of the community are clear on the disproportionate effects environmental degradation has on the most vulnerable citizens (Bowen et al. 2012). Over the past decade health scholars have begun to address these issues, focusing on the interdependence of the health and sustainable development agendas by linking sustainability to health equity (Porritt 2012). In 2010–11 The Sustainable Development Commission in the UK identified five principles of sustainable development, all of which are linked to equity, social justice and good health (see Box 1.2). The Commission's work was intended to promote opportunities to make strategic links between health, wellbeing and sustainable development across organisations, workplaces, recreational facilities and other settings of community life.

Marmot and Bell (2012) argue that to counter inequities, societies need to create and develop healthy and sustainable places and communities. For example, in the workplace, people need a decent living wage, opportunities for developing their capacity for the future, the flexibility of balancing work and family life, and protection from working conditions that are damaging to health. These and other measures require a fair distribution of power, money and other resources to respond to the SDH; the conditions in which people are born, grow, live, work and age (Marmot & Bell 2012).

SOCIAL DETERMINANTS OF HEALTH (SDH)

> ### WHAT IS THE RELATIONSHIP BETWEEN SDH AND EQUITY?
>
> To reduce inequities in health requires people to take action on the social determinants of health (SDH).

The SDH consist of a number of overlapping factors that determine health and wellbeing. These include factors that begin at birth, such as biology and genetic characteristics, gender, culture and various family influences on healthy child development. Family influences include having socio-economic resources for parents to provide for their child, parenting knowledge and skills, a peaceful family life and adequate support systems. Social support networks that are inclusive across genders, cultures and educational opportunities are also social determinants. Support systems influence a person's ability to cope with life's stressors, and to make decisions about personal health practices that either prevent illness or maintain health. Other social determinants are a function of interactions between the individual, family and community, such as having a healthy and supportive neighbourhood with adequate transportation and spaces for recreation, being able to access food and water, and services for health and child care when they're needed, and having employment opportunities with good working conditions and sufficient income. Many of these determinants are embedded in the political and economic environment, where policy decisions affecting community life are made (see Figure 1.1).

Within the SDH are a number of structural conditions. For example, a community's social development needs structures to create employment opportunities, and a physical environment that supports healthy lifestyles and personal health practices. People need access to clean air, water and nutritious foods at a reasonable cost, and affordable, warm, safe housing (Howden-Chapman et al. 2007). They also need to have reasonable working conditions so that they can achieve a work-life balance. Other structures in the social environment that support health and wellbeing include health and social support services such as hospitals, medical practitioners, nurses, and other allied health professionals who are accessible where and when they are needed. Structural supports for health also include government services that provide income protection in the case of unemployment, infrastructure such as safe roads and public transportation, and schools, playgrounds and adult recreational facilities that offer the opportunity for holistic health and wellbeing. Socio-political structures include equitable systems of governance over the community and society, to ensure preservation of resources through wise economic choices and a commitment to conservation; fairness in allocating resources across all groups in the population; and systems that protect people from harm or disempowerment.

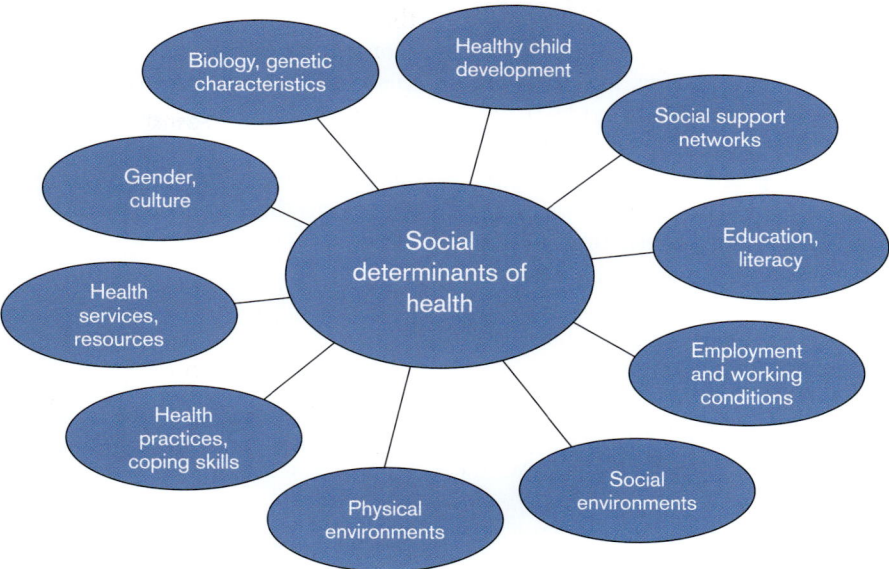

FIGURE 1.1
The social determinants of health

Social determinants of health and primary health care

The 'social determinants' approach to health resonates with the notion of human rights and social justice. Social justice refers to the 'fair distribution of society's benefits, responsibilities and their consequences' (Edwards & MacLean Davison 2008:130). This means that as health professionals, we have an obligation to identify unfairness or inequities and their underlying determinants, advocating for human rights, and working towards just economic, social and political institutions (Edwards & MacLean Davison 2008; Whitehead 2007). The World Health Organization Commission on the social determinants of health (CSDH) contends that equitable, socially just conditions in our communities and society are a matter of life and death, affecting the way people live, their chances of becoming ill, or their risk of premature death (CSDH 2008). This argument is based on the 'McKeown thesis'; that is, the knowledge that the major improvements to health over the past decades have not been due to medical treatments or technologies, but rather to social, environmental and economic changes, smaller family size, better nutrition, a healthier physical environment and a greater emphasis on preventive care (McKeown 1979). These factors are all SDH and they inform the way we use PHC to help communities maintain health and wellness.

> **WHAT IS THE RELATIONSHIP BETWEEN THE SDH AND PHC?**
>
> SDH are the social factors that impact on health.
>
> PHC is a set of principles to guide health professionals in helping people create socially just, equitable conditions for good health.

The WHO commission recommended that governments everywhere take up the challenge of working with health and other organisations to improve health for the world's citizens (CSDH 2008). This involves ensuring sufficient health professionals to provide care, addressing economic issues, overcoming inequitable, exploitative, unhealthy and dangerous working conditions, including restoration of work-life balance for families, and providing social protection for all people across the life course (CSDH 2008). These overarching goals urge us to act in concert with members of our communities, igniting our passion for health and social justice and combining it with research that will build better understandings of what works, where, for what populations, with what outcomes. Public health policymakers have already identified the social sources of many health problems. For example, we know that for some people, an ideal mix of conditions can create a positive start to life that becomes sustained into adulthood and throughout ageing. Improvements to the SDH (housing, employment opportunities, transportation or social services) can provide optimal conditions in which all family members flourish and maintain good health over time. For others, a disadvantaged start to life may not be overcome by sufficient changes in any of the environments affecting their lives, and their disadvantage passes on to the next generation. Another example lies in the disproportionate effects of global warming and natural disasters such as flooding, fires and other weather events that have left entire families at risk of homelessness. For those already disadvantaged by poverty, discrimination or a lack of social support, these events can perpetuate ill health.

THE SOCIAL GRADIENT

Those who earn income at successively higher levels have better health than those who are unemployed or have lower levels of income.

A family's socio-economic status is an important determinant of health. Research studies have shown that there is a 'social gradient' in health, whereby those employed at successively higher levels have better health than those on lower levels (Navarro 2009; Hertzman & Power 2006). This inequity creates disadvantage from birth for some children. A child born into a lower socio-economic family for example, may be destined for an impoverished life, creating intergenerational ill health. This child lives in a situation of 'double-jeopardy', where interactions between the SDH conspire against good health. Without external community supports the family may spiral into worsening circumstances, affecting their child's opportunities for the future. This is the case for many Indigenous people, whose parents have not had access to adequate employment or community supports that would sustain their own health, much less that of their children. They become caught in a cycle of vulnerability where the SDH interact in a way that creates disempowerment across generations. Political decisions governing employment opportunities may hamper the parents' ability to improve finances. A less than optimal physical environment may deprive both parents and the child of a chance to access social groups or gatherings. There may be few opportunities for education, health care or transportation to access services. Parenting skills may be absent for a range of reasons, including younger age, the lack of role

modelling, geographic disadvantage or illness. Discrimination in the immediate environment can worsen the effects of any of these factors. Discrimination and other social injustices have created the impetus for taking a PHC approach to working with families, to foster empowering partnerships between the family and community to cradle children's ability to cope, to grow and to learn (Li et al. 2008).

PRIMARY HEALTH CARE

Primary health care is a philosophy of care based on social justice, and an organising framework for the activities of health professionals.

PRIMARY HEALTH CARE (PHC)

Primary health care (PHC) is a pathway to achieving basic human rights, which is essentially social justice. It is defined in the 1978 Declaration of Alma-Ata as:

Essential health care based on practical, scientifically sound and socially acceptable methods and technology made universally accessible to individuals and families in the community through their full participation and at a cost that the community and country can afford to maintain at every stage of their development in the spirit of self-reliance and self-determination. It is the first level of contact with individuals, the family and community with the national health systems bringing health care as close as possible to where people live and work and constitutes the first element of a continuing care process. (WHO, UNICEF 1978:6)

Primary care (PC) is distinct from PHC in that it is the first point of entry into the health system. PC provides person-focused, integrated, coordinated care over time (Martin-Misener et al. 2012), typically, in Australia and New Zealand, in a general practice or PHC clinic. PC therefore represents an important aspect of care provided within the health sector. PHC is intersectoral which means that, in addition to the health sector, care is planned in collaboration with the many sectors that impact on health and aspects of community life. These include agriculture, and the food industry, education, housing, employment, public works and transportation, communications, natural resources and other sectors. The combination of PC and PHC can help make services more accessible and tailored to community needs (Martin-Misener et al. 2012).

PRIMARY CARE

Primary care is the first line of care when a person is sick or injured. Primary care is an element of primary health care.

PHC is both a philosophy and an organising framework for health professionals. As a framework, PHC guides our activities in illness prevention, health promotion, and structural and environmental modifications that support health and wellness. This does not exclude the important work in caring for those experiencing illness or disability. It does, however, shift the caring agenda to the SDH, in primary care settings such as general practice, in critical or acute care, home care, rehabilitation settings, residential care, or in working to modify the community itself.

PRIMARY HEALTH CARE PRINCIPLES

- Accessible health care
- Appropriate technology
- Health promotion
- Cultural sensitivity
- Intersectoral collaboration
- Community participation

The overarching principles embodied in PHC guide us to work towards equitable social circumstances, equal access to health care, and community empowerment through public participation in all aspects of life. These principles include accessible health care, appropriate technology, health promotion, cultural sensitivity, intersectoral collaboration and community participation. The literature on PHC includes cultural inclusiveness as a common thread in each of these principles. However, we include cultural sensitivity as a separate principle. This acknowledges the important work on cultural safety that has been done over the past two decades, particularly in New Zealand. Being culturally sensitive and enabling culturally appropriate health care that protects cultural safety is one of the most important factors in achieving PHC. The principles are interconnected, but they are examined separately below to underline the importance of each to the overall philosophy of PHC (see Figure 1.2).

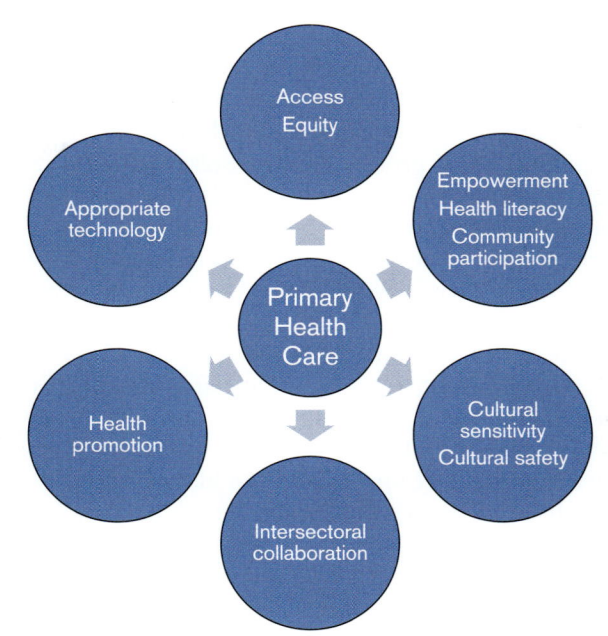

FIGURE 1.2   Primary health care principles

Accessible health care: equity and social justice

In many countries of the world, including those considered highly developed, there is a widening gap in access to health services between genders, cultures, Indigenous and non-Indigenous people, and those living in urban and rural or remote areas (WHO 2008). These factors cause disparity between rich and poor, which is inequitable and socially unjust. The major objective of providing equity of access is to eliminate disadvantage, whether it is related to social, economic or environmental factors. Barriers to access include such things as unemployment, lack of education and health literacy, age, gender, functional capacity, and cultural or language difficulties. These factors prevent an individual from developing personal capacity. Barriers to community capacity include geographical features that isolate people from services or opportunities, civil conflict, or a lack of structures and services that support human endeavour.

Inequity

Unfair distribution of resources and support

(e.g. lack of health professionals in rural areas)

Inequality

Disparity in health status or capacity

(e.g. poorer health among Indigenous people than non-Indigenous people)

As the WHO (2008) reports, a plethora of research evidence has shown that in any country, the greater the gap between the incomes of the rich and poor, the worse the health status of its citizens. This occurs unevenly, as health is distributed differently among different groups. Analysis of population data from 60 million people in 30 OECD countries has confirmed unequivocally that the health of any society is better when wealth is more equally distributed (Kondo et al. 2009). Various interactions among influences also produce different levels of health and illness, and there are also variations in the way different generations respond to events in their social world. Some inequities also affect the community itself. Global warming, overpopulation, the destruction of forests and the harmful effects of globalised industrial processes all add insult to the injurious effects of social policies that keep the wealth at the top of the hierarchy. Decisions for community health should therefore be based on simultaneous assessment of the impact on other people and communities, future generations and the global community. Social justice, or equitable access for all, must supersede individual goals, so that the least advantaged people in a community receive equal opportunity, education, care and service to those who are advantaged by virtue of both tangible (finances) and intangible (knowledge) resources.

Appropriate technology

To some extent, the failure of our health care systems to address inequities in health over the past decades is due to the use of inappropriate technologies in health care. PHC requires efficiency and effectiveness; that is, 'the right care provided to the right people by the right provider, in the right setting and using the most suitable and cost-effective technology' (Besner 2004:352). Although progress has been made in community management of chronic diseases, health systems continue to revolve around services with a medical-technical focus rather than those that support community empowerment and 'distributional equity' throughout all areas, rural and urban (Crooks & Andrews 2009:271). Not all communities can afford the latest and most expensive technologies, so health expenditure on technological supports can sometimes be a barrier to less expensive but adequate care for more people.

WHAT IS THE LINK BETWEEN TECHNOLOGY AND HEALTH?

Inappropriate application of technology in health care leads to inequities in the distribution of health care.

Increased emphasis on health promotion

Health promotion is essentially a political, ecological and capacity-building process, aimed at arranging the social and structural determinants of health in a way that facilitates health. It is the combination of circumstances that enable people to increase control over and improve their health (WHO & Health and Welfare Canada & CPHA 1986). Health promotion activities include global initiatives as well as local community planning activities that develop participative, capacity-building structures for community development (Whitehead 2009). At the local level, strategies may involve working with intersectoral groups to lobby the government for better roads or more parklands, or instituting measures to ensure healthy school lunches or access to workplace-based health services. At the global level, health promotion may involve becoming personally aware of the problems of other countries and making sure their health issues are understood and publicised.

Health promotion should be focused on the community's assets and strengths rather than risks and weaknesses, to enable people to thrive and build resilience rather than just coping with their lives (Hancock 2009). Health promotion actions may be aimed at different population subgroups, such as creating day care centres for the elderly to prevent them from being socially isolated, or working with new parents to ensure they have information and the support systems they need. What these have in common is a commitment to enabling capacity through participation, empowerment and health literacy. However, programs that are limited to a particular group are considered 'selective' rather than 'comprehensive' primary health care.

Selective PHC is a term that was originally associated with the global economic environment. Selective PHC reflects the idea that health services should be aimed at 'best investments in health'; that is, providing health programs on the basis of cost effectiveness, with defined health outcomes linked to specific expenditures (deVos et al. 2009). Comprehensive PHC adopts a whole-of-community approach and an empowerment framework, where community members work in partnership with health professionals to participate fully in health decision-making for the entire community (Baum et al. 2009, deVos et al. 2009, Erickson & Andrews 2011). Although selective PHC has been criticised as creating fragmented services rather than sustainable communities, there are some groups with high-priority needs within the broader context of comprehensive primary health care (Baum et al. 2009). The two types of PHC are therefore important in terms of assessment to identify the breadth of needs and priorities within any given community.

Selective PHC

Health planning aimed at linking outcomes with specific investments

Comprehensive PHC

A whole-of-community approach to participative health decision-making

----

Cultural sensitivity, cultural safety

Culture is the accumulation of beliefs, values and knowledge that are inherited from one generation to another and that determine social behaviour. Cultural sensitivity means being responsive to the way an individual or group's cultural mores and lifestyle habits shape health and health behaviours. Cultural safety is a concept that refers to exploring, reflecting on, and understanding one's own culture and how it relates to other cultures. Understanding and accepting oneself and one's own beliefs and culture is therefore the starting point for culturally safe and sensitive practice, to ensure that no one culture has dominance over another (Ramsden 1993). Importantly, it is not the nurse, midwife or other health practitioner who determines whether practice is culturally safe, but the recipient of care (Richardson & Carryer 2005). We will explore these concepts further in Chapter 13.

Cultural sensitivity requires cultural literacy. This is developed through openness to people's interpretation of their cultural identity and how their expressions of culture shape their behaviour. Cultural sensitivity also requires attention to the way language is used to describe members of different cultures. Being vigilant about language and communication may be as basic as being careful to assess people's needs from their perspective to avoid jumping to conclusions. Describing Indigenous people in relation to non-Indigenous benchmarks may be denigrating. Similarly, describing all Indigenous people, or members of a migrant group or refugees, as if they were a homogenous group without close attention to their particular experiences, may have a detrimental effect on their health and healing.

Intersectoral collaboration

Intersectoral collaboration requires cooperation between different community sectors, including (but not limited to) those managing health, education, social services, housing, transportation, environmental planning and local government. Tapping into the expertise of different sectors and different alliances enables more flexible and collaborative responses to certain needs. Another advantage of intersectoral collaboration is promoting acceptance of the need for a health initiative when all parties involved work together for its success. Collaborative alliances encourage efficient and effective use of resources, with economies achieved from including a range of specialists who, as a collective, may have an interest in long-term continuity of various interventions (Talbot & Verrinder 2010). However, in addressing the allocation of economic resources to health budgets it is important to lobby for national PHC policies that support decentralised control so that communities themselves can participate in health planning.

Public participation

Community participation is one of the central tenets of primary health care. It is also part of a worldwide trend towards client-centred care (Coulter et al. 2008; Wiggins 2011). Effective partnerships see the health care profession and members of the community having equal status, control and reciprocal responsibility for health (Aston et al. 2009). Community partnerships are not only empowering but they enhance capacity for developing social capital with mutual trust and reciprocity as well as cooperative networks for better health. However the major goal of community participation is empowerment itself, which helps people develop mastery and control over the key processes that influence their lives (deVos et al. 2009; Leffers & Mitchell 2010). In this respect, community participation creates a more socially just, inclusive environment where people develop the skills to challenge non-responsive or oppressive institutions to redress power imbalances (deVos et al. 2009).

PHC is focused on redressing social disadvantage by promoting healthy social and structural conditions for good health. We achieve this within an *enabling* role, acting in partnership with people who are empowered to make informed choices to develop their personal and community capacity. The outcome of these community partnerships should be better health, equity, justice and good governance in health services, including appropriate, effective and efficient use of available technologies. However, these outcomes are only achievable where there is the political will to support and sustain good health for all members of the community, which is integral to the notion of social capital.

PRIMARY HEALTH CARE IN PRACTICE

Access and equity: working to alleviate the barriers that prevent equal access to health for all members of the community—identifying any disparities in access to education, health services, employment or other social determinants of health

Appropriate technology: advocating for the right care for the right person or community at the right time, to maximise efficiency and equity rather than the most expensive technologies for all communities

Health promotion: encouraging community capacity through comprehensive promotion of health for the whole-of-community; promoting selective care for those most in need of specific care

Cultural sensitivity: being aware of your own and others' cultural beliefs, values and knowledge and how these shape health and health decisions

Intersectoral collaboration: working in partnership with health, disability services, transportation, education, environment and other sectors to respond to all the social determinants of health

Public participation: ensuring that community members are able to participate fully in making decisions for their health and wellbeing

SOCIAL CAPITAL

When the health of the community is defined from a social perspective we acknowledge its *social capital.* Like *economic capital,* social capital is an accumulation of wealth, but it is the kind of wealth that draws people together as a cohesive force in a climate of trust and mutual respect (Putnam 2005). Putnam (1995) first described the value of social capital in terms of developing civic engagement, trust and norms of reciprocity among community members. Communities become strong when people are connected through networks, associations, and any other means of sharing information and a sense of purpose. Information flows through the community in many directions, people are compelled to help others for mutual benefit and they are more likely to participate in democratic institutions, thereby improving their accountability. Some researchers have drawn a distinction between *bonding* and *bridging* social capital. Bonding social capital refers to the trusting and cooperative

relationships between groups who have similar demographic or social characteristics, whereas bridging social capital describes 'relations between individuals who are dissimilar with respect to social identity and power' (Murayama et al. 2012:180). The importance of understanding social capital in any given neighbourhood or community is in knowing where and how to implement health promotion programs that will have a greater chance of success. For example, where communities have developed a sense of coherence and commitment to one another there is a greater likelihood of mutual support in achieving health goals.

SOCIAL CAPITAL

A sense of trust, civic engagement, participation and belonging.

Communities with high social capital have a better chance of coping with adversity and limitations, as well as being able to build a positive sense of place. A community may have the disadvantage of isolation, or few natural resources conducive to health, yet community attitudes and actions that bring people together can help strengthen *health capacity* (Aston et al. 2009). Community health capacity can also be supported by organisational structures, such as schools, workplaces and community planning mechanisms that include participatory decision-making. Together, members of the community can use their collective voices to lobby for services such as health care, transportation, family friendly education and job re-training, opportunities for physical activities and community policing. With each successful action, there is a greater likelihood of building capacity for the future. In this way communities can work from the ground up to respond to the SDH, addressing inequalities and working toward a more inclusive society (Baum et al. 2010; CSDH 2008; Raphael et al. 2008).

Examples of programs that help build social capital are those that unite people in developing opportunities, those that galvanise community action to preserve the environment, to undertake participatory school reform, support for the homeless, or bring local businesses together to take steps to end discrimination (Baum et al. 2010). When communities draw members together to pursue these types of goals they develop community vitality, a capacity to thrive and change, and greater respect and inclusiveness. This is the key to empowerment. It is based on the premise that if people are prepared for events or circumstances with both information and community support systems, they can control their destiny by participating in decision-making and developing appropriate conditions for living and working (Aston et al. 2009; Baum et al., 2010).

> ## ACTION POINT
>
> Involving community members in activities or projects to pursue common goals will help build social capital.

Social capital and the political ecosystem

In communities with high social capital it is often obvious how interdependent various groups are as they interact with others. To these interactions people bring their own individuality: the combination of genetic predispositions, history, knowledge, attitudes, preferences and perceptions of capacity. Each community, in turn, brings to each of its members a set of distinct environments: physical, psychological, social, spiritual and cultural. As we mentioned at the beginning of the chapter, our socio-ecological interactions are reciprocal. Bandura (1977) called this *reciprocal determinism*, whereby the behaviours of people and the characteristics of their environments are determined by dynamic exchanges between them. These interactions are transformative in that they shape a characteristic community character, which determines the extent to which community members will become a cohesive entity.

> ### RECIPROCAL DETERMINISM
>
> We affect and are affected by the dynamic exchanges we have with the environment. These create both challenges and opportunities for health.

Ecological exchange in the context of particular political influences can yield both constraints and enhancements to personal and community health. Some of the more familiar constraints on health and wellbeing arise from the effects of contaminants in the physical environment, such as air and water pollution, infectious diseases and/or injury. Climate change researchers argue that these effects

disproportionately affect vulnerable populations, with significant impacts not only on personal health, but infrastructure, agriculture and food security, migration and economic development and community resilience and connectedness (Patrick et al. 2011). They see the climate change and environmental agendas in terms of the political ecosystem. Without strong political leaders with policies that include 'footprint thinking', our complacency may perpetuate inequities (Patrick et al. 2011). Footprint thinking is futuristic. It is a way of planning that is mindful of the health impact from all policies across all sectors of society, which, again, underlines the link between sustainable development and health.

> ### FOOTPRINT THINKING
>
> Considering the demands on our ecosystems (consumption) and our biocapacity (regenerative ability)

Our ecological footprint measures both resource consumption demands and the planet's regenerative capacity. In terms of health impact, if the wealthy and powerful control the economic capital and resources, there will be growing inequities in access to the SDH, leading to health inequity on a global scale (Hancock 2011). Citing Aron, Hancock (2011: ii170) argues that if inequality becomes too great, 'the idea of community becomes impossible'. As health professionals we therefore have a dual purpose: to manage the health consequences of environmental problems, and to work towards mitigating the causes and determinants of these problems (Patrick et al. 2011). Although these are often political actions, they are always undertaken with the participation of community members to ensure the acceptability and appropriateness of any changes. To encourage this level of participation requires health literacy.

HEALTH LITERACY

Health literacy is the ability to make sound health decisions in everyday life. Some decisions may be related to health care, but others may be lifestyle choices, decisions that improve quality of life, or that help in understanding civic responsibilities or opportunities. Health literacy is an important element in addressing health inequities, as those at the lower levels of health literacy are often the ones who live in socio-economically disadvantaged

RESEARCH TO PRACTICE: Social capital and health

Murayama et al. (2012) conducted a systematic review of a wide range of studies that were conducted within a social capital framework to investigate whether researchers have found a relationship between social capital and individual health. They reported that both individual social capital and area/workplace social capital had positive effects on health outcomes. These associations led them to conclude that health promotion programs should include consideration of the level and type of social capital in the place they are being conducted. Equally as important is the finding that health promotion and social capital have reciprocal effects. Social capital enhances, and is enhanced by, health promotion interventions and therefore has a continuing impact on the community. Because social capital is shaped by the broader structural forces in a community, developing social capital should be seen as a complement to structural interventions, such as creating appropriate housing or infrastructure. The researchers recommend further research to explore the feasibility of interventions that build social capital as a way of promoting health.

What does this mean for community health research?

Studies linking social capital with health outcomes would make an important contribution to evidence-based community health practice. However, it seems that researchers have used a variety of approaches to measure social capital, including measures of political participation, integration versus isolation, voter turnout, residential mobility and volunteering. Most of these studies have been unable to link health outcomes with their limited notions of social capital (Blakely et al. 2006).

? Can you think of a useful research question that would capture the link between social capital and health outcomes for a population group in your community?

their lives. For many women especially, low literacy prevents them from adequate personal health and from ensuring their family's access to good nutrition, freedom from illness and exercising their own potential.

HEALTH LITERACY

The ability to make sound health decisions in everyday life.

A health-literate person is able to participate in both public and private dialogues about health, medicine, scientific knowledge and their relation to society and culture (Zarcadoolas et al. 2005). It is empowering to be able to make decisions that provide greater control, that help people interact as full participants in clinical situations and preventative care, and navigate the health care system (Coulter et al. 2008; Kickbusch 2008;, White 2008). Since health literacy became part of our research agenda in the 1990s, studies have found strong links between literacy and overall health and wellbeing (Kickbusch 2008). Researchers have also found an association between low literacy and health inequalities, with those having low levels of literacy experiencing poorer health, higher rates of hospitalisation and difficulty in managing chronic diseases than those with higher literacy (Coulter et al. 2008: Smith & McCaffery 2010; White 2008). In addition, people with low levels of health literacy make greater use of emergency care, are less likely to use screening programs, have lower ability to demonstrate taking medications appropriately and have lower ability to interpret labels and health messages (Berkman et al. 2011). Research undertaken by the New Zealand Ministry of Health (NZMOH 2010) showed that less than half of all New Zealanders meet the minimum health literacy requirements for making effective health care decisions.

Having adequate health literacy promotes people's engagement in health care and other aspects of social life, which has clinical and economic benefits to society (Coulter et al. 2008). Clinical benefits include smoother encounters in the processes of diagnosis and treatment of illness, better adherence to prescribed treatments and medications, and better understanding of instructions given by health providers (Smith & McCaffery 2010). When people are engaged with their health services they tend to undertake more self-care and management, select appropriate treatments, and are better at monitoring their health

communities. Being unaware of information relevant to improving their health, or how to access health resources, creates higher levels of disadvantage. For some people, a lack of education and the health literacy that would flow from education prevents them from becoming empowered at any time during and safety issues (Coulter et al. 2008). Understanding how to navigate the health care system provides insight into bureaucratic processes associated with health insurance, admission to or discharge from hospital, and knowing the types of care they can expect to receive from a range of practitioners. Because health literate people tend to have healthier lifestyles they are more likely to engage in preventative activities, which not only improve their quality of life but reduce health care costs (Coulter et al. 2008, Smith & McCaffery 2010, White 2008). In this respect, health literacy is a resource for living; a personal, community and societal asset that is integral to capacity building, citizenship and feelings of self-worth (Green et al. 2007, Nutbeam 2008, Peerson & Saunders 2009).

LEVELS OF HEALTH LITERACY

- Functional
- Communicative (or interactive)
- Critical

Three levels of health literacy have been identified by Nutbeam (2000) and are shown in Table 1.1. *Functional health literacy* means that individuals have received sufficient factual information on health risks and health services, which they also understand, and which allows them to function effectively in a health context (Coulter et al. 2008, Nutbeam 2000). They need to be able to read consent forms, medicine labels and other written health care information. They also need to be able to understand and act on both verbal and written instructions from health care practitioners, pharmacists and insurers (Kickbusch 2001). At a second level, *communicative* or *interactive health literacy* develops personal skills to the extent that community members participate in community life, influencing social norms and helping others develop their personal health capacity. This involves understanding how organisations work, and communicating with others in the context of self-help or other support groups, as well as knowing how to get the services they need.

The third level of literacy, *critical health literacy*, is where people use cognitive skills to improve individual resilience to social and economic adversity. This paves the way for community leadership structures to support community action and to facilitate community development (Nutbeam 2000). At a personal level critical health literacy is an enabling factor, developing capacity for confident, empowered interactions with others, including members of the health professions (Nutbeam 2008). The fundamental element in critical health literacy is the community members' commitment to working together to overcome structural barriers to health, which recognises the role of health literacy in creating awareness of the SDH (Coulter et al. 2008; Nutbeam 2008). Examples of outcomes include workers exerting pressure on workplaces to reduce hazardous risks, or lobby groups gathering support for environmental preservation, or supportive resources for parenting practices or health services. In each of these examples, the community is demonstrating critical health literacy. In some respects, this is also *civic literacy* in that community members actively participate in community life to find collective solutions to health problems. This emphasises the importance of the context for communication (Nutbeam 2008). Progression between the three levels of health literacy depends on a person's cognitive development, exposure to different forms of communication and the content (Nutbeam 2008).

The SDH Commission (CSDH 2008) advocated for the scope of health literacy to be expanded to include the ability to access, understand, evaluate and communicate information on the SDH. de Leeuw (2012:2) extends this notion to *health system literacy*, which she suggests are 'the skills, capacities and knowledge required to access, understand and interact with social and political determinants of health'. This level of health literacy requires in-depth understanding of the political ecosystem, which may be more relevant for political debate and actions to address population level inequities (Kickbusch 2009). The skills to take action at both the individual and community levels are basically the type of advocacy that Nutbeam (2008) defined as critical health literacy (Mogford et al. 2010).

For health professionals, the focus of promoting health literacy is to provide information and education, to encourage appropriate and effective use of health resources, to engage people in health

TABLE 1.1 Health literacy: A continuum of knowledge and skill development			
Functional	**Communicative/interactive**	**Critical**	**Civic**
Knowledge to choose	Ability to influence	Skills for action	Capable of community action

decision-making, and ultimately to tackle health inequalities through empowerment (Coulter et al. 2008; Peerson & Saunders 2009). To help people read, understand, evaluate and use health information requires an understanding of how people learn. This varies according to age, class, cultural group, gender, beliefs, preferences and coping strategies, and experience with the health system. Some differences also emerge as a function of their general literacy level, first language, skills and abilities (Coulter et al. 2008). We revisit these issues in Chapter 4, planning health promotion that will be tailored to people's strengths and needs. These individual and group differences draw into clear focus how communities differ in their populations, resources and capacity to support health and wellness, which is the subject of the chapter to follow.

CASE STUDY: Introducing the Smiths and the Masons, two FIFO families

Australian Family: The Masons

The Mason family lives in Maddington, a suburb of Perth, Western Australia (population 9136). The family consists of Colin (husband, age 44), Rebecca (wife, age 41), Emily (age 6), Caleb (age 4), Joe and Gemma (18-month twins). Emily goes to Maddington Public School, Caleb is about to start pre-primary, Joe and Gemma go to day care two mornings a week. Rebecca attends a mothers group organised through the twins' day care centre. They live in one of the older neighbourhoods, but on a street with a few migrant families. Rebecca's mother lives in the wheatbelt, three hours drive from Perth. Colin, who was previously a bricklayer, flies to a Pilbara mining site every six weeks for four weeks, works 12-hour shifts while he is in the mine, then returns home for two weeks. Rebecca has struggled with her weight since giving birth to the twins and the child health nurse referred her to the GP, where she was diagnosed with metabolic syndrome. She is working with the practice nurse on a program of dietary management and activity. She goes to the gym two mornings a week while the twins are in day care and the rest of the time manages the home and family. Colin is relatively healthy but suffers from poor sleep habits related to his work and lifestyle. He enjoys a drink with the boys. Emily and Caleb are healthy, but Emily is having some difficulties coping with her first year of school. The twins are active but Gemma has eczema, which requires intermittent specialist treatment.

NZ Family: The Smiths

The Smiths live in Papakura, South Auckland. The family consists of Jason (husband, age 34), Huia (wife, age 31), John (age 12), Aroha (age 8), Jake (age 4). Jason works as an engineer in a large mine in the Pilbara and flies to Australia for 6 weeks at a time. He has four weeks at home in between stints in the mine. Huia works as a teacher part time in a local primary school. John attends the local kura kaupapa (Māori language primary school) where he enjoys kapa haka (Māori dance). John has recently been diagnosed with a learning disability. Aroha is 8 and also attends kura kaupapa. John and Aroha catch the bus to kura. Jake is 4 and attends a local Kohanga Reo (Māori language preschool). He is eligible for 20 hours of free preschool education available to all children aged 3 and 4 in New Zealand. Jake also has asthma for which he has been hospitalised several times. Huia spends a lot of her free time at the local marae where she helps run a fitness program for elders.

Jason struggles with high blood pressure which is not helped by his frequent travelling and long hours.

We'll be following the Masons and the Smiths throughout the textbook. We hope you enjoy the journey and find them a stimulating learning experience.

REFLECTING ON THE BIG ISSUES

This chapter outlined several 'big issues' including the following:

- Health is a state of balance between individual, social and environmental factors; the social determinants of health.

- Being healthy includes wellbeing and happiness.

- The SDH have a significant role in determining the health status of people. These include biology/genetics; healthy child development; social supports; education/literacy;

employment/working conditions; social environments; physical environments; health practices/coping skills; health services/resources; gender/culture.

- Healthy communities are the *synthesis* or product of people interacting with their environments when they work collaboratively to shape and develop the community in a way that will help them achieve positive health outcomes and capacities.

- Primary health care is a philosophy aimed at promoting social justice through the principles of accessible health care, appropriate technology, health promotion, cultural sensitivity, intersectoral collaboration and public participation.

- Social capital is created when people feel connected with others, developing mutuality and trust.

- Health literacy is empowering and a vital element of achieving equity in community health.

- Research is an essential part of promoting community health.

REFLECTIVE QUESTIONS: How would I use this knowledge in practice?

1   Explain the role of empowerment in social inclusion and social exclusion.

2   In relation to the 'Happy' research (Box 1.1) what cultural conditions might affect happiness ratings?

3   Explain the link between climate change, social disadvantage and sustainable communities.

4   What is the difference between bonding and bridging social capital?

5   Create a brief map with an overview of the social determinants of health that affect the health and wellbeing of the Smith and Mason families.

6   Identify one research question that would help inform your work with either the Mason or the Smith family.

References

Aston, M., Meagher-Stewart, D., Edwards, N., et al., 2009. Public health nurses' primary health care practice: strategies for fostering citizen participation. J. Community Health Nurs. 26, 24–34.

Baisch, M., 2009. Community health: an evolutionary concept analysis. J. Adv. Nurs. 65 (11), 2464–2476.

Bandura, A., 1977. Self-efficacy: Toward a unifying theory of behavioral change. Psychol. Rev. 84, 191–215.

Baum, F., 2009. Envisioning a healthy and sustainable future: essential to closing the gap in a generation. Glob. Health Promot. 1757-9759 (Suppl. 1), 72–80.

Baum, F., Newman, L., Biedrzycki, K., et al., 2010. Can a regional government's social inclusion initiative contribute to the quest for healthy equity? Health Promot. Int. 25 (4), 474–482.

Berkman, N., Sheridan, S., Donahue, K., et al., 2011. Health literacy interventions and outcomes: an updated systematic review. Evidence report/technology assessment no. 199. (Prepared by RTI International-University of North Carolina Evidence-based Practice Centre under contract No. 290-2007-10056-I. AHRQ Publication Number 11-E006). Agency for Healthcare Research and Quality, Rockville, MD.

Besner, J., 2004. Nurses' role in advancing primary health care: a call to action. Prim. Health Care Res. Dev. 5, 351–358.

Best, A., Stokols, D., Green, L., et al., 2003. An integrative framework for community partnering to translate theory into effective health promotion strategy. Am. J. Health Promot. 18 (2), 168–176.

Blakely, T., Atkinson, J., Ivory, V., et al., 2006. No association of neighbourhood volunteerism with mortality in New Zealand: a national multilevel cohort study. Int. J. Epidemiol. 35, 981–989.

Bowen, K., Friel, S., Ebi, K., et al., 2012. Governing for a healthy population: Towards an understanding of how decision-making will determine our global health in a changing climate. Int. J. Environ. Res. Public Health 9, 55–72.

Bronfenbrenner, U., 1979. The ecology of human development. Harvard University Press, Cambridge, MA.

Coulter, A., Parsons, S., Ashkham, J., 2008. Where are the patients in decision-making about their own care? Policy Brief, WHO and WHO European Observatory on Health Systems and Policies. Regional Office for Europe, Copenhagen.

Crooks, V., Andrews, G., 2009. Community, equity, access: core geographic concepts in primary health care. Prim. Health Care Res. Dev. 10, 270–273.

CSDH, 2008. Closing the gap in a generation. Health equity through action on the social determinants of health, Final report of the Commission on the social determinants of health. WHO, Geneva.

de Leeuw, E., 2012. The political ecosystem of health literacies. Editorial, Health Promot. Int. 27 (1), 1–4.

DeVos, P., Malaise, G., De Ceukelaire, W., et al., 2009. Participation and empowerment in primary health care: from Alma Ata to the era of globalization. Soc. Med. 4 (2), 121–127.

Diener, E., Seligman, M., 2004. Beyond money: Toward an economy of wellbeing. Psychol. Sci. Public Interest 5 (1), 1–31.

Dunn, H., 1959. High-level wellness for man and society. Am. J. Public Health 49, 789.

Edwards, N., MacLean Davison, C., 2008. Social justice and core competencies for public health. Improving the fit. Can. J. Public Health 99 (2), 130–132.

Erickson, D., Andrews, N., 2011. Partnerships among community development, public health, and health care could improve the well-being of low-income people. Health Aff. 30 (11), 2056–2063.

Green, J., 2007. Health literacy:Terminology and trends in making and communicating health-related information. Health Issues 92, 11–14.

Hancock, T., 2009. Act Locally: Community-based population health. Report for The Senate Sub-Committee on Population Health, Victoria BC Canada Online. Available: <http://www.parl.gc.ca/40/2/parlbus/commbus/senate/com-e/popu-e/rep-e/appendixBjun09-e.pdf>; 17 July 2009.

Hancock, T., 2011. It's the environment, stupid! Declining ecosystem health is THE threat to health in the 21st century. Health Promot. Int. 26 (S2), ii68–ii72.

Helliwell, J., Layard, R., Sachs, J. (Eds.), 2012. World happiness report, Available: <www.earth.columbia.edu/worldhappinessreport>; 13 January 2013 New York Online.

Hertzman, C., 2001. Health and human society. Am. Sci. 89 (6), 538–544.

Hertzman, C., Power, C., 2006. A life course approach to health and human development. In: Heymann, J., Hertzman, C., Barer, M., Evans, R., et al. (Eds.), Healthier societies: from analysis to action, pp. 83–106.

Howden-Chapman, P., Matheson, A., Viggers, H., et al., 2007. Retrofitting houses with insulation to reduce health inequalities: results of a clustered, randomised trial in a community setting. BMJ. 334, 460–464.

Kickbusch, I., 2001. Health literacy: Addressing the health and education divide. Health Promot. Int. 16 (3), 289–297.

Kickbusch, I., 2008. Healthy societies: addressing 21st century health challenges. Government of South Australia, Department of the Premier and Cabinet, Adelaide.

Kickbusch, I., 2009. Health literacy: engaging in a political debate. Int. J. Pub. Health 54, 131–132.

Kondo, N., Sembajwe, G., Kawachi, I., et al., 2009. Income inequality, mortality, and self-rated health: meta-analysis of multilevel studies. BMJ 330, b4471. doi:.10.1136/bmj.b4471.

Layard, R., 2005. Happiness. Penguin Books, London.

Leffers, J., Mitchell, E., 2010. Conceptual model for partnership and sustainability in global health. Public Health Nurs. 28 (1), 91–102.

Li, J., McMurray, A., Stanley, F., 2008. Modernity's paradox and the structural determinants of child health and well-being. Health Sociol. Rev. 17 (1), 64–78.

MacQueen, K., McLellan, E., Kegeles, S., et al., 2001. What is community? An evidence-based definition for participatory public health. Am. J. Public Health 91 (12), 1929–1938.

Marmot, M., 2006. Health in an unequal world. The Lancet 368 (9552), 2081–2094.

Marmot, M., Bell, R., 2012. Fair society, healthy lives. Public Health 126, S4–S10.

Martin-Misener, R., Valaitis, R., Wong, S., et al., 2012. A scoping literature review of collaboration between primary care and public health. Prim. Health Care Res. Dev. 13 (4), 327–346.

McKeown, T., 1979. The Role of Medicine: Dream, Mirage or Nemesis? second ed. Blackwell, Oxford.

Mogford, E., Gould, L., Devoght, A., 2010. Teaching critical health literacy in the US as a means to action on the social determinants of health. Health Promot. Int. 26 (1), 4–13.

Murayama, H., Fujiwara, Y., Kawachi, I., 2012. Social capital and health: A review of prospective multilevel studies. J. Epidemiol. 22 (3), 179–187.

Navarro, V., 2009. What we mean by social determinants of health. Int. J. Health Serv. 39 (3), 423–441.

New Zealand Ministry of Health (NZMOH), 2010. Kōrero Mārama: Health Literacy and Māori Results from the 2006 Adult Literacy and Life Skills Survey. Ministry of Health, Wellington.

Nutbeam, D., 2000. Health literacy as a public health goal: a challenge for contemporary health education and communication strategies into the 21st century. Health Promot. Int. 15 (3), 259–267.

Nutbeam, D., 2008. The evolving concept of health literacy. Soc. Sci. Med. 67, 2072–2078.

Patrick, R., Capetola, T., Townsend, M., et al., 2011. Health promotion and climate change: exploring the core competencies required for action. Health Promot. Int. 27 (4), 475–485.

Peerson, A., Saunders, M., 2009. Health literacy revisited: what do we mean and why does it matter? Health Promot. Int. 24 (3), 285–296.

Porritt, J., 2012. No sustainability without health equity. Public Health 126, S24–S26.

Putnam, R., 1995. Bowling alone: America's declining social capital. J. Democracy 6 (1), 65–78.

Putnam, R., 2005. Civic Renewal and Social Capital. Round Table Discussion, Alcoa Research Centre for Stronger Communities, Curtin University, Perth.

Ramsden, I., 1993. Cultural safety in nursing education in Aotearoa. Nurs. Prax. N. Z. 8 (3), 4–10.

Raphael, D., Curry-Stevens, A., Bryant, T., 2008. Barriers to addressing the social determinants of health: insights from the Canadian experience. Health Policy (New York) 88 (2/3), 222–235.

Richardson, F., Carryer, J., 2005. Teaching cultural safety in a New Zealand nursing education program. J. Nurs. Educ. 44 (5), 201–208.

Rossouw, S., Pacheco, G., 2012. Measuring non-economic quality of life on a sub-national level: A case study of New Zealand. J. Happiness Stud. 13, 439–454.

Sachs, J., 2012. Introduction. In: The Earth Institute, World Happiness Report, (Online. Available: <http://www.earth.colunbia.edu>); 11 January 2012.

Smith, S., McCaffery, K., 2010. Health literacy: a brief literature review. NSW Clinical Excellence Commission, Sydney.

Tafarodi, R., Bonn, G., Liang, H., et al., 2012. What makes for a good life? A four nation study. Journal of Happiness Studies 13, 783–800.

Talbot, L., Verrinder, G., 2010. Promoting health. A primary health care approach. Elsevier, Sydney.

Wallerstein, N., 2002. Empowerment to reduce health disparities. Scand. J. Public Health 30 (Suppl. 59), 72–77.

White, S., 2008. Assessing the nation's health literacy. AMA Foundation, Washington.

Whitehead, M., 2007. A typology of actions to tackle social inequalities in health. J. Epidemiol. Community Health 61, 473–478.

Whitehead, D., 2009. Reconciling the differences between health promotion in nursing and 'general' health promotion. Int. J. Nurs. Stud. 46, 865–874.

Wiggins, N., 2011. Popular education for health promotion and community empowerment: a review of the literature. Health Promot. Int. 27 (3), 356–371.

World Health Organization (WHO), 1974. Basic documents, Thirty-sixth ed. WHO, Geneva.

World Health Organization & UNICEF, 1978. Primary health care. WHO, Geneva.

World Health Organization, Health and Welfare Canada, CPHA, 1986. Ottawa Charter for Health Promotion. Can. J. Public Health 77 (12), 425–430.

World Health Organization (WHO), 1992. Health and the environment: a global challenge. Bull. World Health Organ. 70 (4), 409–413.

World Health Organization (WHO), 2008. World Health Report 2008 primary health care, Now More Than Ever. Online. Available: <http://www.who.int/whr/2008/whr08_en.pdf>; 14 July 2009.

Zarcadoolas, C., Pleasant, A., Greer, D., 2005. Understanding health literacy: an expanded model. Health Promot. Int. 20 (2), 195–203.

Useful websites

www.who.int/entity/social_determinants/en—WHO Social determinants of health

www.who.int/social_determinants/themes/socialexclusion/en—WHO Social exclusion

www.euro.who.int/en/data-and-evidence/evidence-informed-policy-making/health-evidence-network-hen—WHO health evidence network

http://nccdh.ca/organizations/entry/social-determinants-of-health-listserv—Social determinants of health listserv

www.healthinsite.gov.au/topics/Health_and_Wellbeing—Australian government site for all health topics

nrha.ruralhealth.org.au—Australian National Rural Health Alliance

http://ihca.com.au—Australian Institute for Healthy Communities

www.canberra.edu.au/faculties/estem/research/institutes/aisc—Australian Institute for Sustainable Communities

uwaterloo.ca/canadian-index-wellbeing—Canadian Index of Wellbeing

www.hsph.harvard.edu/healthliteracy—Harvard School of Public Health, Health and Literacy Website

www.nzliteracyportal.org.nz—New Zealand literacy portal

www.healthnavigator.org.nz/centre-for-clinical-excellence/health-literacy—New Zealand health literacy information

www.footprintnetwork.org/en/index.php/GFN/page/ecological_footprint_atlas_2008—Global Footprint Network

CHAPTER 2

Communities of place

Introduction

The notion of reciprocal determinism, whereby people affect and are affected by their environments, epitomises the relationship between health and place. Place is important to relative states of health because 'it *constitutes* as well as *contains* social relations' (Cummins et al. 2007:1825). Having a geographically bounded 'community of place' where people interact with others can help promote community attachment, cohesion and solidarity (Kilpatrick et al. 2009:285). As we know, certain places are more conducive to health and wellbeing because of their physical features. But places also affect the social and emotional aspects of health and wellbeing. People feel grounded in certain places, but these need not be only defined by a particular geographic boundary or distance or proximity to others. Interacting across multiple places has interesting effects on people's behaviour, particularly in terms of power relationships that allow some people to negotiate access to services and other resources, while constraining others' ability to have equal access. Resources and support systems may also be more readily accessible to those with differing socio-demographic and cultural factors, such as age, gender, employment status, ethnicities and religious beliefs (Cummins et al. 2007). These factors are all integral aspects of the SDH. So in terms of 'place' the effect of older persons being at home rather than in the workplace may create a differential health disadvantage or advantage, just as the neighbourhood may have differential effects on an adult or a young child, depending on the extent to which they are able to spend time in parks or other recreational facilities. In today's world, where there is an increasing concern about our global and local places, there is a need to look more closely at the intersection of health, place, and our personal geographies and how we transit through multiple contexts in the pathways to good health.

One of the most important issues in relation to health and place concerns migration and cultural viability. Just as land and water shortages have caused forced migration, wars, urbanisation and poverty have driven people all over the world to assimilate into foreign cultures. As a result, the world has lost languages and culturally diverse elements that have historically maintained cohesion and trust. In some cases, the fear of protecting borders from refugees and other migrants has had the effect of disempowering some cultures. This in itself is a health hazard, as the disappearance of cultures and traditional ways of life have left whole communities without an understandable means of sustaining health or avenues for communicating with others. Their cultural disempowerment is therefore an important factor in determining the extent to which they flourish in family and community life.

The challenge in all communities is to find local, sustainable solutions and a sense of control or *community comfort*. As health professionals we assume an advocacy role, helping communities construct pathways to change on different levels. As social advocates, we adopt a respectful and culturally sensitive approach, shifting the balance of power to the community. As political advocates, we bring knowledge about the health and welfare systems to the table and help link people together to access resources. As professional advocates, we have an obligation to stay abreast of new knowledge and strategies that will help us maintain professional competence as well as solidarity with others. These processes are developmental in that by working together, people's skills, knowledge and self-confidence are developed, ultimately empowering them to go on to the next undertaking. Facilitating and enabling community empowerment also helps develop the skills of the health professional. Each community and the strategies it uses to strengthen capacity are unique, so every opportunity to work with a community yields new information that the health professional can use to consolidate and refine health promotion skills. In this respect, advocacy is a deliberate two-way process of mutual development, beginning with the global community.

et al. 2010). A further layer of disadvantage has arisen through privatisation of previously public services, which has led to user fees for health care and education. In addition, multinational pharmaceutical companies now dominate the trade in medicines, creating higher costs with no accountability to current and future generations in relation to local development or any social or environmental damage they may cause (Baum 2009; Labonte 2008; Schrecker 2011). The growing number of free trade agreements (for example, the Trans-Pacific Partnership Agreement (TPPA) negotiated between the United States, Canada, Mexico, Peru, Chile, Vietnam, Singapore, Malaysia, Brunei, Japan, Australia and New Zealand, and the Regional Comprehensive Economic partnership (RCEP) between the 10 ASEAN states, together with Australia, China, India, Japan, Korea and New Zealand) further exacerbates these issues, placing the interests of global companies well above the interests of local communities (see Box 2.1).

There is widespread concern about our global community among those attempting to promote the health of local communities. These concerns all converge on the centralisation of decision-making and the effects of these decisions on health. Researchers cite the health effects of excluding some nations from the global market, particularly the developing countries, many of which are already suffering from communicable diseases such as HIV/AIDS, tuberculosis, hepatitis and malaria (Schrecker 2011). These diseases, and the inequities of globalisation have affected women disproportionately, many of whom were already disadvantaged by poverty and discrimination and who, in a competitive global economy, have no hope of improving their situation (Falk-Rafael 2006; Schrecker 2011). In some developing countries the mass migration of health professionals has also eroded the capacity of the remaining workforce to deal with the burden of illness or health promotion. While many Western nations are happy to welcome migrant health professionals to fill workforce shortages, the net loss of these health workers has caused the near collapse of already fragile health systems in their home countries.

WHAT'S YOUR OPINION?

Globalisation has had a significant impact on individuals, families, communities and nations. What negative and what positive impact has globalisation had on you as an individual, your family and your community?

BOX 2.1 The Trans-Pacific Partnership Agreement

The Trans-Pacific Partnership Agreement (TPPA) is a trade agreement under negotiation between Australia, New Zealand, the United States, Canada, Mexico, Japan, Peru, Chile, Vietnam, Singapore, Malaysia and Brunei. However, the TPPA is much more than just a trade agreement. Instead of being simply about freeing up trade in goods and services between countries, the main focus of the TPPA is to create an attractive environment for overseas companies who want to operate in Australia and New Zealand. What this means is Australian and New Zealand laws on environmental protection, public health, intellectual property and economic regulation will be restricted to make it easier for foreign companies who wish to invest in Australia and New Zealand. In particular, US-based pharmaceutical companies are lobbying for provisions that will reduce government regulatory control of pharmaceuticals threatening equitable access to medicines (Faunce & Townsend 2011). The TPPA would also give foreign investors the power to sue the New Zealand or Australian governments in secret tribunals if they think that changes in law or policy have caused a substantial financial loss to their New Zealand or Australian investments. For example, tobacco companies would be able to sue governments if plain packaging has a detrimental effect on profits.

One of the most concerning aspects of the TPPA is that it is being negotiated in secret and there is no opportunity for community members to have their say in whether the TPPA goes ahead. And if it does go ahead, it will bind Australians and New Zealanders to a set of rules designed in the interests of big business, not everyday people. More information on the TPPA in New Zealand can be found at: www.itsourfuture.org.nz and in Australia at: http://aftinet.org.au/cms/.

How is this related to community health?

Commitment to communities requires vigilance and advocacy so that people are aware of the layers of decision-making that affect their lives. In the context of PHC and the goal of social justice it is important to question whether policy decisions are made with equity in mind.

The politics of global health care is clearly an issue for all nations. The global financial crisis of 2008–9 impoverished many people, sweeping the world with new claims on public monies and alarming discussions about resource scarcity. Decisions taken by global leaders led to a reduction in funding for HIV/AIDS, tuberculosis and malaria programs to the extent that in 2010 annual funding for these programs was cut in half to US$9.2 billion (Schrecker 2011). Yet US$1 trillion is spent globally each year on arms and armaments (Schrecker 2011). Surely there is an ethical and moral argument to be made for decentralised decision-making that would allow each community to establish its own priorities based on local needs. In fact, in recognising the need to decentralise their local economies, some developing countries have seen the development of micro-financing at the neighbourhood level, aimed especially at helping impoverished women start their own businesses. This approach has provided small loans, savings, insurance and training to people living in poverty as a just and sustainable solution to alleviate global poverty (10thousandgirl, Online. Available: www.10thousandgirl.com/some-facts/how-microfinance-works/ [accessed 21 December 2013]). Although modest, some of these businesses have helped break the intergenerational poverty chain, helping women become empowered through viable employment that also helps ensure an education for their children. Micro-financing developments are one of the positive outcomes of globalisation, for without global attention and support, poor countries like India and some African countries would not have had these opportunities.

Despite the global attention to poverty in developing countries, another effect of globalisation has been the loss of cultural identities, languages and the right to choice in securing the best level of health for the most number of people. The reality is that even as countries of the West celebrate new wealth, we are all aware that wealth is distributed unequally. So as the global community has continued to develop, there have been greater disparities between rich and poor countries, and between the rich and poor within most countries. Clearly, globalisation has wreaked havoc with the SDH. As Navarro (2009:440) declares, 'it is not *inequalities* that kill, but those who benefit from the inequalities that kill'. This includes the decision-makers who engage in a form of 'predatory capitalism' (Schrecker 2011:205) to control food and tobacco, pharmaceuticals, financial markets and health care (Dickens 2011; Schrecker 2011). The effects of their decisions cascade throughout society, affecting the poor and vulnerable, including women workers, migrants, different cultural groups, and rural and urban dwellers.

URBAN COMMUNITIES

For the first time in history half of the world's population (3.4 billion people) live in cities (WHO 2011). Many of these city dwellers are at the lower end of the social gradient and therefore subject to inequitable living conditions, but even middle-class urban residents can be affected by inequities in relation to those who are better off because they enjoy full employment (CMAJ 2011). Across the global spectrum, many cities have experienced explosive growth over the past two decades, either through personal choice, migration to find employment or to escape wars and civil strife or environmental degradation (Satterthwaite & Mitlin 2011; WHO 2011). In most parts of the world, the major cities are bulging at the seams, trying to accommodate the vast influx of new residents. With growth in numbers there has been a growth in urban poverty, and research has shown that cities contain the largest proportion of those who are malnourished, have poor living conditions, and high maternal and infant mortality (Satterthwaite & Mitlin 2011; WHO 2011). On the other hand, the cost of providing clean water, sanitation, schools, education and health care is more affordable in urban areas because cities enjoy better infrastructure than rural areas (Satterthwaite & Mitlin 2011).

In the city, the layered dimensions of life are played out in daily exchanges of social life and commerce, in celebrations and exploitative acts, through illness and wellness, and across the lifespan from birth to death. Urban life is a microcosm of the many relationships between health, social, cultural and environmental factors, portraying both visible and hidden aspects of family and community life. As population density increases in the cities, the differential effects on health and wellbeing for the rich and poor come into clear focus. For the unemployed or disadvantaged by birth or illness, the risks and hazards of city living include crowding, violence, virus infections, motor vehicle accidents, exposure to harmful subcultures such as substance abusers, environmental pollution and social exclusion (WHO 2011). Yet there is a close connection between what is occurring in rural communities and in the cities. In some cases, the hopelessness seen in impoverished city dwellers reflects the physical and social degradation of rural areas, which has brought many people to the city without their previous support systems.

UP SIDE, DOWN SIDE TO THE CITY

- More services, more jobs, more people
- Higher costs, poverty
- Inequities
- Substandard housing, crowding
- Fewer family supports
- Crime, pollution

Life in the city is increasingly inequitable. As the rich get richer, the divide between the 'haves' and the 'have nots' becomes more entrenched, and this erodes social capital (Hancock 2009; Kawachi & Kennedy 1999). For the 'have nots' life holds few expectations, given the drift of wealthier citizens out of the city and into the suburbs, leaving behind an inflated housing market that is out of reach of many of the working poor. The wealthy also take with them the tax base that might have funded additional services in the core of many cities. Because of declining commerce and conditions in the heart of the city many economically disadvantaged people are relegated to lower paying jobs. At the same time, most urban societies have an unprecedented need to support older citizens and other family members, especially for migrant and refugee families. Many live their lives in substandard housing, which places all family members, particularly children, at risk of ill health. Homelessness, the ultimate marker of disadvantage and inequality in society, is a particular concern, as inadequate shelters struggle to keep up with demand for food, clothing or safety. Many homeless people are the mentally ill who have been left on the streets by deinstitutionalisation and the inadequacy of mental health support services (WHO 2011). Among the homeless is a growing number of adolescents and young families whose wages have not kept up with housing costs, a situation that has been worsened by the global financial crisis. One short-term solution has been house sharing, which has become increasingly common among low-income New Zealand families trying to cope with limited budgets and rising costs. However, this solution has resulted in severe overcrowding, which exacerbates the risk of infectious diseases such as rheumatic fever and respiratory infections—both diseases with marked prevalence in New Zealand (Sharpe 2012; Trenholme et al. 2012).

REMINDER

The socio-ecological perspective argues that everything is connected to everything else.

For some, the vibrancy and energy of urban life serves as a life-sustaining force. For others, city life is a rat race without respite, refusing to soothe the concerns of older or disabled people or, for many workers, to counter the agitation of overwork. The influence of the built environment is more challenging

RESEARCH TO PRACTICE: Access to healthy food in rural and urban New Zealand

Nutrition is one of the most important issues in dealing with population inequities, as some people are disadvantaged by a lack of access to healthy foods. Poor nutrition is one of the most significant risks for chronic illness, particularly diabetes and heart disease. A group of New Zealand researchers sought to map the availability and accessibility of healthy food (low sugar, low fat, high fibre), comparing rural and urban communities (Wang et al. 2009). They found that the weekly family cost of a healthy food basket was 29.1% more expensive than a regular food basket, and the cost difference was greater in urban than rural areas. Their findings concurred with previous studies in other countries, which have shown that healthier eating is more expensive than unhealthy food habits. They concluded that in order to support the NZ Te Wai o Rona: Diabetes Prevention Strategy there must be a vast improvement in the food environment and better strategies to support people in adopting health food choices, especially in the cities. Interventions such as fruit in schools and milk in schools are designed to improve access for children to healthy foods and improve behaviours, but it is important that these are carefully evaluated to provide an evidence base for health promotion. The fruit in schools program shows some success in these areas (Boyd et al. 2009) while the milk in schools program has yet to be evaluated nationally.

So what does this tell us?

The implications of these findings are twofold. First, they indicate that place is very important to health. However, this does not mean that we cannot overcome various obstacles that may exist in one or another geographic location. The study also illustrates some of the impacts of global markets, where suppliers are able to affect health through their purchasing policies.

? How would you go about changing the availability of healthy foods in urban centres, creating more affordable choices, and ensuring sustainability of the food supply?

WHAT IS ... A HEALTHY CITY?

A city where people have choices that can help them reach their maximum potential.

in the city than in rural areas primarily because of concerns about transportation and mobility and the risk of violence in well-concealed spaces. Older people living in cities may be disabled and unable to navigate to essential services. Even for younger people, including workers, human interactions are dictated by streetscapes, and travel to and from work involves difficult manoeuvres through crowded, regulated spaces. However, cities also afford more opportunities to be resourceful in overcoming risks; for example, by developing innovative ways of countering emissions through cycleways or public transport, or cooperative strategies to provide adequate nutrition or to cope with weather events or other effects of climate change (Satterthwaite & Mitlin 2011).

The Healthy Cities movement

The Healthy Cities initiatives have foregrounded the importance of 'place' in health (Hancock 2009). Supported by the WHO, since its beginnings in 1986 the Healthy Cities movement has spanned the globe, drawing support from health professionals, representatives of recreation, police, social services, voluntary organisations, and people of all ages. The model of Healthy Cities is to create awareness of the importance of place in achieving and maintaining health. Healthy Cities initiatives have instigated actions to reduce crime and environmental degradation, increase recreational spaces, and promote connectedness between people for health, education and quality of life. The movement now incorporates thousands of cities worldwide, all with the common aim of using intersectoral collaboration and community participation to respond to the compromises to health that flow from people's everyday lives in the city, to promote a holistic view of health, and to inform policy (Hancock 2009; WHO 1998, 2011). A healthy city is one where people have choices that allow them to reach their maximum potential (see Box 2.2).

The sustainability of Healthy Cities programs relies on continuing political commitment and support. Some cities have been relatively successful in achieving this level of dialogue and health improvements, while others have become mired in inaction and intergovernmental conflicts. The most effective seem to be those linked to other Healthy Cities networks or municipalities in a way that promotes citizen engagement and mutual support.

BOX 2.2 Features of a healthy city

- A clean, safe, high-quality physical environment, including adequate housing
- A stable and sustainable ecosystem
- Strong, mutually supportive and non-exploitative communities
- Public participation in and control over decisions affecting one's life, health and wellbeing
- Meeting basic needs for all, including food, water, shelter, income, safety and work
- Access to a wide variety of experiences and resources within the possibility of multiple contacts, interaction and communication
- A diverse, vital and innovative city economy
- Encouragement of connectedness with the past, with the cultural and biological heritage and with other groups and individuals
- A city form that is compatible with and enhances the above parameters and behaviours
- An optimum level of appropriate public health and sick care services accessible to all
- High health status and low burden of disease for community residents

(Source: WHO 1998)

These networks span the globe, involving municipal leaders in many countries who have pledged to reduce health inequalities and poverty, to promote citizen influence and address social exclusion (Hancock 2009).

An extension of the Healthy Cities movement is the WHO Age-Friendly City concept, designed to provide optimal opportunities for health, participation, security and quality of life for older citizens (WHO 2007). Several initiatives have seen these goals adopted in a number of urban communities, all with a focus on accessibility of city life for people ageing, with or without disabilities, ensuring liveable, walkable communities and ageing in place; that is, in the person's home community rather than in an institution (Plouffe & Kalache 2010). Research indicates that older people are more likely to be socially engaged if the neighbourhood has interconnected street layouts, wide, smooth footpaths, local services, green spaces and opportunities to interact with others (Burton 2012; Parry 2010). These and other factors are being addressed in a number of research studies examining the features necessary for maintaining healthy municipalities, cities and communities as the global population continues to shift to urban environments (Meresman et al. 2010). Each of these strategies will need to be developed on a local or regional basis, to ensure they are responsive to needs and resources of various geographical areas.

RURAL COMMUNITIES

Rural communities have a number of unique challenges that have left many people disadvantaged by poorer health than city dwellers. The most glaring challenge is a lack of appropriate services, and this is the case in both Australia and New Zealand. As we mentioned in the discussion about globalisation, health service planning is no longer undertaken on the basis of need alone; instead many decisions are made on the basis of economic considerations, and this has seen a net outflow of services to those living in rural and remote communities. Even in New Zealand where distances are not as vast as in Australia, there has been a decline in the rural hospital network in favour of centralised services (Tranter 2012). In both countries, small and dispersed populations cannot compete for resident medical, nursing, allied health and specialist services, when the funding for these is based on 'allocative efficiencies'; that is, decisions to allocate resources from revenues that flow to the broader state, national and private health agencies. Yet the core function of health departments under a PHC commitment should be to provide access to health care for all, including preventative services, illness care and a supply of appropriate health professionals (Farmer & Currie 2009; Perkins 2012).

UP SIDE, DOWN SIDE TO RURAL LIFE

- Strong sense of community
- Stable family home
- Few health, social services
- Social, cultural isolation
- Family burden of caring
- Few education, employment, recreational opportunities
- Declining economy

Although the issue of access to care in rural and remote areas has been addressed through a number of innovations, in Australia these have primarily been aimed at flying in health professionals who conduct clinics or community assessments, but are then not able to provide the ongoing attention the

community needs. As a result many rural people have less preventative care—such as screening—than urban residents. The lack of screening affects women in particular, given that there are few gender appropriate medical officers for sexual health screening, which can lead to increased risk for screening preventable disorders such as cervical cancer. Where patients need to travel for treatments such as dialysis, cancer care or treatment for mental health problems, there are not only economic pressures on the family, but problems of social, emotional and cultural isolation (Berends et al.; 2011, Farmer et al. 2012; Francis et al. 2012; NRHA 2012; Wilson et al. 2012). The burden on families to support a person with illness, or even normal maternity care, is substantial and increases with distance. Some medical practitioners are hesitant to treat rural people with mental health problems, instead referring them for specialist treatment, which can create unnecessary treatment delays and add to the family's burden of care (Wilson et al. 2012). Other issues arise when rural clinics or agencies are required to operate across boundaries, with confusion over responsibilities for resources. To date, rural services have been reactive, time limited, poorly coordinated and focused either on service providers or diseases, rather than being based on understanding the rural context and culture, or the specific needs or assets of the community (Farmer et al. 2012; Francis et al. 2012).

Rural communities also have high levels of disadvantage because of restricted access to the range of goods and services that their urban counterparts enjoy. With shrinking economic resources many services such as banks and commercial outlets have left for wider opportunities, and this has led to a decline in the infrastructure for those who remain. Other problems include the lack of educational, employment and recreational opportunities that would enhance health literacy and social interaction. These factors all contribute to higher morbidity and mortality rates for rural people, compared with those who live in cities, which is evident in the significant and unacceptable gradient in health and wellbeing that worsens with distance from capital cities (Humphreys & Gregory 2012). Population ageing has also seen a growing number of rural residents who are ageing, many of whom have chronic diseases. A lack of culturally appropriate services means that these people are not only underserved but often unable to communicate with the health professionals who do make sporadic visits to the community (Humphreys & Gregory 2012). Similarly, those needing mental health services and guidance are often abandoned by the system (Berends et al. 2011). The impact is evident in suicide rates among Australian farmers and rural New Zealanders. Figures from New Zealand, for example, show a rural suicide rate of 15.9 per 100 000 people compared with 10.8 per 100 000 people in cities (NZMOH 2012a). These difficulties of access compromise rural people's empowerment as the lack of resources and support systems means they have little control over their health services or their lifestyles.

Although there are individual differences, rural people tend to be stoical about their lives, perhaps because many have had to be more self-reliant than urban dwellers. Even in terms of the global factors that control their lives some are philosophical about the future. For example, a commentary in the Australian National Rural Health Alliance (NRHA) newsletter suggests that farmers now have to accept that the cost of being able to buy a fair-priced Land Cruiser may also mean accepting that the juice they buy comes from South American and New Zealand fruit rather than their own (NRHA 2012). Stress from the lack of control over markets and the centralisation of so many aspects of rural life is difficult to deal with, particularly the difficulties of competing for government attention (Humphreys & Gregory 2012). Experienced farmers report that the prolonged drought in Australia over the past several years has compounded the stresses of ageing and the pressures of maintaining a farm (Polain et al. 2011). A study of farmers throughout rural New South Wales found that global issues affected them profoundly. Their greatest concerns were rapid social and industry changes, fuel price volatility and the threat of climate change (Polain et al. 2011). Many of these farmers believed there has been a gradual societal erosion of trust in farmers. They felt an overwhelming sense of loss in terms of their ability to compete in the modern world, with diminished profitability and successful professional and personal relationships (Polain et al. 2011). Like farmers around the world, New Zealand dairy farmers feel the impact of global markets acutely. New Zealand's largest dairy company, Fonterra, is a cooperatively owned global company that exports 95% of its products (www.fonterra.co.nz). Like Australian farmers, who also have to sell their milk through cooperatives, the returns to New Zealand dairy farmers are based on world demand, which can vary greatly from year to year, creating unpredictability in the stability of farm income.

Climate change is a particular problem for rural people, with the likelihood that droughts, floods, fires and storms will become more severe in future (McMichael 2011). Forecasters predict that as global warming occurs, the high pressure, low rainfall band running from east to west across Australian farmlands will displace southwards, creating further drought in the north and central regions (McMichael 2011). To cope with this looming crisis requires community-level interventions and careful evaluation of rural people's concerns, including the failures of previous forms of government support for drought-affected farms (McMichael 2011). Intensive farming practices are also impacting on the New Zealand rural environment with water and soil quality particularly affected (Bewsell et al. 2007).

One of the unifying features of rural community life is that, despite the challenges, most people from rural or remote areas have a common belief in the significance of their community, which is a type of cultural bond (Mills et al. 2011). In some cases, being part of the rural culture helps people pull together in the face of difficulties, building collective coping mechanisms and social capital (Farmer et al. 2012). In Canada, which also has vast tracts of rural and remote communities, researchers have found that to overcome health challenges, rural and remote communities need to create conditions conducive to a positive sense of belonging; that is, work towards social capital (Kitchen et al. 2012).

RESEARCH TO PRACTICE: Sense of community for rural people

Kitchen et al. (2012) analysed data from a Canadian national community health survey and found that 'sense of belonging' increased progressively across the urban to rural continuum, especially for young families with children and older people. They found that these two demographic groups are most likely to use social networks and other mechanisms to remain socially engaged and participate in community life (Kitchen et al. 2012). These findings are important in identifying strategic areas of health planning, as a sense of belonging is one of the main constructs of social capital. It is well known that having a sense of attachment to others can lead to positive health outcomes through building mutual respect and self-esteem (Kitchen et al. 2012). Conversely, social isolation has been shown to adversely affect health. This is interesting in light of Kutek et al.'s (2011) population-based survey of rural men in South Australia. The Australian researchers found that, although social support was the most effective predictor of wellbeing, sense of community was only modestly important.

So what does this tell us?

Research into concepts such as 'sense of community' is just gathering momentum as we seek to understand how best to promote the health of various population groups. It is possible that the men in the South Australian study also had higher levels of stress than those in the Canadian study, although these factors were not compared.

 What do you think should be the focus of further research in this area?

In 2012 the Australian National Strategic Framework for Rural Health was developed to articulate five main outcomes that need to be achieved in order to create equal health for urban and rural dwelling Australians (Perkins 2012). The five outcomes include improved access to services, appropriate service and care models, an adequate and appropriate health workforce, collaborative processes for service planning and policy development, and strong leadership and governance (Perkins 2012). Similar recommendations have been made by the National Health Committee in New Zealand regarding rural health (NZ National Advisory Committee on Health and Disability 2010).

An important first step in achieving these outcomes is to ensure adequacy of the research base that could be used for health planning, particularly in relation to meeting comprehensive primary health care goals and an adequate workforce (Gardner et al. 2011; Humphreys & Gregory 2012; NZ National Advisory Committee on Health and Disability 2010; Tham et al. 2010). Tham et al. (2010) identify the need for rigorous evaluations of rural health services and their effectiveness in order to provide the evidence base for appropriate, high-quality planning. As we reiterate throughout this text, expanding the evidence base is crucial to improving services for all communities, especially the rural population. Tham et al. (2010) recommend a number of case study evaluations of existing service structures, processes and outcomes to provide evidence to those implementing health service reforms of what works, in what context and why.

RURAL SOLUTIONS

1   Improved access to services
2   Appropriate service and care models
3   An adequate and appropriate health workforce
4   Collaborative processes for service planning and policy development
5   Strong leadership and governance

RESEARCH REMINDER

We need to continue researching what works, in what context and why (Tham et al. 2010).

FIFO COMMUNITIES

Fly-in fly-out (FIFO) or, in some cases, drive-in drive-out (DIDO) refers to the type of work arrangements that have become common in the mining industry. Since the 1980s under the influence of global economic forces, the resources boom across Australia created a groundswell of high-paying job opportunities for those who were willing to commute to regional or remote sites in Western Australia, Queensland and New South Wales for certain periods of time before returning to their home communities (Carrington & Pereira 2011). Because of the continuous production cycle of 12 hour shifts, 7 days a week and the scarcity of local workers, the mining companies have had to recruit non-resident employees who typically work block rosters and reside in work camps adjacent to existing rural communities (Carrington & Pereira 2011; Storey 2010). Workers include skilled and non-skilled personnel, including miners and the people who support the mining workforce. FIFO employment has spread throughout Australia and New Zealand, with workers flying to the exploration and mining or related infrastructure sites for several weeks at a time, then returning home for a short break. While they are away, working hours are long with minimal time off. Leave can be unpredictable, as it is predominantly dictated by workplace need, sometimes leaving little room for negotiation by the worker.

TRENDING NOW: FIFO

- Substantial wages
- Compressed work schedules
- Numerous family transitions
- Intermittent parenting
- Low sense of community
- Accommodation difficulties
- Lifestyle risks for workers
- Isolation of spouse
- Marital pressures, stress
- Fly-over effects on community
- Low social capital
- Inadequate community services
- Gender discrimination
- Destruction of Indigenous land
- Pressure on infrastructure

Another challenge for workers lies in their choice of residence. Although there is an advantage to living in a place of their choosing (Guerin and Guerin 2009), if this is not a major city, there may be a further burden of travel for the worker. Many companies arrange to fly a worker in and out of the nearest capital city, which can be at a distance from workers living in regional or rural areas. In these cases, additional transportation costs to the capital city are self-funded. An alternative model of mining employment has seen the development of small mining communities that require relocation of the mining family. Advantages of relocating to the mining communities include better family support, higher satisfaction with the employer, and greater capacity to deal with stress (McLean 2012), however most industry employees prefer to maintain their home community in central locations with adequate

education, health and other support services and amenities (Allan 2011; Carrington & Pereira 2011; Pick et al. 2010).

The FIFO lifestyle has an enormous impact on community life in terms of sustainability of the natural environment, local economy and culture (Pick et al. 2010). The mining sites themselves come with environmental disturbances including ground water use, noise, dust, gas emissions and other types of pollution (Storey 2010). These sites also impinge on Indigenous spaces and places with spiritual value as well as the potential for hunting, fishing or other traditional activities (Storey 2010). On the other hand, there have been some benefits to local Indigenous populations, with a deliberate effort to provide training and employment opportunities in mining. However, the industry is also plagued by gender discrimination, with women earning far less for similar jobs as men (Commonwealth of Australia 2013).The main problem in terms of community health is that although the towns adjacent to the mines are a source of resource activity, they are not a major beneficiary. The Australian Commonwealth Government Standing Committee on Regional Australia conducted a national inquiry into the issues, which concluded with a strong indictment of the FIFO style of employment because it has eroded the liveability of many regional communities, hollowing out inland regional towns (Commonwealth of Australia 2013). The pressure on infrastructure in the camps and adjacent towns has made housing, food, fuel and services unaffordable for those who may not have previously experienced these economic hardships. Together, these negative impacts on the community have been called 'fly-over effects' (Storey 2010:1163).

The effects on social and community life are profound. The Australian inquiry revealed disturbing stories of the two different faces of FIFO, depending on whether the perspective was from a 'host' or 'source' community. Residents of the host towns reported being pushed into FIFO schedules where previously they had been given a choice of 'living in' rather than 'flying in'. Children's sporting teams had been disbanded because of a lack of volunteers. Medical practices reported being unable to service local residents because of the influx of FIFO workers. Women said they were fearful of walking the streets at night due to the large number of young men on their streets, and young people expressed a need to leave the town as the price of accommodation had become untenable for them and few training opportunities were available. Because the young people leave to find training and employment, there has been an erosion of community capacity for the future (Pick et al. 2010; Storey 2010).

Men's health has also suffered under the FIFO lifestyle. Many experience personal hardships associated with living in temporary accommodation with little or only intermittent health and social services (Guerin & Guerin 2009). Among workers in both host and source communities interpersonal stress and depression are major problems, particularly in relation to family relationships and social isolation (Commonwealth of Australia 2013). In some cases, these conditions have led to alcohol and substance misuse as well as an increase in occupational accidents. Social problems include male-on-male alcohol fuelled violence, fatigue-related injuries, reduced workplace commitment, and health and relationship problems (Carrington & Pereira 2011; McLean 2012; Storey 2010). Reduced social networks and relationship strain affect the entire family as FIFO workers and their partners struggle with so many entries and exits in and out of family life (Torkington et al. 2011). Some workers reported to the government inquiry that when they are home the family takes extended holidays to make up for lost time together, causing the children to miss school (Commonwealth of Australia 2013).

In some ways, the FIFO lifestyle is similar to that of defence force families during periods of deployment, yet unlike the military, where families have access to extensive training and counselling services, private FIFO employers provide little or no preparation for these transitions. Government services to support the towns are difficult to plan because of the lack of accurate statistics on who resides there, especially with the 'shadow population' of FIFO workers (Commonwealth of Australia 2013:28). During the Commonwealth review community residents put forward strong views, calling FIFO the 'cancer of the bush' (Commonwealth of Australia 2013:42). They decried the decline of social cohesion, a sense of identity, community safety, the degradation of local roads, infrastructure and services, crowding out of local tourism opportunities because the mining companies have taken all available accommodation, and pressures on local council budgets.

Members of the group conducting the inquiry visited Mongolia and Canada, where there is also a proliferation of the FIFO workforce, but with fewer social problems. The group returned with recommendations to adopt the international models of sustainable mining communities, which require the mining companies and their employees to sign a social contract as a condition of working in the community. These agreements are intended to emphasise that the workers are living in a community deserving of their respect. The Commission recommended that a secretariat be established based on the province of Alberta Oil Sands Sustainable Development Secretariat, with responsibility for consulting with state governments and the resources industry to develop cooperative agreements and regional planning. Other recommendations include improving PHC and medical services, family and worker support programs, government funding, training and governance programs for communities with large FIFO populations, a number of taxation and regulatory measures to remove some of the exemptions allowed for FIFO work and a comprehensive program of research into issues related to FIFO employment (Commonwealth of Australia 2013).

Another initiative for the Australian government is to pressure resource companies to demonstrate social responsibility for Indigenous community sustainability through Indigenous Land Use Agreements and legally binding agreements with local communities that will yield economic and social benefits back to the local Indigenous community. For the 'source' communities, where families are coping with FIFO relationships and parenting it is crucial that their needs be understood and that health promotion strategies are aimed at fostering both family strengths and community cohesion.

RELATIONAL COMMUNITIES

A contemporary perspective of health and place sees 'place' as nodes or networks, 'constellations of connections' (Cummins et al. 2007:1827). This approach is appropriate to today's lifestyles where most of us influence and are influenced by multiple places on the web through our virtual networks with others. These places can be described as 'relational', as compared with the conventional view of 'place' as a specific geographical location (see Table 2.1).

ELECTRONIC AND SOCIAL MEDIA COMMUNITIES

We have discussed 'communities of place' in geographical terms—the global, urban and rural communities we inhabit, but in our technological world the networks that bind people together can also be considered as communities, albeit as virtual places. From this perspective, people can enjoy membership in multiple communities. Electronic devices and social media that expedite communication are instrumental to health and wellness because they act as conduits for people to develop health literacy, exchange knowledge on health, become socially engaged with others, and receive information from health professionals or

TABLE 2.1 Conventional and relational understandings of place (adapted from Cummins et al. 2007:1827)

Conventional view	Relational view
Spaces with geographical boundaries	Nodes in networks
Separated by physical distance	Separated by socio-relational distance
Resident local communities	Populations of individuals who are mobile daily and over their life course
Services described in terms of fixed locations	'Layers' of assets available to populations via varying paths of time and space
Area definitions relatively static and fixed	Area definitions relatively dynamic and fluid
Characteristics at fixed time points, e.g. 'deprived' versus 'affluent'	Dynamic characteristics, e.g. 'declining' versus 'advancing'
Culturally neutral territorial divisions, infrastructure and services	Territorial divisions, services and infrastructure imbued with social power relations and cultural meaning
Contextual features described systematically and consistently by different individuals and groups	Contextual features described variably by different individuals and groups

other sources when they need guidance or support. Social and electronic media therefore play an important role in enhancing a community's social capital. Electronic, virtual networks can therefore be seen as enabling places for health (Duff 2011).

RESEARCH TO PRACTICE

Can you identify a research question that would be relevant to studying the effect of health and place in a networked community?

Individuals use the relational space of the web for a variety of health needs, to access information on illness or lifestyle topics, and counselling for psychosocial issues that may be more accessible or acceptable online than in person (Korda & Itani 2013; Verheijden et al. 2008). In addition, nurses and other health professionals are increasingly using the web to promote social engagement (Thielst 2011). Social media can be empowering for community members in that, except in remote areas where there may not be broadband coverage, it is easily accessible at the time and place users prefer (Thielst 2011). Using electronic networks to keep community members engaged with one another may be invaluable in the future, but as yet few studies have been conducted on which population groups would find this most helpful, and whether they would be those with the greatest need. However, virtual spaces can also create risks to health in similar and novel ways to physical communities. Such risks may include cyber bullying and sexual predation, and these issues are examined further in Chapter 9. Other risks are related to eyesight damage from the constant connection to screens, and behavioural effects that see some people become socially isolated or depressed from interacting almost exclusively with online sites rather than individuals. These risks must be managed to ensure virtual networks remain safe environments for all those who choose to use them.

COMMUNITIES OF AFFILIATION

As we discussed above in relation to mining communities, some people are bound by occupation, and this can affect health and social behaviours. Other occupations connect people together by virtue of shared values and attitudes, and this is evident for many nurses who travel throughout the world. Our own experiences have shown that meeting another member of the profession often results in an instant connection based on a common commitment to health and wellbeing. Other occupations may have less of a community connection, and some people prefer to maintain their distance rather than develop a connected relationship with co-workers. So the ties that bind members of an occupational community fall along a continuum of connectedness from very little to very strong linkages. On the other hand, members of religious or faith communities tend to have a strong sense of community, based, again, on a common commitment. Cultural groups may also feel a strong sense of community, but this varies with the particular culture and subgroups within that culture. Community bonds may be based on such things as age, gender, family structure and whether or not people are bound together by social, occupational or religious affiliation. For example, a group of Pacific Island elders who live in a particular neighbourhood and attend a common church may share a close social bond, while another group of seniors from the same region may have a separate, distinctive sense of community outside the group. The children and grandchildren of both groups may not feel part of either community, and instead may create their social bonds in communities bound together by study, sports or recreational activities. These differences caution us against making generalisations about people and their community memberships on the basis of ethnicity, which is important to consider when working with migrant or refugee populations.

HIGH SENSE OF COMMUNITY?

- Physical
- Urban
- Rural
- Communities of affiliation
- Religious
- Cultural
- Virtual
- Professional

Migrant and refugee communities

Migrants include those who move to another country by choice, for economic, education or family reasons; refugees, who have been forced to move because of war, civil unrest or other circumstances that threatened their survival; asylum seekers, who are also refugees, but who claim refugee status upon arrival in another country; temporary workers who may have entered a country under specific employment programs; and undocumented persons, who have no status in their new country either because their visitor or temporary work status has lapsed, or because their refugee claim was refused, or they have chosen to immigrate through irregular channels (Merry et al. 2011a). Migrant communities are growing rapidly, particularly in industrialised regions like our own, which, along with Japan, Europe and North America have accommodated around 127 million people (Merry et al. 2011a). In some cases, the circumstances of migration, such as being a refugee from a country at war, leads to being housed in a common community. However, in these cases, having a common geographic or cultural bond does not translate into better health, especially for

families placed in detention centres. For many years there has been worldwide condemnation of Australian policies that govern the way refugees seeking asylum have been treated. In some cases, those who have been rescued at sea trying to reach the country have lived for years in detention waiting for their migration applications to be processed. The effects on the asylum seekers' mental health have been profound. Children have been deprived of opportunities to grow and develop and sometimes abused in the detention centres. Women have been violated in many ways, by deprivation, a lack of privacy and violent abuse. With large numbers of men from diverse cultures crowded together and little social support there are myriad risks to health and wellbeing. New Zealand, on the other hand, has had a history of tolerant policies toward asylum seekers. Yet, in 2013 the New Zealand Government committed to taking 150 boat people per year from Australia in return for New Zealand having access to Australian detention centres for boat people who may make it to New Zealand. This is a retrograde step for New Zealand, which, for the past twenty years has been held up as a world class example of cultural tolerance.

WHO IS A MIGRANT?

- A person migrating to a new country by choice
- A refugee from difficult to better circumstances
- An asylum seeker claiming refugee status on arrival
- A temporary worker
- An undocumented person

The new Trans-Tasman policy direction is yet another example of how political factors can impinge on health, and highlights the need for health policymakers to advocate for sustainable *human* security rather than *national* security (Labonte 2008). Asylum seekers in detention, as well as refugees in the community, are often affected by a number of issues across the continuum of migration, including the pre-migration, migration and post-migration contexts (Khanlou 2012). Refugees from war-torn countries have pre-migration experiences that are substantially different to those who may have migrated voluntarily. Some have deeply personal experiences such as violence, trauma, and the loss of family members, homes and communities, which can cause post-traumatic stress syndrome throughout the migration and post-migration transitions (Khanlou 2012). Although such people are often thrust together with others in detention centres or temporary accommodation, there may be limited opportunities to develop any kind of communal bond, particularly if the community is organised around incarceration rather than empowerment.

For refugees, the resettlement transition may not resolve health needs, as most have limited access to health and social care because of factors related to finances, discrimination and/or racism, or the appropriateness of services, particularly for women (Khanlou 2012). Many women seeking asylum have endured rape, sexual assault or sexually transmitted diseases as a form of persecution, which can lead to numerous physical and psychological symptoms (Burchill 2012). In cases where asylum is not granted, families sometimes end up homeless because of a lack of access to public funds (Burchill 2011). The enforced destitution can result in the children being taken into care because of the family's inability to look after them (Burchill 2011). The problems are intense for mothers who have arrived in a country illegally, such as occurs when women from Latin American countries cross the border into the United States (Sternberg & Barry 2011). They overcome great odds in being smuggled into the country and then take jobs other women consider too menial or too low-paying. Many end up exploited as indentured servants or sex workers, a situation described as the 'feminization of migration' (Sternberg & Barry 2011:65). A similar situation occurs when organised criminals traffic young women from Asian countries to Australia and New Zealand with the promise of a new life. Although these women are typically elusive to the health care system, when community nurses, health visitors or midwives do encounter them it is because they are experiencing the most serious impacts of disempowerment. Helping creates a dilemma, particularly in assisting them to deal with violence,

which, although tolerated in their original culture, must be carefully dealt with in the host system to safeguard the woman and her family (Burchill 2011). Once abuse is disclosed there can be further recriminations from the community, where lack of awareness and insensitivity can create another level of abusive discrimination (Burchill 2012; Hoban & Liamputtong 2012; Sternberg & Barry 2011).

A number of barriers to achieving health and wellness also exist for those who have migrated by choice. The 'healthy immigrant' effect suggests that because of the criteria for selection, newly arrived migrants tend to be healthier than others in the population. However, the 'transitional effect' indicates that their health advantage declines the longer they live in the host country (Khanlou 2012:10). Resettlement difficulties can be due to language problems, underemployment or unemployment, misunderstandings about the health and social systems, and cultural differences (Khanlou 2012; NZMOH 2012b; Priebe et al. 2011; Perumal 2010; Chan et al. 2009). Age, gender and family issues typically intersect, compounding the effects of each and making it difficult to adapt to a new cultural context. Women may be at risk of being exploited in the workplace, especially those with no legal status whose family members have to rely on them gaining unskilled work in unsafe or unclean environments (Khanlou 2012). Child-rearing behaviours often change, especially with the woman having to work, and adolescents may have to take on roles beyond the capacity of their age group. Young mothers and older people may find themselves isolated, especially if there are also problems with language, culture and mobility (Hoban & Liamputtong 2012; Khanlou 2012; Merry et al. 2011b). Being stereotyped by those in the host community on the basis of religious identity and having a lack of social support can also have a multiplier effect, compromising health and opportunities for the future (Khanlou 2012; Priebe et al. 2011).

CASE STUDY: The Smith and Mason families' communities

In this chapter we present information on the communities where the Smith and Mason families live and work.

Papakura is a working-class suburb of South Auckland with large Māori and Pacific populations. Jason and Huia have recently built a new home on

the outskirts of Papakura approximately 5 minutes' drive to the local shopping centre and a 30 minute drive to Auckland International Airport. Huia's family lives in the Papakura area and, although Jason and Huia could afford to move to more affluent suburbs, she wants to stay close to her extended family.

Maddington is a leafy, older suburb of Perth, with large, comfortable homes and a growing multicultural population. The suburb contains major residential, retail and industrial sections as well as some semi-rural areas. Unusual for a large city suburb, Maddington has several vineyards and orchards from a previous era when it was primarily agricultural. The community has a railway station and is engaged in transit-oriented development planning. The area also has a large shopping centre and a technical college, and it is within 10 km of a major university. The Masons live in a three-bedroom home close to a park and within a short drive to most of the local schools and services. They are only 10 minutes away from the freeway which helps Colin's commute to the airport.

The mining site where both Colin and Jason are employed is in the Pilbara region of Western Australia. The mine operates 24 hours, 365 days a year. It is close to several small communities where some of the mine's service personnel live. The men live in single men's quarters in the mining camp where they have some access to amenities such as a gym, recreation hall and some internet access on most days.

REFLECTING ON THE BIG ISSUES

- Being healthy in any community means having equitable access to resources, empowerment, cultural inclusiveness, healthy environments and participation in decision-making.
- Global factors have an impact on all types of communities.
- Place is important to health because it constitutes as well as contains social relations.
- The reciprocal relationship between health and place means that some places can enhance health potential, while others may create risks to health.

- A relational view of health sees health as dynamic, and created through either virtual or visible networks.
- Social capital means that communities can accumulate social assets.
- Migrant and refugee communities can act as enclaves to develop mutually supportive, empowered lives in the host community.
- Working with FIFO families requires that we are aware of the challenges and potential of two types of communities: the source community and the employment community.

REFLECTIVE QUESTIONS: How would I use this knowledge in practice?

1 Can you identify any influences on the Mason and Smith families from global factors?

2 Which of these factors are evident in their (mining) workplace community?

3 Conduct a web search of the two communities of Maddington WA and Papakura NZ. From the online information describe the relationship between health and place in each community

4 What would constitute social capital in each of these communities?

5 What are the most important assets available to those who live in large cities?

6 Describe a relational community in which you are a member.

7 What are the barriers to empowerment for rural communities?

8 What steps can be taken to help migrant and refugee families acculturate to their new community without losing their cultural identity?

References

Allan, J., 2011. Mining's relocation culture. The experiences of family members in the context of frequent relocation. Int. J. Sociol. Soc. Policy 31 (5/6), 272–286.

Baum, F., 2009. Envisioning a healthy and sustainable future: essential to closing the gap in a generation. Glob. Health Promot. 1757-9759 (Suppl. 1), 72–80.

Berends, L., MacLean, S., Hunter, B., et al., 2011. Implementing alcohol and other drug interventions effectively: How does location matter? Aust. J. Rural Health 19, 211–217.

Bewsell, D., Monaghan, R., Kaine, G., 2007. Adoption of Stream Fencing Among Dairy Farmers in Four New Zealand Catchments. Environ. Manage. 40 (2), 201–209.

Boyd, S., Dingle, R., Hodgen, E., et al., 2009. The changing face of fruit in schools: 2009 overview report. New

Zealand Council for Educational Research & Health Outcomes International, Wellington.

Burchill, J., 2011. Safeguarding vulnerable families: work with refugees and asylum seekers. Community Pract. 84 (2), 23–26.

Burchill, J., 2012. Barriers to effective practice for health visitors working with asylum seekers and refugees. Community Pract. 85 (7), 20–23.

Burton, E., 2012. Streets ahead? The role of the built environment in healthy ageing. Perspect. Public Health 132 (4), 161–162.

Canadian Medical Association Journal, 2011. News. CMAJ 183 (1), E53.

Carrington, K., Pereira, M., 2011. Assessing the social impacts of the resources boom on rural communities. Rural Soc. 21 (1), 2–20.

Chan, W., Peters, J., Reeve, M., et al., 2009. Descriptive epidemiology of refugee health in New Zealand. Auckland Regional Public Health Service, Auckland.

Commonwealth of Australia, 2013. Parliament of Australia House of Representatives Committee, Inquiry into the use of 'fly-in, fly-out' (FIFO) workforce practices in regional Australia. Online. Available: <www.aph.gov.au> 14 October.

Cummins, S., Curtis, S., Diez-Roux, A.V., et al., 2007. Understanding and representing 'place' in health research: A relational approach. Soc. Sci. Med. 65, 1825–1838.

Cushon, J., Muhajarine, N., Labonte, R., 2010. Lived experience of economic and political trends related to Globalization. Can. Public Health Assoc. 101 (1), 92–95.

Dickens, B., 2011. Promoting health near and far. Ed. Am. J. Public Health 101 (3), 394.

Duff, C., 2011. Networks, resources and agencies: On the character and production of enabling places. Health Place 17, 149–156.

Falk-Rafael, A., 2006. Globalization and global health: toward nursing praxis in the global community. Adv. Nursi. Sci. 29 (1), 2–14.

Farmer, J., Currie, M., 2009. Evaluating the outcomes of rural health policy. Aust. J. Rural Health 17, 53–57.

Farmer, J., Bourke, L., Taylor, J., et al., 2012. Culture and rural health. Aust. J. Rural Health 20, 243–247.

Francis, K., McLeod, M., McIntyre, M., et al., 2012. Australian rural maternity services: Creating a future or putting the last nail in the coffin. Aust. J. Rural Health 20, 281–284.

Gardner, K., Bailie, R., Si, D., et al., 2011. Reorienting primary health care for addressing chronic conditions in remote Australia and the South Pacific: Review of evidence and lessons from an innovative quality improvement process. Aust. J. Rural Health 19, 111–117.

Guerin, P., Guerin, B., 2009. Social effects of fly-in fly-out and drive-in-drive-out services for remote Indigenous communities. Aust. Community Psychol. 21 (2), 7–22.

Hancock, T., 2009. Act Locally: Community-based population health. Report for The Senate Sub-Committee on Population Health, Victoria BC Canada. Online. Available: <http://www.parl.gc.ca/40/2/parlbus/commbus/senate/com-e/popu-e/rep-e/appendixBjun09-e.pdf> 17 July 2009.

Hancock, T., 2011. It's the environment, stupid! Declining ecosystem health is THE threat to health in the 21st century. Health Promot. Int. 26 (S2), ii68–ii72.

Hoban, E., Liamputtong, P., 2012. Cambodian migrant women's postpartum experiences in Victoria, Australia. Midwifery <http://dx.doi.org/10.1016/j.midw.2012.06.021>.

Humphreys, J., Gregory, G., 2012. Celebrating another decade of progress in rural health: What is the current state of play? Aust. J. Rural Health 20, 156–163.

Kawachi, I., Kennedy, B., 1999. Income inequality and health: pathways and mechanisms. Health Serv. Res. 34, 215–227.

Khanlou, N., 2012. Migrant mental health in Canada.

Kilpatrick, S., Cheers, B., Gilles, M., et al., 2009. Boundary crossers, communities, and health: Exploring the role of rural health professionals. Health Place 15, 284–290.

Kitchen, P., Williams, A., Chowhan, J., 2012. Sense of community belonging and health in Canada: A regional analysis. Soc. Indic. Res. 107, 103–126.

Korda, H., Itani, Z., 2013. Harnessing social media for health promotion and behavior change. Health Promot. Pract. 14 (1), 15–23.

Kutek, S., Turnbull, D., Fairweather-Schmidt, K., 2011. Rural men's subjective well-being and the role of social support and sense of community: Evidence for the potential benefit of enhancing informal networks. Aust. J. Rural Health 19, 20–26.

Labonte, R., 2008. Global health in public policy: finding the right frame? Crit. Public Health 18 (4), 467–482.

Labonte, R., Schrecker, T., 2007a. Globalization and social determinants of health: Introduction and methodological background. Global. Health 3 (5), doi:10.1186/1744-8603-3-5.

Labonte, R., Schrecker, T., 2007b. Globalization and social determinants of health: The role of the global marketplace. Global. Health 3 (6), doi:10.1186/1744-8603-3-6.

McLean, K., 2012. Mental health and well-being in resident mine workers: Out of the fly-in fly-out box. Aust. J. Rural Health 20, 126–130.

McMichael, A., 2011. Drought, drying and mental health: Lessons from recent experiences for future risk-lessening policies. Aust. J. Rural Health 19, 227–228.

Meresman, S., Rice, M., Vizzotti, C., et al., 2010. Contributions for repositioning a regional strategy for healthy municipalities, cities and communities (HM&C): Results of a Pan-American survey. J. Urban Health 87 (5), 740–754.

Merry, L., Gagnon, A., Hemlin, I., et al., 2011a. Cross-border movement and women's health: how to capture the data. Int. J. Equity Health 10 (1), 56–71.

Merry, L., Gagnon, A., Kalim, N., et al., 2011b. Refugee claimant women and barriers to health and social services post-birth. Can. J. Public Health 102 (4), 286–290.

Mills, J., Lindsay, D., Gardner, G., 2011. Nurse practitioners for rural and remote Australia: Creating opportunities for better health in the bush. Aust. J. Rural Health 19, 54.

National Rural Health Alliance (NRHA), 2012. Partyline 45 NRHA.

Navarro, V., 2009. What we mean by social determinants of health. Int. J. Health Serv. 39 (3), 423–441.

New Zealand Ministry of Health (NZMOH), 2012a. Suicide facts: deaths and intentional self-harm hospitalizations 2010. Ministry of Health, Wellington.

New Zealand Ministry of Health (NZMOH), 2012b. Refugee Health Care: A handbook for health professionals. Ministry of Health, Wellington.

New Zealand National Advisory Committee on Health and Disability, 2010. Rural health: challenges of distance, opportunities for innovation. National Health Committee, Wellington.

Parry, J., 2010. Network of cities tackles age-old problems. Bull. World Health Organ. 88, 406–407.

Perkins, D., 2012. The 2012 Editorial, National Strategic Framework for Rural Health: part of the solution? Aust. J. Rural Health 20, 171–172.

Perumal, L., 2010. Health needs assessment of Middle Eastern, Latin American and African people living in the Auckland region. Auckland District Health Board, Auckland.

Pick, D., Dayaram, K., Butler, B., 2010. Regional development and global capitalism: the case of the Pilbara, Western Australia. Soc. Bus. Rev. 5 (1), 99–110.

Plouffe, L., Kalache, A., 2010. Towards global age-friendly cities: Determining urban features that promote active aging. J. Urban Health 87 (5), 733–739.

Polain, J., Berry, H., Hoskin, J., 2011. Rapid change, climate adversity and the next 'big dry': Older farmers' mental health. Aust. J. Rural Health 19, 239–243.

Priebe, S., Sandhu, S., Dias, S., et al., 2011. Good practice in health care for migrants: views and experiences of care professionals in 16 European countries. B. Public Health 11, 187–200.

Satterthwaite, D., Mitlin, D., 2011. Recognising the potential of cities, Editorial. Br. Med. J. 343, 1–2.

Schrecker, T., 2011. Why are some settings resource-poor and others not? The global marketplace, perfect economic storms, and the right to health. Can. J. Public Health 102 (3), 204–206.

Sharpe, N., 2012. Rheumatic fever: From disease targeting to child-centredness. N. Z. Med. J. (Online) 125 (1365), 7.

Sternberg, R., Barry, C., 2011. Transnational mothers crossing the border and bringing their health care needs. J. Nurs. Scholarsh. 32 (1), 64–71.

Storey, K., 2010. Fly-in/Fly-out: Implications for community sustainability. Sustainability 2, 1161–1181.

Tham, R., Humphreys, J., Kinsman, L., et al., 2010. Evaluating the impact of sustainable comprehensive primary health care on rural health. Aust. J. Rural Health 18, 166–172.

Thielst, C., 2011. Social media: Ubiquitous community and patient engagement. Front. Health Serv. Manage. 28 (2), 3–14.

Torkington, A., Larkins, S., Gupta, T., 2011. The psychosocial impacts of fly-in fly-out and drive-in drive-out mining on mining employees: A qualitative study. Aust. J. Rural Health 19, 135–141.

Tranter, D., 2012. NZ Experience a warning for rural Queensland. NHRA Partyline 45, 35–36.

Trenholme, A., Vogel, A., Lennon, D., et al., 2012. Household characteristics of children aged under 2 years admitted with lower respiratory tract infection in Counties Manukau, South Auckland. N. Z. Med. J. (Online) 125 (1367), 23.

Verheijden, M., Jans, M., Hildebrandt, V., 2008. Web-based tailored lifestyle programs: Exploration of the target group's interests and implications for practice. Health Promot. Pract. 9 (1), 82–92.

Wang, J., Williams, M., Rush, E., et al., 2009. Mapping the availability and accessibility of healthy food in rural and urban New Zealand—Te Wai o Rona: Diabetes Prevention Strategy. Public Health Nutr. 13 (7), 1049–1055.

Wilson, R., Cruickshank, M., Lea, J., 2012. Experiences of families who help young rural men with emergent mental health problems in a rural community in New South Wales, Australia. Contemp. Nurse 42 (2), 167–177.

World Health Organization (WHO), 1998. The Fifty-first World Health Assembly, Health Promotion. WHO, Geneva.

World Health Organization (WHO), 2007. Global Age-Friendly Cities: A guide. WHO, Paris.

World Health Organization (WHO), 2011. Hidden Cities: Unmasking and overcoming health inequities in urban settings. Online Available: <http://hiddencities.org/downloads/WHO_UN-HABITAT_Hidden_Cities_Web.pdf> 21 January 2013.

CHAPTER 3

Assessing the community

Introduction

This chapter addresses community assessment as the first step in working with communities to promote health and wellbeing. We present two sections: Part 1 outlines background information and discussion on assessment in general, and Part 2, called 'Assessment in practice', introduces a new assessment model. Assessment is the foundation for planning to meet the needs of the community. These needs are identified on the basis of any known risks, hazards and strengths, as well as the priorities and preferences of community residents. To plan effective, efficient, adequate, appropriate and acceptable health interventions we need both scientific data gathered by health planners (top-down information) and community perspectives (bottom-up information). As we mentioned in the first two chapters, an 'assets' approach to promoting health focuses on community strengths as well as needs. To generate a list of community assets and needs it is important to create an assessment 'map' of geographic, demographic and social information. Geographic data indicate what features or hazards exist in the natural and built environment, the patterns of health and illness among various groups defined by age or gender, and what social conditions require health promotion interventions for community residents. Simultaneously, the assessment involves finding out from members of the community how they assess their health strengths and needs in terms of personal perspectives and experiences. Once this information has been gathered, the next stage of planning is to develop intervention strategies for improvement, or measures that can be taken to sustain positive aspects of community life. The advantage of conducting a comprehensive assessment is that it allows us to forecast patterns of health or potential changes that may impact on people's lives or the lives of their children in the future. In the final analysis the information should produce a snapshot of strengths, weaknesses, opportunities and threats to community health.

General knowledge of the community has limited usefulness unless it is analysed in terms of subsequent steps that can be taken in partnership with community members to strengthen community resources and enable health and wellbeing. Selecting an assessment strategy should therefore be *goal directed*, so that the assessment information is linked to promoting and sustaining community health and wellness.

COMMUNITY ASSESSMENT— A SUMMARY

1 Map community strengths, resources, needs and risks.

2 Find out from community members what they identify as their strengths and needs.

3 Create a snapshot of strengths, weaknesses, opportunities and threats.

4 Work with the community to develop intervention strategies for improvement or measures that sustain positive community life.

Data—observations, measurements or facts

Information—knowledge of specific and timely events or situations, including data

REMINDER

The role of health professionals in community health involves:

- promoting health and providing care where people live, work and play
- advocating for the community, its people and its physical, social, spiritual environments
- promoting equity, access, social inclusion and adequate resources by assessing community needs and disadvantage and then lobbying for change where required
- encouraging empowerment and health literacy to promote citizen participation in decisions for health and wellbeing
- generating the evidence base relative to community health needs.

OBJECTIVES

By the end of this chapter you will be able to:

1 compare a range of assessment approaches and their usefulness in developing programs and policies to promote community health

2 outline a strategy for assessing an urban community

3 conduct an assessment of a rural or remote community

4 compare the differences in assessment information for an urban and rural community

5 use assessment information to evaluate a community's strengths, weaknesses, opportunities and threats to health and wellbeing

6 apply the Social Determinants of Health Circle to complete a community assessment.

Part 1: Community Assessment Tools

Community assessment tools have evolved over the years in conjunction with changes in the way we see communities and our ability to promote health. Many decades ago, community assessment was predominantly a checklist approach to assessing communities and their ability to support the needs of residents. A number of tools were developed to ensure that assessments took into account vital information on personal as well as community health hazards and risks. This information was then used to predict people's exposure to diseases or the risk of accidental ill health from such things as bushfires, drowning or other events common to the area. Many of these tools focused on the population and age-specific risks (asthma in children, for example), with only cursory evaluation of the relationship between health and place, or the assets (e.g. health services) that could help maintain better health. Some of those tools remain useful in assessing community health and the risk of ill health, but in the context of today's primary health care (PHC) approach, we recognise that people are quite knowledgeable about their needs and the needs of their communities, and community assessment is incomplete without their input.

One of the earliest approaches to assessment was the epidemiological model, which focused on the determinants and distribution of health and disease. The epidemiological approach was embraced by all health professions on the basis that it reflected a whole-of-population approach and included comprehensive assessment of the person, host and environment, called the 'epidemiological triad'. Epidemiological assessments continue to be useful today in developing a base of scientific evidence on health and its determinants in specified populations.

EPIDEMIOLOGICAL ASSESSMENT

The classic model of epidemiology is to examine specific aspects of the host (biology), the agent (a causative factor) and environment (factors that exacerbate or moderate the effects of the agent on the host), to see how each of these affects the spread of a disease or ill health in the population. The objective of epidemiological researchers is to collect data on the incidence of individuals 'at risk' of developing a particular disease in order to inform development of a vaccine or treatment for that disease. Data from epidemiological analyses are presented in terms of *incidence and prevalence*. Incidence is calculated by dividing the number of *new* cases in a population by the population at risk, then multiplying this by a base number (1000 or 100 000). This estimates the likelihood that a condition would occur in the population. The prevalence of a certain condition is the number of *new and existing* cases divided by the population at risk multiplied by 1000 or 100 000 (see Box 3.1).

GROUP EXERCISE: Community assessment

Working in small groups, brainstorm the various ways you think information about a community can be collected. Save your ideas and as you work through the chapter, see if the ways you have identified are discussed in the text. Use your discussion forum or pinboard if working online.

What is … the rate and how is it calculated?

A measure of the frequency of a disease or condition, calculated by dividing prevalence by the incidence multiplied by a population base number (1000 or 100 000).

What is … incidence?

The number of *new* cases of a disease or health issue in a specific period of time, divided by the population at risk multiplied by the base number.

What is … prevalence?

The *total number* (new plus existing) of cases of a disease or health issue in a population at any one time, divided by the population at risk multiplied by the base number.

If an occupational group is exposed to a certain toxic substance, a measure of the 'relative risk' of becoming ill from that exposure can be calculated by comparing a group (called a cohort) who were exposed to the hazard with a cohort who were not exposed. If the group exposed to the risk has a higher rate of the illness, that hazard is declared a risk factor. To confirm that it is a risk factor we would then assess its effect over a longer period of time in the entire population, which would provide greater insight. An example of relative risk in relation to adolescent alcohol-related beliefs was outlined in a systematic review conducted by Australian researchers (Scholes-Balog et al. 2012). The researchers were interested in whether policymakers and health promoters should be advocating for mandatory warning labels on alcoholic beverages. They conducted a systematic review of all available literature in the international databases that addressed warning labels and adolescent knowledge, attitudes, beliefs and behaviours. Analysis of these studies indicated that, with some exceptions, most studies found that the warning labels created awareness of the dangers of

BOX 3.1 **Example of epidemiological rates**

$$Incidence = \frac{No.\ of\ new\ cases}{Population\ at\ risk} \times 1000\ (or\ 100\,000)$$

$$Prevalence = \frac{No.\ of\ existing\ cases\ (new\ and\ old)}{Population\ at\ risk} \times 1000\ (or\ 100\,000)$$

POPULATION AT RISK

The group of people who are susceptible to a disease or condition (e.g. non-immunised children) or who have been exposed to an agent that could cause disease (e.g. occupational dust).

alcohol consumption but generally did not lead to behaviour changes that were sustained over time (5 years). One of the studies they reviewed investigated adolescent characteristics and exposure to the warning labels, which showed differences according to gender, ethnicity, familiarity with alcohol, socio-economic status and individual school grades (Nohre et al. 1999). These researchers found that students with lower school grades were more aware of the warning labels and, although they had exposure to these warnings, they had lower belief in their personal risk than students with higher grades. In another study, the researchers found that adolescents simply avoided drinks with the warning labels (MacKinnon et al. 1994).

RELATIVE RISK

A measure of the extent to which a group exposed to a risk has a higher rate of illness than those not exposed, calculated by dividing the incidence rate among those exposed by those not exposed. If the rate is higher among those exposed, it is called a *risk factor*.

Based on these and other studies in their review, Scholes-Balog et al. (2012) concluded that adolescents generally support having warning labels on alcoholic drinks, with high school students perceiving more overall risks than university students. The findings are important for providing insight into the link between the perspectives of several groups of adolescents in relation to their exposure to warning labels, but without analysing individual and group differences, it is difficult to make generalised statements about relative risk and adolescent behaviours. Still, what can we conclude from this review? In some cases, relative risk is not a helpful statistic. The studies cited in the review demonstrated differences in demographic characteristics, ages and stages, and none included cross-cultural comparisons. Statistical data and statistical comparisons are important tools in health planning, but they must be used with caution in planning whole-of-community interventions.

Because traditional epidemiological measurements of an agent, host and environment are somewhat limited in terms of what we know about the causes of illness, an expanded model, the web of causation, which includes the interconnections between each of these factors, provides a more comprehensive basis for analysis (see Figure 3.1). The web of causation is also inclusive of demographic and social features such as age, gender, ethnicity and social circumstances, which

RESEARCH TO PRACTICE: The epidemiology of malnutrition in an older population

As numbers of older people within communities increase, efforts are being made to assist them to remain living in their own homes longer. This may both decrease health care system costs and promote the health and wellbeing benefits of remaining in the home. However, among the risks facing older people maintaining their place in communities is malnutrition. Factors such as reduced mobility, lower income and cognitive impairment can contribute to this. Nurses in a large metropolitan community nursing service in Victoria, Australia were interested in establishing the rate of malnutrition among their client group. They planned a research study to determine the risk of malnutrition among a sample of community-living older adults receiving home nursing services. Of the 235 participants, 8.1% were identified as malnourished, 34.5% were identified as 'at risk' of malnutrition, and 57.4% were identified as at no risk (Rist et al. 2012).

So what does this tell us?

Findings such as those of Rist et al. (2012) enable the development of programs and policies designed to address such issues in the community.

? What types of programs or interventions do you think may be appropriate for addressing malnutrition risk in the community?

is more closely aligned with a socio-ecological model of health and the social determinants of health (SDH).

WHAT'S YOUR OPINION?

If the rate of asthma in preschool children was increasing in a community, how would you go about investigating whether the cause was a risk factor unique to that community, unique to only certain neighbourhoods, or unique to only certain types of families?

Contemporary methods to support epidemiological and other community assessment approaches enable information to be quickly and accurately compiled, presenting more quantitatively accurate assessments. For example, geographic information systems (GIS) are being commonly used to plan, administer and analyse community assessment information. GIS can enable identification of a population sample and allow for small geographic area analysis of prevalence data (Kazda et al. 2009). The use of GIS is increasingly a requirement in epidemiological analysis; however, its use in assessing needs at the community level has been less popular (Kazda et al. 2009). The risks of the GIS approach mean that some smaller population cohorts within a community may not have their needs identified. For example, the different needs of a small pocket of refugee families in a community or a group of families with children

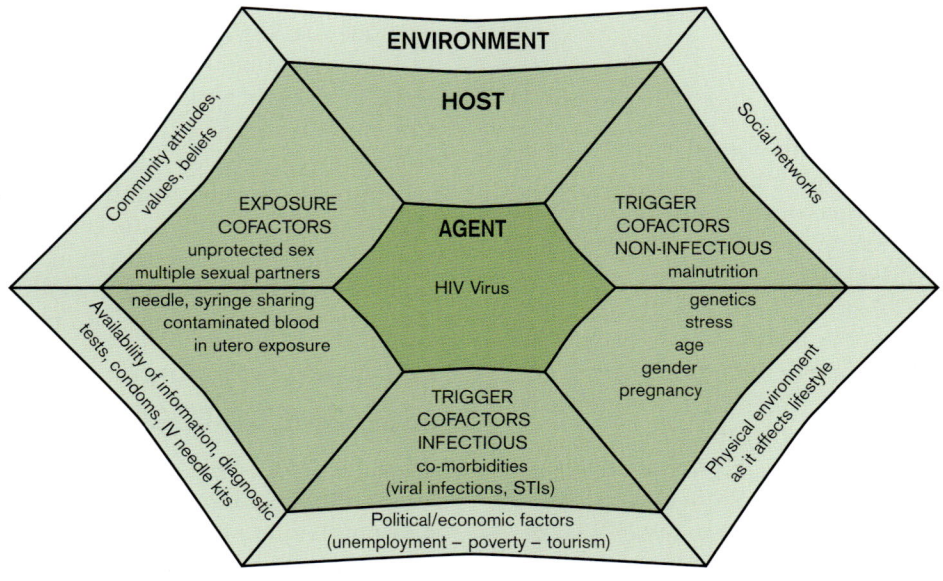

FIGURE 3.1
Web of causation

who have Down syndrome and are spread across a wider geographical area may not have their particular needs identified. Statistics from the geographic analysis reveal what is *typical* and what *trends* exist in the community, rather than what special needs exist for various segments of the population. This aggregated information contributes to the risk of 'ecological fallacy', that is, the risk of misunderstanding individual risk in terms of the overall risk to the majority of the population (Smith 2008). To gain a more realistic picture of the community, a combination of information should be used concurrently, such as combining GIS and traditional epidemiology. GIS can be a useful tool for spatial analysis of communities; for example, in analysing people's patterns of public transportation usage. The United States Environmental Protection Agency's community-focused exposure and risk screening tool (C-FERST) is a good example of this type of approach, providing easy access to maps, locally specific environmental data, and other information in a user-friendly format (Zartarian et al. 2011). But like population trends, it does not capture the breadth of variation in human behaviour, which is a limitation of many systematic approaches.

Epidemiological approaches to community assessment have traditionally struggled to reconcile

WHAT IS ... THE ECOLOGICAL FALLACY?

The risk of misunderstanding individual risk in terms of the overall population risk ... some people's health is determined by unique factors rather than those that are typical of the group or community.

the scientific approach with the broader contextual factors that impact on people's lives and contribute to their health status. Some of the challenges include the struggle to integrate epidemiologically or scientifically determined risk factors with behavioural and social strengths or risk factors; or an inability to identify risk factors whose origins lie in the interactions between individuals, or between individuals and their environment. Epidemiological models are also unable to predict the effects of alternative interventions, which are frequently non-Western in origin (for example, acupuncture), because all interventions tend to be assessed on the basis of traditional Western scientific approaches. Epidemiology also struggles to articulate the experiences of those with multiple co-morbidities, tending once again to focus on an individual disease

rather than the impact of multiple co-morbidities on a person or group. So, for example, a person who has worked in an occupation with a hazardous exposure to dust (such as in a flour mill), and who also has lived in a bushfire area, may develop pulmonary disease. The pulmonary condition may also predispose him or her to a number of other risks (cardiac, renal, stress related diseases). In this case it would be difficult to pinpoint the cause of ill health to the workplace, the natural environment, or the lack of preventative programs that would have provided protection from agents that can cause respiratory problems. The message is that epidemiological data provides only part of the picture. It is also necessary to search for causes of ill health in the social and political factors that also impact on health (Smith 1998).

As researchers have become aware of epidemiological limitations, many have become

LIMITATIONS OF EPIDEMIOLOGY

* No contextual information
* Human behaviour
* People's preferences
* Individual experiences
* Social, political factors ignored

committed to analysing community input in a way that would capture people's experience of certain risks. For example, some epidemiologists have identified that not all people on low incomes experience their life as deprived. This has led them to conclude that using income solely as a determinant of health may not be the most appropriate way to judge needs or risks. In fact, it is more helpful to health promotion planning to understand how people experience deprivation, and the ways deprivation may impinge on their health, than to simply link low income to poor health (Gunasekara et al. 2013). These types of studies provide useful information on population health status contributing to our knowledge of communities and their needs.

THE EVOLUTION OF ASSESSMENT TOOLS

Assessment tools to gather information on community health have evolved over past years to incorporate more appropriate representation of the social characteristics of communities. This refinement of approaches to assessment is useful in prompting nurses and other health professionals to base health policies and programs on knowledge of the SDH and to include community input. As far back as the 1980s several models of assessment were developed to be used in combination with epidemiological data. West (1984) devised an assessment tool based on the interaction between people and their environments in a small community. The tool included analysis of interactions, actions and awareness, and, although it was comprehensive, it was somewhat diffuse and was not validated with larger communities. Its strength was that it was intended to capture extensive information about how people felt about their community, which was helpful in encouraging the PHC principle of community participation. Another community assessment tool of the 1980s was developed to correspond to functional health assessment of individuals living in the community (Fritsch Gikow & Kucharski 1987). However, this tool did not reflect a PHC approach, and instead was focused on structured assessment of community health patterns that corresponded to personal health patterns, such as health perception and management, intersectoral role relationships and social issues. The assessment was very 'top-down', and based on health professionals' presumptions about health patterns among the population. Some of these patterns may be relevant to particular communities, but the assessment approach implied that we could use a 'one-size-fits-all' approach to community assessment. The major limitation of this type of tool is that it is inefficient and ineffective without valuable community input from which planners could predict the relative success of their interventions on the basis of community acceptability. In addition, simply assessing patterns of health and ill health fails to consider inequities between different groups of people, which is important to achieving the PHC goal of social justice.

REMINDER: PHC principles

- Accessible health care
- Appropriate technology
- Health promotion
- Cultural sensitivity
- Intersectoral collaboration
- Community participation

The assessment tool mentioned above, and other assessment tools of the 1980s, reflected nursing's commitment to the systematic approach of the nursing process. The nursing process revolves around making nursing diagnoses, typically described as 'deficits' that nurses can address. Clark's (1984) model of assessment is a comprehensive tool specifically aimed at facilitating a nursing diagnosis. It was originally described as the 'epidemiologic prevention process model', and is now known as the 'dimensions model of community health nursing' because of its later focus on the determinants of health and the dimensions of nursing (Bigbee & Issel 2012:373). Categories of information include general information about the community, epidemiological information such as population characteristics and health status indicators, attitudes towards health, environmental factors and community relationships with society (see Box 3.2 and Box 3.3).

Like Clark's model, Anderson and McFarlane's (1988, 2011) assessment tool is based on the nursing process. Their assessment model is based on their philosophy of 'community as partner', which is congruent with PHC, and a 'systems' approach to the community. Systems approaches are derived from the notion that a community is a living system that is more than the sum of its parts because of numerous and ongoing internal and external interactions that help maintain homeostasis (Neuman 1982, 1989). In Anderson and McFarlane's (2011) adaptation of Neuman's systems model, assessment is guided by an assessment wheel with eight subsystems, which include similar categories of information to those used by Clark with some expansion of the areas assessed (see Box 3.4). Despite the differences, the assessment processes remain the same. Nurses assess each of the categories or subsystems to diagnose the health of the community in order to inform implementation plans based on each.

WHAT'S YOUR OPINION?

Is there any advantage to having fewer rather than more categories of assessment?

What do you see as the strengths and weaknesses of the two models?

Anderson and McFarlane's community assessment wheel has been one of the more widely used models of community assessment in nursing. There are numerous examples in the literature of how the assessment wheel provides the basis for assessment. For example, Springer et al. (2010) used the model to explore the needs of Somali Bantu refugees in Idaho, US; and Huttlinger et al. (2004) explored the health care needs of people living in rural South West Virginia. In addition, Anderson and McFarlane's work has also been used in Australian and New Zealand settings (Francis et al. 2008).

BOX 3.2 Clark's community assessment tool

1 Biophysical

This information maps the demographic profile of the population. Included is the age composition of community members and specific age-related data such as birth rates, deaths, gender distribution, ethnicity and cultural features. Under this category morbidity and mortality are also analysed; that is, which groups in the population are suffering from specific illnesses, disablement or patterns of illness, which groups are dying from certain illnesses, and what indicators of preventative care may be evident, such as child immunisation rates.

2 Psychological

The information in this section of the assessment is aimed at identifying things like significant community events, responses indicating how the community dealt with these events, any future prospects, communication networks and protective services that exist. Communication information includes newspapers and other media that keep people connected, as well as informal networks that foster participation in community life. Information on sources of stress and past responses are also tracked, including economic viability, patterns of community growth and productivity. Patterns of psychological response among different groups are also mapped, including suicide rates, indicators of tension or inter-group conflicts, unrest, and community responses by law enforcement, emergency services or other consumer protection services.

3 Physical environment

The main aspects of the physical environment are whether it is rural or urban, size, topographical features and climate. The type and adequacy of housing are also assessed, as well as air and water quality and availability, sewage and other waste issues, nuisance factors and any potential for disaster. Environmental hazards should be identified, including risks emanating from climate change, stress-related conditions such as overcrowding, substance abuse problems, violence, motor vehicle accidents, and noise. Other environmental information may be

(Source: Clark 2003)

factors related to the causes of infectious diseases such as insect-borne diseases, or industrial hazards.

4 Socio-cultural

Social, cultural and psychological factors may show some overlap in relation to community patterns of language, leadership, education, income, occupations, marital status, family composition and religion. Transportation and availability of goods and services are also part of this aspect of assessment. Community decision-making for resource allocation is important to assess, as is the role of education and health leaders. Cultural factors may be unique to particular communities, and these are assessed with the distribution of various cultural groups, such as new migrants or older citizens. The extent of poverty in the community should also be identified, as well as accessibility of various groups to outside communication through the internet, newspapers or other media.

5 Behavioural

Behavioural factors include community consumption patterns, leisure pursuits, opportunities for physical activity, ethnic nutritional patterns, indicators of alcohol and drug misuse, or tobacco smoking, seatbelt use, entertainment and safe patterns of sexual behaviour. Behavioural factors could also reveal patterns such as attitudes towards certain groups, including visible indicators of discrimination.

6 Health system

Data collected on the health system includes not only available services but their level of performance, and which population groups use which services, including preventative and illness services. Issues surround equity and access of services, distribution of health professionals, including GPs, alternative carers, and sources of information for crisis or ongoing care, including the homeless or transient members of the community. Health financing is also assessed in this category and the extent to which government health budgets provide adequate coverage in relation to needs.

While providing a useful framework for community assessment, the model is limited by its 'top-down', deficit approach; that is, the identification of community problems rather than strengths, and seeking community input after problem identification. An existing concern with many community assessment approaches is a lack of community involvement in the early stages of the process. Communities should be involved as early as possible, as we underline throughout the chapter.

Although the early assessment tools were devoid of community input, they did help advance nursing's

BOX 3.3 The evolution of a community assessment tool

Clark's assessment tool arose from having to undertake an assessment of health needs at a summer day camp in 1995. She began the task by categorising the various needs of campers, then identifying a set of primary and secondary interventions designed to address these needs. The process was intended to identify a series of nursing diagnoses that would illuminate the physical risks and service deficits that could potentially impact on camp participants. As was accepted practice at the time, there was no dialogue with staff or campers regarding their perspective on needs and means of addressing these. Nearly 10 years later, Clark (2003:457) critiqued the model in terms of new ideas on community health, following feedback from a research project she was undertaking, where community members reported feeling '... researched to death'. She and her colleagues recognised the need for a community engagement process to round out the assessment information (Clark et al. 2003). By using focus groups with community members, the researchers identified a range of community health needs and assets. The major needs identified by community members were housing, environmental and safety needs followed by access to health care. The major assets included the proximity of the community to the larger metropolitan area, its mild climate and recreational opportunities. From the findings of this research Clark and her colleagues were able to identify a number of community-led initiatives to address some of the needs.

So what does this tell us?

The development of models help guide nursing practice with communities, and this case study demonstrates how models evolve over time as new knowledge is gained. Being aware of the history of model development helps nurses understand past practice in the context of contemporary practice and encourages us to explore new models and practices based on our previous experiences and knowledge.

? What do you see as the next phase in community assessment model development?

(Source: Clark 2003, Clark et al. 2003)

BOX 3.4 A comparison of community assessment: Anderson and McFarlane, and Clark

Anderson and McFarlane (1988, 2011)	Clark (1984, 2003)
Physical environment	Physical
Economics	Biophysical
Education	Socio-cultural
Safety and transportation	Behavioural
Health and social services	Health system
Politics and government	
Communication	
Recreation	

WHAT'S YOUR OPINION?

Early assessment models included person-environment interactions and were not always inclusive of what we now call the SDH. They were also intended to provide a nursing diagnosis as a basis for systematic health planning.

What are the strengths and weaknesses of these early approaches?

scientific agenda, by systematising the processes of assessment. Over time, those using the tools began to recognise the importance of social and interactive factors that are so important to community health. However, by being prescriptive about categories of assessment data, sometimes critical information was overlooked, including the need to assess cultural factors within various community neighbourhoods and groups. Subsequent community assessment models have contributed to a deeper understanding of the cultural domain of assessment, following the lead of Leininger (1967) and other nursing theorists (Giger & Davidhizar 2002; Leininger & McFarland 2006; Jirwe et al. 2006; Tripp-Reimer et al. 1984). Cultural assessment is now a major focus in community assessment, integrating cultural information with other assessment information. Cultural assessment strategies are intended to provide the depth and breadth of locally identified information that is crucial to ensuring their acceptability in the context of the nurse–client relationship.

Cultural assessment information can include community members' perspectives on their worldview, relevant issues related to ethnicity, values, beliefs, history and social orientation (Springer et al. 2010). For migrant groups, information on pre-movement, migration and post-migration events is also collected to assess the combination of social, environmental, cultural and medical factors that determine health. In the case of many refugees this information is significant in assessing the impacts of conflict, torture, stress and a variety of traumas, and how these experiences help or hinder their transition to community life (Merry et al. 2011). Samarasinghe (2011) argues for a more comprehensive model of cultural assessment for refugee populations, which includes detailed information on family factors, family reactions to the transition to a new country, the impact of changes, and aspects of the host community that cause or exacerbate the trauma and stress of dislocation. An important element of the cultural assessment involves assessing caregivers, as some researchers have found that accessibility and use of services is dependent upon cultural and language competencies of staff members (Bourgeault et al. 2010; Habersack et al. 2011). Including cultural assessment in all community assessments is congruent with the work of Ramsden (1993) in highlighting cultural safety in all professional interactions. Cultural information also provides a more realistic picture of the community and its socio-cultural environment, and shifts the emphasis from the deficit model of the nursing process to the more positive 'asset mapping' model of assessment.

ASSET MAPPING

WHAT IS ... ASSET MAPPING?

Assessing the community strengths and assets that will help develop community capacity.

Deficit models of assessment such as the nursing process can be helpful in identifying needs and priorities for health service provision; however, this type of assessment is incomplete without assessing positive community features or 'assets' (Morgan & Ziglio 2007). Asset mapping is a more resourceful, inclusive approach that can help identify health inequities in the community, particularly if the assessment includes information on the capability of communities to identify problems and activate solutions (see Figure 3.2). This approach to assessment is therefore responsive to the goals of PHC and the SDH. An asset map is intended to build an inventory of community strengths in relation to

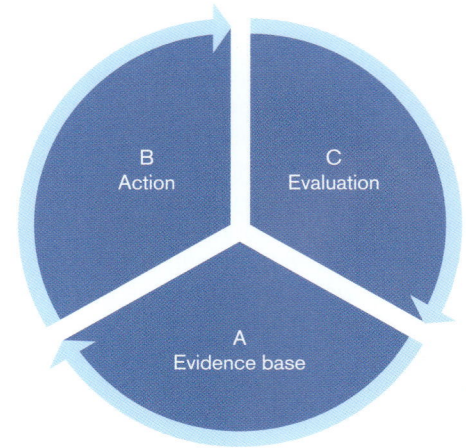

FIGURE 3.2
The asset model

(adapted from Morgan & Ziglio 2007)

the SDH. Data consists of epidemiological information on the population, their key assets at each stage of life, and the links between these assets and health outcomes (Morgan & Ziglio 2007). This assessment information can provide a foundation for planning strategies to reduce health inequities. Categories of information include primary building blocks (assets and capacities of residents, their skills, talents, experiences, associations, under neighbourhood control); secondary building blocks (assets in the community controlled primarily by outsiders, such as physical resources, land, waste, energy, public institutions and services); and potential building blocks (resources outside the community controlled externally, such as public capital and expenditures) (Kretzmann & McKnight 1993). From this base of evidence members of the community can work with health professionals to identify actions to improve health that will be evaluated for their effectiveness. However, in using this approach to assessment, consideration must be given to the way data are aggregated. As noted earlier in the chapter, if the information represents an epidemiological approach that focuses only on the total assets within each of these building blocks, it would be difficult to identify pockets of inequity among subgroups, even within a particular neighbourhood. As a guide for planning to meet the goals of PHC, it would be necessary to ensure that information was *stratified*, or categorised according to groups such as the homeless, young people, older citizens and those with disabilities.

The strength of asset mapping is that it is a community-based approach to assessment intended

WHICH ASSETS TO MAP?

- Primary—resident controlled features
- Secondary—externally controlled features
- Potential—external resources that could be mobilised

to respond to the SDH, and it continues to evolve. A related assessment approach is encompassed in community-based participatory research (CBPR), which is designed to assess community needs from the perspective of residents (Israel et al. 1998; Cook 2008). CBPR uses focus group interviews to foster collaborative identification of community needs as a basis for plans to improve health and wellbeing (Cook 2008). This type of approach has been shown to be effective in a number of contexts, particularly for occupational and environmental health planning, but increasingly, as a strategy for conducting research with cultural groups (see Box 3.5). Together, asset mapping and CBPR represent a goal-directed approach to assessment that is particularly useful for program planning. It is important to remember that most programs are aimed at addressing a specific health problem, which is important, but they are usually confined to a particular population group or health issue rather than the whole of the community. The program planning approach is therefore more closely aligned with *selective* rather than *comprehensive* PHC.

REMINDER: Selective and comprehensive PHC

Selective PHC is aimed at health programs for certain groups.

Comprehensive PHC is a whole-of-community approach.

One of the key elements of CBPR as an approach to community research is the engagement of the community at the earliest possible moment in the process. This ensures that community members are involved in identifying the most appropriate approach to data collection, analysis and reporting, they have a say in how the information is interpreted, they are encouraged to share their knowledge and skills with the researchers, and can

BOX 3.5 **CBPR in action**

CBPR is a collaborative research approach that specifically focuses on the equitable involvement of community partners in the research process (Israel et al. 1998). CBPR should always begin with a research topic of importance to the community and be based on the principles of co-learning and community partnerships in investigating inequities, which is intended to address health from both positive and ecological processes, and promote sharing of findings (Israel et al. 1998).

Evaluations from CBPR studies have found that the approach allows a good understanding of a community, participants feel ownership of a study, the voice of community members is heard, trust is built, and challenges acknowledged (Kobeissi et al. 2011). Some of the challenges of a CBPR approach include increased cost associated with the time it takes to do the research, and the need to ensure that appropriate communication with community members can take place—particularly if language and cultural barriers exist (Williams et al. 2009; Israel et al. 1998). It is important to work with informal as well as formal leaders to assess needs and strengths from a balanced perspective that goes beyond only the views of those in authority.

An Australian study that developed a framework for a planned school-based health promotion program to encourage healthy computing behaviours among middle school students offers a good example of how CBPR can work in practice (Soares et al. 2012). In this study, the school principal and head of the middle school, concerned about the health implications of introducing a 1:1 notebook computer program for year 7 students, approached the research team to develop and implement a health promotion program that would mitigate these concerns. Using the unique strengths of each research partner, the study considered epidemiological risk factors, attitudes of the entire school community towards health-enhancing behaviours, and environmental factors such as the physical and cultural learning environments as they developed the program. The evaluation will be interesting in terms of the impact of the program on the children's health once the study has been completed.

gain increased knowledge and skills in return. This reciprocal process contributes to community and individual improvements in health literacy, and reflects the PHC principle of community participation.

ASSESSMENT TOOLS SPECIFIC TO HEALTH EDUCATION PLANNING

Among the most specific, goal-directed tools is the PRECEDE-PROCEED tool for health education planning (Green & Kreuter 1991) (see Figure 3.3). The objective of the tool is to identify the multitude of factors related to specific health behaviours among members of the community or group (Tramm et al. 2011). Like the nursing process models, Green and Kreuter's model revolves around gathering diagnostic information: first, a social diagnosis, including such issues as education, community crime, population density, unemployment and other variables similar to the SDH. This phase is followed by an epidemiological diagnosis, intended to reveal rates of morbidity, mortality, disability and fertility. This phase is aimed at determining the extent and nature of determinants of health (Green & Kreuter 2005). Next, a behavioural and environmental diagnosis is undertaken to identify factors related to actions people might take and how interactions with their physical and social environments might affect these (Green & Kreuter 2005). Included are indicators such as dietary patterns, preventative actions such as safe sexual behaviours, self-care indicators and coping skills.

THE PRECEDE-PROCEED MODEL

What are predisposing, reinforcing and enabling factors?

Predisposing: knowledge, attitudes, values and perceptions

Reinforcing: attitudes and behaviours of others

Enabling: skills resources and barriers to change

How do these factors contribute to our understanding of communities?

The environmental diagnosis includes economic and geographic indicators of community health and services and how people interact with these services. Analysis of these factors is complemented by an educational and organisational diagnosis to reveal Predisposing, Reinforcing and Enabling factors that could lead to behavioural and environmental change. Predisposing factors include knowledge, attitudes, values and perceptions that may hinder or facilitate motivation for change, so health literacy is important to assess at this stage. Reinforcing factors include the attitudes and behaviours of others that affect behaviour and the environments for change (Green & Kreuter 2005). Enabling factors are those skills,

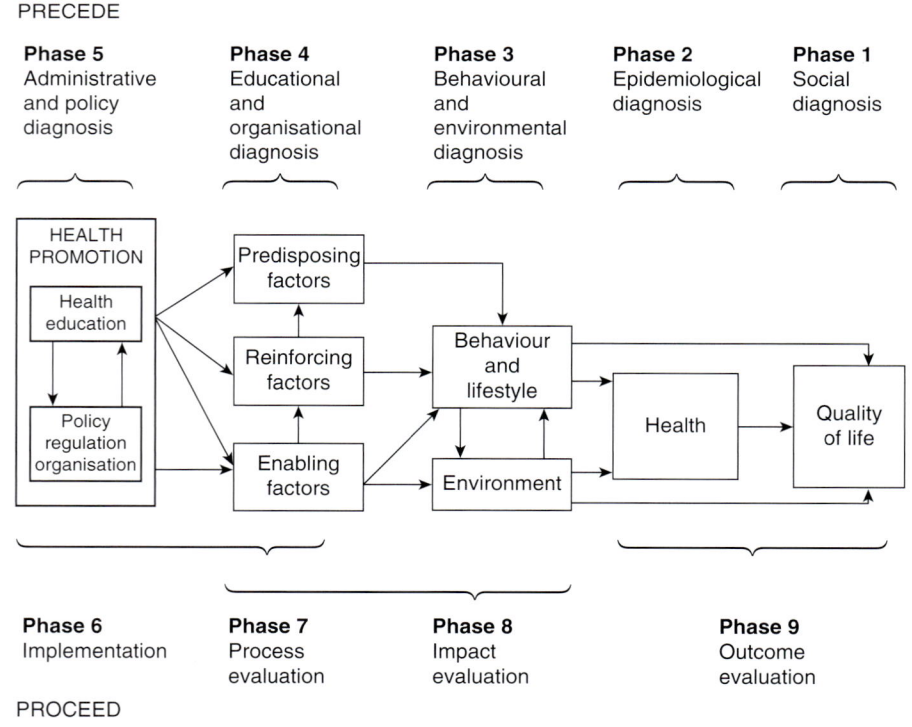

FIGURE 3.3
PRECEDE-PROCEED model

resources, assets or barriers that could help or hinder the desired changes. Following this phase, an administrative and policy diagnosis is conducted to examine the community's capabilities and resources to respond to needs. With this level of assessment, implementation of changes can begin, based on careful evaluation of each of the previous aspects of the model (Green & Kreuter 1991, 2005). The PRECEDE-PROCEED model has been used for many years to make a community diagnosis, but like some of the other models, it is limited by the top-down perspective of the health professional on what a community needs or prefers. In this respect, it is limited in providing a comprehensive assessment that includes input from community members who feel empowered to participate in charting the course of community health.

WHAT'S YOUR OPINION?

What are the strengths and weaknesses of the Precede-Proceed model of assessment?

Would it provide sufficient information to work with community members to meet their needs?

SOCIAL EPIDEMIOLOGY, CBPR, PHC AND THE SDH

In a comprehensive PHC context, assessment information should reveal where inequities exist in the community, what levels of disadvantage exist for which groups in the community, what links there are between community attitudes, local and centralised decisions and health outcomes, and a myriad of other relationships relevant to the SDH. One approach to collecting this information is to adopt a 'social epidemiological' approach. The goal of social epidemiology is to test associations between the socio-ecological aspects of community life and population health outcomes (Wallerstein et al. 2011). This approach is closer to the goals of both PHC and the SDH than the type of assessment outlined above, in that it is aimed at resolving issues of inequity. Used in conjunction with CBPR, social epidemiology yields a depth and breadth of information that can be helpful for planning.

WHAT IS ... SOCIAL EPIDEMIOLOGY?

Assessing associations between the socio-ecological aspects of community life and population health outcomes

How is this process linked to the SDH?

A social epidemiological assessment begins with demographic and epidemiological data, mapping the main indicators of community life. Concurrently, a CBPR study can provide information on what people believe community life is like, what could be done to improve the community, what would improve health, how the health department could help, and how the community nurse and other health professionals can effectively participate in enabling health and wellbeing (Clark et al. 2003, Wallerstein et al. 2011). Next the social epidemiological data will show the balance between resources and demand, strengths and needs. Among the information collected would be indicators of social capital such as indicators of cohesiveness and bonding, health behaviours, illness indicators and community perceptions. Integral to the process is evaluation of the power structures and how they affect certain groups, to provide policy planners with the information to challenge these conditions, including issues of racism, discrimination or other forms of social exclusion (Wallerstein et al. 2011). A social epidemiological approach is therefore similar to asset mapping. Identifying community assets or strengths can help community members develop empowering strategies to gain mastery and control over health decision-making. In this way, information can be inspiring, helping people participate fully in their community and expand their ability to negotiate, influence, control and hold accountable the institutions and decision-makers that control their lives (Wallerstein et al. 2011). This social epidemiological approach to assessment comes closest to the ideal of an SDH approach.

STREAMLINING COMMUNITY ASSESSMENT

It should be evident from the assessment models described above that most community assessment tools combine epidemiological data with psychological, socio-cultural, and environmental indicators, including information about the health system and its use. The most useful tools are those that combine the multidimensional and dynamic nature of community life as well as capturing individual and family strengths and constraints (McMurray 2013). Community assessment does not need to be a complex process, although the more information that is included in the assessment, the more likely it will be that the interventions will be appropriate and acceptable to the community. The following steps provide a simple process for undertaking a community assessment and capture the varying sources of information required.

1.   Approach key community members to identify how you can work with their community to

undertake a community assessment. Gain their consent to work in and with the community and work with them to identify how they appraise and assess their health strengths and needs along with their perceptions, priorities and understanding of community assessment.

2. Map community strengths, resources and risks by a) talking with everyday community members about their perceptions, priorities, and relationships within and external to the community and b) collecting information using the SDH Assessment Circle (see Box 3.6) as a framework for organising the data.

3. Analyse the information in collaboration with community members using a SWOT analysis.

4. Share the findings with community members and work with them to develop intervention strategies for improvement or measures that sustain positive community life.

WHY DO A SWOT ANALYSIS?

To identify community:

Strengths

Weaknesses

Opportunities and

Threats to health

Key community members are those who hold positions of respect and/or authority in the community, either through formal or informal leadership. These people may be community elders, local health care providers, teachers, social workers, town council or community board members, and/or others who may provide services in the community. While speaking with some of these people may simply be a formality, speaking with community elders and gaining their consent to work with you in the community is an essential first step to community assessment. Talk to them about what you want to find out, what they want to find out, and let them tell you where to find the information. They will know who to talk to, where to look for information, and what not to do as you undertake your community assessment. This process will also help establish trust between you and the community and keeps everyone 'in the loop' as you go about your assessment.

The next step is to map the community's strengths, resources and risks. This is a two-step process (although both steps can occur concurrently). Firstly, talking with community members yields a wide range of information that shows the demographic 'mix' in the community—how many people in which population groups may require certain specific services (e.g. older persons, young children); the mix of cultures in the community; what people think about their lives; opinions about environmental strengths that may support healthy lifestyles, or barriers to health. Find out about people's perceptions, priorities and relationships— these are the relationships that exist between people, and between people and their environment. Once this information is gleaned, the second part of this step involves mapping resources—trying to understand the capacity for supporting health, the assets and support systems that may be mobilised for certain interventions. The SDH Assessment Circle provides a framework for mapping these resources and is outlined in Box 3.6.

The third step is to analyse the information— this can take the form of a SWOT analysis to identify strengths, weaknesses, opportunities and threats to community health. Included in the SWOT analysis will be a deeper level of analysis of the community that provides information on the SDH. This analysis should be done in collaboration with community members to ensure the way you interpret and make sense of the information is aligned with community members' understanding of the data. This action will help build trust with the community and serve to facilitate the development of the community-led interventions that make up the final step in the process.

SOURCES OF ASSESSMENT INFORMATION

For nurses who are new to a community, comprehensive assessments can be daunting, and the sources of information a bit confusing. Some information will be available online in government documents. For example, Australian data on morbidity, mortality and age-related conditions are included in the document 'Australia's Health', which is updated every 2–4 years. Australian Government Census reports and health department reports on a variety of topics are also available online. Health Insite (www.healthinsite.gov.au) has a wealth of information on Australian health indicators. The New Zealand Ministry of Health has a range of publications that provide background data on the health status of New Zealanders. The New Zealand Health Survey is now a continuous study and provides the most up-to-date information on population health in New Zealand. Findings are published on the Ministry of Health website: www.health.govt.nz. Statistics New Zealand

BOX 3.6 **The SDH Assessment Circle**

1   Biological or genetic population indicators
2   Groups defined by culture and gender
3   Physical environments, including geographical factors such as climate change or transportation barriers to care, or activity-friendly neighbourhoods
4   Social environments, indicators of social inclusion or exclusion
5   Indicators of child health and development
6   Education and literacy indicators
7   Employment and financial status of the population, including unemployment rates,

working conditions, types of employers, availability of workplace support
8   Social support networks, access for vulnerable groups, volunteer networks
9   Health services and resources and patterns of accessing these by various population groups
10   Health practices, coping skills in the context of recreation and leisure, which may support or compromise health, such as drop in centres, places that encourage health literacy and capacity, or drug and alcohol misuse

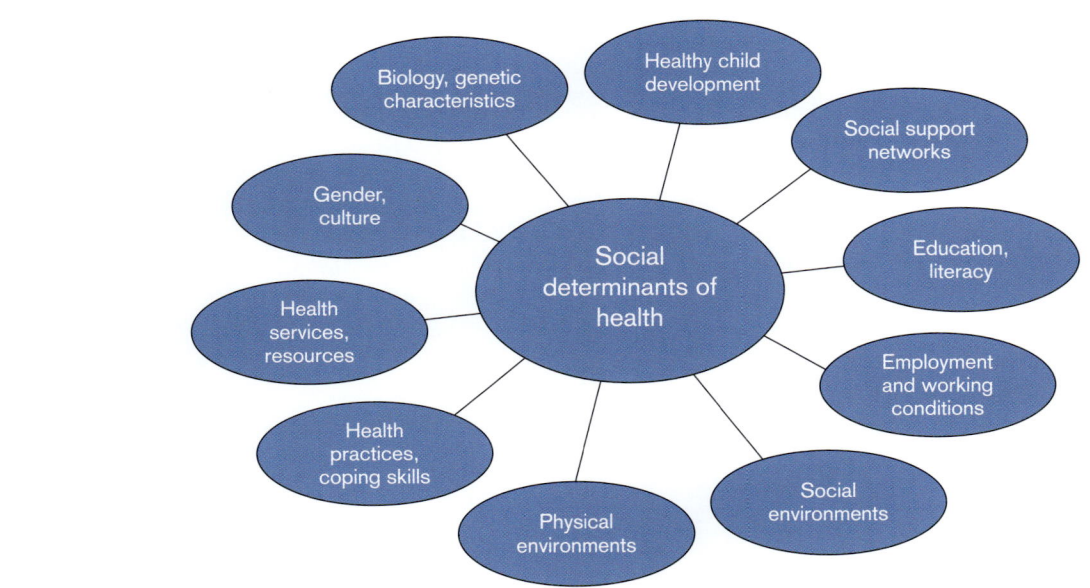

(www.stats.govt.nz) is also a useful portal for accessing any statistical data on communities and publishes many existing community profiles developed from census data. For the more enthusiastic nurse, it is also possible to manipulate excel data tables to find the specific statistics required for a geographic area. The Christchurch earthquake in February 2010 occurred only a few days before the scheduled five yearly census of populations and dwellings. As a result, the census was delayed until 2013. This means there was an eight year gap between censuses. The much-awaited data from the 2013 census became available throughout 2013 and 2014, and provides New Zealand nurses with the most up-to-date information on populations and communities.

WHAT IS ... A WINDSCREEN SURVEY?

Placing a paper survey under a windscreen wiper blade?

Counting the number of cars in a community?

Driving around to gain a good understanding of the 'lay of the land' in a community?

The Yellow Pages are another source of community information, as are community business directories. Some of the most useful information for community assessment comes from local surveys that may have been conducted in recent years, or from observations of community life. A search of websites like Google or PubMed, or any of the research databases (see Chapter 15) may also reveal whether there have been any research studies in the community, which may provide additional information.

Most community nurses have their own strategies for collecting various types of information, depending on whether they are responsible for the whole community, or practising in specific areas, such as general practice, child, school or occupational health, or in a visiting nurse service. In the first instance nurses can become familiar with a community by conducting a 'windscreen survey', driving around to gain a sense of the community—a big picture of life in that context. Such a survey can yield information about spaces for recreation, transportation and access, child care services, the location of schools, clinics, hospitals and other health services, places of employment, the state of available housing such as whether there are affordable homes, or whether certain sections of the community seem to be in decline. This type of information can also be confirmed by speaking to various community groups or by analysing records of community activities such as immunisation rates, public health indicators and data from other policy documents that indicate activities of the local council or other authorities (fitness programs, elder day care facilities). Community assets, strengths and risks can also be identified by being attentive to people's visible health behaviours such as observing people out walking, older persons engaging in Tai Chi, and/or parent get-togethers.

Part 2: Assessment in Practice

The SDH Assessment Circle shown in Box 3.6 and Figure 3.4 below gathers information within the ten categories of the social determinants of health. This framework incorporates all of the elements of community assessment, epidemiological data and social epidemiological information in one cohesive framework. Using the information in Figure 3.4 as a guide, the following group exercise demonstrates the SDH Assessment Circle in practice. We then use the SDH approach in the case study of the Smith and Mason families to describe the families' communities.

Group exercise: SDH assessment

Working in groups of two to three, undertake a windscreen survey in your local community. Make notes on what you observe. Consider how the notes you have made (the data you collected) fit into the SDH Assessment Circle and where. Make some notes on how useful you found this exercise and what you learned. Share your findings with the wider group.

'The SDH Assessment Circle' - Please refer to the diagram on previous page.

1. Assessing biological, genetic factors

Assessment prompts	Sources of information
What is the demographic mix of population by age, gender, ethnicity? What is the birth rate among the various groups? What is the death rate and the leading causes of death? What patterns of health and disease exist in the community? What is the prevalence and incidence of the most common conditions in the community? Which groups in the community are more prone to certain genetic or biological conditions? What is the mix of dual and single parent households? What proportion are single dweller households?	www.healthinsite.gov.au (search Western Australian Health Report, Statistics, Life Stage, Women's health, Men's health), Australian Institute of Family Studies (AIFS) (search www.aifs.gov.au) Department of Health Western Australia (search www.health.wa.gov.au) Australian Bureau of Statistics (www.abs.gov.au) Church groups (search www.touristradio.com.au/pages/church.htm Ministry of Health (search www.health.govt.nz) Statistics New Zealand (search www.stats.govt.nz for census data) Ministry of Social Development (search www.msd.govt.nz)

FIGURE 3.4
The SDH Assessment Circle

2. Assessing gender and culture

Are there any indicators of gender inequity in the community?
What languages are spoken?
What cultural or special needs groups are visible in the community?
To what extent are gender relations protected through a women's health and men's health policy (see Chapter 14)?
Is there equal support for fathers and mothers in the education, health, childcare and social support systems?
How are the rights of LBGTI people supported in the community (see Chapter 12)?
Are there groups in the community with particular spiritual needs?
How are these addressed?
(search www.touristradio.com.au/pages/church.htm)

3. Assessing the physical environment

Is the community disadvantaged by remoteness or distance from health and social supports?
What steps are taken to ensure the community has clean air, water, and sufficient environmental supports for health?
How is the link between climate and health outcomes measured and disseminated to the population?
What health literacy initiatives help develop knowledge of environmental risks? For which groups of people?
What green spaces are available for people to engage in recreation and for children to play?
Do all population groups have access to, safe, efficient and affordable public transportation?
What types of systems are in place to ensure healthy food and safe water is available?
Are food bank and budgeting services available where needed in the community?
How are pollution and waste managed?

4. Assessing the social environment

What supportive programs are available to promote healthy lifestyles? For which groups of people?
Are houses adequate, safe, warm or cool enough and protective from crowding?
Which areas in the community have substandard housing? Is emergency housing available when needed? Are any community groups excluded from this type of help?
What policies and programs are available to support those with difficulties in finding housing?
What are the indicators that the social environment is inclusive? How are different groups encouraged to participate in community life?
What special programs are available to support cultural diversity?
What types of social support is available for different age groups?
What local council initiatives support families?
Do most citizens of all ages have access to the internet?

5. Assessing child health and development

What reproductive choices are available to women in the community?
What is the distribution of antenatal services and other forms of pregnancy support? To what extent are these available to all parents?
What is the rate of child and maternal mortality? VLBs? Stillbirths? What is the variability of these rates for various groups in the community?
What supports exist for postnatal depression and other postpartum issues?
Do all families have access to neonatal and ongoing child care?
What programs are available to support parenting?
Is there access to early childhood education (ECE) and child care for everyone who wants these services?
Do ECE and child care services accommodate cultural diversity? Are they inclusive of the needs of disadvantaged children?

6. Assessing education, literacy

What is the distribution of publicly subsidised schools in the community? To what extent do these serve all neighbourhoods?
What initiatives exist to encourage adolescents to complete high school?
How do schools support the health and wellbeing of children and their families?
How are schools involved in community life?
What literacy programs are available for new migrants, NESB groups?
What supports are in place for vulnerable and disadvantaged people to undertake education and/or skills retraining?
How is health literacy addressed in the community? To what extent are health literacy programs inclusive?

7. Assessing employment and financial status

What is the rate of employment/unemployment for various groups (young people, adults)?
What are the more predominant occupations in the community?
What is the rate and type of occupational injuries, diseases and exposure to hazards?
What policies exist to support those who are unable to find work?
To what extent do workplaces support parental leave arrangements?
How does the workplace support workers' rights at work, especially for migrants, casual employees, and those disadvantaged by illness or distance?
What physical and psychosocial supports exist for workers to minimise the risk of illness, injury and work related stress?
What are the indicators of gender and cultural equity in the workplace?

8. Assessing social support networks

Are there sufficient voluntary agencies and volunteers to help those in need?
How does the community support those who are impoverished?
What disability supports are provided for the disabled and their families?
How are community members encouraged to engage in partnerships for health and wellbeing?
How do community organisations reduce social exclusion?

FIGURE 3.4 cont'd

9. Assessing health services and resources

What are the indicators that health and other services are governed by a 'health in all policies' program?
What is the distribution of acute and community services?
Are these appropriate for all population groups?
Does the community provide equal access to affordable care?
What evidence is there that health services are well governed?
What evidence-based clinical and management practices are used?
What is the distribution of culturally appropriate services for Indigenous people and those who have language or communication difficulties?
What limitations exist on access for older or disabled residents?
What indicators are there that community services are client-centred, promoting self-care and choice?
What health promotion initiatives exist to reduce alcohol, tobacco, fat consumption and other hazardous lifestyle factors? What is the prevalence of these lifestyle factors in the community?

10. Assessing health practices and coping

What are the indicators of community advocacy initiatives to promote health literacy?
What is the distribution of health professionals? To what extent is this adequate for the population?
Does the community provide access to a variety of health practices, including alternative practices, and is access to alternative practitioners available?
Are working people able to access appropriate health and social services outside working hours?
How are people made aware of local resources?
Which mental and emotional support services are available to all?
How are the needs of the mentally ill accommodated?
How are family support centres made available for those in crisis?

FIGURE 3.4 cont'd

On completion of an SDH assessment, presentation of your work to the community and/or to your colleagues and peers is a useful way of disseminating the information you have gathered. These groups may have useful ideas on where further information can be obtained, how the information can be used, and what the next steps in the process may be. In the context of community placements, discussion of assessment information with community nurses or the teaching staff supervising your placement can also provide locally relevant information for health promotion.

CASE STUDY: Assessing community needs for the Mason and Smith families

We now return to the Smith and Mason families to provide an example of some of the information you may collect as part of assessing their communities' strengths, weaknesses, opportunities and threats to health. There are distinctive differences in the three communities that influence health and wellness for the Mason and Smith families. The mining camp where Colin and Jason work is sparse and functional, approximately 1000 km from Perth, the capital of Western Australia and the epicentre of the 'resources boom'. In the area surrounding the mining camp are several small towns, where each community is comprised of a mix of long-term residents and newcomers. Many of the townspeople live in caravan parks because of the shortage and high cost of housing. Some are service workers who service the mine and the local population. The physical environment is challenging, with extreme dry, dusty heat during the day and little rainfall.

Maddington is known as a family-friendly but diverse community with many young families, some of them migrants, and older residents. The Smith family has ready access to the train station and the shopping centre, which they can reach by bus from the stop on their street. There is moderate unemployment in the suburb because there are so many opportunities across a range of jobs to work in the mines, and access to the airport is ideal, within 10 km of Maddington. The Smith's neighbourhood has a large number of FIFO families, and an informal mining wives' club which meets regularly at the community centre. There is a shortage of GPs in the area, but several child health clinics, and a school health nurse attends the public school. The day care is staffed by accredited early childhood educators.

Papakura is a low socio-economic community with moderate levels of unemployment and a high multicultural population. The area has a large number of young families, single parent households and older retired people. There are also a large number of state houses, private rental properties and some home ownership. While FIFO families are not common in New Zealand it is a growing response to a lack of employment opportunities. The community has a local integrated family health centre which offers general practice, pharmacy and physiotherapy services. There is a local Plunket room and a playground near the shops.

REFLECTING ON THE BIG ISSUES

- Community assessment includes mapping strengths, resources, risks and needs with input from members of the community.

- Epidemiological data provide information on the determinants and distribution of risks and diseases in the population, usually defined as incidence and prevalence rates.

- Quantifying rates of health risks and diseases is useful in some ways, but is not inclusive of community perspectives and preferences or the particular needs of subgroups in the population.

- Socio-ecological assessment tools have evolved over the years to reflect an increasing emphasis on the SDH.

- Asset mapping is a tool for assessment that outlines primary, secondary and potential features and resources that can be mobilised for community health.

- Community-based participatory research (CBPR) can be combined with asset mapping to provide a realistic assessment of community health needs.

- Social epidemiological assessment integrates demographic and epidemiological assessment data with information from the community, often in the context of CBPR.

- The SDH Assessment Circle is an ideal way to ensure data are collected on all the social determinants of health in a community.

REFLECTIVE QUESTIONS: How would I use this knowledge in practice?

1. Using the SDH assessment model identify the most important priorities for promoting health in the mining community.

2. What information will you use to assess the Maddington community in relation to its strengths, weaknesses, threats and opportunities for socio-ecological support for the Smith family?

3. What strengths, weaknesses, threats and opportunities are readily identifiable in Papakura?

4. What information do you need to glean from Rebecca and Huia on their family and community needs? Compile a list of questions to prompt your assessment interview with both of the women.

5. What gaps in assessment data did you find from your assessment interviews?

6. What extra sources of information did you use to complete the assessments in both communities?

7. From the assessment data of all three communities, what provisional plans would you put in place for health promotion?

References

Anderson, E., McFarlane, J., 1988. Community as partner: Theory and practice in nursing. JB Lippincott, New York.

Anderson, E., McFarlane, J., 2011. Community as partner: Theory and practice in nursing, sixth ed. Lippincott, Williams & Wilkins, New York.

Bigbee, J., Issel, M., 2012. Conceptual models for population-focused public health nursing interventions and outcomes: The state of the art. Public Health Nurs. 29 (4), 370–379.

Bourgeault, I., Atanackovic, J., Rashid, A., et al., 2010. Relations between immigrant care workers and older persons in home and long-term care. Can. J. Aging 29 (1), 109–118.

Clark, M., 1984. Community nursing: Health care for today and tomorrow. Reston Publishing, Reston.

Clark, M.J., 2003. Community health nursing: Caring for populations, fourth ed. Pearson Education, Upper Saddle River NJ.

Clark, M., Cary, S., Diemert, G., et al., 2003. Involving communities in community assessment. Public Health Nurs. 20 (6), 456–463.

Cook, W., 2008. Integrating research and action: a systematic review of community-based participatory research to address health disparities in environmental and occupational health in the USA. J. Epidemiol. Community Health 62, 668–676.

Francis, K., Chapman, Y., Hoare, K., et al., 2008. Australia and New Zealand community as partner: Theory and practice in nursing. Lippincott Williams & Wilkins, New South Wales.

Fritsch Gikow, F., Kucharski, P., 1987. A new look at the community: Functional health pattern assessment. J. Community Health Nurs. 4 (1), 21–27.

Giger, J., Davidhizar, R., 2002. Culturally competent care: emphasis on understanding the people of Afghanistan, Afghanistan Americans, and Islamic culture and religion. Int. Nurs. Rev. 49, 79–86.

Green, L., Kreuter, M., 1991. Health Promotion Planning: An Educational and Environmental Approach. Mayfield Publishing Company, Mountain View.

Green, L., Kreuter, M., 2005. Health Promotion Planning: An Educational and Environmental Approach, fourth ed. McGraw Hill, New York.

Gunasekara, F., Carter, K., Crampton, P., et al., 2013. Income and individual deprivation as predictors of health over time. Int. J. Public Health doi:10.1007/s00038-013-0450-9.

Habersack, M., Gerlich, I., Mandi, M., 2011. Migrant women in Austria: difficulties with access to health care services. Ethn Inequal Health Soc Care 4 (1), 6–15.

Huttlinger, K., Schaller-Ayers, J., Lawson, T., 2004. Health care in Appalachia: a population-based approach. Public Health Nurs. 21 (2), 103–110.

Israel, B., Schultz, A., Parker, E., et al., 1998. Review of community-based research: Assessing partnership approaches to improving public health. Annu. Rev. Public Health 19, 173–202.

Jirwe, M., Gerrish, K., Emami, A., 2006. The theoretical framework of cultural competence. J. Multicult. Nurs. Health 12 (3), 6–16.

Kazda, M., Beel, E., Villegas, D., et al., 2009. Methodological complexities and the use of GIS in conducting a community needs assessment of a large U.S. municipality. J. Community Health 34 (3), 210–215.

Kobeissi, L., Nakkash, R., Ghantous, Z., et al., 2011. Evaluating a community based participatory approach to research with disadvantaged women in the southern suburbs of Beirut. J. Community Health 36 (5), 741–747, doi. <http://dx.doi.org/10.1007/s10900-011-9368-4>.

Kretzmann, J., McKnight, J., 1993. Building communities from the inside out: a path towards building and mobilising community assets. Institute for Policy Research, Evanston Ill.

Leininger, M., 1967. The culture concept and its relevance to nursing. J. Nurs. Educ. 6 (2), 27–39.

Leininger, M., McFarland, M., 2006. Culture care diversity and universality: A worldwide theory of nursing, second ed. Jones and Bartlett, Sudbury, MA.

MacKinnon, D., Nemeroff, C., Nohre, L., 1994. Avoidance responses to alternative alcohol warning labels. J. Appl. Psychol. 24 (8), 733–753.

McMurray, A., 2013. Healthy communities: The evolving roles of nursing. In: Jackson, D., Daly, J., Speedy, S. (Eds.), Contexts of Nursing, third ed. Elsevier, Sydney.

Merry, L., Gagnon, A., Hemlin, I., et al., 2011. Cross-border movement and women's health: how to capture the data. Int. J. Equity Health 10 (1), 56–71.

Morgan, A., Ziglio, E., 2007. Revitalising the evidence-base for public health: an assets model. Promot. Educ. (Suppl. 2), 17–22.

Neuman, B., 1982. The Neuman systems model. Appleton-Century-Crofts, Norwalk.

Neuman, B., 1989. The Neuman systems model, second ed. Appleton-Lange, Norwalk.

Nohre, L., MacKinnon, D., Stacy, A., et al., 1999. Generality and specificity in health behaviour: Application to warning-label and social influence expectancies. J. Appl. Psychol. 16 (3), 245–259.

Ramsden, I., 1993. Cultural safety in nursing education in Aotearoa. Nurs. Prax. N. Z. 8 (3), 4–10.

Rist, G., Miles, G., Karimi, L., 2012. The presence of malnutrition in community-living older adults receiving home nursing services. Nutr. Diet. 69, 46–50.

Samarasinghe, K., 2011. A conceptual model facilitating the transition of involuntary migrant families. International Scholarly Research Network. doi:10.5402/2011/824209.

Scholes-Balog, K., Heerde, J., Hemphill, S., 2012. Alcohol warning labels: unlikely to affect alcohol-related beliefs and behaviours in adolescents. Aust. N. Z. J. Public Health 36 (5), 524–529.

Smith, M., 1998. Community-based epidemiology. J. Health Soc. Policy 9 (4), 51–65.

Smith, B., Keleher, H., Fry, C., 2008. Developing values, evidence and advocacy to address the social determinants of health. Health Promot. J. Austr. 19 (3), 171–172.

Soares, M., Jacobs, K., Ciccarelli, M., et al., 2012. Promoting healthy computer use among middle school students: A pilot school-based health promotion program. Work 41, 851–856.

Springer, P., Black, M., Martz, K., et al., 2010. Somali Bantu refugees in Southwest Idaho. Adv. Nursi. Sci. 33 (2), 170–181.

Tramm, R., McCarthy, A., Yates, P., 2011. Using the Precede-Proceed model of health program planning in breast cancer nursing research. J. Adv. Nurs. 68 (8), 1870–1879.

Tripp-Reimer, T., Brink, P., Saunders, J., 1984. Cultural assessment: content and process. Nurs. Outlook 32 (30), 78–82.

Wallerstein, N., Yen, I., Syme, L., 2011. Integration of social epidemiology and community-engaged interventions to improve health equity. Am. J. Public Health 101 (5), 822–830.

West, M., 1984. Community health assessment: The man-environment interaction. J. Community Health Nurs. 1 (2), 89–97.

Williams, K., Gail Bray, P., Shapiro-Mendoza, C., et al., 2009. Modeling the principles of community-based participatory research in a community health assessment conducted by a health foundation. Health Promot. Pract. 10 (1), 67–75. doi:10.1177/1524839906294419.

Zartarian, V., Schultz, B., Barzyk, T., et al., 2011. The Environmental Protection Agency's community-focused exposure and risk screening tool (C-FERST) and its potential use for environmental justice efforts. Am. J. Public Health S286–S294. doi:10.2105/AJPH.2010.300087.

Planning and promoting community health: principles and practices

CHAPTER 4

Introduction

Health promotion is essentially a political, ecological and capacity-building process, aimed at arranging the social and structural determinants of health in a way that facilitates health. To help people build health capacity requires awareness of both global and local conditions that affect health. Global influences on health include the type of trade relations and employment constraints that impact on local economic and social conditions, as we outlined in Chapter 2. At the local level, health promotion extends across the continuum from prevention to intervention. Activities revolve around preventing illness and/or injury, promoting healthy living, responding to place-based conditions that affect health, advocating for structural conditions to support people's choices for health, and ensuring there is appropriate care for those who need it.

As a fundamental element of primary health care (PHC), health promotion is multidimensional and inclusive. Health promotion actions achieve the best outcomes for health when they involve intersectoral collaboration. Intersectoral activities can involve working with various non-health sectors of the community to lobby the government for safer roads, for more parklands to support physical activity, or to ensure equitable access to child care. These collaborative actions advocate for the whole community, either directly or by supporting those who may have a voice in lobbying for change; for example, at the political or local council level. In the various settings of people's lives health promotion activities can include selective or program advocacy, working with caregivers, teachers, volunteers and employers to reduce threats to health or to develop programs for better health. At the level of the individual, health promotion includes supporting community members' empowerment by helping them become confidently health literate. This type of action typically involves health education, a planned strategy for teaching and guidance so that people are well informed about health issues and have the capacity to make choices for improving their health and the health of their community.

Specific health promotion actions begin with community assessment. From this basis of knowledge, plans are developed in partnership with community members to maximise assets, reduce risks to health, and plan for a sustainable future for current and future generations. The role of nurses and other health professionals in promoting community health includes advocating, teaching and enabling health based on local knowledge and understanding of the community's health goals. Central to this type of analysis is assessing the interplay of the social determinants of health (SDH), how these are interacting with the environment in

OBJECTIVES

By the end of this chapter you will be able to:

1   explain the challenges involved in global health promotion

2   outline the difference between health promotion and health education and the significance of each in community health

3   explain how knowledge of health and place can be used in promoting health

4   analyse the usefulness of the Ottawa Charter as a basis for health promotion

5   develop a comprehensive strategy for enabling health literacy among residents of a given community

6   plan a community-wide health promotion intervention that includes primary, secondary and tertiary prevention.

the local context, and what influences are exerting pressures on the community and its residents along their social, cultural and developmental pathways. This is a more inclusive, comprehensive view of health promotion than simply seeing the community in terms of a single issue or health problem at a discrete moment in time. Conducting an assessment of the SDH is an ideal place to begin.

TERMINOLOGY AND HISTORY: PUBLIC HEALTH, POPULATION HEALTH, PRIMARY HEALTH CARE AND HEALTH PROMOTION

Public health

Public health is aimed at preventing disease and promoting the health of populations. Public health initiatives are based on population-level data and typically involve measurement and surveillance, and development of evidence-based strategies to either prevent or overcome diseases. This involves collecting and analysing epidemiological information on the distribution and determinants of health and ill health in a particular community or country, and linking this information to what is known in other populations. Comparisons are sometimes helpful, but one of the problems with a traditional public health approach is that by aggregating this type of information, the assumption is made that all community members develop or behave in similar ways, thereby creating stereotypes of communities that are actually diverse and changing (Abbott et al. 2008).

Population health

Population health is similar to public health in that its focus is health and disease in the community, but population health programs tend to address disparities in health status between different groups. In Australia, the Commonwealth Government adopts a population health approach to establish the priority groups for intervention in an effort to provide timely and accurate information for health promotion planning. (AIHW, Online. Available: www.aihw.gov.au/population-health/ [accessed 18 February 2013]). In New Zealand, the Ministry of Health has oversight of all population health programs, with population health being identified as a key health priority in the New Zealand Health Strategy (NZMOH 2000) and the New Zealand Primary Health Care Strategy (NZMOH 2001). The Ministry of Health New Zealand website has the most up-to-date information on New Zealand's population health strategies: www.health.govt.nz.

Primary health care

As we explained in Chapter 1, PHC is both a philosophy and an organising framework for care. PHC guides our activities in illness prevention, health promotion, and structural and environmental modifications that support health and wellness. However, priorities are not established by health professionals alone; instead members of the community help define the goals of health promotion. This partnership approach is embodied in the overarching principles of PHC, which guide us to work towards equitable social circumstances, equal access to health care, and community empowerment through public participation in all aspects of life.

The distinctions between public health, population health and PHC illustrate how the ideas of health planners and policymakers have changed over time. Although the focus of public health has always been to ensure the highest level of health for the greatest number of the population, historically, public health has been about illness, not health. From the 19th century, public health authorities adopted a regulatory approach of surveillance and control to overcome infectious diseases. They tracked epidemics or potential epidemics, and ensured that government regulations were in place for monitoring illness in the population and responding quickly when it was required. Public health was therefore defined according to a biomedical model where the emphasis was on understanding the causes of illness in order to apportion resources appropriately. In the biomedical model the public health focus is primarily on interventions and rehabilitation activities to protect people and manage threats to health, such as epidemics or other potential risk factors.

Problems with the 'old public health'

In the biomedical public health era, public health experts were guided by current medical knowledge, political factors and the availability of financial and personal resources. So, for example, in those parts of the world where health personnel and resources were plentiful, people were expected to have higher levels of health. Where vaccines were available and where the politics of the day encouraged medical research through generous funding schemes, it was expected that diseases would be curtailed. Members of the public rarely questioned the medical experts on any of these public health matters. Yet, analysis of information on the prevalence of diseases found no relationship between good health and the provision of services. Clearly, there was a need to look for a broader set of criteria for good health.

In 1978 an important international meeting among members of 189 countries culminated in the Declaration of Alma-Ata, named after the city in the former USSR where the meeting took place. The Declaration was the first global proclamation that a broader perspective of health was needed to galvanise the efforts of health planners around the world to meet current and future challenges. PHC was declared as a roadmap to achieving better health for all populations. The architects of the Declaration were supported by numerous health professionals, who also believed the answers to good health were to be found in the social and structural conditions of people's lives.

Four years earlier, the *Lalonde Report* in Canada had suggested a more socially contextualised definition of health, including strategies for achieving health that placed less onus on individuals and more emphasis on creating the right environments for health (Lalonde 1974). PHC embodied this idea. It was not only a vision for health, it was seen as a philosophy permeating the entire health system, a strategy for organising care, a level of care (primary or 'first line' of care) and a set of activities (Chamberlain & Beckingham 1987).

The Declaration of Alma-Ata represented a watershed in public health. Its focus was on empowering people to have control over decisions that affected health in their own families and communities. Health was conceptualised as a fundamental right for all people, an individual and collective responsibility, an equal opportunity concept and an essential element of socio-economic development (Holzemer 1992). This represented a stark contrast to the historical 'top-down' approach to planning for public health in that people at the grassroots level of societies were now to have a greater say in planning from the 'bottom-up', or 'inside out' instead of 'outside in' (Courtney 1995). The bottom-up or grassroots approach shifts the balance of power to the people, so that health professionals are 'on tap' rather than 'on top'; acting as a resource to the community rather than telling them what they should do (Baum 2007).

HEALTH PROMOTION AND THE NEW PUBLIC HEALTH

The Lalonde Report, the Declaration of Alma-Ata and several reports that followed, such as the Black Report in the UK, were all important milestones in our evolving policy and research agenda. Collectively, they signalled a shift in thinking from the 'old public health', wherein health professionals decided what was best for the community, to the 'new public health', where communities themselves decide

HEALTH PROMOTION

The process of enabling people to increase control over, and improve their health (WHO 1986).

priorities and preferences for health from where people live, work and play. This PHC vision placed collective action by the community at the centre of health decision-making. Another significant shift was a strong focus on health promotion. Placing health promotion at the centre of public health activities can be linked back to the leadership of Ilona Kickbusch, then Head of Canada's Health Promotion Directorate, who convened the first WHO International Conference on Health Promotion, in 1986 in Ottawa, Canada. The conference embodied PHC as the 'new public health', focusing the health promotion discussions on lifestyle factors, living conditions, and the environments where people lived, rather than health services (Kickbusch 2003). The conference defined health promotion as the process of enabling people to increase control over, and to improve their health (WHO, Health & Welfare Canada & CPHA, 1986). The objective of the Ottawa Charter was to clarify the conditions and resources required to provide health for all people and to define the prerequisites for health. These included peace, a stable ecosystem, social justice and equity, and resources such as education, food and income (WHO, Health & Welfare Canada & CPHA 1986).

GROUP EXERCISE: Health promotion

Working in groups of three or four, brainstorm as many examples of health promotion activities that you can think of (for example, smoking cessation campaigns). As you work through the chapter, keep adding to your list of examples and make a note of which campaigns have been most successful and why. How have these health promotion campaigns helped or would they help in your work with individuals in the home or in community clinics?

THE OTTAWA CHARTER FOR HEALTH PROMOTION

The Ottawa Charter emphasises the importance of promoting health at a global level and identifies the fundamental conditions and resources for community health. Five major strategies for health promotion are circumscribed within the public health activities of disease control and resource allocation, yet activities are guided by the PHC approach of grassroots community development and an ecological view of health (see Figure 4.1). The five strategies are as follows:

1 Build healthy public policy

This strategy is aimed at encouraging all those involved in health care to ensure that health becomes incorporated into all public policy decisions. The Charter suggests intersectoral collaboration where there is mutual recognition that the policies of other sectors, such as education, housing, industry, social welfare and environmental planning, also affect and are affected by, those that guide the health of our communities.

2 Create supportive environments

This strategy embodies the socio-ecological approach to health. The Charter encourages all people to recognise the importance of conserving and capitalising on those resources that enable people to maintain health, including physical or social resources.

3 Strengthen community action

Information and learning opportunities are seen as the focus for empowering communities to work together to make informed choices for better health. This type of community action exemplifies what is meant by community capacity development.

4 Develop personal skills

This strategy guides communities to provide adequate and appropriate education and opportunities for skills development so that people can influence their communities to make local decisions for effective use of resources in order to attain health.

5 Reorient health services

Those involved in decisions affecting community health should operate from a base of evidence on what best works to foster the health of people. Included in this strategy is the need for research and the dissemination of knowledge from the multiple perspectives of those concerned with social, political, economic and physical resources as well as health.

The Second International Conference on Health Promotion was hosted by Australia in 1988, with an emphasis on healthy public policy. Next, the Third International Conference on Health Promotion was held in Sundsvall, Sweden in 1991, focusing on supportive environments for health. The fourth took place in Jakarta, Indonesia in 1997, culminating in the Jakarta Declaration on Leading Health Promotion into the 21st Century. By this time, the influence of economic rationalism had shaped global politics and the language of health promotion. The Indonesian meeting focused on health promotion as an investment in overcoming poverty as a major cause of ill health. The Fifth Global Conference on Health Promotion, in Mexico City in 2000, was called 'Bridging the Equity Gap'. The recommendations from this conference revolved around positioning health promotion as a fundamental political priority in all countries, across all sectors, with information shared freely between nations (Catford 2000, 2011). As the new century dawned, the United Nations (UN) convened a summit of 191 nations to discuss strategies for overcoming the conditions that were causing serious disadvantage for many people throughout the world, especially in developing countries. Their discussions produced the Millennium Development Goals (MDGs) (see Figure 4.2).

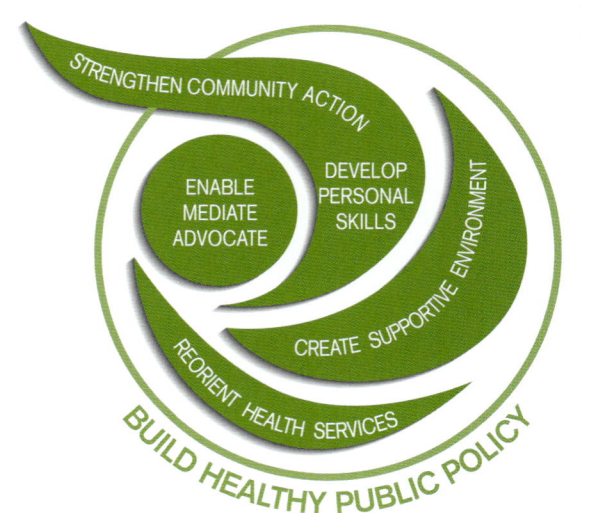

FIGURE 4.1
The Ottawa Charter for Health Promotion (WHO, Health and Welfare Canada & CPHA 1986)

WHAT'S THE POINT?

The five strategies of the Ottawa Charter and other health promotion statements are aimed at overcoming inequalities (bias and disadvantage) and inequities (unfair distribution of health care and other resources) through action on the SDH at all levels of society.

The ultimate goal is social justice.

Millennium Development Goals

Eradicate extreme poverty and hunger — reduce by half, the proportion of people living on less than a dollar a day; reduce by half the proportion of people who suffer from hunger.

Achieve universal primary education — ensure that both boys and girls complete a full course of primary schooling.

Promote gender equality and empower women — eliminate gender disparity in primary and secondary education preferably by 2005 and at all levels by 2015.

Reduce child mortality — reduce by two-thirds the mortality rate among children under five.

Improve maternal health — reduce by three-quarters the maternal mortality ratio.

Combat HIV/AIDS, malaria and other diseases — halt and begin to reverse the spread of HIV/AIDS, halt and begin to reverse the incidence of malaria and other major diseases.

Ensure environmental sustainability — integrate the principles of sustainable development into country policies and programs; reverse the loss of environmental resources; reduce by half the proportion of people without sustainable access to safe drinking water.

Develop a global partnership for development — develop further an open trading and financial system that is rule-based, predictable and non-discriminatory. This includes a commitment to good governance, development and poverty reduction nationally and internationally. Address the least developed countries' special needs. This includes: tariff and quota-free access for their exports; enhanced debt relief for heavily indebted poor countries; cancellation of official bilateral debt; and more generous official development assistance for countries committed to poverty reduction. Address the special needs of landlocked and small island developing states. Deal comprehensively with developing countries' debt problems through national and international measures to make debt sustainable in the long term. In cooperation with the developing countries, develop decent and productive work for youth. In cooperation with pharmaceutical companies, provide access to affordable essential drugs in developing countries. In cooperation with the private sector, make available the benefits of new technologies — especially information and communications technologies.

FIGURE 4.2
The UN Millennium Development Goals

THE MILLENNIUM DEVELOPMENT GOALS

The MDGs, to be achieved by the year 2015, addressed the effects of extreme poverty, hunger, disease, lack of adequate shelter and exclusion, and were designed to promote education, gender equality and environmental sustainability for developing countries (Sachs 2005). Under the auspices of the Director-General of the UN, the Millennium project that introduced the goals was based on the conviction that sound, proven, cost-effective interventions can ameliorate and often eliminate extreme poverty, especially where it is most needed, such as in the countries of sub-Saharan Africa.

Achieving the goals would require major investment from wealthy countries to help poorer nations develop capacity in education, the environment, health care, nutrition and social programs, especially those that foster equity.

The intention of the MDGs was to save the lives of 30 million children and 2 million mothers by 2015, to provide safe drinking water and sanitation to hundreds of millions of people, and to send hundreds of millions of women and girls to school to prepare them for economic and political opportunities and a safer and more secure life (Sachs 2005). Yet to date, there have been only modest gains in achieving the goals. The World Health Organization (WHO, Online. Available: www.who.int/

mediacentre/factsheets/fs290/en/index.html [accessed 13 February 2013]) reports that by 2010, 80% of the targets have been reached. Some countries have made impressive gains, while others are falling behind, especially those affected by high levels of HIV/AIDS, economic hardship or conflict. Globally, from 1990 to 2011, there was a significant decline in the percentage of underweight children and child deaths under age 5. Worldwide, new cases of HIV and tuberculosis infections continue to decline. The proportion of births attended by a skilled health worker has increased, but fewer than 50% are attended in the African countries. The MDG targets for safe drinking water will be met by 2015, but the sanitation goal is unlikely to be achieved.

Criticisms of the MDGs focus on the lack of equity and inclusiveness of the goals in terms of human development. Sachs, who was instrumental in establishing the goals, argues that the focus should shift in future to Sustainable Development Goals (SDGs) (Sachs 2012). He advocates continuing the crucial work of the MDGs in trying to end extreme poverty, given the successes in countries such as China. But, in his view, sustaining the environment to support development opportunities, social inclusion and good governance are equally as important (Sachs 2012).

At the same time as the MDGs were established, eight non-government groups came together in Bangladesh as the First People's Health Assembly. The meeting culminated in the People's Health Charter, which demanded that the WHO eliminate their links with the corporate interests of economic globalisation that had influenced its activities, and focus instead on comprehensive PHC and protection of the natural environment (Baum 2007). This charter resonated with the sustainability agenda, which had become a major focus throughout the world.

The next major development in global health promotion occurred in 2005, when the Bangkok Charter was produced from the Sixth Global Conference on Health Promotion in Bangkok, Thailand. The conference's discussions sought to highlight the global development agenda as a core responsibility for all governments, a key focus of communities and civil society, and a requirement for good corporate practices (Catford 2011). The Bangkok meeting was followed in 2009 with the Seventh Global Conference on Health Promotion, convened in Kenya, culminating in the Nairobi Call to Action. The Nairobi document drew attention to the urgent need to strengthen leadership and workforces, mainstream health promotion, empowerment of communities and individuals, participatory processes and the need to build and apply knowledge (Catford 2011). In 2013, the Helsinki statement on health in all policies called for governments to systematically take into account the health implications of public policy decisions across all sectors of government. The statement also called for improved accountability of policymakers for health impacts at all levels of policymaking (Helsinki Statement, Online. Available: http://www.healthpromotion2013.org/images/8GCHP_Helsinki_Statement.pdf [accessed 28 June 2013]).

In 2008 the WHO (2008) and the Commission on the SDH commemorated the 30th anniversary of the Declaration of Alma-Ata by recommitting to the PHC agenda in the report: 'Primary health care—now more than ever' (WHO 2008). 'Now more than ever' referred to the state of global health care, which continues to this day to be plagued by inequitable access, impoverishing costs and erosion of people's trust in governments. Together, these factors constitute a threat to social stability. The report underlined the need for PHC at a time when the global financial crisis was compromising people's quality of life, and when our failure to create an equitable world impinges on human rights (WHO 2008). The WHO statement clearly refocused our attention to the original Declaration of Alma-Ata and the Charters that followed to consider progress in meeting their goals.

All of the declarations and charters (listed in Box 4.1) have drawn global attention to the health effects of widespread inequalities (unequal distribution of health resources) and inequities (the moral aspect of health inequality in terms of decisions taken on health care and the distribution of resources) (Baum & Sanders 2011; Catford 2011). These important statements and the declarations from subsequent international meetings and policy deliberations have been unequivocal in their goal to address the SDH, and they have been extremely powerful in shaping PHC thinking today. In the 21st century, mainstream thinking in the promotion of health takes the view that without equal access to education, health care, transportation, nutritious food and social support, the world will never have health for all. In 2012, Professor Ilona Kickbusch, who convened the group that developed the original Ottawa Charter for Health Promotion, declared that all societies need to address 'the political, the commercial, the social, the environmental and the behavioral determinants of health' (Kickbusch 2012:427), a view echoed by many other global scholars (Sparks 2009).

PROMOTING GLOBAL HEALTH

Global health promotion is a central tenet of global development, and therefore a core responsibility of

BOX 4.1 Charting global health promotion

Declaration of Alma-Ata (USSR) (1978)

1st International Conference (Canada): Ottawa Charter for Health Promotion (1986)

2nd International Conference (Australia): focus on healthy public policy (1988)

3rd International Conference (Sweden): focus on supportive environments (1991)

4th International Conference (Indonesia): focus on global politics and Jakarta Declaration (1997)

5th Global Conference (Mexico): focus on equity, information sharing (2000)

Millennium Development Goals (UN) (2000)

People's Health Assembly (Bangladesh) (2000)

People's Health Charter to refocus on PHC and environment (2000)

6th Global Health Conference (Thailand): focus on development and corporate practices (2005)

WHO/Commission on SDH: 'PHC now more than ever' focus on global equity and financial responsibility (2008)

7th Global Health Conference (Kenya) Nairobi Call to Action: focus on leadership, empowerment, participation, knowledge (2009)

8th Global Health Conference (Finland) The Helsinki statement on health in all policies (2013)

(see Appendices B–F)

governments and the business community (Catford 2011; Sparks 2009; Kickbusch 2012). Labonte (2008) suggests that promoting health at the global level requires major changes in how we deal with globalisation to manage social risks. The reality is that many crises are created by global forces and affect the most vulnerable disproportionately. A major element of shifting goals and shifting focus is to blunt the negative impact of the global marketplace by critically appraising the health problems that have inherently global causes and consequences. In his view, there are many ways to think about health. It can be seen in terms of security, as development, as a global public good, as a human right and as a commodity (Labonte 2008). Health as commodity is a convoluted way to view health. It represents the worst of globalisation, in reducing the notion of health to goods (drugs, new technologies) and services (private health insurance, facilities and providers), and maximising profits

rather than promoting health. The other four concepts embody a type of 'transnational health activism' which is central to the global development agenda (Labonte 2008:467).

WHAT'S YOUR OPINION?

Fear of epidemics that may influence global trade, finance or travel has been used as a means of privileging high-income nations, particularly the industries that create the drugs to prevent or treat such epidemics.

As a health professional how would you go about dealing with this mix of politics and business to achieve equity?

The political orientation of a country can also determine the outcomes of health promotion rhetoric. Raphael (2013a, b) has found that despite a country's explicit commitment to health promotion in public policy, this commitment does not necessarily result in implementation of such concepts in practice. Liberal welfare states such as Canada, Australia and the UK have all been seen to provide leadership in health promotion, yet are less successful at providing the prerequisites for health and addressing the SDH than conservative countries such as France, where health promoting public policy is less apparent. Social democratic nations such as Finland, Norway and Sweden have achieved the greatest success in both articulating health promotion concepts in policy, implementing these in communities, and improving health outcomes. These examples demonstrate the importance for those involved in health promotion to understand that health promotion is inherently a political activity and that gaining knowledge of the broad policymaking process is essential, especially given that not all health promoting public policy is identified as such (Raphael 2013a). Advocacy is required in many different places within the health system and other sectors.

GLOBAL HEALTH, GLOBAL DEVELOPMENT

Health as security

When health is seen as security it conjures up fear of bio-terrorism, terrorists, and the general inclination towards border protection, 'whether the invaders are pathogens or people' (Labonte 2008:468). This idea has helped prevent some diseases from crossing borders, but it is also associated with 'repressive political measures' (Labonte 2008:468). Instead of encouraging high-income nations to help those less fortunate, some countries have focused on those diseases most likely to inconvenience global trade and finance or travel. Fear of new epidemics has also proven a major windfall for the pharmaceutical industry. The SDH approach indicates that instead of *national* security we should be working towards *human* security; that is, securing food, income, health care, housing, education, peace and a viable and sustainable environment. As health professionals, we can contribute to these high-level activities by being well informed and vigilant about global conditions. At each opportunity it is our mandate to help shift ideas, attitudes, resources and power to focus on strengthening the health and wellbeing of the population (Sparks 2009).

Health as a global public good

One approach to promoting global health that has gained momentum since the 1990s is the notion that when wealthy nations provide health assistance to the less fortunate it is not only humanitarian aid, but a selfish investment in protecting health in their own population (Smith & MacKellar 2007). This notion of selfishness may not be as negative as it first sounds, as the emphasis is on the community, and stable, sustainable systems that support health and nation building. Globally, this idea of sharing would see a broader perspective where all countries become concerned about risks (risk pooling) and work towards developing common financial regulations to benefit everyone, not just those in positions of wealth and power (Baum et al. 2009; Labonte 2008).

Health as a human right

The People's Health Movement that originated in the Bangladesh meeting on health promotion clearly situated health as a human right, which is congruent with PHC. The movement has created the momentum for a global health ethic which would entrench rights, regulations, redistributive justice and a concern with the inequality of persistent poverty. The strategies for achieving this type of ethical, socially just approach is on a bottom-up mobilisation of action through training, capacity building, documenting health rights violations, and lobbying governments for policy change.

Promoting global health clearly requires diplomacy, based on the need for ethical, rights-based public good, development, and foreign policies that promote security for all people (Labonte 2008). These are lofty goals, but they are achievable with grassroots or bottom-up pressure combined with top-down policy action (Baum et al. 2009). Policies

---

ACTION ON HUMAN RIGHTS

The Australian Human Rights Commission (www.humanrights.gov.au) and the Human Rights Commission New Zealand (www.hrc.co.nz) work towards identifying and finding solutions to human rights inequities in a range of areas to overcome discrimination and promote social justice. A visit to their websites indicates current priorities. Do you agree with these or would you add others?

---

that create employment or other conditions that improve the SDH at the population level are critical. Previously unconsidered contributors to improving health include union density and the presence of collective employment agreements that help preserve human rights in the workplace. Countries that have employment policies that support union membership and/or collective bargaining have better population health outcomes (Raphael 2013a). These population level policies are shaped by three key forces which need ongoing attention (Kickbusch 2012). They include the power of markets and business, particularly the transnational companies that have emerged from globalisation; the strong voice of civil society; and financial pressures being experienced by many countries and agencies. As health professionals, we should have a say in the type of decisions made by governments and health planners. We can also encourage our respective nations to invest in the health literacy of parliamentarians as well as the citizens who elect them (Kickbusch 2012). Although we cannot all be involved in formal policy development, there is a major role for nurses and other health professionals in examining how existing policies affect health, and in identifying the issues that require new or modified policies to maintain health and community capacity. Health impact assessment (HIA) is a useful tool for in-depth analysis of the impact of a policy on health outcomes and is advocated by the World Health Organization as an important method for maximising health promotion at the local, national and global levels (Winkler et al. 2013). The New Zealand Ministry of Health offers a range of resources to support people who wish to undertake HIA. (See www.health.govt.nz/our-work/health-impact-assessment for further information.) Australian resources are less comprehensive; however, some useful resources may be found here: www.health.gov.au/internet/main/publishing.nsf/content/health-pubhlth-publicat-document-metadata-env_impact.htm.

Becoming closely involved in the global and local policy environment can often be the first step in mediating, enabling and facilitating the processes, people and systems that can be mobilised to achieve health goals. Being aware of the wider global issues poses a number of questions for health promotion (see Box 4.2).

Health promotion at any level requires a broad understanding of human development and behaviour, the ability to communicate well, and commitment to community empowerment and participation. In addition, we must be sensitive to people's knowledge needs at different stages of their development and help fill the gaps in their understanding through health education.

HEALTH EDUCATION

Health education is an integral strategy in promoting community health. The process begins by building the knowledge base, then working with community members to identify strengths, weaknesses, assets, inequities, vulnerabilities or other aspects of community life that may impinge on health. This knowledge is gained through assessment, and maintaining a receptive and resourceful attitude towards new ideas and local approaches to thinking about problems or areas that need to be strengthened.

In previous times, there was a view that health education was about changing people's lifestyle habits. Throughout the developed world, the 1970s and 1980s approach to community health promotion was focused on broad media campaigns to promote behaviour change using social marketing techniques (Egger et al. 1983; Lasater et al. 1988; Maccoby & Solomon 1981; McAlister 1981; Nutbeam & Catford 1987). Social marketing is a process of using the marketing techniques of business to achieve behavioural goals that are considered a social good (Reynolds 2012). As community-wide programs, social marketing campaigns were widely advertised and improved general population awareness of health risks and the benefits of exercise, good nutrition and managing a range of stressors. Some were criticised as generating fear; for example, the

'Grim Reaper' campaign that threatened HIV/AIDS from unsafe sexual behaviours. However, the programs have also been effective in some ways, contributing to a number of positive changes as follows:

- policy change—legislating seatbelts, introducing disability insurance, parental leave, child care subsidies, bans on television advertisements for unhealthy food targeting children
- socio-cultural change—restricting smoking, anti-discrimination, wages and working conditions
- environmental change—reducing car emissions, pesticides, food safety
- behavioural change—safe sexual practices, crime prevention
- technological change—public access to wi-fi, Australian National Broadband network
- economic change—micro-financing in poor countries that has allowed collective purchasing power.

Although creating awareness of healthy lifestyles and healthy communities has been beneficial to many people, in most cases the social marketing campaigns 'preached to the converted', in that they provided the impetus for lifestyle changes among those who were already planning to improve their health. When researchers began looking a little more deeply at the differential effects of the campaigns it became evident that the 'reach' of the information and the uptake of the message had not been consistently received across the population (Dyer 2005). Another outcome of this approach was 'victim blaming', where in many cases, people were made to feel that if they became ill it was because they failed to follow the advice of the experts. The major conclusion from the approach of this era was that health promotion campaigns actually widened health disparities across broad population groups, because the messages tended to be better understood and had a greater uptake by the upper and middle classes in society (Green 2008).

HEALTH EDUCATION

knowledge + capacity

As a health promotion strategy health education facilitates empowerment by showing people where to access appropriate, relevant information on health, and how to use it to build health capacity.

By the 1980s the Ottawa Charter focused the health promotion agenda on an advocacy and enabling role to promote supportive environments and policies, access to information, life skills and opportunities for making choices (Green 2008). Health education continued to be seen in a negative light, because the messages had become somewhat coercive in trying to persuade people to lead healthy lives. This situation required a shift in thinking about health education. Several health promotion scholars began to recognise how important the social, environmental and political conditions of people's lives were in terms of their ability to make healthy choices (Green & Kreuter 1991).

Tones (1986, 2002) also supported the idea of a comprehensive and systematic approach to health education, but he argued for a more radical model of community empowerment that would focus on people having both knowledge of the fundamental causes of ill health and the capacity to address them. His work foreshadowed the move towards health literacy, and today health education is clearly entrenched as a strategy to foster health literacy, which is another integral element of health promotion (Green 2008).

The approach of knowledge plus capacity is the 'new health education', which is oriented towards empowerment rather than persuasion. When health education is delivered in an empowering way, knowledge nurtures the self-esteem and self-confidence that is essential for developing and using health literacy (Wiggins 2011). Health literacy is therefore not an end in itself, but a tool for participation, community activism and health decision-making (Cambon et al. 2012; Nutbeam 2008). Health education can provide people with substantive information and processes for accessing health knowledge. This can include access to information on health issues and the structures and processes that help them use this knowledge for self-management (functional health literacy). Health education can also provide people with helpful techniques for influencing determinants in the local community and society (communicative health literacy), skills and mechanisms for developing coalitions and networks for change (critical health literacy), and political skills to engage in community action and work with others for health capacity building. While it is important that levels of health literacy are assessed and addressed, it is also important that strategies identifying and addressing health literacy are included in organisational and governmental policy. Clearly, a multi-faceted approach to health literacy will be the most successful (Coulter et al. 2008; NZMOH 2010).

REMINDER: Health literacy

1   Functional
2   Communicative
3   Critical

Nutbeam (2008), who has undertaken significant work in the area of health literacy, has developed a conceptual framework for practice, education and research that revolves around the notion of health literacy as an asset. This conceptual model is presented as an example of community participation and empowerment in health promotion. The value of this model will lie in its application across settings and across different population groups, including those with different starting points in progressing through the various levels of health literacy (see Figure 4.3).

Understanding the level of health literacy of an individual, family or community is useful for developing appropriate health education interventions. Health literacy measures such as the test of functional health literacy in adults (TOFHLA),

RESEARCH TO PRACTICE: Why participate?

Why participate? This question has yet to be fully addressed in the health promotion research agenda. We understand that participation is a pathway to empowerment, but what motivates community members to participate in capacity development? A group of Dutch researchers decided to try to identify the factors that motivate citizens to actively engage with health educators in a diverse array of programs. They planned their study on the basis that, despite participation being a core principle of health promotion, little is known of what motivates people to become involved at various levels of participation; consultative, functional, interactive and/or self-mobilising activities. They conducted in-depth interviews with 24 people who were involved in at least one of six community projects. Participants explained their reasons for being involved as one or more of the following: purposeful action (wanting to produce tangible results or advancement of the group or health issue); personal development (a felt need to develop or advance oneself mentally, socially and/or occupationally); exemplary status (to be recognised as an example to others for achievements and ability); service and reciprocity (wanting to 'do one's bit' for the community) (Fienieg et al. 2011).

So what does this tell us?

These are interesting findings because the knowledge of motivating factors may lead to strategies for sustaining community participation in other contexts, particularly if the research findings are replicated in other settings.

? Do you think knowledge of motivating factors in those who are already engaged in health promotion will help with recruitment of other community members to help develop plans for health education or health promotion?

health literacy capacity, which can be identified through screening tools.

Assessing health literacy capacity is particularly important given the growing focus on involving people in health decision-making. Partnership approaches such as shared decision-making, client-centred care, self-care, self-management and patient-centred professionalism place greater onus on people to be well informed and take an active part in decision-making about their health care. However, this can be challenging for people who have lower levels of literacy. Smith et al. (2009) have found that patients with higher levels of education and functional health literacy characterise their engagement with health professionals as sharing the responsibility for decision-making, helping others with their decision-making, and acting as information resources, whereas those with lower levels of education and lower functional health literacy characterised their involvement as consenting to a decision made by the health professional and relying on friends and relatives for support. Both higher and lower level participants in Smith's (2009) study wanted respect from health professionals but those with higher levels sought respect as equals and those with lower levels sought respect for who they were and empathy for their situation. Building health literacy to achieve equal partnership with people is a goal of the health professional, but it is important to remember that partnership is both a process and an outcome, and the process may be tempered by differences in knowledge and power between the health professional and the patient.

The differential effect of knowledge and power is a consideration in *motivational interviewing*, one of the techniques currently being used in health education, which encourages people to examine their actual and ideal health behaviours (Abramowitz et al. 2010). Motivational interviewing is intended to support the partnership approach to health education as a way of building people's confidence in their ability to change (Abramowitz et al. 2010; Chittendon 2012; Huffman 2010).The technique is a type of health coaching, which engages people to discover and address their ambivalence about changing health behaviours (Huffman 2010). The nurse or health professional integrates health teaching into the process of actively discovering why a person is ambivalent about change through active listening and change talk (Huffman 2010). Active listening requires accurate empathy; that is, understanding what it is that keeps people stuck in old behavioural habits and empathising with them about the difficulties of changing. Change talk simply revolves around posing questions about what people would like to change about their health and

rapid estimate of adult literacy in medicine (REALM), and the US health activity literacy scale (HALS) have been used by clinicians and researchers to categorise the literacy and health literacy levels of individuals and help us understand the difficulties groups may have in understanding health-related material (Nutbeam 2009). Most important for the health practitioner is the recognition that every individual, family and community will have differing

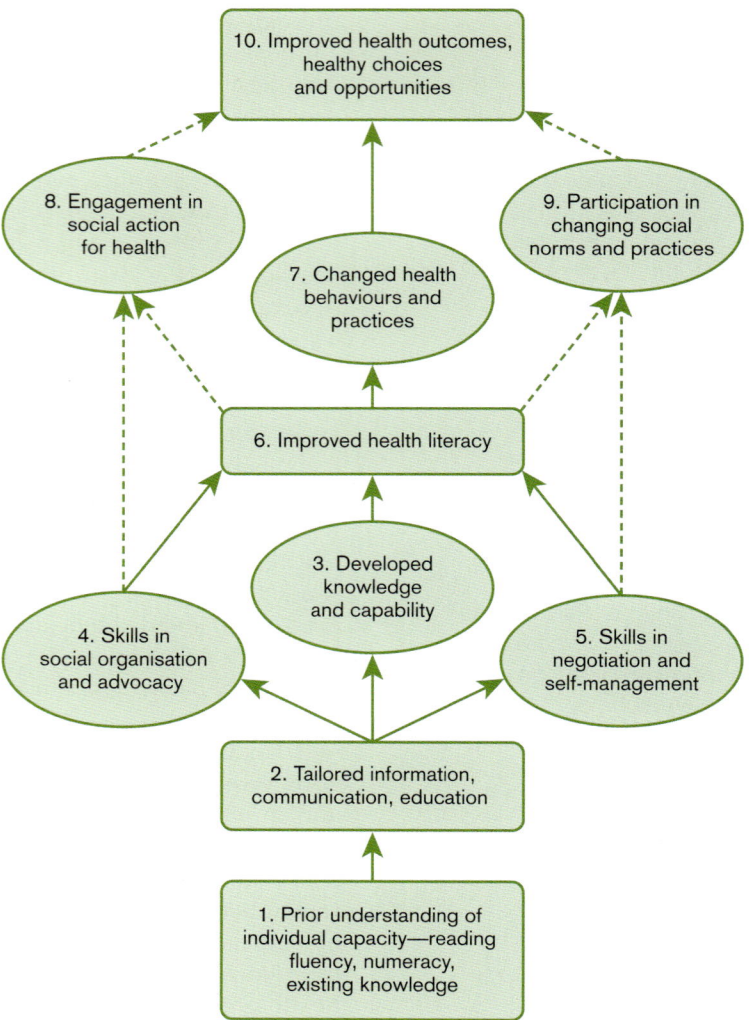

FIGURE 4.3
Conceptual model of health as an asset (Nutbeam 2008)

which aspects of these changes are preventing change (Huffman 2010). Being able to acknowledge the barriers to change conveys the message that their issues are important and their right to make decisions about change are respected (Chittendon 2012). A four-step model guides the process of motivational interviewing as illustrated in Box 4.3. Further information on health coaching can be found online (www.nshcoa.com/site/).

Techniques such as health coaching and motivational interviewing play an essential role in raising people's awareness of personal healthy lifestyle choices, such as physical activity, smoking cessation, and food and alcohol consumption (Abramowitz et al. 2010; Huffman 2010). However, the socio-ecological model also includes emphasis on access to healthy environments to support individual changes (Barter-Godfrey et al. 2007). According to the

Ottawa Charter, healthy environments are designed to make the healthy choice the easiest choice (WHO, CPHA, Health & Welfare Canada 1986). But there is a need for caution in the way health education programs are framed to ensure empowerment and choice rather than coercion. For example, recent programs have returned to social marketing to pair up people's concern for the environment with healthy lifestyles. Proponents of this approach, called behaviour change by 'stealth', believe that popular, collective causes can instigate personal preferences for such things as healthy foods and physical activity (Skouteris et al. 2013). This approach has been used to encourage children to replace passive entertainment that uses non-renewable energy (TV, electronic games) with active leisure activities (riding a bike), and to encourage adults to ride their bikes to reduce their carbon footprint (Egger 2007; Skouteris

BOX 4.3 Motivational interviewing

- Step 1 Engaging—simple reflections, open-ended questions, affirmations of client strengths or past successes, summarising, reflecting back what the client has stated
- Step 2 Focusing—creating a balance between satisfying the client's needs and expectations and the health education agenda
- Step 3 Evoking—responding to change talk, or indications of readiness to change
- Step 4 Planning—strengthening commitment and support for change (Chittendon 2012)

et al. 2013). The motivation for behaviour change is presumably to capitalise on people's commitment to behaving consistently with their collective identity as someone who is concerned about environmental sustainability, rather than simply benefit the individual personally. For children, tapping into their self-identity in this way is seen to establish values that will endure throughout their lives (Skouteris et al. 2013). This approach to health education, along with the motivational interviewing approach may be beneficial in some ways, but both need to be undertaken in such a way that is non-coercive or intrusive.

WHAT'S YOUR OPINION?

Should we engage in health education 'by stealth' to achieve desirable outcomes?

Like all health promotion activities, health education should be based on evidence of what works, for whom, in what context. This type of evidence, translated into the practicalities of various contexts, can be helpful in tailoring messages to specific elements of the population. A study of cyclists' attitudes towards encouraging bicycle travel in New Zealand provides an example of how specific, targeted information can be used to inform policy development. New Zealand has one of the highest levels of car ownership in the world, and poorly developed public transportation systems. Yet there has been a declining rate of cycle commuting to work, despite the fact that using cycles instead of cars can save fuel and reduce urban air pollution (Tin Tin et al. 2009). The researchers canvassed the views of participants in the 2006 Wattyl Lake Taupo Cycle Challenge to investigate their attitudes toward

environmental and policy factors that would encourage them to use bicycles to travel to work (Tin Tin et al. 2009). The study revealed many useful ideas about the constraints and facilitating factors that might lead to greater bicycle travel, including better bicycle paths, better security, reduced motor vehicle speed, bike-friendly public transport, shower facilities at work, rising fuel costs, fewer car parks, having a bike designed for commuting and a rise in the cost of car parking (Tin Tin et al. 2009). These factors are all important, but because the study captured the view of a group of regular cyclists, it is difficult to know the extent to which poverty (lack of a bicycle), distance, type of employment or other SDH would affect the total population. Although it is helpful to understand the evidence of what works for this group of cyclists in the context of their lives, further research with other groups may reveal a more complete picture of what could be done to discourage car travel and encourage alternative means of commuting to work.

Research on the cyclists illustrates the importance of 'agency' and 'structure' (Barter-Godfrey et al. 2007:346). *Agency* refers to individual capacity, a person's disposition and preference for health behaviours, while *structure* includes the context, resources and social factors that contour these choices. The combination of agency or disposition towards healthy lifestyles and health literacy can be powerful assets for addressing the structural conditions for maintaining health and wellness in the physical, economic, socio-cultural and political environments (Signal et al. 2012). Current trends in health education combine facilitative strategies (safe, accessible bike paths), communicative strategies (teaching people about the merits of reducing air pollution and exercising daily), and regulatory or legislative strategies (providing bicycle lanes, road rules and drop-off points in the city) (Allender et al. 2011). Messages are based on the premise that the starting point for change is where people have sufficient knowledge, and there are realistic options for supportive policies that could support healthy lifestyles (Allender et al. 2011).

SUSTAINING HEALTH PROMOTION INITIATIVES

An important consideration in evaluating the viability of health promotion initiatives is to determine whether, and to what extent, they can be sustained. In some cases, population health outcomes will not be evident in the short term, but success may be measured in terms of strengthening community capacity for future developments. This is an important distinction between simply promoting behaviour change and taking a more holistic, socio-ecological

Sustainability

- Continuing, effective functioning of a program or project
- Coverage for all those intended by the program
- Integration with existing services
- Strong community ownership
- Local resources mobilised by the community (Leffers & Mitchell 2010)

Sustainable development

- Human wellbeing
- Social inclusion
- Environmental sustainability (Sachs 2012)

view of health promotion. An integrative review of nurses' roles in health promotion revealed that, in the context of providing health care, they tend to focus on the provision of information rather than adopt a broader community-oriented approach (Kemppainen et al. 2012). In the studies examined for the review, empowerment was not embedded in practice, which

limited client participation (Kemppainen et al. 2012). Enabling and sustaining community capacity to support individuals is an important health promotion goal, one that can multiply health gains (Lovell et al. 2011). Sustainability of health promotion requires assessment in context, reviewing any infrastructure needs for the longer term, alignment of health promotion goals with those of stakeholders, integrity and effectiveness of the innovation, and the potential to transfer ownership of the program or project to community control (Leffers & Mitchell 2010) (see Box 4.4).

PROMOTING HEALTH AT THE LOCAL LEVEL

In enabling community health we use the word 'primary' in several ways. As mentioned in Chapter 1, primary health care means working towards equitable social circumstances for all people, equal access to health care and community empowerment. Primary care is the first line of care when people seek help for injury or illness. Another aspect of promoting health in the community involves three distinct levels of prevention, one of which is 'primary'.

BOX 4.4 A conceptual model for global health promotion partnerships

For many years nurses have been undertaking dynamic health promotion activities. However, global health promotion initiatives are often contextualised to a single situation or country and not always shared. Leffers and Mitchell (2010) argued that to advance our knowledge base and share strategies for developing partnerships, the profession needs to build a theoretical base to frame global practice. They interviewed 13 global nurse experts on their views of the most important elements for sustainable partnerships. These were woven into a conceptual framework of lessons learned to guide others.

Partnership

1. Two-way engagement—listen and learn with humility, foster equal participation in decision-making, building on the community's history, culture, assets and needs.
2. Cultural bridging—cultural safety and sensitivity, being open to and valuing differences, cultures, and ways of thinking and doing, being willing to learn a new language.
3. Collaboration—precede any intervention by learning what people are doing. Discover partners' goals, knowledge, limitations and

perspectives. Maintain an attitude that you learn more than you bring.

4. Capacity building—promote not only education but the capacity of the profession to empower others through leadership, local structures and champions, and policies and procedures that contribute to positive health outcomes.
5. Mutual goal setting—establish and revise goals as the exchange goes along.
6. Partnership—view partnership as both a process and an outcome. Empowerment means sharing knowledge and opportunities so that the community controls future outcomes.

Sustainability

1. Undertake comprehensive community assessment to provide a community map of assets and needs.
2. Secure financial and material resources.
3. Work within the social and political climate that influences community participation.
4. Enlist the help of a 'champion' who will show commitment, value community perspectives, and provide energy and stability.
5. Encourage local empowerment to identify ongoing goals.

Primary, secondary and tertiary prevention

As one of the major elements of health promotion, preventing ill health or injury is an instrumental goal of PHC. Leavell and Clark's (1965) three levels of prevention are widely accepted as encompassing the range of activities involved in preventing illness or injury. These levels, primary prevention, secondary prevention and tertiary prevention, distinguish between strategies aimed at maintaining health and wellbeing and preventing illness (primary), treating and limiting illness or injury (secondary), and rehabilitative or restorative actions (tertiary). The aim of primary prevention is to promote health by removing the precipitating causes and determinants of ill health or injury. This can include vaccinating children against communicable diseases, health education, and promoting healthy lifestyles in areas such as personal nutrition, rest, exercise and companionship, and protecting the physical, social and cultural environments. Secondary prevention usually refers to steps taken to recover from illness, to guard against any deterioration in health, screening for early detection and treatment of disease, and any measures to limit disability. Tertiary prevention is restorative. Programs revolve around rehabilitation, transitions to community care and providing support programs (Leavell & Clark 1965).

Conceptualising health professionals' activities across these three levels indicates a holistic, PHC approach that can be applied across the lifespan. The metaphor of a waterfall illustrates this concept. Primary prevention activities at the community level are 'upstream' actions, such as developing educational

> **Primary health care**: working towards equitable social circumstances for all people, equal access to health care, and community empowerment
>
> **Primary care**: the first line of care when people seek help for injury or illness
>
> **Primary prevention**: strategies aimed at maintaining health and wellbeing and preventing illness

materials to portray the benefits of nutrition or regular exercise to help individuals become health literate and make healthy choices. Besides offering encouragement for healthy individual choices, primary prevention includes lobbying the local council or government agencies to create the conditions that support these choices. This type of activity might include helping secure cost-effective foods or safe spaces for children to play. Secondary, or 'midstream', prevention includes such preventative activities as screening for skin cancer, conducting mammography clinics, or establishing drop-in centres for adolescents or isolated older people. Tertiary prevention occurs 'downstream' and typically involves providing assistance or information to help people cope with a potentially disabling condition. This could involve the establishment of walking programs for those who have had a cardiac incident, support groups for family members coping with a loss, or any measure that helps ensure continuity of care and health literacy, such as access to timely health advice (see Figure 4.4).

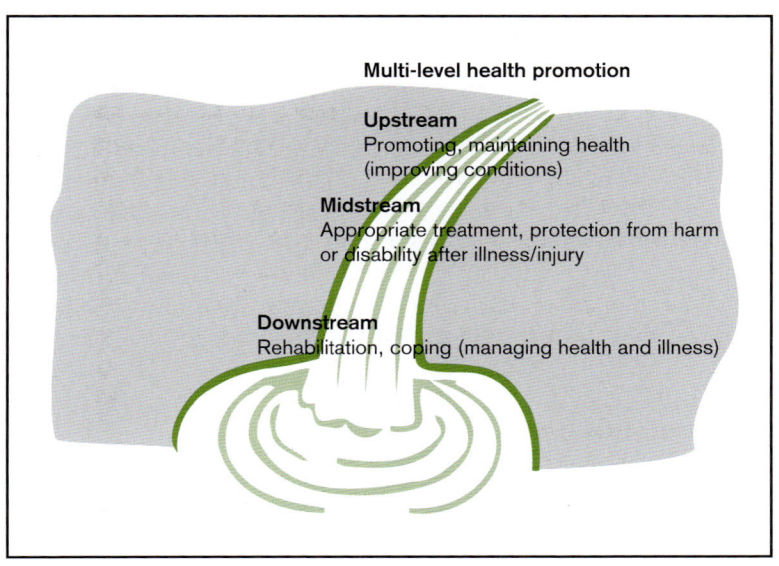

FIGURE 4.4
Primary, secondary and tertiary prevention

Nurses typically play an important role at all three levels of prevention. At the primary prevention level, it is common to see practice nurses immunising children against common vaccine-preventable diseases and public health or community nurses working with a community to secure funding for a safe playground. At the secondary prevention level, a nurse practitioner may be seen running a youth drop-in centre (see for example, www.vibe.org.nz), while a practice nurse may be found undertaking Pap smear tests to screen for cervical cancer. At the tertiary level, a specialist nurse may run a 'cardiac club' for people who have suffered a heart attack or a district nurse may do the same for people who have leg ulcers. Chapter 5 will explore these roles in greater detail, exemplifying further how health promotion is both a core skill and a theoretical underpinning of nursing practice.

PROMOTING HEALTH IN COMMUNITIES OF PLACE

Promoting health at the local level extends across the continuum from prevention to intervention. It is also important to 'think global' and 'act local', considering global concepts such as human security and human rights when developing plans for local capacity building. These plans can involve a range of approaches, as a group of Canadian researchers found. They conducted a study of capacity-building in several different communities to identify the major processes involved (Montemurro et al. 2013). Their study was based on the premise that when there are limited resources it is crucial to maximise existing community assets, and to understand how community groups can be encouraged to define, assess, analyse and act on health. The findings from all communities studied revealed six primary categories of capacity-building activity: networking, partnering, information exchange, prioritising, planning/implementing and supporting/sustaining (Montemurro et al. 2013). These activities resonate with Leffers and Mitchell's (2010) conceptual framework for guiding community partnerships (Box 4.4). Both sets of guidelines reflect health promotion activities at the three levels of prevention (see Box 4.5).

Effective health promotion plans begin with knowledge of the local context, the SDH that either enhance or constrain health and wellbeing in that environment, and individual or family factors that may be influencing personal choices. Place is where people share meanings and understandings of their lives based on experiences and the extent to which they can engage with others in that particular place (Nykiforuk et al. 2012). Some places are more

> ### BOX 4.5 Primary, secondary, tertiary capacity-building activities
>
> 1 **Primary prevention**—networking, partnering, information exchange to provide guidance on preventing illness and/or injury, and to promote healthy living through health literacy and support for community decision-making.
>
> 2 **Secondary prevention**—collaborating with other sectors and agencies as well as with the local community to prioritise, plan and implement short- and long-term projects. Included are plans to respond to structural, place-based conditions that affect health.
>
> 3 **Tertiary prevention**—Ensuring there are appropriate resources to support and sustain community activities. Included are strategies for maintaining and extending funding to accommodate the needs of capacity-building initiatives, maintaining the integrity of the social and cultural contexts, and embedding projects within existing community agencies.

conducive to good health than others. For example, some communities enable and sustain health and wellbeing by virtue of their therapeutic or restorative landscapes; places where illness and/or stress can be alleviated by the healing air of the sea or the forest, or by spaces for physical activity and other family leisure pursuits, all of which can buffer the stresses of everyday life (Duff 2011).

Comprehensive assessments of the links between person and place will reveal those community characteristics that can be relied upon to support health and wellbeing and those that inhibit healthy choices. For example, recognising that work, study, child care or safety fears may be discouraging people from participating in lifestyle improvements is as important as knowing where people can access affordable venues, programs, information and other resources that facilitate participation (Barter-Godfrey et al. 2007). Understanding people's place-based social and cultural supports is also critical in

> ### HEALTH PROMOTION: A SUMMARY
>
> Step 1—Assessment
>
> Step 2—Identify mutual goals
>
> Step 3—Planning in partnership
>
> Step 4—Evaluating progress
>
> Step 5—Sustaining health

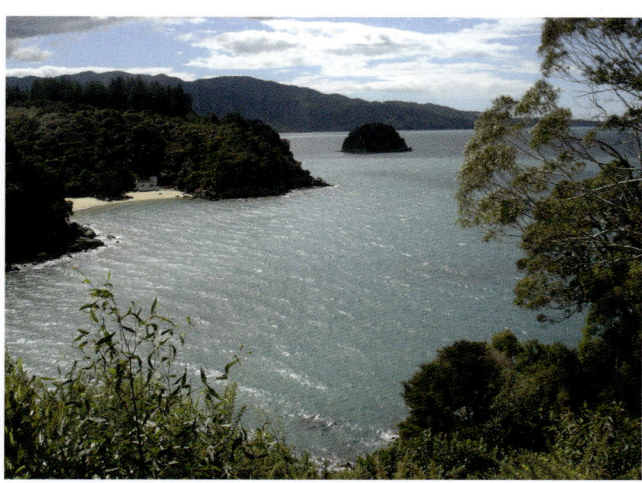

Healing landscapes (Jill Clendon)

assessing their needs (Wainwright et al. 2007). In some cases, intergenerational family influences that shape health beliefs, knowledge and the way people use spaces and structures may also need to be explored and acknowledged (Taylor et al. 2012). Once programs or interventions are established for primary, secondary or tertiary prevention, these can be evaluated to provide input for future programs.

HEALTH PROMOTION EVALUATION

Health promotion evaluation is essential for developing the evidence base for practice; however, implementation remains problematic. How would you make evaluation a priority in your health promotion activities?

Evaluation of the effectiveness of health promotion activities is an essential step to ensure effectiveness and appropriateness of interventions. Where change is expected, evaluation strategies help to provide mutual feedback to all involved so that barriers and facilitating factors are identified, as well as whatever lessons can be taken away from one situation and applied to another. Evaluation continues to be problematic in developing the evidence base for practice. Many programs and projects simply conduct an internal review of general and immediate outcomes, without sustainability indicators or breaking information down for different segments of the population according to social or cultural characteristics (Jolley et al. 2007). Careful, thorough evaluative information on processes and outcomes can be invaluable to future planning by indicating which groups or

contexts are receptive to various health education strategies, how best to access community resources, and how partnerships can be developed to help build community capacity. Evaluation should be integral to health promotion practice, even where evaluation is not mandated by funding bodies.

HEALTH PROMOTION IN THE CITY

Promoting the health of urban communities begins with the global commitment to healthy cities, which have made important inroads into health in numerous cities throughout the world (WHO 2011). Locally, many healthy city initiatives begin at the neighbourhood level, particularly in those neighbourhoods where there is a high concentration of poor and socially excluded people due to unemployment, low education or fear of crime (Froding et al. 2011). The major health promotion challenges lie in helping people improve liveability of their neighbourhood and in helping marginalised residents become socially integrated (Froding et al. 2011). These two goals reflect the combination of place-based and people-based approaches that are so important to healthy neighbourhoods (Erickson & Andrews 2011). The challenge is substantial, given what is known about people's motivation for participating in community life (Fienieg et al. 2011). A group of Swedish researchers found that with encouragement, many neighbourhood residents who have participated in one small activity will be encouraged to participate again, to contribute for the greater good of the neighbourhood (Froding et al. 2011). Adopting a small steps approach can help build the type of solidarity that can be used to foster incremental change and ultimately, social capital. Motivating factors for participation are similar to those that influence volunteerism. Volunteers are typically those who have a sense of obligation (I ought to get involved), importance (I have to), demand (I am needed), effectiveness (I can make it work), and meaningfulness (I get back in return) (Froding et al. 2011). These findings are similar to those of the Dutch researchers mentioned previously who found that people participate in community life out of a desire to be involved in purposeful action, personal development, recognition of their contributions and wanting to 'do one's bit' for the community.

Knowledge of what motivates people to participate is relevant to promoting health in a range of settings, in the city as well as in rural or regional areas. One of the crucial areas for citizen participation is in hospitals, especially where health promotion programs are in place. Throughout the past two decades the health promoting hospitals (HPH) concept has been used to encourage acute care staff to engage in health promotion and health education. However, HPH has been more popular in Europe than in Australia, where only 11 Australian health services are registered (McHugh et al. 2010) or in New Zealand where none are registered. International standards for these programs include having a management policy for promoting health among staff, patients and families; including health promotion as an aspect of patient assessment, providing patients with health education materials, promoting a healthy workplace, and collaborating with other health services, organisations and sectors to promote health (WHO 2004a). There is also growing evidence that there is a link between the health of the health professional and the health of the patient, with calls for physician wellness to become an indicator of health system quality (Wallace et al. 2009). Health promotion among those who provide health care is essential to ensure optimal messages regarding health are given (Kemppainen et al. 2012).

> ### TIPS FOR HEALTH TEACHING
>
> - Start where the people are—literacy level, location
> - Essential information first
> - Be consistent, accurate
> - Combine verbal, written information
> - Keep it simple
> - Right information, right time, right place, right person
> - Tailor information to individual needs
> - Communicate trust, respect

Health Promoting Schools (HPS) are also place-based settings for health promotion, developed around a whole-of-school approach to engaging students and staff in promoting their health and that of their school. Nurses in both Australia and New Zealand are actively engaged in promoting health in schools (Lovell et al. 2011), but not always in the context of a HPS program (Senior 2012). In those schools that do work within the HPS framework, there have been some successes in engaging school members to work towards improving children and adolescents' physical and mental health (Senior 2012). The HPS model begins with healthy policies that promote a healthy physical and social environment, which can support the development of healthy individual skills and actions for health in the context of providing both health and education

services (Senior 2012). The HPS is also closely linked to the external community and home environment, to provide an integrated set of values for mental and physical health, respect for learning and social justice (WHO 2004b).

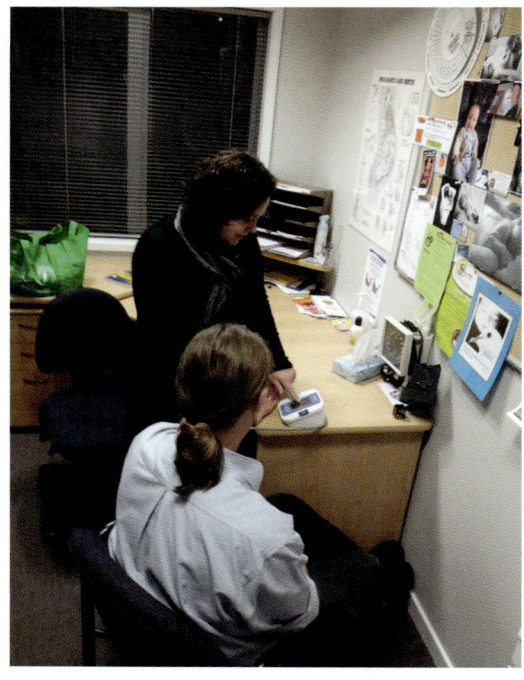

Chris Gaul (RN) working with a client at a school-based evening health clinic (with permission)

Other settings for promoting urban health include neighbourhood PHC centres, where people can access many types of health-related information and services, and mobile clinics (see Box 4.6). These are effective because of their accessibility, which can make health education more efficient (ANF 2009; NZMOH 2001). Although hospitals and clinics are an ideal source of health education, the first source of health information for many community residents is in primary care, such as general practice. In addition to receiving information the primary care visit often provides the impetus for empowerment, especially where people are provided with a range of options for citizen engagement. Sometimes this is as simple as knowing where they, and their family, can access resources, or being treated as a partner by health professionals in helping their neighbourhood or community. Referrals to various networks and support groups can encourage people to take a more active role in community capacity building. Researchers have found that consumer health organisations also play an important role in engaging people in health promotion, especially

BOX 4.6 Promoting health in the city—The Coachstop Caravan Park

The health promotion program established in Maitland, New South Wales is one of the most exemplary health promotion projects initiated and sustained by Australian community nurses in collaboration with other health professionals and community stakeholders.

Identifying the problem

In 2000 the nurses ran an unfunded pilot project to document what they saw as a large number of referrals to health services from the Coachstop Caravan Park. They realised that many of these cases were from women at risk who had a range of special needs. They successfully secured funding in 2002 from the Hunter Area Health Service and Women's Health Outcomes (NSW Health) for a two-year project that was to be organised around the principles of the Women's Health Outcomes Framework, PHC and the SDH. Their preliminary audit revealed a large number of single mothers were living in the caravans with their children, relying on social benefits and having no family or community support. Many were frequent victims of domestic violence, had poor levels of literacy, high substance abuse and high rates of hepatitis C. Most avoided mainstream health services such as child immunisation programs, dental and antenatal care. The women were socially isolated with poor self-esteem, and often had been evicted from public housing or women's refuges. Their children had poor school attendance. A number of male residents of the park had criminal records.

Planning and advocacy

Loretta Baker, the project coordinator, is a nurse with experience in community, midwifery and psychiatric nursing. She is immunisation accredited and has qualifications in alcohol and drug dependence. Other team members include a clinical psychologist and adolescent counsellor, an Aboriginal liaison officer and early childhood nurses. All have a passion for helping people. Loretta and her colleagues realised that something had to be done for this unique neighbourhood and those who inhabited it, even in transition. In Loretta's words 'once seen their collective plight could not be ignored'. They developed a plan for intervention that consisted of the following:

- development of trust, advocacy and reorganised, accessible services
- identification and engagement of collaborators from established organisations and agencies

- facilitation of collaborative partnerships in care with existing service providers
- demonstration of the effectiveness of positive life choices, nurturing friendships, social support and health literacy
- fostering community capacity building to help the women establish priorities and strategies to address them.

In the first instance, the nurses borrowed a mobile clinic from the Aboriginal Health Team to provide access fortnightly to drug and alcohol counselling, stress management, advocacy for housing, access to health services, health education and health promotion, women's health services, child immunisation programs, adolescent counselling, assistance with legal and court matters and enrolment in education and training courses. Through the outreach van, they established a needle and syringe program, the first ever on a residential property. Their van became a venue and the centre of activity in an area of the park that was acceptable to everyone, offering a non-threatening environment, opportunities and hope. In addition to providing health care, they established a mentorship program for residents who were undertaking education and training programs, helping them enrol in and progress with their studies.

Strategy and success

Within the first two years of the program, some of the residents enrolled in TAFE courses, and some secured employment. Others commenced drug detoxification programs, exercise and swimming classes, participated in antenatal and postnatal care programs and stress counselling. Some of the children began to attend preschool, others ballet and tennis classes. The local primary school included children from the park into their Breakfast Club, which provides a nutritional start to the day. Teachers began to liaise with the project coordinator to discuss the children's progress at school. Families began to buy healthier food, reducing their intakes of Coca Cola and alcohol. Some moved out of the park into government or private housing.

In 2013 they are proud to report on a decade of success for 'Women in the Park'. The keys to success include community participation in decision-making, holistic, comprehensive, community-oriented services, multi-level advocacy and intersectoral collaboration. They still immunise children in the chook shed of the caravan park, and they try to help

Continued

BOX 4.6 **Promoting health in the city—The Coachstop Caravan Park—cont'd**

the homeless who come to the van when it is parked there. The team has negotiated a partnership with the St Vincent de Paul organisation and together they engage in fundraising to try to provide services for people who fall outside the guidelines of any organised program, such as homeless non-Indigenous people. The partnership has yielded a number of benefits, including provision of resources such as medications and housing, with some members being able to influence the highest levels of government to secure ministerial support for what

they are trying to accomplish together. The team carefully charts progress, and is currently lobbying for a PHC nurse to undertake surveillance, assessment and treatment of some of the residents in the Emergency Department of the local hospital, where many park residents attend when necessary. There are many reasons to believe this program could be replicated throughout those caravan parks and neighbourhoods where layers of disadvantage trap many people in a vicious cycle of vulnerability. It is what we mean by PHC in practice.

(Source: Loretta Baker, personal communication; Ridgway, B. 2003 Interim report on the Coachstop Caravan Park Outreach Project. NSW Health)

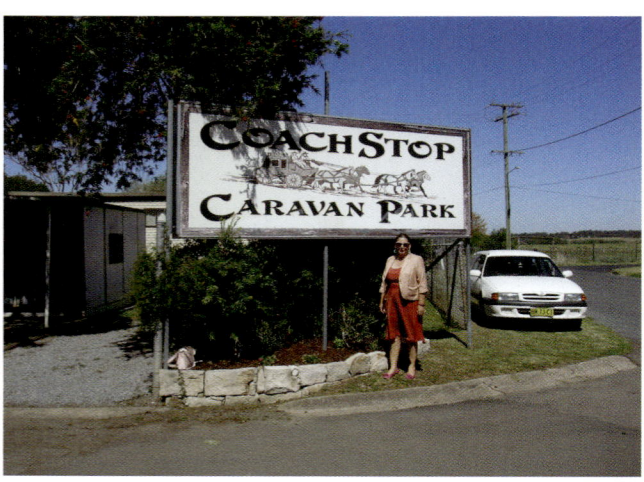

Loretta Baker, Coachstop Caravan Park (with permission)

where they are interested in self-management of chronic conditions (Boyle et al. 2011).

The effectiveness of health education strategies varies not only with the place where they are conducted, but also according to the level of understanding of community members. Health professionals can help people who may be only minimally health literate by understanding the scope of the problem. Those with low levels of literacy don't always reveal this, as they may be ashamed at their lack of understanding or reading skills. For this reason, health teaching should be sensitive to those who may have lesser understanding than others. Yet current research shows that printed health materials remain difficult for most people to understand, which may prevent them from active participation in their care and use of health services (Shieh & Hosei 2008;

van der Ploeg & Towle 2012). A large systematic review identified a range of specific interventions that have been demonstrated to improve comprehension for low-health-literacy populations (Berkman et al. 2011). These include presenting essential information by itself or presenting essential information first, being consistent and accurate when presenting risk and treatment benefits, and adding video to verbal narratives.

Irrespective of a person's literacy level, anticipating their needs at specific decision-making milestones is also important, especially the type of material a person might access in a health care setting (Coulter et al. 2008). Information should be not only appropriate, but timely, relevant and reliable. In many cases, people come to clinics or hospitals only to be given handouts with complex information and low readability (van der Ploeg & Towle 2012). Information that is not aimed at the most fundamental reading level is often ignored, preventing people from accessing services that may be crucial for their health (van der Ploeg & Towle 2012). The lesson for those developing printed material for health education is to use proven guidelines such as the SMOG index to ensure the usefulness of the material (SMOG, Online. Available: www.wordscount.info/wc/jsp/clear/analyze_smog.jsp [accessed 18 February 2013]).

ACTION POINT

Because people with low levels of health literacy may not reveal this to the health professional it is important to ensure accurate assessment of their health literacy before providing any health teaching.

The SMOG process involves checking written material according to a formula that has been used since the 1960s to reduce the number of sentences and the number of polysyllables (words of more than three syllables). In verbal as well as written information, appropriate communication means providing the right information at the right time, in the right situation, with the right point of entry for guidance. The message conveyed should be transparent and aimed at empowering people for decision-making. Interactions should communicate trust, respect, participation by all involved and have realistic expectations.

Written health information tailored to individual needs has been found to help reinforce professionals' explanations of health problems, but used alone, it is not always understood. Computer-based information may be more helpful than written instructions, as it is more readily tailored to different needs. However access to computers can be a problem for disadvantaged people (Coulter et al. 2008). A review of the research has found that when they do have access, those from disadvantaged groups tend to benefit more from computer-based support interventions (Coulter et al. 2008).

STRATEGY FOR ACTION

Have you ever accessed health information on the web that is incomplete or incorrect? How do you think you could help community members judge the adequacy and appropriateness of the information they access electronically?

One of the challenges of health education is to help maintain integrity in the type, level and appropriateness of information they are accessing from the internet. We can fulfil an enabling role by providing access to expertise, research evidence, and contextual information that will assist people in making healthy choices and finding the resources they need. However the information they receive from the web may need additional guidance and some degree of filtering to assure its credibility. Of course, many rural residents do not have internet access and their place-based health promotion may involve alternative approaches.

RURAL HEALTH PROMOTION

Like health promotion in the city, promoting health in rural communities is dependent on understanding people and place factors. Rural culture provides a structure for what is valued and how people experience their lives (Farmer et al. 2012). This is not to imply a homogenous culture in rural and regional areas, but there are some shared cultural norms among rural people that are evident in the particular way they express their beliefs and health challenges. Feelings of disempowerment are common, primarily because of the disadvantage of distance and a lack of services and personnel (Bourke et al. 2012). Many rural people are self-reliant—often as a result of years of realising that support systems are not forthcoming. It is typical for rural people to feel a sense of ownership of services in their local area, and this often creates a closer pattern of interaction with health professionals than in the city (Farmer et al. 2012). Like other communities of place, rural areas contain subcultures, however, members of these distinct groups often share a strong sense of belonging to the rural area. They tend to look out for each other. Even in farming communities where homes are at a distance from each other, people are mindful if someone has not been to town for some time, or has not picked up their mail. These are protective attitudes, as if helping one another from within the community makes up for the lack of external supports. This commonality of purpose means that health promotion personnel from outside the community may have to be clear that their message is one of collaboration and partnership rather than dominance in planning services.

ACTION POINT

People who live in rural or remote regions frequently have poorer access to health promotion programs. What specific role could you see a nurse undertaking to improve access to health promotion for rural families?

In many rural and regional areas, there is often closer collaboration between acute and PHC services, both with an interest in integration of services (Humphreys & Gregory 2012). Although many health promotion programs are multidimensional, in some cases it is important to develop selective PHC programs, particularly where the demographics of a community are distinctive. So, for example, health promoters in an area that has predominantly young families, or retired families, or transient workers would find that the best use of scarce resources would be to develop programs to respond to the unique issues of the particular community. In many rural areas one of the greatest needs for engaging local communities is in enabling mental health literacy and supports. With the decline of the rural economy, young people often feel isolated from their peers at a time when social connections are most important. Adolescents may be receptive to health education messages that encourage responsible alcohol consumption, or other healthy behaviours, but in rural areas even when programs or services are available, they may not access these because of the stigma of the entire community knowing their reasons for attending a clinic or service. McMichael (2011) suggests that school-based mental health programs, often developed as part of the Healthy Schools initiatives in urban areas, should be adapted for use in rural schools.

As with other health promotion interventions, the key to success lies in encouraging participation by the rural community to develop viable programs appropriate to the context (Berends et al. 2011). At times, programs will require external personnel, and this may be the case with some counselling services. A partnership approach to establishing the health promotion agenda can help ensure that people have access to information that is appropriate for them. One way of working towards community acceptability is through networking ideas and plans. For example, the FarmLink program in rural New South Wales (www.farmlink.com.au) and in Western Australia (www.farmlinkrural.com) provides networks of rural services and supports for rural workers. In addition to connecting farm families, these resources also provide valuable forums for information exchange so that they are all informed of the best way to partner with the community (Berends et al. 2011). A similar international network is accessible from Canada (www.farmlink.net.). Other sources for information for rural and regional communities are the Australian National Rural Health Alliance (www.nrha.org.au) and in New Zealand, the Institute for Rural Health (www.nzirh.org.nz).

The viability of rural and regional communities is an important consideration for health promotion and this involves the accessibility and acceptability of structural supports. This is problematic in a number of Australian rural and regional communities that have been overwhelmed by the FIFO workforce, especially where there has been a deterioration of the SDH in the local community. In these cases, health promotion plans must be multidimensional, working towards empowering local citizens to secure and sustain resources to support family and community life, and to provide health education and guidance for community-identified needs.

PROMOTING HEALTH IN RELATIONAL COMMUNITIES

As we have reiterated throughout the chapter, health promotion activities begin with assessment of assets and risks, strengths and needs, and the influence of people and place relationships. In urban and rural communities, this type of information is essential for planning to build healthy public policy, create supportive environments, strengthen community action, develop personal skills and reorient health services. We use these five major strategies of the Ottawa Charter in relational communities too, for supportive strategies that are appropriate to the situation, the people and the environment. So in promoting health in FIFO communities, plans would include consideration of structures, resources and relationships between the workers and the employers in the mining camps, their relationships with the local community, and the workers' concerns about what may be occurring in their home communities. For the families of FIFO workers, health promotion activities will be determined by issues such as their particular health needs and various social and parenting challenges. Environmental concerns would feature across all of these settings. Some of the FIFO workplace and family concerns are common to all occupational groups, as we discuss in Chapter 5, but in their situation, there are additional needs to ensure the intermittent nature of family life and the social isolation of both partners does not have adverse effects on health. Like FIFO families, other groups of affiliation have distinctive needs, whether they are affiliated through faith, culture or group commitment. In all cases, the Ottawa Charter guides us toward a comprehensive approach to helping each community create and maintain health. The examples below address the special health promotion needs of migrant communities and those brought together as a virtual or media community.

PROMOTING HEALTH IN MIGRANT COMMUNITIES

The most visible 'health and place' issue for migrant communities is the notion of 'transition'. Regardless of their reasons for migrating, people transitioning to a new country have significant issues in establishing or re-establishing a lifestyle that will see them sustain their health and that of their family. Making a successful transition is based on dealing with the stressors at each stage of migration (Samarasinghe 2011). In the case of involuntary migration because of war or civil unrest, migrants may have to deal with a sudden, unplanned move coinciding with the loss of home, relatives, friends and homeland. The loss of familiar, communal and culturally determined patterns of behaviour is also a cause of psychological stress, as is the pressure to adapt to another country's cultural values and norms. This can involve transitioning from a collectivist culture, where the family and community are pre-eminent, to individualistic cultures that emphasise individual autonomy (Samarasinghe 2011). Another problem lies in the fact that mental health services in the new country are often inadequately prepared to help with the intense issues of migration. Cultural or language difficulties can result in increased personal suffering, detrimental effects on the family, and increased costs on the health care system through inappropriate or unnecessary investigations and/or poor treatment options (Cross & Singh 2012). In some cases, women are prevented from attending English classes because of family norms. Their language difficulties also pose a dilemma for their children, who, like other children, need to be helped through their adjustment to school. Medical care is sporadic, often leaving new migrants to rely on charities for assistance. Like other community members, migrants need to be supported through developing a sense of wellbeing, mastery of new behaviour and positive interpersonal relationships (Samarasinghe 2011).

> ## REMINDER: Cultural sensitivity and cultural safety
>
> **Cultural sensitivity** means being responsive to the way an individual or group's cultural mores and lifestyle habits shape health and health behaviours.
>
> **Cultural safety** is a concept that refers to exploring, reflecting on, and understanding one's own culture and how it relates to other cultures.

Developing health literacy in the new context is critical, especially when health and social service structures are difficult to understand or access, and are organised around the dominant culture (Merry et al. 2011). Access to interpreter services is one of the keys to addressing the problems of health care access, but interpreters need to be well-informed, professional, sensitive to cultural norms and consistent, to ensure that information is not selective or inadequately translated (Bauer & Alegria 2010; Habersack et al. 2011; Henderson et al. 2011; Komaric et al. 2012; Priebe et al. 2011). Appropriate interpreter services can reveal the extent to which culture shapes people's awareness of health and illness and indicate areas of particular concern (Komaric et al. 2012). Ensuring access to professional interpreters can be particularly challenging in smaller communities where only a few people may speak the required language. These concerns may require nurses to create safe spaces to express spiritual practices in conjunction with the social, gendered, cultural,

historical, economic and political contexts (Pesut & Reimer-Kirkham 2010). For example, some people, despite having diabetes mellitus may maintain the need to fast during Ramadan; others may refuse to be shaved in hospital because of religious traditions; and for many women, there are cultural constraints on having male medical practitioners. These issues create the need to negotiate care through the transitions in a way that does not further marginalise members of various cultural groups, and that has positive health outcomes (Komaric et al. 2012; Pesut & Reimer-Kirkham 2010). Migrant people also tend to resettle in 'ethnic enclaves' where there are others in the community from similar backgrounds (Cross & Singh 2012:157). These communities can be seen as assets for health, particularly when they provide mutual support that can mobilise people to consider their strengths and feel empowered for decision-making (Rotegard et al. 2010). Living in neighbourhoods with others who have had similar experiences can help build a sense of community and help buffer some of the pre-migration and post-migration stress, especially if health professionals develop in-depth understanding of and sensitivity toward their particular risks and strengths (Cross & Singh 2012).

> ## REMINDER: Reciprocal determinism
>
> People both affect and are affected by the environment in which they live.

Successful transition to the new culture involves a process of *acculturation*, the biological, economical, political, social and psychological changes that are developed in adopting a new lifestyle, new values and often, a new language (Khanlou 2010; Samarasinghe 2011). Acculturation can require adjustment in food, dress, language and manner of interacting, which often involves rejecting a previous identity and attempting to develop a new one (Samarasinghe 2011). The process can be traumatic in itself, causing stress, eroding self-esteem and self-efficacy, which increases vulnerability to further cycles of psychological distress and physical illness (Merry et al. 2011; Samarasinghe 2011). Successful acculturation occurs when the individual and the family develop a sense of belonging and participation in both the old and the new culture, which can take many years (Khanlou 2010; Samarasinghe 2011). Ultimately the most important assets to emerge from acculturation may be resiliency, resourcefulness and reconciliation between the old culture and the new.

Biculturalism—being able to maintain two different cultures at once—is often a successful outcome of the acculturation process (Buscemi 2011).

STEPS IN FOSTERING ACCULTURATION

- Conversations to share stories
- Norms, behaviours in host country
- Addressing cultural differences
- Cultural comfort

Nurses and other health professionals can assist acculturation using an incremental approach to help people work through the issues related to their family's experience of migration (Samarasinghe 2011). The first step involves conversations with the family that encourage them to tell their stories and share what they wish to share (Millender 2011). In the context of these conversations people should be encouraged to focus on their perception of differences between the two cultures, with the health professional making an effort to honour their story (Millender 2011; Samarasinghe 2011). Second, it is helpful to discuss prevailing norms and behavioural patterns in the host culture, including the health care system and how it works (Samarasinghe 2011). The third stage revolves around addressing specific differences, including family functions and roles, gender roles, culture shocks and misunderstandings (Samarasinghe 2011). Some believe that the end point of acculturation is cultural competence (Khanlou 2010) but this contention may not be congruent with an empowerment approach, given the dilemma of judging competence from anything but a dominant cultural approach. Although cultural competence is identified by the NHMRC (2005) as a health promotion goal it may be more appropriate to think of this stage as *cultural comfort*. Feeling comfortable in the new environment allows a person to straddle two or more cultures at once, without pressure to be 'competent' in either. To help foster cultural transitions we outline the guidelines developed by the Ministry of Health in New Zealand for working with refugees (see Box 4.7). Basically, the intention for promoting health should be to focus on maintaining open and meaningful communication with all migrant communities; increase trust in the health system; guide people toward greater knowledge about health and services in their communities; and expand cultural understandings among those who work in the health system (Henderson et al. 2011).

BOX 4.7 Tips for working with refugees

- Get to know the client, their background, the community they live in and their needs.
- Focus on the strengths of the client—don't ask them to repeat their story.
- Don't assume clients obtain support from their ethnic community or are linked to their community.
- Arrange for the services of a professional interpreter where necessary—obtain the consent of the client first.
- Don't leave clients waiting (being made to wait is often used as a form of torture).
- Be clear that you are there to help and explain confidentiality.
- Avoid early morning appointments as sleeping problems may be common among this population group.
- Be aware that clients may be under financial pressure when arranging follow-up appointments or referrals.
- Encourage clients to bring a support person where appropriate.

(Source: NZMOH 2012; NSW Refugee Health Service & STARTTS 2004; Victorian Settlement Planning Committee 2005).

PROMOTING HEALTH IN VIRTUAL COMMUNITIES

Virtual communities, linked through electronic communication networks, are a rapidly evolving context for health education. Internet-based tools and aids that constitute social media provide two-way messaging platforms that can be used to reach people whose physical location varies. Social networking sites such as Facebook, Twitter, Flickr, YouTube and Linkedin have been rapidly growing worldwide, with 800 million users as of 2011 (Randolph 2011). With as many as 80% of adults and around 90% of adolescents worldwide accessing health information online, social media can be effective in conveying messages about health, providing current information on services and, sometimes, encouraging behaviour change (Baum et al. 2012: Crutzen & de Nooijker 2010; Korda & Itani 2013; Monshat et al. 2011; Verheijden et al. 2008). Clearly, the internet is a major factor in promoting health literacy. Delivering guidance on mental health issues online is particularly helpful for adolescents, as this is a time when mental health problems that may track into adulthood first emerge (Crutzen & de Nooijer 2010). For example, an online cognitive behavioural therapy (CBT) computer game developed for adolescents demonstrating symptoms of depression has been found to be equally as effective as traditional face-to-face CBT (Merry et al. 2012). According to Crutzen and de Nooijer (2010) chat rooms where young people have access to mental health professionals have been used extensively around the world (Trimbos, Online. Available: www.trimbos.org/projects/e-health/master-your-mood-online [accessed 12 March 2013]). Paradoxically, some of these sites are designed to help with problems such as bullying that have been perpetrated through the media. Some internet sites are designed to provide peer support, which can act as a gateway to seeking professional help (Crutzen & de Nooijer 2010). Mindfulness training is one specific approach that Australian health professionals are using online to help Australian young people with their emotional development (Monshat et al. 2011).

TRENDING NOW

- Social media for health information
- Smart phones
- Digital divide
- Online peer support

Question: how would you measure the effectiveness of health promotion messages online?

Connecting young people with emotional or mental health issues in this way can help enhance personal capacity, the built environment, and social capital by dissolving the geographic and social barriers caused by stigma, marginalisation or loss of privacy (Hallett et al. 2007; Monshat et al. 2011). Being in control of the amount, type and timing of information can be both empowering and efficient in providing access to the information or peer group when, how and where users prefer (Thielst 2011). However, there are also access problems for some people which create barriers to participation. In some cases, a lack of access to readily understood information can affect culturally and linguistically disadvantaged (CALD) people and those with low literacy (O'Mara 2012). The 'digital divide' can therefore be a cause of social exclusion, exacerbating existing inequalities (Baum et al. 2012). Although 79% of Australians enjoy home internet, there is a

digital gradient, similar to the gradient effect on health, whereby disadvantaged groups, particularly rural and Indigenous people, have less access than those at the higher end of the socio-economic scale (Baum et al. 2012). There is also a caution for nurses in using the internet for health education. Because information placed on the internet is publicly accessible for perpetuity nurses must be careful that any postings maintain client confidentiality, and that they are accurate and represent best available knowledge at the time they are disseminated (Randolph 2011).

HANDLE WITH CARE!

Internet information is never confidential.

All information must be carefully evaluated for accuracy before being recommended to community members.

Studies of social media use show that more than half of older adults use the internet to find treatment information, many of whom are also interested in using electronic access for their health records (Korda & Itani 2013; Thielst 2011). Although it is relatively easy to ascertain who is using the sites, evaluation data are not always available on the impact or efficacy of these sites in terms of behaviour change. Clearly, there is a need for further research into how and why they are being accessed by various population groups and the link between these factors and health outcomes (Crutzen & de Nooijer 2010). Some of the challenges inherent in evaluating the impact of social media on health include trying to understand whether people are just accessing information on a superficial level or whether they are engaging with content to maintain health (Korda & Itani 2013; Verheijden et al. 2008).

WHAT'S YOUR OPINION?

Do you know a website or app that may be insensitive to issues of gender or culture?

What would be a first step to take in monitoring the influence of health information on the web?

Robinson and Robertson (2010) suggest that we should promote e-Health Literacy to empower people to seek out and use electronic information to solve health problems. How could you encourage this process?

A major advantage of promoting health and health literacy through web-based applications is that they provide an opportunity to reach those who may be hesitant to access information elsewhere. Young men, in particular, tend to ignore health information provided in 'feminised spaces' such as General Practitioners' offices (Robinson & Robertson 2010:363). Many use the internet for a wide range of information, such as sporting, gay, music or entertainment sites, which could be used as spaces for promoting health literacy (Hallett et al. 2007; Robinson & Robertson 2010). Blogs or wikis are particularly useful tools as they have flexible access, a participative structure and personalised support and feedback from mentors. One such site is www.dadtalk.co.uk, which filters out commercial advertising and invites expert contributions on parenting, health, work-life balance and building self-esteem (Robinson & Robertson 2010). Other sites encourage young people to discuss health topics (such as www.youthhealthtalk.org, www.healthtalkonline.org and www.netdoctor.co.uk). Some sites include commercial content (www.menshealth.com), while others exclude expert participation, providing avenues for men to have a say on topics of concern to them.

Robinson and Robertson (2010) consider whether online networks can be conceptualised as social capital, with benefits potentially accruing to the network, and relationally, to individuals in terms of building trust, norms and motivation. They argue for more research to investigate whether those accessing information through social media are able to avoid commercial manipulation and critically interpret messages. In terms of men's health they believe the research could help illuminate young men's socially contingent health practices and how 'discourses around masculinity and health might confirm, contradict or transform each other' (Robinson & Robertson 2010:369). Baum et al. (2012) argue that this type of media access should now be considered an SDH (Baum et al. 2012). Another electronic application for health promotion is the use of smartphones to reach people (Thielst 2011). Tailored text messages sent from health professionals can be used to reinforce health information or healthy behaviours. These messages serve as cues to action, particularly for those who are actively seeking advice or guidance (Korda & Itani 2013). Other media create a range of opportunities for social connectedness where it is most needed. For special groups such as migrants and refugees, a combination of peer-led self-empowerment programs using digital video in their native language and online viewing in communal spaces can be effective (O'Mara 2012). Photo-novella, photovoice techniques that request people to take digital videos or photos of their community can be uploaded onto YouTube or social media to share with others, either in their homelands or local communities. These help people record images of their daily lives in a way that can help build a participatory culture, effectively creating bonding and bridging social capital. The technologies are therefore invaluable in alleviating the social isolation of migration, often encouraging people to participate through digital storytelling in their native language. This type of endeavour is empowering by providing a forum for information exchange, which can help promote personal and group agency (O'Mara 2012). The technological platform effectively provides a critical space where feedback, concerns and dialogue can be shared between community members, health service providers and others (O'Mara 2012).

CASE STUDY: Promoting health for the Smiths and Masons

Strategies for promoting health in the three communities of the Smiths and the Masons are planned around the Ottawa Charter; that is, promoting healthy public policies, creating supportive environments, strengthening community action, developing personal skills and reorienting health services. For example, in the mining community we may want to debate the creation of wealth from the mining companies that provide employment versus the distribution of resources and services that may disadvantage some members of the community. The mining camp has a dearth of supportive services for Colin and Jason's health and wellbeing, especially as both suffer from isolation and a lack of work-life balance. They are also not included in the local community, and in some cases when they go to town they are made to feel the resentment of the locals. Colin and Jason both need support for healthy ways of coping while they are up at the site, which involves some personal skill development and support from the mine site health service.

Maddington has assets and resources to support families, and several social networks for miners' wives. However, there is considerable stress on family life, with Rebecca having to get the children to child care, school and the child health nurse. Like Maddington, Papakura has a range of services available for families but not all are considered culturally appropriate by local families. Rebecca enjoys the social support of a group of FIFO wives, but in New Zealand, as one of only a handful of FIFO wives Huia has few friends who understand the loneliness and isolation of her family's lifestyle, despite being relatively well off.

REFLECTING ON THE BIG ISSUES

- Being healthy in any community means having equitable access to resources, empowerment, cultural inclusiveness, healthy environments and participation in decision-making.

- Health professionals undertake primary, secondary and tertiary prevention, using health promotion, appropriate technology and intersectoral collaboration.

- Health promotion is a combination of health education and helping people arrange the social and structural circumstances of their lives to maintain health.

- PHC principles focus on capacity building and empowerment of communities and those who reside in them.

- The relationship between health and place is a major consideration in promoting health and advocating for the community.

- The greatest issue for migrant communities is in making the transition to a new community, preserving their culture while adapting to the new one.

- The Ottawa Charter provides a guideline for health promotion across all communities.

REFLECTIVE QUESTIONS: How would I use this knowledge in practice?

1 How would you deal with the tensions in the mining town in such a way that would promote the health of both the townspeople and the mining employees?

2 In what ways are the experiences of migrant families similar to those of a family who chose to move to the mining town?

3 What do you see as your role in: building healthy public policy, creating supportive environments, strengthening community action, developing personal skills and reorienting health services in each of these communities?

4 Do you think these five strategies of the Ottawa Charter can yield health improvements for the host communities of Papakura and Maddington?

5 What level of advocacy could you engage in to make visible the need for community resources in the mining community?

6 Identify the primary, secondary and tertiary steps that can be taken to promote health in a relational community, such as one connected by social media.

7 How will you know if your strategies for health promotion are helpful?

References

Abbott, S., Bickerton, J., Daly, M., et al., 2008. Evidence-based primary health care and local research: a necessary but problematic partnership. Prim. Health Care Res. Dev. 9, 191–198.

Abramowitz, S., Flattery, D., Franses, K., et al., 2010. Linking a motivational interviewing curriculum to the chronic care model. J. Gen. Intern. Med. 25 (Suppl. 4), 620–626.

Allender, S., Gleeson, E., Crammond, B., et al., 2011. Policy change to create supportive environments for physical activity and healthy eating: which options are the most realistic for local government? Health Promot. Int. 27 (2), 261–274.

Australian Nursing Federation (ANF), 2009. Primary health care in Australia. A Nursing and Midwifery Consensus View. ANF, Canberra.

Barter-Godfrey, S., Taket, A., Rowlands, G., 2007. Evaluating a community lifestyle intervention: adherence and the role of perceived support. Prim. Health Care Res. Dev. 8, 345–354.

Bauer, A., Alegria, M., 2010. Impact of patient language proficiency and interpreter service use on the quality of psychiatric care: A systematic review. Psychiatr. Serv. 61 (8), 765–773.

Baum, F., 2007. Health for all now! Reviving the spirit of Alma Ata in the twenty-first century: an introduction to the Alma Ata Declaration. Soc. Sci. 2 (1), 34–41.

Baum, F., Begin, M., Houweling, T., et al., 2009. Changes not for the fainthearted: reorienting health care systems toward health equity through action on the social determinants of health. Am. J. Public Health 99 (11), 1967–1974.

Baum, F., Newman, L., Biedrzycki, K., 2012. Vicious cycles: digital technologies and determinants of health in Australia. Health Promot. Int. doi:10.1093/heapro/das062.

Baum, F., Sanders, D., 2011. Ottawa 25 years on: a more radical agenda for health equity is still required. Health Promot. Int. 26 (S2), ii253–ii257.

Berends, L., MacLean, S., Hunter, B., et al., 2011. Implementing alcohol and other drug interventions effectively: How does location matter? Aust. J. Rural Health 19, 211–217.

Berkman, N., Sheridan, S., Donahue, K., et al., 2011. Health literacy interventions and outcomes: an updated systematic review, Evidence report/technology assessment no. 199. (Prepared by RTI International-University of North Carolina Evidence-based Practice Centre under contract No. 290-2007-10056-I. AHRQ Publication Number 11-E006) Agency for Healthcare Research and Quality Rockville, MD.

Bourke, L., Humphreys, J., Wakerman, J., et al., 2012. Understanding drivers of rural and remote health outcomes: A conceptual framework in action. Aust. J. Rural Health 20, 318–323.

Boyle, F., Mutch, A., Dean, J., et al., 2011. Increasing access to consumer health organisations among patients with chronic disease—a randomised trial of a print-based intervention. Prim. Health Care Res. Dev. 12 (3), 245–254.

Buscemi, C., 2011. Acculturation: state of the science in nursing. J. Cult. Divers. 8 (2), 39–42.

Cambon, L., Minary, L., Ridde, V., et al., 2012. Transferability of interventions in health education: A review. BMC Public Health 12, 497–510.

Catford, J., 2000. Mexico ministerial statement for the promotion of health: from ideas to action. Health Promot. Int. 15 (4), 275–276.

Catford, J., 2011. Ottawa 1986: back to the future. Health Promot. Int. 26 (S2), ii63–ii67.

Chamberlain, M., Beckingham, A., 1987. Primary health care in Canada: in praise of the nurse? Int. Nurs. Rev. 34 (6), 158–160.

Chittendon, D., 2012. A concept analysis of motivational interviewing for the community practitioner. Community Pract. 85 (10), 21–23.

Coulter, A., Parsons, S., Ashkham, J., 2008. Where are the patients in decision-making about their own care? Policy Brief, WHO and WHO European Observatory on Health Systems and Policies, Copenhagen, Regional Office for Europe.

Courtney, R., 1995. Community partnership primary care: a new paradigm for primary care. Public Health Nurs. 12 (6), 366–373.

Cross, D., Singh, C., 2012. Dual vulnerabilities: Mental illness in a culturally and linguistically diverse society. Contemp. Nurse 42 (2), 156–166.

Crutzen, R., de Nooijer, J., 2010. Intervening via chat: an opportunity for adolescents' mental health promotion? Health Promot. Int. 26 (2), 238–242.

Duff, C., 2011. Networks, resources and agencies: On the character and production of enabling places. Health Place 17, 149–156.

Dyer, O., 2005. Disparities in health widen between rich and poor in England. Br. Med. J. 331, 419.

Egger, G., 2007. Personal carbon trading: a potential 'stealth intervention' for obesity reduction? Med. J. Aust. 187, 185–187.

Egger, G., Fitzgerald, W., Frape, G., et al., 1983. Results of a large scale media anti-smoking campaign in Australia: the North Coast Healthy Lifestyle Program. Br. Med. J. 287, 1125–1187.

Erickson, D., Andrews, N., 2011. Partnerships among community development, public health, and health care could improve the well-being of low-income people. Health Aff. 30 (11), 2056–2063.

Farmer, J., Bourke, L., Taylor, J., et al., 2012. Culture and rural health. Aust. J. Rural Health 20, 243–247.

Fienieg, B., Nierkens, V., Tonkens, E., et al., 2011. Why play an active role? A qualitative examination of lay citizens' main motives for participation in health promotion. Health Promot. Int. 27 (3), 416–426.

Froding, K., Elander, I., Eriksson, C., 2011. Neighbourhood development and public health initiatives: who participates? Health Promot. Int. 27 (1), 102–116.

Green, J., 2008. Health education—the case for rehabilitation. Crit. Public Health 18 (4), 447–456.

Green, L., Kreuter, M., 1991. Health Promotion Planning: An Educational and Environmental Approach. Mayfield Publishing Company, Mountain View.

Habersack, M., Gerlich, I., Mandi, M., 2011. Migrant women in Austria: difficulties with access to health care services. Ethn. Inequal. Health Soc. Care 4 (1), 6–15.

Hallett, J., Brown, G., Maycock, B., et al., 2007. Changing communities, changing spaces: the challenges of health promotion outreach in cyberspace. Promot. Educ. 14 (3), 150–154.

Henderson, S., Kendall, E., See, L., 2011. The effectiveness of culturally appropriate interventions to manage or prevent chronic disease in culturally and linguistically diverse communities: a systematic literature review. Health Soc. Care Community 19 (3), 225–249.

Holzemer, W., 1992. Linking primary health care and self care through management. Int. Nurs. Rev. 39 (3), 83–89.

Huffman, M., 2010. Health coaching. A fresh approach for improving health outcomes and reducing cost. AAOHN J. 58 (6), 245–250.

Humphreys, J., Gregory, G., 2012. Celebrating another decade of progress in rural health: What is the current state of play? Aust. J. Rural Health 20, 156–163.

Jolley, G., Lawless, A., Baum, F., et al., 2007. Building an evidence-base for community health: a review of the quality of program evaluations. Aust. Health Rev. 31 (4), 603–610.

Kemppainen, V., Tossavainen, K., Turunen, H., 2012. Nurses' roles in health promotion practice: An integrative review. Health Promot. Int. doi:10.1093/heapro/das/034.

Khanlou, N., 2010. Migrant mental health in Canada. Can. Issues/Themes Canadiens Summer 98–102.

Kickbusch, I., 2003. The contribution of the World Health Organization to a new public health and health promotion. Am. J. Public Health 93 (3), 383–388.

Kickbusch, I., 2012. Addressing the interface of the political and commercial determinants of health, Editorial. Health Promot. Int. 27 (4), 427–428.

Komaric, N., Bedford, S., van Driel, M., 2012. Two sides of the coin: patient and provider perceptions of health care delivery to patients from culturally and linguistically diverse backgrounds. BMC Health Serv. Res. 12, 322–346.

Korda, H., Itani, Z., 2013. Harnessing social media for health promotion and behavior change. Health Promot. Pract. 14 (1), 15–23.

Labonte, R., 2008. Global health in public policy: finding the right frame? Crit. Public Health 18 (4), 467–482.

Lalonde, M., 1974. A New Perspective on the Health of Canadians: a Working Paper. Government of Canada, Ottawa.

Lasater, T., Carleton, R., LeFebre, R., 1988. The Pawtucket heart health program: utilizing community resources for primary prevention. R. I. Med. J. 71, 63–67.

Leavell, H., Clark, A., 1965. Preventive Medicine for the Doctor in his Community, third ed. McGraw-Hill, New York.

Leffers, J., Mitchell, E., 2010. Conceptual model for partnership and sustainability in global health. Public Health Nurs. 28 (1), 91–102.

Lovell, S., Kearns, R., Rosenberg, M., 2011. Community capacity building in practice: constructing its meaning and relevance to health promoters. Health Soc. Care Community 19 (5), 531–540.

Maccoby, N., Solomon, D., 1981. The Stanford community studies in heart disease prevention. In: Rice, R., Paisley, W. (Eds.), Public Communication Campaigns. Sage, Beverly Hills, CA.

McAlister, A., 1981. Anti-smoking campaigns: progress in developing effective communications. In: Rice, R., Paisley, W. (Eds.), Public Communication Campaigns. Sage, Beverly Hills, CA.

McHugh, C., Robinson, A., Chesters, J., 2010. Health promoting health services: a review of the evidence. Health Promot. Int. 25 (2), 230–237.

McMichael, A., 2011. Drought, drying and mental health: Lessons from recent experiences for future risk-lessening policies. Aust. J. Rural Health 19, 227–228.

Merry, L., Gagnon, A., Hemlin, I., et al., 2011. Cross-border movement and women's health: how to capture the data. Int. J. Equity Health 10 (1), 56–71.

Merry, S., Stasiak, K., Shepherd, M., et al., 2012. The effectiveness of SPARX, a computerised self help intervention for adolescents seeking help for depression: randomised controlled non-inferiority trial. BMJ 344, doi: <http://dx.doi.org/10.1136/bmj.e2598>.

Millender, E., 2011. Using stories to bridge cultural disparities, one culture at a time. J. Contin. Educ. Nurs. 42 (1), 37–42.

Monshat, K., VElla-Brodrick, D., Burns, J., et al., 2011. Mental health promotion in the Internet age: a consultation with Australian young people to inform the design of an online mindfulness training programme. Health Promot. Int. 27 (2), 177–186.

Montemurro, G., Raine, K., Nykiforuk, C., et al., 2013. Exploring the process of capacity-building among community-based health promotion workers in Alberta, Canada. Health Promot. Int. doi:10.1093/heapro/dato08.

National Health and Medical Research Council, 2005. Cutlural competency in health: A guide for policy, partnerships and participation. NHMRC, Canberra.

New Zealand Ministry of Health (NZMOH), 2000. New Zealand Health Strategy. MOHNZ, Wellington.

New Zealand Ministry of Health (NZMOH), 2001. The Primary Health Care Strategy. MOHNZ, Wellington.

New Zealand Ministry of Health (NZMOH), 2010. Kōrero Mārama: Health Literacy and Māori. Results from the 2006 Adult Literacy and Life Skills Survey. Ministry of Health, Wellington.

New Zealand Ministry of Health (NZMOH), 2012. Refugee Health Care: A handbook for health professionals. Ministry of Health, Wellington.

Nutbeam, D., 2008. The evolving concept of health literacy. Soc. Sci. Med. 67, 2072–2078.

Nutbeam, D., 2009. Defining and measuring health literacy: what can we learn from literacy studies? Int. J. Public Health 54, 303–305.

Nutbeam, D., Catford, J., 1987. The Welsh heart program evaluation strategy: progress, plans and possibilities. Health Promot. 2 (1), 5–18.

Nykiforuk, C., Schopflocher, D., Vallianatos, H., et al., 2012. Community health and the built environment: examining place in a Canadian chronic disease prevention project. Health Promot. Int. doi:10.1093/heapro/dar093.

O'Mara, B., 2012. Social media, digital video and health promotion in a culturally and linguistically diverse Australia. Health Promot. Int. doi:10.1093/heapro/das014.

Pesut, B., Reimer-Kirkham, S., 2010. Situated clinical encounters in the negotiation of religious and spiritual plurality: A critical ethnography. Int. J. Nurs. Stud. 47, 815–825.

Priebe, S., Sandhu, S., Dias, S., et al., 2011. Good practice in health care for migrants: views and experiences of care professionals in 16 European countries. Br. Public Health 11, 187–200.

Randolph, S., 2011. Using social media and networking in health care. AAOHN J. doi:10.3928/21650799-20111227-14.

Raphael, D., 2013a. The political economy of health promotion: part 1, national commitments to provision of the prerequisites of health. Health Promot. Int. 28 (1), 95–111.

Raphael, D., 2013b. The political economy of health promotion: part 2, national provision of the prerequisites of health. Health Promot. Int. 28 (1), 112–132.

Reynolds, L., 2012. 'No decision about me, without me': a place for social marketing within the new public health architecture? Perspect. Public Health 132 (1), 26–30.

Ridgway, B., 2003. Interim Report on the Coachstop Caravan Park Outreach Project. NSW Health, Maitland.

Robinson, M., Robertson, S., 2010. Young men's health promotion and new information communication technologies: illuminating the issues and research agendas. Health Promot. Int. 25 (3), 363–370.

Rotegard, A., Moore, S., Fagermoen, M., et al., 2010. Health assets: A concept analysis. Int. J. Nurs. Stud. 47, 513–525.

Sachs, J., 2005. Investing in Development. A Practical Plan to Achieve the Millenium Development Goals. United Nations, New York.

Sachs, J., 2012. Introduction. In: The Earth Institute, World Happiness Report. Online. Available: <http://www.earth.colunbia.edu> 11 January 2012.

Samarasinghe, K., 2011. A conceptual model facilitating the transition of involuntary migrant families. ISRN Nursing doi:10.5402/2011/824209.

Senior, E., 2012. Becoming a health promoting school: key components of planning. Glob. Health Promot. 19 (1), 23–31.

Shieh, C., Hosei, B., 2008. Printed health information materials: evaluation of readability and suitability. J. Community Health Nurs. 25, 73–90.

Signal, L., Walton, M., Ni Mhurchu, N., et al., 2012. Tackling 'wicked' health promotion problems: a New Zealand case study. Health Promot. Int. 28 (1), 84–94.

Skouteris, H., Cox, R., Huang, T., et al., 2013. Promoting obesity prevention together with environmental sustainability. Health Promot. Int. doi:10.1093/heapro/dat007.

Smith, S., Dixon, A., Trevena, L., et al., 2009. Exploring patient involvement in healthcare decision making across different education and functional health literacy groups. Soc. Sci. Med. 69, 1805–1812.

Smith, R., MacKellar, L., 2007. Global public goods and the global health agenda: problems, priorities and potential. Global. Health 3 (9). doi:10.1186/1744-8603-3-9.

Sparks, M., 2009. Acting on the social determinants of health: health promotion needs to get more political, Editorial. Health Promot. Int. 24 (3), 199–202.

Taylor, J., Price, K., Braunack-Mayer, A., et al., 2012. Inter-generational learning about keeping health: a qualitative regional Australian study. Health Promot. Int. doi:10.1093/heapro/das068.

Thielst, C., 2011. Social media: Ubiquitous community and patient engagement. Front. Health Serv. Manage. 28 (2), 3–14.

Tin Tin, S., Woodward, A., Thornley, S., et al., 2009. Cyclists' attitudes towards policies encouraging bicycle travel: findings from the Taupo Bicycle Study in New Zealand. Health Promot. Int. 25 (1), 54–62.

Tones, B., 1986. Health education and the health promotion ideology. Health Educ. Res. 1 (1), 3–12.

Tones, B., 2002. Reveille for radicals! The paramount purpose of health education. Health Educ. Res. 17, 1–5.

Van der Ploeg, W., Towle, N., 2012. The readability of patient handouts from an inner regional hospital emergency department. Aust. J. Rural Health 20, 226–227.

Verheijden, M., Jans, M., Hildebrandt, V., 2008. Web-based tailored lifestyle programs: Exploration of the target group's interests and implications for practice. Health Promot. Pract. 9 (1), 82–92.

Wainwright, N., Surtees, P., Welch, A., et al., 2007. Healthy lifestyle choices:could sense of coherence aid health promotion? J. Epidemiol. Community Health 61, 871–876.

Wallace, J., Lemaire, J., Ghali, W., 2009. Physician wellness: A missing quality indicator. Lancet 374 (9702), 1714–1721.

Wiggins, M., 2011. Popular education for health promotion and community empowerment: a review of the literature. Health Promot. Int. 27 (3), 356–371.

Winkler, M., Krieger, G., Divall, M., et al., 2013. Untapped potential of health impact assessment. Bull. World Health Organ. 91, 298–305.

World Health Organization (WHO), Health and Welfare Canada & CPHA, 1986. Ottawa Charter for Health Promotion. Can. J. Public Health 77 (12), 425–430.

World Health Organization (WHO), 2004a. Standards for health promotion in hospitals. WHO, Geneva.

World Health Organization (WHO), 2004b. The physical school environment: an essential component of a health promoting school. WHO information on school health. WHO, Geneva.

World Health Organization (WHO), 2008. World Health Report 2008 primary health care. Now More Than Ever. Online. Available: <http://www.who.int/whr/2008/whr08_en.pdf> (accessed 14 July 2009).

World Health Organization (WHO), 2011. Hidden Cities: Unmasking and overcoming health inequities in urban settings. Online Available: <http://hiddencities.org/downloads/WHO_UN-HABITAT_Hidden_Cities_Web.pdf> 21 January 2013.

Useful websites

www.unicef.org/saotome/health.htm—United Nations Children's Fund (UNICEF) Primary Health Care Programme

www.un.org/en/rights/index.shtml—United Nations human rights organizations and issues www.who.int/en/—World Health Organization

www.phmovement.org/en/resources/charters/peopleshealth—People's Health Charter

www.phmovement.org/en/node/798—Cuenca Declaration, People's Health Movement

www.who.int/healthpromotion/conferences/previous/ottawa/en/—Ottawa Charter

www.who.int/healthpromotion/conferences/6gchp/bangkok_charter/en/—Bangkok Charter http://www.SDOH@YORKU.CA—social determinants of health Website and archives

www.un.org/millenniumgoals/—Millennium Development Goals

www.healthinfonet.ecu.edu.au—General health information

www.health.gov.au—Commonwealth Department of Health and Aged Care

www.healthinsite.gov.au—Health Insite (Commonwealth Government)

www.aihw.gov.au—Australian Institute of Health and Welfare

www.phaa.net.au—Public Health Association of Australia

www.healthpromotion.org.au—Australian Health Promotion Association

www.hreoc.gov.au—Human Rights and Equal Opportunity Commission

www.ceh.org.au—Centre for Culture, Ethnicity and Health

www.msd.govt.nz/about-msd-and-our-work/publications-resources/research/nz-families-today/—New Zealand Families Today

www.plunket.org.nz—Royal New Zealand Plunket Society

www.moh.govt.nz—Manatu Hauora New Zealand Ministry of Health

www.nzhis.govt.nz—Te Parongo Hauora New Zealand Health Information Service

www.kidshealth.org.nz—New Zealand Child Health

www.hc-sc.gc.ca/hppb/phdd/pdf/perspective/pdf—A New Perspective on the Health of Canadians—the Lalonde Report http://www.canadian-health-network.ca—Canadian health facts and figures

www.moh.govt.nz/hiasupportunit—New Zealand Ministry of Health—Health Impact Assessment Support Unit

www.hauora.co.nz—Health Promotion Forum of New Zealand

5

Community health nursing roles

Introduction

This chapter is aimed at exploring the various roles from which nurses promote health and wellbeing in their communities. As you will see throughout the chapter, despite having common PHC goals, they use a variety of approaches to community health that are influenced by the context of community care, the population they assist, diverse and changing regulations, policy imperatives, employer requirements, and their specialised preparation for practice. For example, some nurses are employed as nurse practitioners (NPs) in a particular specialty (gerontology, for example), others as child, school or practice nurses, and some are attached to primary health care (PHC) clinics that may serve a range of populations, or specifically defined needs (women's health, family services, aged care, remote area nursing). Despite the differences, initiatives to enable community health are guided by the PHC principles: *accessible health care, appropriate technology, health promotion, intersectoral collaboration, community participation, cultural sensitivity and cultural safety.* Enabling health in any given community is based on the understanding of the social determinants of health (SDH). Practice is holistic, encompassing the notion that health is created and maintained in the context of the settings of people's lives, where they work, play, study, worship, engage in recreational pursuits and access care. In each of these settings the community itself is at the centre of care, and members of the community are empowered by knowledge and the expectation that they will be full participants in health decision-making. Because the models and processes of care differ between settings and between different groups of people we describe both generalised and specialised practice in response to changing needs and different contexts.

> ### REMINDER
>
> All nursing roles in promoting community health are guided by the principles of primary health care: accessible health care, appropriate technology, health promotion, intersectoral collaboration, community participation, cultural sensitivity and cultural safety.

The chapter begins with a description of the changing nature of professional roles to respond to the global mandate for PHC. Although PHC and the goal of health for all people have been in place for the past three decades, midway through this second decade of the 21st century they are reaffirmed as lighthouse concepts, guiding the way toward global, national and local health promotion and illness prevention. The descriptions of current and potential practice provided in the sections to follow demonstrate how the SDH are embedded in practice.

OBJECTIVES

By the end of this chapter you will be able to:

1. describe the global re-orientation of practice roles toward primary health care

2. explore a variety of professional nursing and nurse practitioner roles in relation to populations and the links between health and place

3. explain the importance of settings in the practice of child and family health, school health, rural and remote area practice, community mental health, and occupational health nursing

4. outline the current and potential role of nurses in managing chronic disease in the community

5. identify primary, secondary and tertiary prevention strategies in each of these settings.

THE ROLE OF NURSES IN PROMOTING SOCIAL JUSTICE

As health professionals, many of us are aware that we hold enormous potential to change the world and help make it a fairer place. This is not blind ambition, but rather a moral imperative to help people change and develop in ways that would see them live the lives they choose (Sen 2000). We know that social inequities and unequal access to resources exist in communities throughout the world, but our health care systems and those responsible for allocating public resources often fail to see the importance of social inclusion, community empowerment and culturally sensitive engagement in creating and sustaining health. The World Health Organization (WHO) has been unequivocal in identifying nursing practice in the community as essential to achieving the goals of PHC in the global community (Chiarella et al. 2010).

> ## REMINDER
> Social justice is the fair distribution of society's benefits, responsibilities and their consequences.

A WHO sponsored compendium of case studies from throughout the world showed that the key element of success in implementing PHC is nurse-community partnerships that foster culturally sensitive, community empowerment (Chiarella et al. 2010). However, despite endorsement by WHO, and being the largest group of health professionals worldwide, nurses continue to practise under a set of constraints imposed externally by the systems in which they are employed. In some cases, these systems present barriers to keeping the focus on the community, rather than the health professionals. For example, shorter hospital stays, acute and palliative care in the home, and greater complexity in managing care have led to more highly organised, top-down systems of care that leave community nurses with a broader scope of practice but less discretion over their work (Hallett & Pateman 2000; Pulcini et al. 2010; Underwood et al. 2009). This situation runs counter to the bottom-up, community-empowered and culturally appropriate model of care we mentioned in Chapter 3. Community nurses have had a long tradition of working relatively autonomously, but they also have the safety net of supervision by employers and colleagues who help ensure that they are engaging in best practice informed by the most recent, relevant and rigorous

evidence to support their work. Support and mentoring of community practice can take place through intermittent monitoring of activities, face-to-face individual or group meetings with peers, supervisors or managers, or online resources.

In contemporary society the mandate for nursing is to protect, promote and maintain dignified, respectful client-centred care (Kitson et al. 2010). As the health professionals most visible in working with communities, nurses are often best situated to lead the shift from provider-driven to client-driven models of care (Schofield et al. 2011). This is not always readily achieved, given the constraints of health systems. Nurses who have been successful in helping communities participate fully in their health care have tended to use a number of deliberate strategies. They are inspired by knowing their work can make a difference, especially from intervening 'for the collective good, using levers for change such as advocacy, policy change and social interventions' (Edwards & MacLean Davison 2008:130). They are committed to evidence-based practice and translation of evidence into practice (Schofield et al. 2011). This commitment is illustrated in studies that show 'how' and 'why' people participate in improving their health. For example, research findings have shown that honest, direct relationships with people based on trust and sincerity can promote community participation (Clancy & Svensson 2010). Sharing this type of knowledge can be helpful to other clinicians as well as policymakers. When nurses promote common understandings they gain a feeling of collegiality, which promotes a sense of professional belonging. We know from research into practice relationships that community nurses thrive where they enjoy strong community relationships and an atmosphere that supports collaborative, creative approaches to practice (Underwood et al. 2009). The sense of identity and belonging shared by community nurses enhances the profession, particularly when they are vocal about embedding PHC principles into curriculum development for the next generation of nurses (Schofield et al. 2011).

> ## PROMOTING CLIENT-CENTRED CARE
> - Advocating for the collective good
> - Policy change
> - Acting on the SDH
> - Evidence-based practice
> - Collegial relationships
> - Collaborative, interprofessional care

As a profession, nurses practising in any setting have a unifying conceptual basis for practice, which revolves around care (Kitson et al. 2010). In advancing the evidence base for practice some of the greatest challenges lie in researching the effectiveness of various caring interactions from the perspectives and experiences of diverse roles. This will continue to be a challenge for community nurses, as roles evolve beyond what has been prescribed by other professions (Nugus et al. 2010). To date, nursing roles are subjected to a 'culturally and organizationally-sanctioned pattern of role-domination' by medical doctors' (Nugus et al. 2010:901). Ideally, to promote client-centred care, roles should be determined by collaborative, interprofessional processes rather than by vested interests of one or another professional group. The imbalanced power relationship sanctioned by current systems inhibit the ability of nurses to collaborate with other health professionals to make decisions for the good of the community (Nugus et al. 2010; Villegas & Allen 2012). Clearly, this runs counter to the goals of PHC, which becomes clear in tracing the evolution of nurses practising as nurse practitioners (NP) or advanced practice RNs (APRN).

WHAT IS … CLIENT-CENTRED CARE?

Client-centred care is the mandate of all health professionals. It should inspire **interprofessional collaboration** so that community needs, rather than the needs of any one professional group, determines care.

GROUP EXERCISE: Community nursing roles

Working in groups of two to three, list as many different types of nursing roles that you can think of that are based in community settings. As you work through the chapter, keep adding to your list. You may identify roles that have not been included—add these to your list as well. At the end of the chapter, discuss your list as a class considering the depth and breadth of community nursing roles.

ADVANCED PRACTICE NURSES AND NURSE PRACTITIONERS

Advanced practice registered nurses (APRN), including nurse practitioners (NP) have been identified as ideally prepared to provide primary health care, particularly for vulnerable populations,

and those living in areas inadequately served by other health care services (Coyle et al. 2010; Lenthall et al. 2011; NZMOH et al. 2009; Parker et al. 2013; Pulcini et al. 2010; Villegas & Allen 2012). A global survey conducted by the International Council of Nurses (ICN) found that the NP-APRN roles have been expanding throughout the world since the turn of the century, which has led to establishment of the International Nurse Practitioner-Advanced Practice Nursing Network (Pulcini et al. 2010). Reasons for the expansion include changes in health care systems where care is shifting to PHC in the community, global shortages of medical professionals, and research showing the safety, effectiveness, cost efficiency and population satisfaction with APRN and NP care (Gagan & Maybee 2011; Newhouse et al. 2011; Pulcini et al. 2010; Underwood et al. 2009; Villegas & Allen 2012). ICN defines the role as follows:

A nurse practitioner-advanced practice nurse is a registered nurse who has acquired the expert knowledge base, complex decision-making skills and clinical competencies for expanded practice, the characteristics of which are shaped by the context and/or country in which s/he is credentialed to practice. A master's degree is recommended for entry level.

(ICN 2001. Online. Available http://icn-apnetwork.org [accessed 26 March 2013])

The first advanced practice role, the nurse anaesthetist, emerged in the United States late in the 19th century (Villegas & Allen 2012). From the 1960s and throughout the 20th century the American NP role was expanded to include a number of general and specialist NP roles (Villegas & Allen 2012). ICN reports that many other countries including Australia, Belgium, Botswana, Canada, Fiji, New Zealand, Sweden, Thailand and the United Kingdom, have now developed the NP role. Other countries, such as South Korea, Singapore and Switzerland refer to the advanced practice nurse (APN) rather than the NP for a similar role (Pulcini et al. 2010). The variable nomenclature used in different countries, including Australia and New Zealand, has created confusion over the scope of practice.

According to ICN (2005) the scope of practice for the NP-APN includes advanced health assessment, diagnosis, disease management, health education and promotion, referrals, prescribing diagnostic procedures, medications and treatment plans, admitting and discharging privileges, patient caseload management, collaborative practice, evaluation of health care services, and research.

Although this description provides clarity on what should be expected of those undertaking advanced practice roles, other nursing roles and position titles in Australia and New Zealand have influenced perceptions and expectations of the role or position (Cant et al. 2011; Duffield et al.; Roberts et al. 2011). For example, the advanced practice nurse role is not equivalent to the NP in that there is no endorsement or standard qualification for the APRN role (Cant et al. 2011). Advanced practice is defined by the Nursing Council of New Zealand (NCNZ 2008) as a role that reflects highly developed clinical skills and judgements acquired through a combination of nursing experience and education (Roberts et al. 2011). A growing need to define the role of the advanced practice nurse in New Zealand led to the development of the NP scope of practice with New Zealand's first NP registered in 2001 (Jacobs 2007). An NP is registered under the NP scope of practice by the Nursing Council of New Zealand. RNs seeking to become NPs in Australia and New Zealand must present a portfolio to the ACN or the NZ Nursing Council respectively, and go through a rigorous assessment process prior to being admitted to the scope of practice. In both countries, the NP role has steadily evolved over the past two decades, gradually gaining acceptance as a viable contribution to the health care systems. Advanced practice in Australia is described by the RCNA (now the Australian College of Nursing [ACN]) as a role that uses extended and expanded skills, experience and knowledge in assessment, diagnosis, planning, implementation and evaluation of care (RCNA 2006). The advanced practice nurse is an RN who has acquired an expert knowledge base, complex decision-making skills and clinical competencies for expanded practice, which is shaped by the context of care. The RCNA description is clear on the contention that advanced practice is related to a *level of practice* rather than a specific role (RCNA 2006).

The context of care is an important determinant of how NPs practise. In New Zealand NPs are responsible for diagnosing and managing care. Around one-third are employed in primary health care settings, which allows the NPs, like their colleagues, to practise in a way that is responsive to local needs (Wilkinson 2012). In New Zealand, primary health organisations (PHOs) are responsible for funding primary health care services. The PHO distributes capitation funding to those who hold contracts for health service provision in the community. Most providers who hold contracts with PHOs are general practices. Some PHOs employ practitioners directly but mostly a PHO acts as a contracting body. Because those who hold contracts with PHOs are funded on a per capita basis rather

than in terms of a specifically designated role, there is an incentive for them to use health professionals in a way that best meets the needs of the population they serve (Wilkinson 2012). This means that where it is appropriate to the goals of PHC, there should be no constraints on NPs or other advanced practice nurses (such as PNs) adopting an advanced practice role, especially in cases where the financial benefit to the practice is similar for a medical and nursing service (Wilkinson 2012). Despite the framework in place to enable NP practice in primary health care, barriers remain; in particular a lack of employment opportunities due to both a lack of understanding of the role in some regions and concerns regarding the cost of employing NPs (Carryer 2012). General practice has been particularly slow to employ NPs with only one or two out of a total of 36 NPs practising in primary health care working in this environment (Wilkinson 2012). Most NPs working in PHC settings are employed by third party providers (non-governmental organisations). In contrast, the role of Australian NPs is determined by geographical, organisational or industrial jurisdictions rather than by professional expectations or patient outcomes (Duffield et al. 2011). The Australian NP was originally developed to improve PHC in the rural and remote regions of Australia where nurse-initiated care was often the only source of health care for communities (Harvey et al. 2011). However, as the role has evolved throughout Australia there are major inconsistencies in the NP role, with disparities between states and territories, and complicated endorsement processes that have restricted NP mobility and caused role confusion (Harvey et al. 2011).

> ### ADVANCED PRACTICE IN AUSTRALIA AND NEW ZEALAND
>
> - Expert knowledge base
> - Education and experience
> - Highly developed clinical judgement skills
> - Clinical competencies, shaped by context of care

The outcome of role confusion is a major problem for the nursing profession and population groups, especially in Australia, and to a lesser extent, in New Zealand. Consistency may be more readily achieved in New Zealand, with a single regulatory authority, but Australia continues to have the difficulty of many 'divergent and somewhat convoluted practices driven by the local agenda in

Australian nursing regulation' (Harvey et al. 2011:2485). Both Australian and New Zealand NPs have prescribing rights and conduct diagnostic tests. The majority of Australian NPs do not practise in PHC, but rather in a wide range of specialist areas of practice with variability in the requirements for endorsement. Even rural and remote NP is considered an area of specialty, albeit geographically determined (Duffield et al. 2011). This minimises the opportunity for the NP to choose alternative settings or to transfer her/his endorsement as an NP across states or territories or across the Tasman. Ironically, only around 18% of endorsed Australian NPs practise in rural and remote regions, with the majority working in metropolitan areas (Mills et al. 2011). Some have withdrawn completely from the NP role in frustration at the endorsement processes (Harvey et al. 2011). Nurse leaders tend to believe that the move in 2010 towards national regulation of the Australian nursing and midwifery professions could eventually prove helpful in standardising the roles of NPs, but to date, national regulation of NPs has not occurred (Duffield et al. 2011). Nursing organisations and academic institutions in Australia are vocal advocates for this type of change, but thus far have been unable to control the national and cross-national politics that maintain inconsistencies (Duffield et al. 2011; Harvey et al. 2011).

The terminology and blurred boundaries between NP, APRN and other roles can be misleading, which has consequences for the nurses, the profession, the public and the health care system (Duffield et al. 2011; Roberts et al. 2011). In New Zealand, the role of the clinical nurse specialist (CNS), is described in similar terms as an APRN role. Distinct from the responsibility for diagnosing needs, the CNS typically cares for patients with already identified health problems, often in specialised, acute settings. The New Zealand Nurses Organisation (NZNO) defines the CNS role as 'having a focus on patient care delivery, providing specialist care and expertise, supporting nursing staff to provide expert care, and having a role in research and policy procedure development' (Roberts et al. 2011:27). The New Zealand CNS role is therefore similar to the specialist expert CNS in the US, who is attached to a specialty or subspecialty. In Australia, the CNS is not described in terms of specialised practice, but designated as a particular position in a clinical career pathway (Duffield et al. 2011). This is further confused by the Clinical Nurse Consultant (CNC) (Bloomer & Cross 2011) and, in some states, Nurse Unit Manager (NUM). These positions are also considered 'advanced' in relation to other RN roles, but the scope of their practice is largely determined by their position in the health care organisation.

In the US and Canada similar problems plague the profession in trying to achieve consistent titles and role descriptions. Even after nearly a half century of experience with the role, nurses are subjected to varying titles and scope of practice regulations in each of the American states and Canadian provinces and territories (Underwood et al. 2009; Villegas & Allen 2012). To some extent, the barriers to national professional regulation of the role is due to the influence of some health professionals opposing the status of NPs, which has perpetuated the notion of nurses as subservient in the health care order (Harvey et al. 2011; Underwood et al. 2009; Villegas & Allen 2012). This is a common view among international nurse researchers who have found that opposition to NP-APNs comes from domestic physician organisations and individual physicians (Pulcini et al. 2010).

NPs IN AUSTRALIA AND NEW ZEALAND

NPs are advanced practitioners with masters degrees who practise in a range of settings according to their specialist area of expertise and the needs of the employer.

Despite the inconsistencies, there is widespread agreement on the impact of NPs in the populations they serve. Historically, researchers have been examining NP practice and outcomes for many years. A Cochrane review undertaken in 2004 determined that that there were no discernible differences in patient outcomes between doctors and nurses (including NPs) providing similar care in primary care settings although patient satisfaction was higher with nurse-led care (Laurant et al. 2004). More recently, a comprehensive review of advanced practice outcomes has found that care provided by NPs and certified midwives in collaboration with physicians is similar and in some cases, better than that provided solely by medical practitioners (Newhouse et al. 2011). Researchers have drawn this conclusion by comparing outcomes of care provided by NPs, CNSs, CNMs, and certified nurse anaesthetists (CRNAs) in the US with medical care. Their findings include similar or better outcomes for patient satisfaction, patient health status, functional status (better glucose, lipid and BP control, and efficient use of the emergency department (Newhouse et al. 2011). A review of studies also found lower mortality rates and decreased Length of Hospital stay (LOS), and lower health care costs under NP care (Newhouse et al. 2011). The research also includes a Cochrane review of midwifery care outside the US which also supports the viability of advanced practice (Hatem et al. 2008). The Cochrane review showed that midwifery care was associated with reduced risk of losing a baby before 24 weeks, reduced use of regional analgesia, fewer episiotomies or instrumental births, increased spontaneous vaginal birth, and increased initiation of breastfeeding (Hatem et al. 2008). Australian researchers have also found that NPs providing PHC are seen as providing a feasible alternative to general practitioners (GPs) in managing minor acute illness and injury as well as stable chronic conditions (Parker et al. 2012). Likewise, researchers have begun to study the safety, efficacy and financial viability of the NP role in New Zealand, beginning with the gerontology NP, with a view toward expanding this avenue for research (Gagan & Maybee 2011). With extended and expanded skills, clinical experience, and a Masters level of education, NPs are capable of functioning autonomously and collaboratively as fully functioning members of the health care team (Driscoll et al. 2012; Parker et al. 2012). Importantly, the general public has been described as overwhelmingly in favour of NP care (Gagan & Maybee 2011; Parker et al. 2012). This finding is consistent with American research, where NPs have found vocal support from the community through the American Association of Retired Persons, who have lobbied politicians for eliminating barriers to consistency for NPs and advanced practice nurses, to date, but with little success (Villegas & Allen 2012). Boxes 5.1 and 5.2 describe some unique NP roles in Australia and New Zealand.

WHAT'S YOUR OPINION?

If NP care has been demonstrated to be as good as, and in some situations better than care provided by physicians, why has it taken so long for NPs to become embedded within the health care system in Australia and New Zealand?

NPs and Advanced Practice Nurses throughout Australia and New Zealand have forged important links with the communities they serve especially in creating models of PHC practice. In rural and remote areas, cities and general practices, what each of these have in common is a commitment to social justice through PHC.

BOX 5.1 Unique Australian NP roles: dive medicine in the ADF, Aboriginal NP in the cape

Nursing Review (www.RCNA.org.au 2012) reports that Lieutenant-Commander Morag Ferguson is Australia's first military NP with the Royal Australian Navy (RAN). She is based at HMAS Stirling in Perth and, as a specialist in dive medicine, she has responsibility for the care and safety of all submariners and divers during their pressurised escape training. The escape and rescue centre is the only submarine escape training facility in the southern hemisphere, one of six worldwide. She works closely with a medical officer in controlled scenarios that replicate responses that they might use in rescuing a diver from an ascent from the 20-metre deep vertical escape tower. When necessary they put the diver straight into one of two hyperbaric chambers. Her training for such an important role included twenty years' experience as an RN, and three years as a NP attached to the base medical centre. Her role has been so successful, the Australian Defence Force (ADF) has appointed an additional NP. She has reported immense enjoyment from the role, unlike any other nursing role in her civilian or military career (Nursing Review 2012).

A second milestone in the Australian NP movement was the appointment of the first Indigenous NP. Nicole Ramsamy is attached to Weipa, the largest community in Cape York. She works from the hospital and conducts regular visits to all of the local small towns, managing clients' needs, and ensuring that they have access to timely comprehensive care when necessary. She described the strength of her role as being able to do the simple things within a legal scope of practice, providing health services where people need them and being able to discuss their health needs where they're most comfortable (Nursing Review 2012).

RURAL AND REMOTE AREA NURSING PRACTICE

Although the context may differ, practising in rural and remote areas holds many common challenges for nurses around the world. Most of these challenges are related to the need to provide both primary care (PC) and PHC to a geographically defined community that is disadvantaged by distance from services and support. The notion of 'remoteness' varies in different countries, which is an

BOX 5.2 Unique New Zealand NP roles: Māori NPs in practice

Janet Maloney-Moni was endorsed as the first Māori NP in New Zealand in 2003. She works in her home town of Opotiki on the East Coast of the North Island supporting people to self-manage their conditions and providing preventative health care to whānau (families). Janet says it was 'the opportunity to work more autonomously in the community delivering health care that motivates people to take care of themselves' that encouraged her to pursue an NP pathway. Janet has a long history of working to improve Māori health outcomes and is happy to be back among her own people to give back to her community (Online. Available: www.ngamanukura.co.nz/Janet_Maloney-Moni [accessed 17 April 2013]).

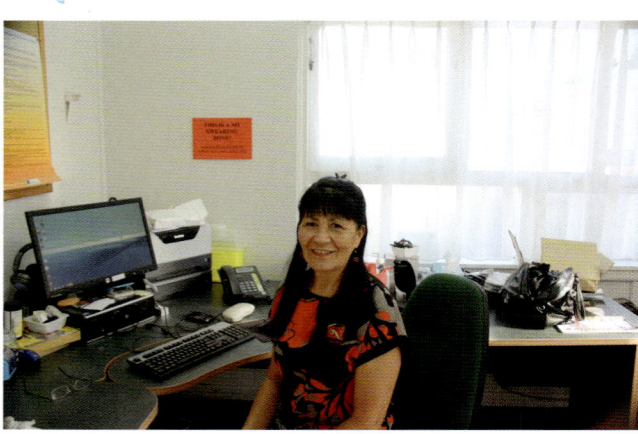

Janet Maloney-Moni, Nurse Practitioner (photo courtesy of Janet Maloney-Moni)

TABLE 5.1 Potential social justice core competencies for public health

Domain of core competencies	Potential competency reflecting social justice
Public health sciences	Describe role of public health in righting social injustices
	Understand relationship between social determinants of health and inequities
Assessment and analysis	Use data to differentiate inequities, inequalities
	Work with marginalised population for research-based action on inequities and disparities
Policy and program planning, implementation evaluation	Identify policy role in reducing or increasing inequities
	Recognise differential effects of interventions on population subgroups
Partnerships, collaboration, and advocacy	Support government and community partners to build just institutions
	Solicit input from individuals and institutions
Diversity and inclusiveness	Understand, apply Universal Declaration on Human Rights
Communication	Develop strategies for historically oppressed subpopulations
Leadership	Integrate social justice in organisational mission and strategic plans
	Identify how redistributing public health resources may alter or reinforce inequities

(Edwards & MacLean Davison 2008:131)

issue for defining rural and remote practice (Coyle et al. 2010). In Australia, remoteness is interpreted across a continuum of physical distance from service centres, from 0 (very accessible) to 15 (very remote) (Coyle et al. 2010). Some researchers describe remoteness in terms of 'distance decay', which refers to the lower access to services with increased distance from a regional centre (Wong & Regan 2009:2). Because of substantial differences in resources and access to other health professionals, the degree of remoteness is therefore significant in determining the breadth of the nursing role, which can range from being part of a team to being a sole practitioner. In New Zealand, the definitions of rural are complex with four levels of rurality defined not

by population but by how much influence there is from main or satellite urban areas (NZ Health Workforce Information Programme 2009). These definitions can make it difficult to determine who is and who is not a rural nurse; however, Health Workforce New Zealand (the New Zealand agency set up to provide national leadership on health and disability workforce development) define rural nurses as either rural-area nurses who usually live and work in rural areas and rural-outreach nurses who tend to live in independent urban areas and travel to rural areas to provide services (NZ Health Workforce Information Programme 2009).

Remote area nurses (RANs) work in outback and isolated town, islands, tourism settings, railway, mining, pastoral and Indigenous communities (CRANA 2003). Like outpost nurses in Canada and the US, most remote area nurses work in community single nurse clinics, but some are also attached to health facilities where there may be two or more nurses and occasionally, other health professionals (Lenthall et al. 2011). Some are employed by the Royal Flying Doctor Service (RFDS), as part of the fly-in fly-out (FIFO) workforce who travel to remote locations to conduct clinics or medical evacuations. The role and scope of practice for most rural nurses is generalist, rather than specialist with many working part-time (Francis & Mills 2011).

The 2006 census showed that most Australian remote area nurses practise in single nurse PHC clinics employed by state or territory governments, a large majority of which are remote Indigenous communities (Lenthall et al. 2011). Only 5% have postgraduate qualifications and there are few NP prepared nurses in remote areas (Lenthall et al. 2011; Mills et al. 2011). Whereas in the past most of the nurses held midwifery qualifications, and often child health certificates, the number of nurses with extra qualifications has gradually declined (Lenthall et al. 2011). To some extent this is due to a lack of opportunities for ongoing professional development, which are often limited because of health departments' lack of commitment to the community and a lack of access to workplace-based education (Francis & Mills 2011). Although scholarships are provided by the Australian government to encourage further education, there is often no access to locums for relief to accept these opportunities (Francis & Mills 2011). Child care and needing to accommodate a partner's employment can also be a problem for RANs (Francis & Mills 2011).

In New Zealand, 327 nurses were identified as working in rural settings in 2011 with 57% of these aged over 50 (Nursing Council of New Zealand 2012a). Rural nurses face similar challenges to those in Australia despite the geographical and demographic differences. For example, rural nurses seeking to become NPs are challenged by the lack of a clear pathway to support their transition, and internship-type programs are recommended to facilitate this (Carryer et al. 2011). Scholarships are available for rural nurses to undertake postgraduate study and provide payment for locum cover, but as is the case in Australia, locums are frequently not available. Increased funding for some rural nurse services in New Zealand has been demonstrated to advance rural nursing practice, improve access to health services for rural communities, and strengthen the links between rural nurses and the nursing profession (Connor et al. 2009), but this funding has yet to extend to other rural nurse services.

In general, the rural and RAN roles include providing clinical care, health education and promotion across the lifespan, administering the clinic or service, and performing a myriad of general, non-nursing duties (Coyle et al. 2010; Francis & Mills 2011). In some cases, the part-time nature of GP practice has supported the development of advanced nursing roles (Parker et al. 2012). Rural and remote area nurses have demonstrated effective management of some acute illness and injury as well as chronic conditions and have attracted positive feedback and the confidence of the community (Gardner et al. 2011; Parker et al. 2012). For all rural and remote area nurses clinical responsibilities cover emergency care; antenatal and midwifery; infant, child and adolescent health; women, men's and family health; mental health and aged care, which may also include palliative care and chemotherapy (Coyle et al. 2010). In preparation for such an extensive clinical role Australian rural and remote practitioners are provided with the Central Australian Rural Practitioner Association's (CARPA) Standard Treatment Manual (STM), which provides culturally appropriate guidance for a wide range of conditions and issues, and is updated regularly (Coyle et al. 2010). Queensland nurses are also given a Primary Clinical Care Manual (PCCM) and guidelines to ensure they practise within the relevant act governing drugs and poisons (Coyle et al. 2010). The New Zealand Primary Care Handbook 2012 (New Zealand Guidelines Group 2012) is available to all practitioners working in primary care in New Zealand and offers useful guidelines on a range of commonly experienced conditions. Most nurses working in rural areas in New Zealand also receive specialist training in primary response to medical emergencies (PRIME) training.

The health promotion role of rural and remote area nurses ranges from whole-of-community initiatives to health teaching to foster health literacy for certain individuals or groups. Administrative tasks include maintaining client records, coordinating patient transport or retrieval and monitoring of supply and storage of equipment and medicines (Coyle et al. 2010). As a care coordinator, the nurse is also responsible for maintaining good relationships with other health professionals, mentoring Aboriginal, Māori, and other health workers and, occasionally, community volunteers. In both New Zealand and Australia this extends to providing direction and delegation of tasks to health care assistants and enrolled nurses.

Preparation for the role includes orientation programs in occupational health and safety, advanced clinical practice, PHC, and organisational systems and support. One aspect of occupational health and safety lies in understanding the nature of rural work and the difficulties of farmers who are at risk of losing their lifestyles because of economic circumstances. Because nurses in rural and remote areas typically work with a range of cultural groups, cultural safety training is another important consideration, and a mandatory component of orientation to the role in Queensland, the Northern Territory (Coyle et al. 2010), and New Zealand. In those cases where rural or remote area nurses are NPs, the role is governed by the state which has endorsed their capabilities. In all countries and regions, rural and remote area nurses take their responsibilities for culturally competent care seriously. Over the last century, there has been a worldwide professional focus on cultural considerations, particularly ensuring culturally safe care. As we explained in Chapter 1, cultural safety is a process of exploring, reflecting on, and understanding one's own culture and how it relates to other cultures with a view toward promoting partnership, participation and cultural protection. Culturally safe care enhances the effectiveness of nursing interactions, promotes better community participation (Starr & Wallace 2011) and fosters health literacy. Nurses learn to relate to people of

different cultures in a way that recognises their values, ideas and identity, and how these are reflected in their health and wellbeing. In some cases, this can be easier for health professionals from diverse cultural backgrounds (Benkert et al. 2011). It is also more effective when there is organisational cultural competence; that is, when the system or agency shares congruent attitudes, practices, policies and structures that enable health professionals to work more effectively in cross-cultural situations (Olavarria et al. 2009). However, when all health professionals reflect on cultural considerations there is a greater likelihood of appropriate, effective and acceptable strategies to promote health.

REMINDER: Cultural safety

Cultural safety begins by reflecting on, and understanding one's own culture and how it relates to other cultures.

Like Aboriginal Australians, Māori in New Zealand are more likely to live rurally and face the compounded challenge of inequities of ethnicity, income and rurality (NZMOH 2012). Recent research has found that Māori utilisation rates for nursing consultations are 1.68 times greater than non-Māori (Mills et al. 2012) suggesting that nurses have a significant role in addressing health disparities using culturally safe approaches—particularly in rural areas. Maloney-Moni (2006) describes the work she does as a NP with a rural Māori population using a Kaupapa Māori model (Māori-centred model), demonstrating improving health outcomes for the families/whānau she is working alongside. Maloney-Moni's research, and research by Litchfield (2004) and Connor et al. (2009), have demonstrated how rural nurse-led clinics have improved access to health care for those from lower socio-economic groups and Māori, by creating nurse-community partnerships. It is vital that rural nurses in New Zealand and Australia continue to extend this type of research to demonstrate that these nurse-led models, which we outline in Chapter 14, are clearly linked to improvements in the health of the people with whom they are working.

PARTICIPATION IN RURAL HEALTH

Because of their close connection with the communities in which they live and work, rural and remote area nurses are in an ideal position to promote inclusive, empowered health decision-making.

Research conducted in the US in the late 1980s and 1990s by leaders in rural health such as Long and Weinert (1989) and Bushy (2000) established some commonalities in rural nursing. As these researchers have established, rural nursing is shaped by the way rural people perceive health, which is by being able to work and feel productive, carrying on their lives in the usual way. Rural people also have a common belief in the significance of their community, which is a type of cultural bond (Mills et al. 2010). As we mentioned in Chapter 2, they are also typically more self-reliant and stoical than urban dwellers and tend to resist outside help, preferring to care for one another within the family unit. Other issues that pose challenges for rural populations include their higher morbidity and mortality rates, some of which is related to lack of access to services, particularly those that provide early screening and prompt treatment for a range of diseases. Rural residents are also ageing like the rest of the population, and many have chronic diseases. They are physically and socially disadvantaged because of restricted access to goods, services and opportunities for social interaction. In addition, the current state of the world's economy has seen the withdrawal of services as economic and infrastructure decline, and in most rural areas there are limited educational, employment and recreational opportunities, limited choices for health care and low levels of health literacy, all of which are of concern to nurses (Coyle et al. 2010; Francis & Mills 2011). Shortages of health professionals are also a significant problem, and the strategic directions of the Australian Rural Health Alliance reflect the urgent need for governments to deal with recruitment and retention issues (Humphreys & Gregory 2012). Similarly in New Zealand, demand for rural nurses is projected to grow by over 37% between now and 2026 (NZ Health Workforce Information Programme 2009). As noted previously, the rural nurse population is also older and there are calls to increase recruitment of nurses under 35 into rural positions to ensure there are sufficient nurses to meet demand in the future (NZ Health Workforce Information Programme 2009). Despite work in 2009 to develop a rural nursing workforce strategy for New Zealand, this has yet to come to fruition.

Declining local services can also be mediated by appropriate transportation, social networks and the informal care of families, which are challenges for all rural health professionals. These challenges can be personally stressful. Geographically dispersed nurses report higher levels of work stress, few opportunities for replacement leave, longer working and on-call hours than nurses in urban areas, and a lack of support for new staff (Francis & Mills 2011;

Henwood et al. 2009). For remote area nurses (RANs) stress is a major issue because of the isolation and responsibilities, and the fact that they are too frequently subjected to violence in the community and workplace (Lenthall et al. 2009). Another source of stress is that they are often the only way of providing a stable workforce given the disruption of medical practitioners rotating through the areas, and the unevenness and skill level of other health professionals (Searle 2007).

PRACTICE STRATEGY

Nurses can foster horizontal ties between members of the community, groups and health services and vertical ties between health services and society.

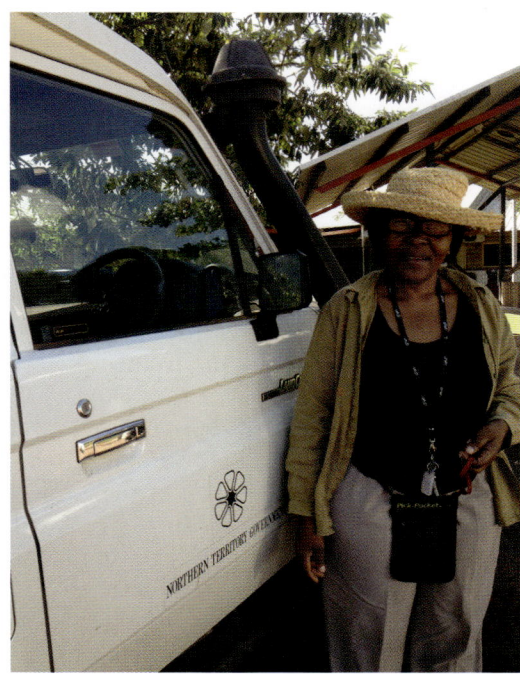

RAN Tshepiso (Daisy) Mojapelo—Wurrimiyanga NT (photo courtesy Daisy Mojapelo)

The advantages of rural and remote area nursing include feeling closely connected with the community on a social as well as professional level. As a member of a community of place, nurses can facilitate horizontal ties between people, groups and organisations such as hospital or district boards, community clinics and medical practices. Their relationships can be interdisciplinary, multi-institutional or intersectoral. As community residents as well as health professionals, they can also provide vertical ties between hospital and health departments and the wider society, to connect people with external resources and centres of power (Kilpatrick et al. 2009). This tends to attract greater local public awareness of the potential of their role compared with public perceptions of nursing in non-rural communities. Rural and remote practitioners also have a strong sense of the need for ecological sustainability in their communities, which arises from their close relationships with people on the land. This broader perspective connecting the local and global issues is important in supporting the PHC goal of promoting health and social justice, which connects all rural nurses in our globalised world (Grootjans & Newman 2013).

Rural and remote practitioners also have greater role diffusion than nurses working with non-rural populations, where the boundary between personal and professional life is porous (McCoy 2009). Some describe their lives as 'living their work', where maintaining relationships with colleagues outside of work has an effect on the work dynamic as well as social relationships (Mills et al. 2010:33). This type of role diffusion has both negative and positive effects: it can be difficult for the nurse to maintain anonymity in the community, which can lead to role strain; on the other hand, their closeness to the community may also make them more effective because of the level of trust they have established (McCoy 2009). This community embeddedness and engagement at a personal level can also create challenges for nurses seeking to advance their nursing practice (Carryer et al. 2011). However, Ross's (2011) development of a place-based practice model for rural nursing can help rural and remote nurses understand the complexity of their role. Ross describes three aspects of rural nursing practice relative to 'place'. These are 'location'—the rural context in which the nurse works; 'locale'—the setting and the relationships which nurses form within the rural setting; and 'sense of place'—where the nurse develops a sense of belonging and is able to blend professionally into rural culture and society (Ross 2011).

PRACTICE NURSING

Practice Nursing (PN) is one of the most pervasive nursing roles in PHC. The role includes caregiving, organising, maintaining quality control and improvement, problem-solving, educating and connecting people, and bridging the gap between clinical and administrative staff in general practice (APNA 2012 Online. Available: www.apna.asn.au/ [accessed 20 March 2013]; Phillips et al. 2009). Many

PN roles revolve around the *primary care* activities that are common in general practice, such as chronic illness management (Halcomb & Hickman 2010; Holden et al. 2012; Merrick et al. 2012). However, PNs are also considered part of the PHC workforce, and in 2013 their professional group, the Australian Practice Nurses Association (APNA), changed its name to the Australian Primary Health Care Nurses Association Incorporated. The change of name reflects the importance of the broader PHC agenda in their work, which includes advocacy on broader PHC and nursing issues as well managing chronic conditions in the community. In Australia, the focus on chronic care has emerged from the health sector reforms of 2009–10, which have seen decreasing reliance on hospital care and a strengthening of general practice capabilities and continuity of care between hospitals and the community (Australian Government DoHA 2010). The focus on chronic care was a response to the growing prevalence of chronic conditions, with almost half of all general practice consultations involving a chronic condition (Joyce & Piterman 2011). The reforms have strengthened and expanded the role of nurses in managing people with chronic conditions, particularly with the government's introduction of the Practice Nurse Incentive Program (PNIP) (Australian Government, DoHA 2011). The program offers financial incentives to general practitioners (GPs) to employ PNs who have a major focus on prevention, patient education and chronic disease management. In response to the incentives there has been a substantial increase in PNs employed by GPs to nearly 60% of Australian medical practices (Hart et al. 2012; Merrick et al. 2012). Like the New Zealand situation, the ratio of PNs to GPs is approximately one nurse for every 2.3 medical practitioners (Joyce & Piterman 2011).

DETERMINANTS OF PN SCOPE OF PRACTICE

- Nurse's expertise and experience
- Practice arrangements with GP
- Population needs, understanding
- Policies governing reimbursement

Practice nursing in Australia

As a rapidly growing component of the Australian nursing workforce it is interesting to reflect on the PN role and activities. In Australia, practice nursing is a specialist practice strand of the generalist PHC role, complementary to the role of the GP (National Nursing and Nursing Education Taskforce 2006). The

PN role is expanding and becoming more diverse, incorporating the NP role in some cases. Despite rapid expansion of PN practice across the country, the scope of practice continues to vary according to the nurse's expertise and experience, practice arrangements, the GP's understanding of the role, and the needs and understanding of the role by the local population (Halcomb et al. 2010; Keleher et al. 2007; Mazza et al. 2011). The role is also responsive to government policy. One of the important policy changes has been the addition of eight specific Medicare reimbursements for nursing activities in general practice (Australian Government DoHA 2011). Merrick et al.'s 2012 analysis of these rebates shows the direct influence of changes to the Medicare scheme on practice activities, with increases in nurse immunisations and wound care, Pap smears, chronic disease management items and antenatal care corresponding to the Medicare items. However, without further research it is unknown whether the increases reflect an actual increase in nurses undertaking these activities, or simply a change in the way they are being reported to Medicare (Merrick et al. 2012). The Medicare changes for chronic disease management include reimbursement for PNs and Aboriginal health workers (AHWs) to monitor and support people with chronic conditions on behalf of a general practitioner (GP) (Halcomb et al. 2010). This change has led to an increase in the uptake of the chronic disease Medicare item, albeit inconsistently across the country, and Halcomb et al. (2010) recommend further research to examine the reasons for the differences and the effect on the overall PN role. What is evident is that the role is expanding in tandem with growth in the PN workforce (Halcomb et al. 2010).

There is also a need for in-depth research into service delivery by PNs, especially in terms of disease prevention and health promotion (Halcomb & Hickman 2010). These researchers conducted a Delphi study of PNs to identify their perspectives on priorities for research that would advance the PN agenda. They found that most nurses in general practice would like to see evidence that would support their role development, but many had little time, knowledge or access to supports for evidence-based practice (EBP) (Halcomb & Hickman 2010). This finding suggests that there may be a role for academic institutions in supporting PNs. Existing research studies have focused on the outcomes and acceptability of PN practice. A systematic review of the PN role in chronic disease management indicates that where they are employed, GPs acknowledge the capabilities of PNs, especially in providing longer consultations and appropriate referrals to other health professionals, such as dietitians (Parker et al.

2012; Phillips et al. 2009). The Parker et al. (2012) review found that nurse-led care in general practice can improve the clinical outcomes of blood pressure and cholesterol management for people with Type 2 diabetes. Research into the different aspects of the PN role revealed that approximately 30% of all patient encounters involved giving people advice (Joyce & Piterman 2011). Another study of PN perspectives on their potential role with young people indicates that PNs may also be ideally placed to provide the link between GPs, school nurses and other resources for dealing with mental health issues (Hart et al. 2012). Public satisfaction with nurse-led care in general practice has also been reported, primarily because nurses tend to develop closer relationships with patients by spending more time with them than medical practitioners (Keleher et al. 2009).

Practice nursing in New Zealand

Practice nursing in New Zealand is also growing in strength and numbers. When the New Zealand Primary Health Care Strategy was released in 2001, it was clearly indicated that nurses were seen as crucial to its implementation (NZMOH 2001; Joyce & Piterman 2011; Keleher et al. 2009). In 2003 the Expert Advisory Group on Primary Health Care Nursing created a framework for activating PHC nursing practice in New Zealand in order to realise the potential of nurses to achieve the goals of the PHC Strategy (Expert Advisory Group on Primary Health Care Nursing 2003). The framework provided a definition of PHC nursing and a set of corresponding goals. PHC nurses were defined as registered nurses with knowledge and expertise in PHC practice. They work autonomously and collaboratively to promote, improve, maintain and restore health, in roles that encompass population health, health promotion, disease prevention, wellness care, first-point-of-contact care and disease management across the lifespan. Their models of practice are determined by the setting and the ethnic and cultural grouping of their clientele. They practise in partnership with people—individuals, whānau, communities and populations—to achieve the shared goal of health for all, which is central to PHC nursing. The goals of practice therefore include aligning nursing practice with community need, innovative models of nursing practice, governance, leadership and career development (Expert Advisory Group on Primary Health Care Nursing 2003:9).

PNS AND PHC IN NEW ZEALAND

Practice nursing in New Zealand is integral to the implementation of the Primary Health Care Strategy.

Many nurses practising in PHC settings have grasped the framework as a guide for developing their PHC nursing practice including district nurses, public health nurses and practice nurses. Practice nurses in New Zealand were originally employed in the mid-1970s in GP practices, largely to provide support to general practitioners. Since that time, the role of the PN has evolved substantially. The Primary Health Care Strategy and subsequent framework for activating primary health care nursing were seen as providing opportunities for practice nurses to demonstrate the impact they could have on population health. However, by 2007 the New Zealand Nurses Organisation and the College of Nurses (Aotearoa) suggested that significant work was still required to achieve the potential of PHC nursing in line with the original framework suggested by the Expert Advisory Group (New Zealand Nurses Organisation & The College of Nurses Aotearoa 2007).

Evaluation data indicated that there were ongoing barriers to enacting the PN role, such as hierarchical employment structures, limited access to education, and poor funding of nursing initiatives, all of which continue to require urgent attention (New Zealand Nurses Organisation & The College of Nurses Aotearoa 2007). Professional development of PNs has largely been initiated and implemented by the NZNO. The organisation developed a strategic plan for PNs in 1996–98, identifying a career pathway, a marketing plan to enhance the professional profile and adequate employment conditions. The College of Primary Health Care Nurses (a College under NZNO and previously known as the College of Practice Nurses) now offers a comprehensive professional development program for members, a journal and various other publications and support processes (New Zealand Nurses Organisation, Online. Available: www.nzno.org.nz/groups/colleges/college_of_ primary_health_care_nurses [accessed 20 April 2013]). The College of Primary Health Care Nurses has a broad membership that includes PNs, district nurses, public health nurses, school nurses, occupational health nurses and any other nurse who identifies as working in primary health care. Professional development programs for PNs are also available through PHOs and DHBs although the College program remains popular.

Formal evaluation of nursing developments in PHC in New Zealand from 2001 to 2007 demonstrated that the barriers identified by the NZNO and College of Nurses did indeed exist, and their recommendations included a need for leadership, mentoring, governance, and recruitment and retention of practice nurses (Finlayson et al. 2009). Despite the barriers, the profession was able to demonstrate examples of excellence in PN, including substantial growth in the development of nursing roles and capability within PHOs. Particular strengths of the PNs included the management of long-term conditions (Finlayson et al. 2009). This has been supported by subsequent research into nurses providing care to people with diabetes under the government funded Get Checked program. The research found that the program had a substantial impact on the practice of nurses, enabling the development of new models of nursing care, improved education levels among nurses (and doctors), improved confidence in the management of diabetes and increased satisfaction with their work (Clendon et al. 2013). A further strength of PNs is the ability to work with under-served and vulnerable population groups (Finlayson et al. 2009). Among these vulnerable populations are older persons in residential care settings, who too often are overlooked in the PHC agenda. This is being redressed through ongoing discussion of models of PHC in Australia and New Zealand, especially in the evolution of nurse practitioner roles. The care of older persons, like that of younger population groups, should be included in the PHC agenda, with appropriate needs assessment, care coordination, health promotion and disease management. An example of work in this area is a pilot trial by a PHO that employed a gerontology nurse specialist to work across three general practices to provide comprehensive assessment, referral and intervention for older people in their own homes. The pilot has proved successful for all concerned and calls are now being made for the pilot to be extended to more locations (King et al. 2011).

The education needs of practice nurses and primary health care nurses are also unique and it is critical that relevant professional education is provided to nurses. While ongoing clinical education is assumed to be essential, recent research has demonstrated that leadership education and career mentoring are considered just as important by nurses working in primary health care settings in New Zealand (McKinlay et al. 2012). In 2013, the Nursing Council of New Zealand consulted on the introduction of a community nurse prescribing model. When approved, it will enable appropriately educated nurses working in primary health care settings to prescribe from a formulary of commonly prescribed medicines including antibiotics, anti-virals and anti-fungals among others (Nursing Council of New Zealand 2013). This will enhance the capacity of primary health care nurses to more comprehensively meet the needs of the populations they work with.

MANAGING CHRONIC CONDITIONS IN THE COMMUNITY

The number of people with one or more chronic conditions continues to escalate in our communities and throughout the world. Chronic illnesses are the leading cause of mortality, responsible for 63% of deaths worldwide and therefore a great burden on all health care systems (WHO 2012). As of 2010 there were over 7 million Australians and over 2 million New Zealanders suffering from one or more chronic conditions (AIHW 2010; Holt 2010). Population ageing, combined with risk factors such as obesity, poor nutrition and inadequate levels of physical activity have led to an increase in conditions such as cardiovascular disease, diabetes, stroke, arthritis and depression (Abramowitz et al. 2010; Boyle et al. 2011; Signal et al. 2012). Helping people manage these conditions in their home and communities is now a major element of community health practice, for PNs, NPs and all nurses who do home visits.

> ## CHRONIC CONDITIONS
>
> Helping people manage chronic conditions is a major element of many community health nursing roles. The main goal is to work within models of care that enable health literacy and client-centred decision-making.

Home visiting

Home visits are undertaken by nurses in many roles. In addition to midwives, who visit new parents in their homes, child and family health nurses, school nurses, community mental health nurses, public health nurses and occupational health nurses conduct home visits when there is a need for home based assessment or care. PNs may also undertake home visits, particularly where the nurse's role may be to assess and monitor chronic disease self-management strategies that have been planned during the practice visit. Home visiting is integral to the role of the family nurse practitioner, many of whom care for families where there are one or more members with a chronic condition (New Zealand National Health Committee 2007). While opportunities for PNs to extend their role into the home under New Zealand's PHO structure exist, few PNs have been able to extend their practice in this area. PNs remain employed directly by GPs who limit their practice in many situations to clinic-based care due to funding constraints—a major source of tension in terms of enabling PNs to take on more complex roles. The barriers outlined by the College of Nurses Aotearoa and NZNO in 2007 and reiterated by Finlayson et al. in 2009 remain. PHOs employ very few nurses directly and usually only specialist nurses in areas such as diabetes and asthma. These nurses do undertake home visits. District nurses (DNs) also undertake home visits providing wound care, palliative care, continence management, IV management, oxygen management and other 'hospital in the home' activities. DNs do provide some support for people with long-term conditions such as diabetes where needed but generally don't case manage chronic conditions. There are opportunities for DNs to extend their role in this area.

Home visits are also undertaken in the context of a relatively new role; that of the PN attached to a specialist service. These nurses practise between hospital, GP practices and clients' homes. Most are employed by a specialist surgeon to assist them with pre-surgical or post-treatment assessments and follow-up. Their roles do not have specific designations; instead they tend to be negotiated by the nurse and the employing medical practitioner or surgeon. Cardiac and orthopaedic surgeons are among those who are adopting this model of practice in Australia, employing a nurse or, in some cases an NP, to conduct a pre-operative home visit to prepare the client for surgery, assess their home environment to ensure adequate support for them on returning home post-operatively, and provide any health education and guidance required by the client and family. Other nurses may be employed by a hospital, government health department or private agency to undertake domiciliary nursing, where care is provided either in a person's home or a group residence, such as an aged-care facility. The objective of this type of nursing role is to maintain continuity of care, beginning prior to hospital admission and following the client and family from surgery to hospital discharge and home care. A major objective is to ensure rehabilitation (tertiary prevention) and prevent readmission to hospital for those at risk of exacerbation of illness (Baker Laughlin & Beisel 2010). Continuity of care, which focuses on communication between acute and community services, should be part of all nursing roles; however, in many cases, it is the community nurse who assumes responsibility for this level of coordination, with the goal of maintaining client-centred self-management (Johnston et al. 2012; Kawi 2012). Although this model is less widely adopted in New Zealand, it is growing. Most specialist nurses in New Zealand are currently employed by District Health Boards (DHBs) to provide follow-up clinic care for people with chronic diseases such as diabetes, respiratory disease, cardiac disease and rheumatic conditions. DHB specialist nurses, employed by PHOs run clinics in the community and only infrequently conduct home visits. Research into the impact of nurse specialists working in the home and the community on patient outcomes is urgently required to support this model of care.

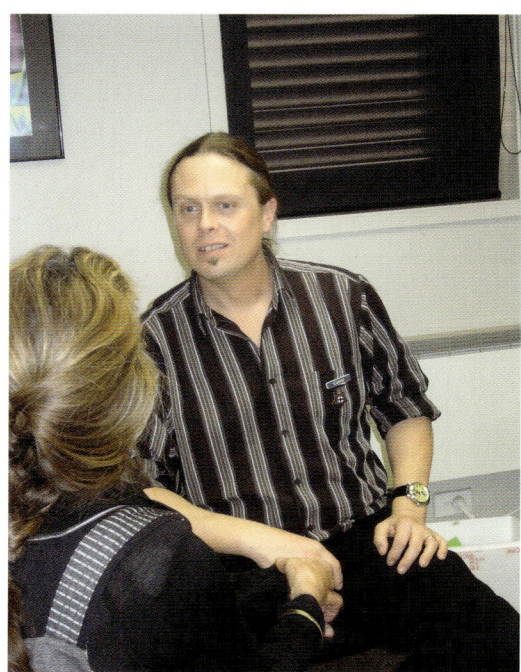

Carter Storman (PN) visits a client at home (with permission)

Nurses working for Māori and Iwi providers (by Māori for Māori) in New Zealand use home visiting as a core element of PHC practice. Those who work with chronic disease are often called disease state management (DSM) nurses. DSM nurses are doing exemplary work with their communities to help people manage chronic disease with most chronic disease management programs targeted at Māori, run by Māori DSM nurses (Sheridan et al. 2011). Nurses working for Māori and Iwi providers number around 508 throughout NZ (Nursing Council of New Zealand 2012a) and usually do a mixture of DSM and child health nursing.

Home visits to promote client-centred self-management require understanding the person's stage in life, their family situation, and any environmental risks and assets that may help them in managing their health (Kawi 2012). Appropriate assessment of client and family needs is essential to assist people across all age groups, including new parents, their infants and/or other children, adolescents, adults and older persons (Mitchell & Ellis 2011; O'Connor & Alde 2011). In some cases, it is necessary to assess and monitor the needs of caregivers, whose burden is often substantial, particularly where a family member is in the latter stages of chronic disease (Ward-Griffin et al. 2012).

Since the move towards PHC in both New Zealand and Australia, the role of home visiting nurses has also been extended to include a greater emphasis on the diagnostic role and provision of acute care in the home. Many home visiting agencies provide programs such as Hospital in the Home (HITH), and offer a range of services from diagnostic tests to a range of complex treatments including intravenous injections, pump infusions and specialised wound care (Duke & Street 2003). The breadth and protracted nature of these programs have shifted the focus from the public health orientation of surveillance and monitoring in the home to treatment and extended PHC planning. However, many nurses working in HITH programs do not recognise their work as PHC, which suggests the need to create greater awareness and appreciation for the many dimensions of their practice. To provide this type of care adequately requires advanced practice skills, a comprehensive knowledge of health behaviour change strategies, and technological skills, including expertise in information technologies.

Some home visits involve some degree of autonomous decision-making in planning to meet client and family needs. However, most home visiting nurses have a daily caseload based on the mix of clients assigned to their care by their employers. Both require time management techniques to integrate planning, needs identification and careful documentation of the goals of the visit (St John et al. 2007). Entering a home also requires sensitivity to the family's personal space and consideration of the client's preferences for the entire interaction from monitoring needs to the provision of care. This information can then be communicated to others who may be visiting the home, or other team members who may be involved in the overall plan for care. Plans are typically developed within a model of care specific to helping people manage their chronic condition.

A further issue that the nurse must consider when home visiting is the risk to self, particularly if visiting alone, as is often the case. A brief risk assessment will assist in identifying any potential risks to self and enable the nurse to put in place steps to ensure their own safety. Table 5.2 provides a brief risk assessment that can be completed prior to undertaking a home visit. It is important to realise that risks may arise from the neighbourhood being visited, a family member, dogs on the property or unexpected visitors at the home.

Chronic disease models of care

Most models for managing chronic conditions are based on the PHC principle that the client is the centre of the health care system. This places the

TABLE 5.2 Brennan's rapid risk assessment tool for home visiting

1 Do you know the client/customer/service user and their family? Yes = 1 No = 3
Explanation: The more or better somebody is known to you, the better you are at making judgements regarding their future behaviour. The less you know the more you should be concerned.

2 If not, are you able to access information from other services, e.g. police, social services, local authority, colleagues? Yes = 1 No = 3
Explanation: Making predictions about a person's future behaviour needs to be as informed as possible, other sources of information can provide answers to facilitate better judgement.

3 Is there a known history of violence or harassment from the client/service user/customer? Yes = 6 No = 1
Explanation: The best predictor of future behaviour is past behaviour. The fact the person has a history of violence must be acknowledged, and as such this one factor is of cardinal importance. A 'yes' to this question in itself should be a decisive factor—hence the reason it scores 6. This immediately means that visiting the person alone should not happen.

4 Is the area where the person lives known to be unsafe (e.g. poor lighting, high-rise flats, isolated, gangs, vandalised lifts, history of robberies)? Yes = 3 No = 1
Explanation: Sometimes it isn't the person who is the problem, but the area where they live. High-risk areas should also be treated as significant. Visiting an address at 10.00 am may be safer than going at 4.00 pm in the winter when it is dark.

5 Do you have a tracking system to ensure colleagues know of your whereabouts or time of anticipated return to the office/home? Yes = 1 No = 3
Explanation: There is a clear need for employees who work alone to be accessible through the use of a 'snail trail' recording where they are going to be, at what time and for how long. Technology exists today enabling dedicated systems to be introduced using mobile telephones in the form of identity badges which carry a signal and use satellite tracking technology to almost pin-point a person's location to within 3 metres. Do you and your colleagues have an agreed 'code word' to alert them of a potentially dangerous predicament without arousing suspicion in the client?

6 Do you have a mobile telephone and personal alarm? Yes = 1 No = 3
Explanation: Once possibly viewed as luxury items. Today such items should be viewed as essential pieces of personal protective equipment. Even having a personal alarm that emits a loud screech may distract a potential aggressor to allow for escape through another route.

7 Can you call on a colleague to accompany you on the visit? Yes = 1 No = 3
Explanation: The fact is, working in pairs is safer. Increasingly it is becoming standard practice that all FIRST visits should be conducted by two people. Once the risk has been identified as low, then future visits may be done individually.

8 Do I have training in de-escalation skills? Yes = 1 No = 3
Explanation: Good training in calming angry people is just one measure employers need to introduce for staff safety. Being able to calm and soothe somebody's anger is a skill which can be easily learned, practised and implemented.

9 Do I have the ability to break away from a violent person? Yes = 1 No = 3 Not sure = 3
Explanation: Having skills in breakaways or disengagement allows for a victim to use fast, effective techniques to escape a risky situation and make themselves safe. But if the skills are not used, they rapidly disappear unless they are updated on a regular basis. It is important that staff who feel unsure about whether or not they can implement such skills should score the issue as highly as they would a definite 'No'.

10 Is the task I am about to undertake likely to trigger violence? Yes = 3 No = 1 Not sure = 3
Explanation: Some tasks by their very nature are simple and easy to deliver, while others are almost certain to prompt a negative response. It is important to recognise that certain visits may increase the danger to the employee. An example may be a district nurse who is visiting a patient who lives with an angry relative, or a health visitor who may become involved in a child-safeguarding issue.

Scoring: 10–15 = low risk, 16–23 = medium risk, above 24 = high risk

(Brennan 2010, with permission)

emphasis on patient choice, shared decision-making and the psychosocial and health promotion aspects of care delivery (Abramowitz et al. 2010; Kawi 2012, Commonwealth of Australia 2009). The major goal of chronic disease management programs should be empowering people towards self-management (Abramowitz et al. 2010; Kawi 2012). Self-management applies across the continuum from primary prevention and early risk identification to managing the chronic condition in daily living activities, with the patient care plan tailored to individual needs. A variety of models have been developed to guide nurses in helping people manage their chronic conditions in their home and community. What all of these models have in common is that they are multidimensional and comprehensive. The nurse acts as coordinator and collaborator, working horizontally; that is, with everyone concerned including the patient, family and other members of the health care team; and vertically, coordinating care from the top (the health system) to community systems for support and education that will foster health literacy, to case management for the patient and family support people, including provision of any therapeutic interventions. Chronic illness management therefore includes health promotion activities at primary, secondary and tertiary levels of care.

REMINDER

Primary prevention—strategies to maintain health and wellbeing and prevent illness

Secondary prevention—treating and limiting illness or injury

Tertiary prevention—rehabilitative or restorative actions

Although there are a variety of self-management support programs for chronic illness the one that is used widely throughout Australia and New Zealand is the Flinders Program (formerly the Flinders model) (Flinders University, Online. Available: www.flinders.edu.au/medicine/sites/fhbhru/self-management.cfm [accessed 30 March 2013]). The program has been used in a variety of settings and countries, with research data reinforcing its viability and adaptations for special populations. The program exemplifies PHC. The objective is to enable partnerships for self-management of chronic conditions through informed choices. Participants using the program are expected to learn new skills and ways of thinking about their condition so that they can manage current and new problems as they arise, practise new health behaviours, and maintain or

regain emotional stability (Flinders University 2013). As Table 5.3 illustrates, the program has five functions.

The latter function (health professional change) can be a challenge for clinicians who have not been involved in PHC, with its emphasis on empowered participation in care planning. Self-management means that people have knowledge of their condition, follow the care plan, participate in decision-making, monitor and manage their condition and its effect on their physical, emotional and social life, adopt a healthy lifestyle and have confidence, access and the ability to use support services (Flinders University 2013). This philosophical approach to chronic condition self-management has been reinforced by a number of research studies and adopted in many countries throughout the world (Abramowitz et al. 2010; Johnston et al. 2012; Kawi 2012). The common understanding shared by clinicians and researchers alike is that self-management strategies have to be based on research evidence, a systematic, sustainable approach and where necessary, upskilling health professionals in communication and change management approaches (Abramowitz et al. 2010; Kawi 2012). Nurses and other health professionals supporting self-management have to be mindful of the social ecological context and accommodate diversity and innovativeness in the way that education is provided to clients and their families (Johnston et al. 2012; Kawi 2012). At times there is a need to combine strategies for client teaching, which can include verbal discussions, written material,

TABLE 5.3 Functions of the Flinders program for managing chronic conditions

1 **Generic and holistic chronic condition management**—the semi-structured client-centred frameworks can be used in planning for any chronic condition.

2 **Case management**—a 'Partners in Health' Scale is used to screen clients to identify the appropriate role of the health professional and the client.

3 **Self-management support**—The client's self-management knowledge, behaviours and barriers are assessed as a basis for education and support.

4 **Systemic and organisational change**—an integrated, longitudinal care plan is tailored for each person.

5 **Health professional change**—use of the program can change the health professional's understanding of the importance of client engagement and self-management.

phone, email or other electronic media, telehealth systems, and thorough follow-up interviews (Abramowitz et al. 2010; Kawi 2012). Abramowitz et al. (2010) contend that our curricula should teach health professionals the techniques of motivational interviewing and health coaching so that they are better able to counsel clients and work with them on goal-setting and health literacy. This approach is also important for families trying to help a child manage chronic conditions, where they experience multiple transitions through different stages of the child's illness, each with its own need for specific knowledge. As we mentioned in Chapter 4, these skills are essential for health promotion. Table 5.4 below outlines the skills required by all health professionals adopting a PHC approach in all roles and settings to assist people in self-managing chronic conditions. Box 5.3 provides an example of good/best practice by the NP. The section to follow describes a number of nursing settings and roles for PHC in practice.

CHILD HEALTH NURSING PRACTICE

Child health nursing is a specialised area of nursing in the community. In different Australian states and territories, the role has been variously designated 'child health nurse', 'community child health nurse',

'child and youth health nurse', 'maternal and child health nurse', 'child and family health nurse', child health and parenting service nurse, or maternal, child and family health nurse' (Kruske & Grant 2012). Also varying across the different states and territories are position titles that add another layer

BOX 5.3 The family NP as advocate for self-managing chronic conditions

Several years ago an opportunity arose for a New Zealand advanced practice nurse to participate in a joint initiative of the Lake Taupo PHO and Lakes District Health Board (DHB) aimed at improving care to families with high needs and chronic conditions in that area. As a former hospital nurse, she and her colleague had become alarmed at the 'revolving door' that sees many people with chronic conditions admitted and readmitted to hospital. The area targeted by the DHB (now the Midlands Health Network) is rural, has a high Māori population, and many low socio-economic families, some who had been avoiding general practice checks because of cost and because they had no relationship with the locums, a situation that had resulted from the shortage of local GPs. After some time in the role, the nurses realised that their work with the families captured the essence of PHC. Both decided to undertake their NP masters degrees to continue this important work. They adopted the Flinders Program as a way of structuring their practice with the families needing help to self-manage chronic conditions. They run a mobile service to the community and work as a team, with others who provide pharmacy support, a social worker, dietitian, lifestyle coaches, mental health nurse and a smoking cessation practitioner. As recommended by the Flinders Program, they share knowledge and strategies that allow them to tailor their activities to family needs. Among their challenges is the need to allay concerns of other health professionals beyond the team about their role and its effectiveness in providing a consistent, systematic approach to managing chronic conditions. They have found the family NP role satisfying and interesting in terms of accepting a leadership role with clients, their interprofessional colleagues, and other nurses such as PNs, with whom they have developed relationships focused on the common goal of eliminating inequalities in the population by improving the health of the most disadvantaged (Dawson 2011).

? If you were in such a role, how would you go about evaluating the impact of your practice?

TABLE 5.4 Core skills for the PHC workforce to promote capabilities

Patient-centred	Behaviour change	Organisational/ systems
Health promotion	Change management	Multidisciplinary learning and practice
Risk assessment	Motivational interviews	Information, communication systems
Communication skills	Collaborative problem defined	Organisational change techniques
Collaborative planning	Goal setting, achievement	Evidence-based knowledge
Peer support	Structured problem-solving	Practice research, quality improvement
Cultural awareness	Action planning	Awareness of community resources (psycho-social assessment, support)

(Commonwealth of Australia 2009)

of ambiguity, some as early childhood nurses, women's and children's health nurses, mothercraft nurses and school nurses (Duffield et al. 2011). The wide variability in roles and titles has created havoc with parents who, as Duffield et al. (2011), suggest would be utterly confused as to the best source of assistance for their child. Specialised education for child health nurses is also inconsistent in Australia. In the current climate of financial constraint universities tend to provide generic rather than specialised courses to increase postgraduate enrolments (Kruske & Grant 2012). This has led to only a small proportion of universities offering child health courses, again, with a variety of titles. Some educational programs provide a graduate certificate and others a graduate diploma, the latter course being generally one year, twice the duration of the graduate certificate (Kruske & Grant 2012).

Although all Australian child health nurses aspire to a PHC philosophy as prescribed by the Australian Association of Maternal, Child and Family Health Nurses (AAMCFHN) (Kruske & Grant 2012), confusion has arisen from years of inconsistent nomenclature and role descriptions, which has been influenced by the service structure within which they practise as well as their different credentials and levels of preparation. Because only the NP role is considered advanced practice in Australia, the Australian Nursing and Midwifery Accreditation Commission (ANMAC) does not accredit child health or any of the other specialised nursing roles. The lack of national regulation is a problem in the context of shrinking state and territory health department budgets and subsequent decisions to reduce child and family nursing positions. Paradoxically, at the same time as state and territory governments have reduced positions, national policies such as the National Early Childhood Development Strategy (Australian Government DEEWR 2011) have created an increased need for child health specialists. There is a need to address recruitment and retention issues in child health given the impending retirement of many current child health nurses who represent only 2% of the nursing workforce (Australian Government Productivity Commission 2011). With only limited opportunities for specialist education or employment of new nurses there are doubts over the extent to which the workforce will meet future demands (Australian Government Productivity Commission 2011). As concern for the specialty has grown, the professional association has lobbied across states and territories for a common title (Maternal Child and Family Health Nurses Australia [MCaFHNA]) that is expected, in future, to be recognisable nationally to child health nurses, their employers and their clients.

MATERNAL, CHILD AND FAMILY HEALTH NURSES, PLUNKET NURSES, TAMARIKI ORA NURSES

- Primary, Secondary, Tertiary prevention
- Child and Family case management
- Postnatal Home Visiting
- Care Coordination
- Parenting group work
- Telephone support

The impact of poorly coordinated services and fragmented policy development at state, territory and Commonwealth Government levels is felt most by vulnerable families (Australian Government Productivity Commission 2011). Currently, some jurisdictions do not employ sufficient child health nurses to deliver the recommended health checks to young children, especially in rural and remote areas. Variation in services means that some families receive home visits unnecessarily, while others continue to draw on other professionals such as practice nurses (PNs) for ongoing support and assistance where no child health nurses are available (Australian Government Productivity Commission 2011). Continuity of care is also problematic, especially given the incompatibility of data systems. With only some states and territories attracting sufficient funding for electronic health records and timely transmission of child health information between health professionals and across jurisdictions, there are inequities in the type and level of care provided, especially for rural and remote families, many of whom are Indigenous (Ridgway et al. 2011). A proposed national electronic health recording system may help connect families and services in future, but this initiative is also fraught with numerous, divergent views about recording and disseminating health information.

The lack of standardisation in child health nursing is not a problem in countries like Canada, New Zealand, the US, the UK and the Scandinavian countries, which maintain national standards and educational requirements. In Canada, child health nurses have a baccalaureate degree in nursing, belong to a professional regulatory body, and have qualifications in either community health nursing or public health. In the UK, health visitors complete a one-year postgraduate program in community nursing following a Bachelor of Nursing or Midwifery. In New Zealand, child health nurses practising as 'well child' or 'Tamariki Ora' nurses or within the Royal New Zealand Plunket Society (RNZPS) as Plunket nurses often have both nursing and midwifery qualifications as well as a graduate certificate in PHC (Kruske & Grant 2012). Many child health services in New Zealand are also provided by public health nurses (PHNs). Most PHNs work with school-aged children up to the age of 12 years but some also work with preschoolers, bridging the gap between child health nurses and school nurses. Some PHNs also provide health services to secondary schools either in support of existing school nursing services or, where these are not present, providing the entire school nursing service. Recent work has been undertaken to develop an education framework for PHNs that is intended to improve PHN career pathways. PHNs also undertake the B4 School Check outlined in detail below. Traditionally PHNs have provided home care to vulnerable families and children, while Plunket nurses have focused on those less needy. There is some regional variability so where PHNs do not work with under-fives, Plunket nurses do, and where PHNs do work with vulnerable children and families under five, Plunket steps back. Plunket has worked very hard to improve services to vulnerable families but are sometimes limited by government contracts as to the number of visits they can make to vulnerable families. PHNs generally have no such limits. PHNs, Plunket and also Tamariki Ora/well child nurses working for Māori and Iwi providers offer home visiting services to new mothers. After the first two or three visits depending on need, mothers using Plunket will then visit a Plunket clinic, whereas PHNs and Tamariki Ora nurses will continue to home visit.

What all of these nurses have in common is an expanding role, which is a global trend in child health nursing. In the UK there has been a move towards universal provision of health visiting for early interventions and a continuum of support for families as partners in dealing with social and developmental issues (Hogg et al. 2012). New Zealand child health nurses provide family parenting support in home visits, and undertake an expanded PHC role with families, particularly disadvantaged groups (Comino & Harris 2003; Yarwood 2008). The New Zealand Well Child Framework provides the policy framework for child health service provision for under-fives in New Zealand (NZMOH 2010). The framework outlines a universal service that all New Zealand families can access and provides for a minimum of 11 visits with a child health nurse up until the child turns five. At the age of four, as part of the framework, all children have access to a screening program called the B4 School Check. The B4 School Check is a screening and education visit with a child health nurse introduced to promote health and wellbeing in preschool children and identify any behavioural, developmental or other health concerns that may be detrimental to the child's ability to learn at school (NZMOH 2008). Evaluation of the B4 School Check program has found that more boys than girls were identified with behavioural problems and these children were likely to come from more deprived households. Parents and caregivers expressed high satisfaction with the outcomes of the B4 School Check including referrals for support (Hedley et al. 2012).

In Australia, child health nurses undertake universal home visits for all families with new babies and, in some cases, enhanced and sustained home visiting for families with additional needs (Paton et al. 2013; Schmied et al. 2011). In addition to the newborn and ongoing home visiting role, many child health nurses run well-child clinics, and some provide a range of PHC activities in primary schools, especially where there is no designated school nurse. This type of role is typically undertaken in New Zealand by PHNs. These activities include student screening, health education for teachers and parents, and community engagement activities. This PHC aspect of practice promotes the idea that the school should be seen as a resource for the community's health as well as its education.

PHC IN PARENTING

Child and family health nurses interact with parents in a way that can encourage their health literacy and participation in health decisions that will sustain their family's health and wellbeing throughout the family lifecycle.

Another more specialised type of child health practice involves acting as the expert resource person in special schools for children with disabilities. In this context, the nurse's health promotion activities extend from primary and secondary care of the child to ongoing tertiary care for the entire family. On occasion, this includes hospital visiting and grief counselling for family members and fellow students.

Some child health nurses practise within a case management model; for example, working with social workers and other disciplines to provide counselling, consultation and referrals for children in foster care (Schneiderman 2006). Others practise as generalist public health nurses, rather than as specialists, focusing on health promotion and family guidance, promoting health literacy and empowerment for all family members. In all cases, developing a sense of connectedness with the family is paramount, and this is typically based on a close and trusting relationship in which information and support is freely shared (Paton et al. 2013; Shepherd 2011). Child health nurses can also be employed by government or non-government agencies to deliver specific programs, such as comprehensive parenting programs or those conducted at early learning centres that function as a referral point for parents. Some programs are aimed at assisting migrant and refugee families or those with culturally specific needs (Borrow et al. 2011). Others are part of outreach programs such as the Community Mothers program (in Western Australia) or the NSW, South Australian and New Zealand Family Partnership Training programs, all of which are aimed at developing parenting capacity. The model of child health care in these and other programs is comprehensive and enabling, in that nurses provide anticipatory guidance, education and skills development to parents simultaneously with their surveillance and monitoring of the child's health status (Downie et al. 2004; Wilson & Huntington 2009; Paton et al. 2013).

EVIDENCE-BASED CHILD HEALTH

Child health nurses in Australia and New Zealand have an opportunity to collect information from parents and other members of the community linking their interactions with child and family health and wellbeing.

This information could be used to demonstrate the dimensions and viability of their roles.

An important child health nursing role lies in providing advice through telephone support lines for parents, currently available as a 24 hour service. These systems have become an important aspect of child health nursing practice in Australia, New Zealand and other countries. Both the Plunket Society and the New Zealand Ministry of Health provide telephone support lines for parents of young children (NZMOH, Plunket, Online. Available: www.healthline.co.nz and www.Plunket.org.nz [accessed 8 April 2013]). Twenty-four hour telephone support is also available for children and their parents in all Australian states and territories (Commonwealth Youth Health, Online. Available: www.cyh.com, and Kids helpline, Online. Accessed: www.kidshelpline.com.au [accessed 8 April 2013]).

The Australian website healthinsite also has numerous online resources for children and parents, including information about post and antenatal depression (www.healthinsite.gov.au/lookup/PANDA), SIDS (www.healthinsite.gov.au/lookup/SIDS), and a wide range of information on children's issues as well as adult health. Telephone access is available in both Australia and New Zealand (Australian Parent helpline 1300 364 100 and Youth helpline 1300 13 17 19; New Zealand Healthline 0800 611 116). These telephone services provide immediate response for children, youth and parents with a range of needs, particularly those relevant to new parents.

To some degree, the extension of child health practice into family nursing is linked to the complexity of family life. Knowledge of the SDH and their effect on the family, recognition of the importance of early childhood development and greater understanding of the ecology of child health has led to a multifaceted, family-oriented, PHC role (Borrow et al. 2011). As a result, contemporary practice has become more aligned with global PHC goals, focusing on family strengths and assets as well as risks. As in other countries, child health nurses in Australia and New Zealand adopt a partnership approach with parents to empower their choices for ongoing care, and maintain interdisciplinary, evidence-based practice to help enable family and community capacity to support children (Kruske et al. 2006; Schmied et al. 2011).

Child health nursing research continues to evolve throughout Australia and New Zealand. In some cases, child health nurse interactions with the family is the major focus; for example, in demonstrating the viability and effectiveness of child health nursing practice. The 'Parent Advisor Model' currently used by Plunket nurses in New Zealand, UK Health Visitors and Australian child and family nurses has been shown to improve the knowledge of helping and listening skills of nurses, sensitising them to the needs of families, and improving outcomes for parents and children (Bidmead et al. 2002; Keatinge et al. 2007). Shepherd's (2011) research into the nurse-mother relationship in the context of home visiting in Australia underlines the importance of a trusting and therapeutic relationship in maintaining mothers' emotional health and parenting skills. Similarly, Clendon and Dignam's (2010) study on how nurses interact with New Zealand mothers keeping the 'Plunket Book' has shown how these interactions can foster strong and enduring relationships. Focusing on the baby provides a safe and legitimate way for women to accept support from the nurse, especially at the most stressful times in a woman's life. This support is often intangible in the context of interactions with the mother, and somewhat hidden from view, as it is not always reported in the documentation systems required by employers (Shepherd 2011).

The increase in research conducted by practising child health nurses is a strong indication that the profession is gathering important evidence that can be translated into practice. Evidence generated by Belle and Willis (2013), Paton et al. (2013), and Shepherd (2011) illustrates that child health nurses are ideally placed to incorporate the research role into their practice. Their studies show that home visits can help restore a sense of control to women following childbirth, which has an important impact on their emotional health. Studies conducted internationally indicate that the advantages of home visits by child health nurses include improvements in parenting, helping parents with children's cognitive and developmental issues, assessing and detecting risks related to postnatal depression, reducing accidental injuries among children, and improving breastfeeding (Australian Government Productivity Commission 2011; Kitzman et al. 2010). This research agenda should be extended to studies that link the role to the more latent outcomes for parents, and studies that would help differentiate various practice strategies that will best suit the needs of families in different circumstances, particularly the most vulnerable (Australian Government Productivity Commission 2011; Nelson et al. 2011). Two significant research studies are outlined in the 'Evidence for practice' box.

EVIDENCE FOR PRACTICE: Child health

Nelson et al.'s (2011) research in New Zealand investigated a range of strategies used by Plunket nurses to help high need or 'stretched' families in Wellington. They used a 'bottom-up' partnership approach to identifying some of the most pressing issues and then worked with the community to identify appropriate solutions. The study revealed a number of positive outcomes that sowed the seeds for ongoing community health and development. These were attributed to having taken a partnership approach with the community to build relationships, linking services through cross-program networking, and helping people make sustainable choices for ongoing healthy behaviours as well as community development to support these changes (Nelson et al. 2011). This is an example of research that revolves around the SDH, which is an ideal focus for extending the child health research agenda.

South Australian child health nurses also focused on relationship building in their study of intensive home visiting for vulnerable mothers. In the context of normal home visits they identified mothers most at risk of poor outcomes. Included were women who had previous child protection issues; children with developmental difficulties, mental health, substance abuse or family violence issues; children with abnormalities or other issues assessed by the nurses to imperil their parenting. Guided by the Family Partnership Model they offered intensive visits to the women. The research involved a number of interviews to explore the women's perspectives of the program of home visiting. The women went through a cyclical process that changed from initial apprehension, to trust, respect, support and challenging experiences. All believed the program had helped them gain control over their lives.

These valuable insights, and those of the Wellington families, illustrate the importance of discovering how families feel about child health services and their close and enduring interactions with child and family health nurses. As a PHC practitioner child health nurses often 'walk with people on some of their most intimate and difficult life journeys' (Jackson & Saltman 2011:58). Where family life is difficult because of social exclusion, lack of access to services or other risks to family health, activism and advocacy by the child health nurse can often make a difference in giving voice to the family's needs (Jackson & Saltman 2011). Further research into these important interactions would help elevate the profile of this important specialty area of nursing families and the community, particularly in providing evidence for appropriate policies and practices.

SCHOOL HEALTH NURSING

The school nurse (SN) is a PHC practitioner who combines the roles of public health liaison or community nurse, health promotion professional, primary care provider and collaborator in maintaining children's health and educational achievement (Baisch et al. 2011). Many SNs apply their substantial knowledge of child and family nursing to the school setting, working within local regulations and structures, providing screening and monitoring of children's health as well as providing first aid and subacute care for minor conditions (Guzys et al. 2013). Combining primary and secondary prevention, SNs manage safety and protective strategies in the educational environment, which can include detecting infectious diseases and administering immunisations, treating and where necessary, transporting sick and injured students, screening children for developmental and medical conditions, and environmental surveillance of the school community. For example, in New Zealand, PHNs have an important role in schools in preventing rheumatic fever, a preventable disease that can occur following an infection of the throat with Group A Streptococcus (Litmus Ltd 2013). It is virtually unknown in other developed countries, but the prevalence in New Zealand is high with a total rate of 17.2 per 100 000. Rheumatic fever is disproportionately prevalent among Māori and Pacific children who account for 95% of cases— prevalence among Pacific children is 81.2 per 100 000 and among Māori children 40.2 per 100 000 (Milne et al. 2012). PHNs are funded to run 'sore throat clinics' in high need schools as a means of preventing rheumatic fever. Although this program is effective in identifying and treating children who are already infected (secondary prevention), the narrow focus of the program does not enable PHNs to address the broader social determinants of health that contribute to disease prevalence (primary prevention) (Litmus Ltd 2013), an issue that frustrates many PHNs working in the role.

SCHOOL NURSING ROLES

- Primary, secondary, tertiary prevention to enable children's capacity for academic achievement and their ongoing health and wellbeing,
- Health promotion for students, staff and the school itself

In some cases, SNs also provide tertiary prevention for students with chronic illnesses or injuries who require monitoring and support as they readjust to the school environment. The SN role is therefore complex, a specialised advanced practice role that revolves around promoting students' wellbeing, their academic success, normal development and lifelong achievement, and intervention for actual and potential health problems (Downie et al. 2002; JOSN 2008; Smith & Firmin 2009). The comprehensiveness of the role requires a broad knowledge and skill set related to child and adolescent development, human behaviour and learning.

The way SNs' roles are organised depends on whether the SN is employed in a primary or secondary school, and whether the employer is a health or education service, either private or publicly funded. What all SNs have in common is a role as the 'navigator' (Brooks et al. 2007:226) who helps the child along the school journey, collaborating with teachers and other support personnel in the process (Guzys et al. 2013). Some Australian school nurses working in the primary school setting undertake developmental screening for conditions affecting learning, such as vision and hearing. The major focus of their role is to ensure students are safe, healthy, able and ready to learn. Priorities change daily, especially where there is a need to help a child manage medications for a chronic condition such as asthma, which can not only cause distress to the child and family, but be responsible for episodes of absenteeism and therefore decreased school performance (Baisch et al. 2011). Liaising with and supporting families and caregivers is an important part of SN practice in primary schools.

Other SNs may be required to help teachers with routine care for children with special needs related to developmental disability (Seigart et al. 2013). Like child health nurses, SNs working in schools where young people have disabilities often act as the mediator between the health and education systems. This includes liaising with teachers, parents, peers and others affected by the child's journey along the health and development continuum. In some cases the nurse is the first person to provide early detection of children with developmental disabilities, which requires sensitive communication between parents, other health professionals and education staff (Wallis & Smith 2008). Where the school accommodates children with disabilities, the SN role extends to helping them with independent living needs and ensuring they have opportunities to participate in the educational experience, including field trips. To help students take advantage of these opportunities the SN has to ensure that educational staff as well as parents are fully apprised of the students' needs and potential, and help them plan for both the home and learning environment to accommodate their needs.

In some primary school systems nurses also provide immunisation services. Researchers have found that where this service is provided at school immunisation rates have tended to improve (Baisch et al. 2011). SNs also respond to children's needs for support in relation to diet, behaviours at school, issues related to the home environment and coping with stress, even in very young children. The scope of SN practice includes maintaining health records, and promoting the efficient dissemination of information to other clinicians when necessary; for example, in the case of allergies or other clinical history that would affect the management of child health out of school (Baisch et al. 2011). As a PHC provider, the SN is often the person who is able to detect the health effects of social disparities in the child's family and community that may undermine the child's educational achievement (Basch 2011).

High school nurses also provide care for students and staff, but their role tends to deal more with students' social and emotional needs, many of which revolve around adolescent 'acting out', problems with parental relationships and other issues that affect students' mental health (Weist et al. 2012). These can include issues related to sexuality, risky behaviours or other areas where peer pressure causes conflict between the young person's struggle for identity formation and family or group norms. SNs in high schools have to maintain current knowledge of adolescent behaviours, and the changing nature of their social world. For example, the immediacy of young people's communication tools means that the school day is extended through computers, texts, mobile phones and social networking, and some return to school the next day with no respite from the troubling relationships of the previous day. One of the most important interactions SNs have with adolescents is in helping them develop health literacy, particularly in navigating through web-based information (Ghaddar et al. 2012). Students may access online information that is incomplete or even inaccurate, which places the onus on the SN as a credible source of information, to help ensure that they are better informed and using appropriate sites for future searches (Ghaddar et al. 2012). Another common issue in young people's lives is stress. The busyness of their lives can be problematic, especially for children whose after-school times are filled with difficult encounters with friends or other commitments. For young adolescents in particular, the stresses of significant amounts of homework on top of a highly scheduled daily routine can result in activity-based stress, which has an effect on their ability to concentrate on learning (Brown et al. 2011). These insights are crucial for the SN to maintain strong and trusting relationships with students but they often inflate the SN role beyond the scope of practice expected.

Many SNs are experiencing a rapid increase in helping students manage mental health issues and chronic conditions, particularly with growing rates of childhood obesity, stress-related illnesses and bullying (Maslow et al. 2012; Shi et al. 2013; Mehta et al. 2013; Weist et al. 2012). Students can bring to school a wide range of vulnerabilities and social issues such as family crises, immigration or refugee-

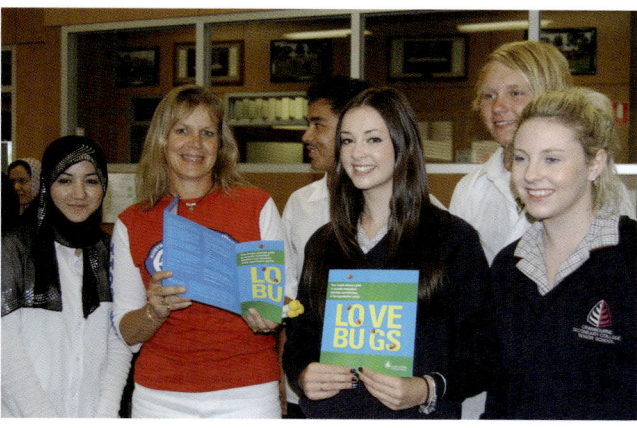

Victorian School Nurse Gina Harrex with 'love bugs' (STI) program group (photo courtesy of Gina Harrex, VSNA, with permission)

related problems, poverty and violence (Barnes et al. 2004a; DeBell 2006; JOSN 2008). Adolescents in particular can have serious mental health needs, sometimes requiring early detection of and intervention for substance abuse, family relationship challenges, adolescent pregnancy and/or sexually transmitted infections, or a risk of suicide (Brooks et al. 2007). Poverty and family disadvantage also affect the social context of their education, for which they need a continuum of learning supports (Weist et al. 2012). In 2012, the New Zealand Government announced an extra $10 million dollars to extend secondary school nursing services. Currently government-funded school nurses provide care in decile one and two secondary schools (the most highly socio-economically deprived schools) but the new funding will see this extended to decile three secondary schools. The focus of these new nurses will be particularly on mental health issues (National Party 2012), although given the evidence to support 'one stop shop' type services in schools (Bagshaw 2011), it is anticipated that these nurses will provide comprehensive care.

STRATEGY FOR ACTION

School nurses must carefully balance the need to build effective relationships with students to promote health, responding quickly to any health needs arising in the school.

Body image problems are a common issue, especially for girls, many of whom are overweight or obese. Other mental health interventions include the nurses' involvement in de-escalating reactive situations between students, school staff and parents

(Weist et al. 2009). Tertiary prevention may include periodic monitoring of a student or staff member's health condition or establishing a close engagement with groups or classes. The main objective of these relationships is empowerment, which requires the SN to bridge transitions between the family and school environment. This is done in an atmosphere of support and acceptance, a safe haven where young people can disclose their concerns, feel acknowledged and protected, receive nonjudgemental help, and build resilience (JOSN 2008; Smith & Firmin 2009). In many cases, administrators are unaware of students' need for rehabilitation and have little idea of the breadth of the SN role. This is because most activities are confidential and oriented towards building a trusting relationship with members of the school community (Green & Reffel 2009). As a result mental health services may become marginalised as 'extra' services, and poorly resourced (Weist et al. 2012). SNs need to be supportive of teachers, helping them deal with medically fragile students and their treatment requirements. Their support role with the school or education system is often expressed in bringing expert information to the school planning committee in areas such as emergency management and health protection (DeBell 2006; Green & Reffel 2009).

SNs also need a working knowledge of education systems and the processes and protocols of their school. They often work towards maintaining a boundary between themselves and the teaching staff, but some find that they are more effective when they work as part of the school resource team, becoming an integral part of the school culture. Within this culture SNs try to balance the proactive part of their role that focuses on relationships and student capacity development, with the need to respond quickly to any immediate health needs of students, teachers and school administrative staff. Another challenge in SN is the immediacy of demands on their time because of unscheduled student access and the fact that many SNs work part-time (Smith & Firmin 2009). Their role can be a careful balancing act, one that requires strong leadership and management skills, as well as extensive networks for liaising with a wide range of personnel, advocating for family members and community resources (Basch 2011; Seigart et al. 2013; Smith & Firmin 2009). The diversity of the SN role can cause role strain from a combination of emotional fatigue and frustration at being unable to provide sufficient services for students or staff, in some cases because of excessive waiting lists, and in others because of the lack of services (Guzys et al. 2013).

Health promotion is a significant element of the SN role, particularly in meeting the learning supports and strategies appropriate to adolescent needs (Guzys et al. 2013; Weist et al. 2012). In this role SNs negotiate primary prevention initiatives on the basis of their understanding of the SDH, promoting positive parenting, providing advice, support and counselling and maintaining a student-centred, partnership approach (Brooks 2007). Many see their role as helping young people become resilient adults by encouraging them to develop self-awareness and the ability to find solutions and options to the issues that challenge them. This often requires the nurse to make the first overture toward students who seem to need support for a physical or emotional issue. Their approach is one of deliberate engagement, building trust, taking advantage of the 'teachable moments' and whatever opportunities arise to convey the message that they are there to help. One of the main challenges is the vast number of students, many of whom have multiple issues that require a number of supportive interventions and resources. In addition to guiding students and staff with emotional health problems, some SNs also engage with educational staff in planning and delivering health-related curriculum components, which can overwhelm the nurse's workload (Barnes et al. 2004a, b; Green & Reffel 2009; JOSN 2008).

The Health Promoting Schools (HPS) framework developed by the WHO in 1995 (WHO 1996) was intended to strengthen health promotion in schools at local, regional, national and global levels using a whole-of-school approach (St Leger 1999). However, the HPS model is often poorly understood, with education authorities expecting a behavioural, healthy-lifestyle approach rather than a broader focus on school and student capacity building (Bruce et al. 2012; Ryan 2008; Whitehead 2006). The guidelines for health promotion were developed on the basis of the socio-ecological approach to health, to address the school, its policies, social environment, community and health service relationships as well as personal health skills (Bruce et al. 2012). The HPS model is therefore intended as a guide to connecting the school community to the wider environment and its resources (Barnes et al. 2004a, b, Moses et al. 2008). However, most HPS programs have retained the focus on changing students' behaviours rather than developing an empowering approach to promoting the health of schools and students. Most SNs practise relatively autonomously, but not in isolation from others, which creates an additional pressure to stay abreast of new developments and current research. Maintaining knowledge of physical and mental health issues, PHC, school and community organisational systems and role expectations can sometimes be daunting. In some cases, there may be different expectations of the SN role by principals, teachers or Department of Health employers, which can create barriers to maintaining the focus on students and the school community. Guzys et al. (2013:5) suggest that a process of 'critical companionship' replace models of clinical supervision of SN practice, to provide a mechanism that is 'supportive, focused on developing evidence-based, person-centred care, practitioner effectiveness, and expertise'. A strategy for critical companionship is the Community of Practice (CoP), which American SNs have begun to use to provide supportive communications and group resourcefulness in school health by mutual sharing, deepening their knowledge base, and support for health promotion in schools (Weist et al. 2012). One such group is co-sponsored by the IDEA Partnership (Online. Available: www.ideapartnership.org [accessed 6 April 2013]). This group and others emerging among SNs are aimed at providing the most up to date information on adolescent mental health promotion. Websites are also a way of sharing information to overcome some of the difficulties of practising in isolation. These are also helpful in making the SN role more visible for policy and planning. Several sites are available to SNs including the Victorian School Nurses ANF Special Interest Group (www.anmfvic.asn.au/sigs); The Independent School Nurses' Association of Western Australia (www.ais.wa.edu.au), and the Auckland School Nurses Group (www.schoolnurse.org.nz). Through their web-based interactions and a number of meetings, the Victorian School Nurses ANF Special Interest Group (SIG) have developed the National Standards for School Nursing in Australia (see Appendix G). The Auckland group has also drawn attention to the need for 'work stories', a set of case studies that would help capture the role in more detail for the District Health Boards (DHBs). This suggestion could also help advance the research agenda for school health. To heighten visibility of the role, there remains a need for research that would demonstrate the paradigm shift away from the exclusive focus on school health services, towards promoting health and its social determinants. Kool et al. (2008) suggest that SNs using an embracing pattern of health care provision rather than a 'band aid' pattern provide more effective school-based services. An example of the efficacy of an 'embracing' pattern of health care provision is in the improved health outcomes demonstrated among children attending a nurse-led clinic based in a primary school in Central Auckland (Krothe & Clendon 2006; Clendon 2004/5). An initial community assessment process and ongoing community involvement in the clinic have been integral to its success, demonstrating the importance of involving community members as partners at the outset of any health project.

> ## WHAT'S YOUR OPINION?
>
> Websites provide a good opportunity for school nurses to connect and find the professional collegiality they need to ensure safe practice. However there are risks to web-based communication. Can you think of any of these potential risks?

The importance of a career pathway for school nurses has been identified by Buckley et al. (2012). The ad hoc way in which school nursing services have developed, the relatively autonomous way in which school nurses practice, as noted above, and the limited understanding of the role by policymakers and funders has created a practice environment with little or no career pathway and few opportunities for advancement. This combined with inconsistent funding streams challenges school nurses to ensure they advocate for the role at all levels, providing evidence for the efficacy of the school nurse role in improving health outcomes.

COMMUNITY MENTAL HEALTH NURSING PRACTICE

The prevalence of mental health issues in our societies has created renewed awareness of the importance of community mental health nursing (CMHN). Deinstitutionalisation, early discharge for patients hospitalised with mental illnesses, and an ageing population living at home with conditions such as dementia have led to substantial increases in the number of mental health nurses working in the community rather than acute care settings (Happell et al. 2012a). In Australia and New Zealand, CMHNs have recognition in the respective legislative acts, and are registered to act as responsible clinicians within their scope of practice (Hurley & Linsley 2007). CMHN is a complex, specialised, multidimensional role; one that combines primary, secondary and tertiary prevention with individual and family case management for all age groups. This breadth of activities and age groups distinguish the role of community mental health nurses (CMHNs) from that of community nurses whose practice is focused on young children in the context of child or school health; the adult working population in the context of occupational health; or domiciliary services with a primary responsibility for older people. In some cases, there is considerable overlap between the role of the CMHN and other specialist areas. For example, CMHNs can be employed in postnatal child and family health to work with children whose parents suffer from mental illness (Foster et al. 2012), in conducting clinics or programs for postnatal mental health (Harvey et al. 2012), or in working with those suffering post-traumatic stress syndrome, such as war veterans (Allan et al. 2012). Others work in general practices, as a PN specialist in a team-based program to coordinate clinical care for those with severe mental illness (SMI) (Chamberlain-Salaun et al. 2011), or in New Zealand as a primary mental health care nurse—providing brief intervention for minor to moderate mental health issues (Clendon 2010).

COMMUNITY MENTAL HEALTH NURSE ROLE

- Primary, secondary, tertiary prevention
- Specialised case management
- Integration of physical, mental health
- Counselling
- Care Coordination
- Home Visiting for clients across the lifespan
- Family teaching, support, health literacy
- Community support for vulnerable people

The number of PN mental health nurses has increased, which is a trend worldwide. In Australia, their role has expanded as a result of the Australian Mental Health Nurse Incentive Program, which has increased funding for their positions to respond to a growing need that can't be met by general practitioners (GPs) (Chamberlain-Salaun et al. 2011). Their role is crucial for the estimated 75% of people who access care from their GPs, who may not have the time for adequate therapeutic engagement (Chamberlain-Salaun et al. 2011), or who prefer to attend general practice rather than encounter the stigma associated with mental health services (Machado & Tomlinson 2011). In the context of GP practice the CMHN may undertake home visiting. Home visits are a feature of practice in most models of care, whether the nurse is employed by a public or private agency in a targeted project or program that requires assessment and intervention in the home. Home visits can be aimed at assisting young families or older people deal with specific mental

health issues, all of which tend to be family focused and combine strategies to meet both mental and physical health needs (Callander et al. 2011; Happell et al. 2012a; Hardy 2012; Harvey et al. 2012; McCloughen et al. 2011).

Medication management is an important part of the role of CMHNs, especially for those with severe mental illness (SMI) (Happell et al. 2012b). The CMHNs' level of clinical decision-making, especially in relation to medications, is distinctive in being beyond the scope of practice of most other nurses working in the community. CMHNs also order diagnostic tests, referrals to specialists, recommendations for involuntary treatment and authorisation of sick certificates (Elsom et al. 2009). Other areas of responsibility include careful management of chronic mental health conditions, especially for those who have become the victims of deinstitutionalisation. Their role in chronic illness management extends to coordinating supports to enhance client and family quality of life. One of the major issues for those who have experienced mental illness is securing affordable, secure housing. As an SDH, housing security is instrumental in their recovery and rehabilitation, with many acutely ill people getting caught in a revolving door of homelessness and substance abuse, which can compound their vulnerability to further ill health (Hamden et al. 2011). The coordination role of the nurse is therefore significant. In many cases, it is up to the CMHN to ensure timely referral to emergency accommodation, specialist care, community supports such as self-help or advocacy groups, and help people plan for the future (Hamden et al. 2011). This continuum of PHC activities revolves around the SDH. In mental health terms it is called Assertive Community Treatment (ACT), which is focused on keeping people undergoing treatment out of hospital and in their home community (Hamden et al. 2011). Achieving community treatment involves major challenges; advocating for ongoing community support while helping people cope with acute episodes of illness (primary prevention), maintaining adequate screening and assessment strategies that may prevent a relapse of illness (secondary prevention); and helping people plan for the future in the face of limited employment opportunities, and often limited family assistance (tertiary prevention). These challenges are magnified in rural and regional areas, where the lack of access to mental health services adds another layer of disadvantage (Happell et al. 2012b). The nurse's role is particularly difficult in rural and regional areas, as s/he is often the only mental health nurse available, with few backup resources that can help out when s/he is unavailable. In recognition of this type of professional isolation, the Mental Health Professionals' Network (MHPN) has been developed to help maintain connections between mental health professionals practising in rural areas (Tyrell 2013). Some of these networks meet online (www.mhpn.org.au) while others are able to organise face-to-face meetings, albeit infrequently.

> **Primary prevention**—treating acute episodes, advocating for community supports
>
> **Secondary prevention**—screening and needs assessment to prevent relapse
>
> **Tertiary Prevention**—helping clients, families plan for the future, accessing appropriate supports

Ideally, the CMHN works collaboratively, in partnership with the client, family and other carers to help with the development of skills for daily living, problem solving, health literacy and forward planning (Happell et al. 2012a; McCloughen et al. 2011). Collaborative practice with a focus on community participation has been sanctioned by the New Zealand Government (NZMOH 2006) and the Australian Health Ministers (Australian Health Ministers 2009), which reflects the commitment of both health policies to PHC. Collaboration takes many forms. In some cases, clients with mental illness may prefer to exclude the family, because of their need for autonomy and confidentiality, or because of the stress and trauma resulting from early childhood experiences (van de Bovenkamp & Trappenburg 2012). This situation can be resolved through authentic communication that honours the client's wishes, and helps empower them for decision-making. Maintaining a broad base of resources and networks helps the nurse empower people to access appropriate and acceptable resources and supports that are an alternative to relying on the family. In cases where treatment of mental illness is mandatory, other issues arise. When this occurs it is up to nurses to identify the specific issues a client may want to collaborate on, and how they prefer to collaborate. McCloughen et al.'s (2011) study of collaboration in these cases revealed that successful shared decision-making relies on communication, trust, respect and consistency. However, there are some cases where the challenges of collaboration are insurmountable, particularly where organisational systems operate on the basis of controlling, rather than partnering with people who need mental health services. McCloughen et al.'s (2011) findings suggest that effective collaborative relationships require mutual valuing of goals, active

sharing of knowledge and expertise, responsiveness and flexibility as well as the type of organisational support one would expect in a PHC system.

The collaborative approach to working with mental health clients is an essential element of the CMHN's health promotion role. Health promotion has historically been a relatively uncharted aspect of the role; however, the New Zealand PHC approach and Australian health reforms that shift the focus to community-based care have seen this role become more prominent (Happell et al. 2012b). Health promotion is also entrenched in the shift from a mental illness focus to the positive health and wellness 'asset-based paradigm' (Wand 2013:2012). Historically, the role of mental health nurses was more narrowly focused on psychiatric disorders and illness, whereas contemporary practice focuses on promoting both individual and community competencies, resources, attributes and abilities (Wand 2013). This approach is congruent with the strengths-based approach that focuses on assets rather than risks as we outlined in Chapter 4. In mental health the overriding goal is to promote resilience, positive adaptation in the face of adversity and a sense of mastery (Wand 2013). This is achieved when people become health literate, when they become aware of the importance of the social determinants of their lives, and where they are encouraged to identify their strengths, abilities and hopes for the future (Wand 2013).

> ## CMHN PRACTICE FOCUS
> * PHC for all age groups
> * Physical and mental health
> * Addressing stigmatisation
> * Meeting needs of most vulnerable
> * Health promotion
> * Interdisciplinary collaboration
> * Sustaining workforce

The health promotion role in CMHN has also been shaped by the close association between physical, social and personal mental health issues, and the need to assess these comprehensively in order to help individuals, families and community access supports (Coombs et al. 2012; Hardy 2012; Nardi 2011; Pope 2011). Health education activities in the CMHN context therefore integrate physical and mental health goals, based on the strong links between these aspects of health as established from the research evidence (Hardy 2012; Holm & Severinsson 2012). Chronic care models are used to help those suffering from depression, which is often co-morbid in those with cardiovascular disease, arthritis and metabolic disorders (Holm & Severinsson 2012). Exercise is frequently included in these approaches, as the efficacy of exercise programs in preventing death or disablement from the combination of these conditions has been well established (Weber 2010). Physical activity programs have also been combined with various therapies, such as cognitive behavioural therapy for young mothers with mental health issues such as perinatal depression (Harvey et al. 2012), and in anti-bullying programs (Jones Warren 2011). These programs are most successful when they are available locally, at low cost to participants and where people have the option to participate at the level and duration of their choice.

The challenges of CMHN include work intensification caused by mental health nursing and psychiatrist shortages, increasing levels of unstable clients in the community for long periods of time prior to admission to psychiatric facilities, a large burden of administrative responsibilities, legal considerations in all cases they deal with, and changing models of service provision (Henderson et al. 2008). The emotional demands of the role create inordinate stress, especially in the broader, PHC role where there is a focus on such SDH as discrimination, poverty, family relationships and education. The responsibility of coordinating care in general practice can also be stressful, creating interdisciplinary blurring of roles, and add additional layers of administration and documentation on top of a heavy case load, as referrals are organised, liaison systems put in place, and competing ideologies are dealt with (Crawford et al. 2007; Henderson et al. 2008). The research agenda is gradually evolving, with CMHN charting the course of their practice changes and strategies (Happell et al. 2012a; Wand 2013). What remains is to extend nursing research to show how the changes in service initiatives and models of practice can be translated into better health outcomes for this group of disadvantaged, vulnerable people.

Since implementation of the Primary Health Care Strategy (NZMOH 2001) in New Zealand, ongoing work has focused on the needs of people with mild to moderate mental health issues in community settings. While it is recognised that most people with mild to moderate mental health issues can be effectively cared for in PHC settings, this care has frequently been dependent on their health provider's interest and expertise in the area of mental health (NZMOH 2002). Funding to establish primary mental health initiatives across New Zealand has seen the development of a variety of models of care designed to meet the needs of these groups, including a model of shared care between GPs and mental health nurses (Dowell et al. 2009). However, the business model of general practice is seen to be inadequate in allocating sufficient time to those with mental health needs (O'Brien et al. 2006). With the inception of primary mental health coordinators (often CMHNs) who have been appointed in many communities across New Zealand, a more collaborative approach has been achieved with greater potential for the future (O'Brien et al. 2006). These specialised nurses provide needs assessment and service coordination for service users, mentoring of general practice staff, stronger links between primary and secondary services, advocacy for service users, case management and counselling services, and advice to general practice staff on referral options (Dowell et al. 2009). Evaluation indicates that up to 80% of service users benefited from the variety of interventions offered in PHC settings (Dowell et al. 2009).

Despite such developments designed to use general practice more effectively for primary mental health care, an analysis of the PN role within interdisciplinary general practice teams providing primary mental health care found that attitudinal, structural and professional barriers existed that limited PN engagement with mental health patients in the general practice setting. The study recommended that the PN workforce be substantially developed in order to meet the demand for primary mental health care (McKinlay et al. 2011). Importantly, a new credentialing process for nurses working in primary mental health care has been established by Te ao Māramatanga New Zealand College of Mental Health Nurses Inc. that will support PNs as well as CMHNs to demonstrate their competence in this area (NZCMHN, Online. Available: www.nzcmhn.org.nz/Credentialing [accessed 26 April 2013]). In addition, curriculum changes at some institutions were implemented to allow undergraduate students greater experience in primary mental health (Spence et al. 2012).

Evaluation of curriculum changes at one institution has shown that more graduates were intending to take up positions in mental health after the curriculum change than had indicated prior to the change. Student and staff satisfaction with the curriculum had also improved (Spence et al. 2012).

OCCUPATIONAL HEALTH NURSING

Occupational health nursing extends the goals of PHC to the workplace. It is a specialist area of community or public health nursing, with a scope of practice that includes 'worker and workplace hazard detection, health education and promotion, disease management, regulatory compliance, emergency preparedness, research, and program management' (Thompson & Wachs 2012:128). Occupational health nurses (OHNs) practise in partnership with workers, worker groups and employers to plan health care that is accessible, empowering, and part of a comprehensive and continuing health conservation process. When required they also provide primary care for injuries and illnesses, administering over-the-counter medications and undertaking minor procedures such as removing sutures (Strasser 2011). The uniqueness of OHN is manifest through a bilateral advocacy role, where the health, safety and business interests of both employee and employer may all be priorities in health planning. On occasion, balancing these challenges can be daunting, requiring diplomacy, high-level communication skills, understanding of interpersonal and industrial relations, and familiarity with professional and government standards and legislation. Other factors influencing OHN practice include the need for specialised knowledge of environmental issues, the context and expectations of the employing organisation, employer and union philosophy and policies, budgetary restraints, and the nurse's scope of practice, professional supports and educational opportunities.

THE SCOPE OF OHN PRACTICE

- Worker and workplace hazard detection
- Health education and promotion
- Disease management, regulatory compliance, emergency preparedness, research and program management

OHN practice has changed considerably since the 'industrial nurse' role was developed as a subset of the public health role early in the 20th century (Schwem 2009). At that time, where industries were localised to small communities, the objective of occupational health was often to ensure containment of illness in the workplace to prevent any workplace infections spreading to the community, and to monitor employees' adherence to doctors' orders (Burgel & Childre 2012; Schwem 2009). Since mid-last century, rapid industrial expansion and globalisation with its multi-national, highly competitive corporations, have created occupational health environments that are more systematic and focused on cost-containment, worker productivity and return on investments (Burgel & Childre 2012; Marinescu 2007). The changes have seen the OHN role shift from a medical agenda for onsite diagnosis and treatment of illness and injury, to autonomous, specialty practice within which health care services are based on independent nursing judgements (Strasser 2011). At the global level the WHO has developed a global plan of action on workers' health 2008–17, which includes five major objectives (WHO 2007). These are to devise and implement policies for workers' health; to protect and promote health at the workplace; to improve the performance and access to occupational health services; to provide and communicate evidence for action and practice; and to incorporate workers' health into other policies. Australian and New Zealand policymakers are challenged, along with OHNs, to implement these objectives in their practice.

Although OHNs practice within a broad scope of practice they are not credentialed as a specialty in Australia or New Zealand. In Australia OHNs are regulated by the Australia Nursing and Midwifery Accreditation Council and in New Zealand by the Nursing Council of New Zealand. The New Zealand Occupational Health Nurses Association represents the interests of OHNs professionally, developing professional standards, holding conferences, and providing support and networking for OHNs across the country (NZOHNA, Online. Available: www.nzohna.org.nz/page.php?id=105 [accessed 27 April 2013]). Many OHNs work as part of a workplace health and safety team, in some cases working alongside physiotherapists, occupational therapists and safety officers in health promotion and injury prevention (Mellor & St John 2009). A distinctive aspect of the OHN role is the technical skill required to combine assessment of the workplace with assessment of workers. In addition to assessment skills this requires extensive knowledge of the workplace itself and its particular hazards. Ergonomic knowledge is essential in understanding the fit between the worker and their interface with the work environment. Ergonomic risks can include boredom, glare, repetitive motion, poor workstation-worker fit, lifting heavy loads or tasks that require the worker to assume an abnormal position. Physical hazards can include such things as extremes of temperature, noise, radiation or poor lighting. Biological hazards include exposures to chemical or various biological agents. Psychosocial hazards are those that produce inordinate stress, such as shiftwork, or negative interpersonal relationships on the job.

> ### ERGONOMIC ASSESSMENT
>
> Assessing the interface between the worker and their work environment.

Stress is a major workplace hazard, particularly with company reorganisation and downsizing often affecting management staff as well as those whose jobs are under threat (Wallace 2009). The OHN can help monitor worker stress, providing education, counselling, worksite stress reduction programs or referrals to specialist services (Wallace 2009). Another aspect of the role is in maintaining accurate documentation and communicating sufficient information to management for planning and implementation of workplace initiatives. For example, a hazard survey may be conducted as part of the OHN's primary prevention activities. Where such a survey exists, it is usually up to the OHN to make it readily accessible to all members of the workforce. Most companies also have a disaster plan, which may have been developed with input from the OHN, who then takes a leading role in disseminating it to the workforce and assuming responsibility for intermittent updates. Disaster planning requires close collaboration with emergency services, other health professionals, and workplace health and safety personnel (Lobaton Cabrera & Beaton 2009).

Secondary prevention requires knowledge of the workforce and any pre-existing conditions that may place their health or wellbeing in jeopardy. This information is often garnered during the pre-employment health examination and updated during periodic health assessments. To respond to any injuries or illness episodes in the workplace the OHN typically needs to be skilled in primary care such as first-aid procedures, crisis intervention and trauma management. Workplace violence is another issue that arises in many places, including threats, physical or emotional abuse, stalking or sexual harassment (Olszewski et al. 2007). The risk of violent incidents and high levels of workplace stress create the need for nurses to maintain counselling skills and an extensive referral network for both physical and mental health issues. Case management is also integral to the role, especially in working with employees with a chronic illness or disability to help

them manage their condition and prevent acute episodes in the workplace (Aziz 2009).

Tertiary prevention in the workplace is aimed at minimising any compromises to health, or helping restore workers' health following any injury or illness. Included are strategies to help people in their transitions back to work after a workplace incident, or counselling to help people resolve any issues surrounding job restructuring or retraining. Recovery and rehabilitation following illness or injury often requires ongoing liaison with the worker's family physician and may also involve family members, depending on the circumstances. In this role the OHN is typically the care coordinator, providing the collaborative link between the employee, their GP, PN, specialists, social worker, physiotherapist or other health professional (Aziz 2009). Many OHNs maintain a range of health intervention programs to engage workers while they are recovering from an illness episode or injury. These include employee assistance for those with substance abuse problems, corporate smoking cessation, and workplace health and fitness programs. Parallel with these in-house programs the OHN usually maintains a database of agencies that can help workers offsite. The information network required for all of these activities is extensive, and a major part of the OHN role.

A new level of OHN has gained prominence in the US; that of the OH Nurse Practitioner (Burgel & Childre 2012; Haag 2013; Thomas 2011). Nurse practitioners in the workplace tend to take a higher level of responsibility for service improvements, particularly in relation to the convergence of occupational health and safety and human resources issues (Thomas 2011). Some NPs take responsibility for helping workers manage acute pain following illness or injury, while managing the company's direct and indirect costs related to the injury (Ferriolo & Acree Conlon 2012). For all OHNs, pain management can be a major element of the role, with musculoskeletal pain or muscle spasms occurring as a residual effect of overuse, or workers experiencing inflammatory or neuropathic pain, which needs to be assessed and treated (Ferriolo & Acree Conlon 2012). NP OHNs typically work from a formulary to administer pain treatments, while other OHNs tend to use over-the-counter medications or massage therapy and guidance to prevent deterioration and discouragement that can lead to depression or other problems related to dealing with pain (Ferriolo & Acree Conlon 2012).

NP OHNs also are required to be skilled in leadership and management techniques. Their role often involves making a rational business case for health promotion programs on the basis of increased efficiency and evidence-based change management strategies (Haag 2013). This level of strategic leadership is described as enabling OHNs to 'question, reflect, anticipate, predict and make decisions, ensuring the viability of quality-driven and cost-effective occupational health programs and services' (Randolph 2012a:52). Some occupational NPs have developed an entrepreneurial approach to their role, using business strategies and negotiation skills to develop their own organisations to manage occupational health and safety (Haag 2013). Box 5.4 outlines the major trends that have transformed OHN practice over recent decades.

PHC for the working population

The demographics of the working population have an impact on the OHN role, even though the common basis for nursing interventions is PHC and consideration of the SDH for both workers and employers. Changes to family life have created an increase in the number of women in the workplace, some of whom have gravitated to traditional male jobs, including those in the mining industry, which are physically demanding and can be difficult for women juggling home and work responsibilities. With increases in global migration, today's

workplaces also have high proportions of migrant workers, some of whom may not speak or understand English, which carries a risk of misunderstanding safety instructions. Along with farmers and construction workers, they may be unskilled in the jobs they are asked to do, which tend to be lower level jobs with higher risks of accidents with machinery or respiratory conditions from poor air quality (Thompson & Wachs 2012). Many migrant workers experience occupational downgrading and limited opportunities to use their actual skills and education in the host country, a situation even more common among refugees (Crollard et al. 2012). Although there is limited

---

BOX 5.4 Trends in occupational health nursing

Current practice	rather than	Historical practice
Evidence-based practice		tradition
Worker performance		absenteeism
Economic outcomes		health care costs
Employee prevention		treatment
Population		individual focus
Health focus		disease or illness
Multiple risk factors		single factors
Employee-centred interventions		program-centred
Creating a culture of workplace health and safety across the organisation		enforcements
Focus on communication, management, leadership skills		worker v management

(Source: Marinescu 2007)

BOX 5.5 Wellington City Council's OHN

In 2011, Trish Knight won the Practitioner of the Year Award at the New Zealand Occupational Health Nurses Association awards for her work in implementing a heart health program across Wellington City Council's workforce. Trish started by collecting medical data from employees on a voluntary basis throughout all business units. She undertook measures of blood pressure, blood sugar, total cholesterol, waist measures, BMI, and waist to hip ratios. Using statistical data obtained from the Employee Assistance Programme (EAP) report, wellness leave and the organisation's existing heart health programme, Trish then developed a workplace wellness strategy that was able to target the diverse employee groups she was working with.

Key interventions with employees have included: running a men's health day with the men in charge; implementing the 'Climb a mountain challenge' with 250 staff including the CEO climbing the equivalent of Mt Everest in three weeks by walking up stairs; entering 14 employees in the Global Corporate Challenge—a 16 week web-based walking challenge; entering two teams in the 'Iron Māori' (more information on 'Iron Māori' can be found at www.oneheartmanylives.co.nz/iron-maori.html); and running a parks staff health day. Participants in many of the programs have achieved weight loss and better blood pressure control. Future plans include developing nutritionally focused plans for Council-controlled café contracts, recreational settings and vending machines and adaptation of current health days to suit other business units, recognising their individual workforce needs.

(Source: Adapted from Knight 2012)

research into the difficulties they face in the workplace, studies conducted thus far conclude that their employment is one of the most significant social determinants of their health, as they tend to suffer stress, anxiety, depression, irritation and frustration linked to conflicting social expectations and feelings of injustice or deprivation (Crollard et al. 2012). Understanding their plight is relevant to OHNs working with migrant workers in New Zealand and Australia, given the steady flow of migrants to both countries. One Australian study found that 32–49% of non-native English speakers were overeducated for their employment compared to 7–22% of Australian natives (Green et al. 2007). The OHN, human resources and other safety personnel must maintain vigilance for these workers, as they are often placed in hazardous jobs and suffer more occupational illnesses and injuries than other workers (Crollard et al. 2012). Some employers provide cultural competence training and, where possible, community-based participatory research (CBPR) to engage with migrant workers so they can become empowered to overcome the challenges of their diminished role and status in the workplace (Crollard et al. 2012). This is an important role for the OHN, as advocate for the workers and liaison between them and other employees as well as the employer. With increased duration of residence as a migrant, many become upwardly mobile (Crollard et al. 2012). Their successful transitions in the workplace, supported by the OHN, can help with transitions in the community. Even skilled migrants can face significant challenges in the workplace. Up to 50% of new registrations with the Nursing Council of New Zealand are from internationally qualified nurses (Nursing Council of New Zealand 2012b) and yet research has shown that many face discrimination, undervaluing of their skills and dissatisfaction with their work (Walker & Clendon 2012a) in similar ways to other migrants. OHNs can play an important role in supporting new colleagues to settle into their roles.

Workers suffering mental health issues are another challenge in the workplace. The OHN often has to mediate between the worker, work colleagues and employers to prevent any stigma from other workers creating stressful conditions at work that might interfere with their capabilities. In these cases, the OHN may liaise with carers or family members as well as the employee to help reduce their vulnerability to physical or psychosocial risks (Callander et al. 2011). Nurses are another group with significant occupational health and safety needs. Nursing is a high-risk profession, due to lifting and other physical demands, exposure to infectious agents in the workplace, and, for shift

workers, sleep deprivation, and poor exercise and nutrition habits (Clendon & Walker 2013; Buss 2012; Thompson & Wachs 2012). Recent New Zealand research has revealed that 11% of New Zealand nurses had required time off in the past two years due to a workplace-acquired injury or infection (Walker & Clendon 2013). Stress is also a major concern for nurses. Research by the US National Institute of Occupational Safety and Health (NIOSH) shows that stress has 'deleterious effects on physical and mental health, including cardiovascular and gastrointestinal systems, and leads to muscle tension, headaches, sleep disturbances, irritability, anxiety and depression' (Zeller & Levin 2013:85). Workplace stress has been linked to high job demands, low control, effort-reward imbalances, characteristics of the job, low social support at work, and individual coping abilities (Reineholm et al. 2011). Many nurses would recognise these characteristics of their workplace, where they are constantly required to have technical expertise, vigilance and judgement to provide safe, high-quality patient care (Zeller & Levin 2013).

The important issue for OHNs in hospital and health agencies is to treat the nurses suffering from stress, to guard against burnout and compassion fatigue, which may cause nurses to leave the profession, and prevent stress from interfering with their ability to deliver patient care. Nurses aged under 30 have been identified as at particular risk from workplace stress due to the high emotional challenge of nursing work—12% indicated in a recent survey that they intended to leave the profession within the next year (Clendon & Walker 2011). Researchers have found that work engagement can help workers in stressful, high-demand jobs, which suggests a role for the OHN in promoting a positive workplace culture of mutual respect that is considerate of the demands of the role (Torp et al. 2012). In addressing the psychosocial issues in nursing workplaces, OHNs will have the advantage of familiarity with the work, but they may also need to develop advanced mental health skills to create treatment and support networks and programs that can be empowering (Zeller & Levin 2013).

PRACTICE STRATEGY

Nurses aged under 30 identify the emotional work of nursing as particularly challenging. What support mechanisms do you think may be helpful for younger nurses in the workplace?

Population ageing and the global financial crisis of 2009 has also meant that more older persons continue to work longer, and many of these older workers also suffer from chronic conditions. Some have taken jobs in the resources sector, where there is an abundance of work in mining. Mining jobs are hazardous for all workers, but for older workers increased monitoring can be necessary to prevent injuries. Many mining employees have also come from other industries with different work practices, requiring retraining. Among the older workforce are many people with co-morbidities such as hypertension, diabetes, hyperlipidemia, and respiratory conditions such as asthma (Thompson & Wachs 2012). These conditions may be affected by the working environment, particularly air quality as it affects asthma or other respiratory illnesses. Although generally, older workers are valued for their knowledge, education, wisdom, dependability and loyalty to the company, they also need careful guidance about their personal risks, as many have slower reflexes, diminished sensory abilities and slower recovery time from illness (Rogers et al. 2011; Thompson & Wachs 2012).

The most recent estimates indicate that 40% of the Australian nursing workforce is over age 50, and approximately 3.5% of the New Zealand nursing workforce is aged over 65 (Graham & Duffield 2010; Nursing Council of New Zealand 2012a). Recent research exploring the experiences of nurses aged over 50 in the New Zealand workplace has found that many nurses need to continue working into older age due to financial imperatives—many noted divorce, loss of financial independence due to the collapse of finance companies, the impacts of the Christchurch earthquake, and having to take on the care of grandchildren as impacting on their financial capability to retire (Walker & Clendon 2012b). These nurses experience many of the same health issues as other older workers and in some cases, the OHN becomes involved in helping older workers with retirement planning. This can include helping them facilitate a smooth transition to flexible work by encouraging policies and practices amenable to their needs; helping the workers themselves develop a realistic concept of their future health; encouraging self-discovery of what they value, and helping them evaluate needs in their living environment as well as the workplace (Zinner 2006). Some OHNs provide chronic self-management programs for those living with conditions such as diabetes (McCarver 2011; Miller 2011). These programs include promoting workplace programs and structural supports for self-management, providing primary care (primary prevention), assessment, monitoring and periodic examinations, managing complications and administering medications as well as maintaining documentation systems (secondary prevention), and follow-up evaluations and referrals for ongoing care where necessary (tertiary prevention) (Burgel 2012; McCarver 2011; Randolph 2012b) (see Box 5.6).

Health literacy is a major goal of OHNs working with chronically ill employees, as well as employers whose interests lie in balancing the need to maintain productivity while improving employee health (Wong 2012). OHNs have coined the term 'occupational health literacy' to refer to 'the degree to which workers can obtain, communicate, process and understand occupational health and safety information and services to make appropriate health decisions in the workplace' (Wong 2012:364). Occupational health literacy is a social responsibility for employers who seek to retain their workforce and promote a culture of quality, safety and productivity (Wong 2012). Developing a health literate workplace culture can be of enormous help to migrant workers, and it is also crucial for those who are vulnerable to accidents or illnesses because of low general literacy or other risk factors such as age or lack of specific

---

BOX 5.6 Primary, secondary, tertiary prevention in the workplace

Primary prevention

- Activities to promote a healthy workplace—corporate health literacy, cultural competency, flexible work arrangements (job sharing), ergonomic analysis, hazard surveillance, interdisciplinary planning and liaison
- Programs to promote healthy choices—smoking cessation, weight loss, nutrition counselling, stress reduction, corporate fitness programs, immunisations for older workers, health coaching

Secondary prevention

Assessment, monitoring of chronic conditions, periodic assessments for work readiness after illness or injury, case management, hazard communication, medication management, occupational health literacy, managing documentation and communication between employers and employees

Tertiary prevention

Follow-up evaluations, referrals, liaison and ongoing care for chronic conditions, securing ergonomic aids and protective devices for working.

skills. Table 5.5 outlines the attributes of a health literate organisation (Wong 2012).

Research in OHN practice

Like school nursing, and rural and remote area nursing, the OHN is primarily a place-based role. It is unique in its 'community', which is the worker and employer workforce and the industry within which they perform their duties. Yet the knowledge base for practice remains under-researched (Mellor & St John 2009). The dearth of research, especially evaluation studies in the Australian and New Zealand contexts, has delayed development of models to guide good and best practice in OHN. However, American OHN researchers report major advances in the knowledge base for OHN. Lusk et al. (2004) have conducted a program of research throughout the past decade demonstrating the relationship between acute noise exposure and blood pressure and heart rate, finding that workers who used hearing protection had lower blood pressure and heart rate than those without protection (Lusk et al. 2004). Lipscomb et al. (2009) have investigated the effects of extended work schedules and work organisation on the health of health care professionals, including nurses. They have also researched the effects of bloodborne pathogen risk and pandemic influenza preparedness among home health care workers, finding that there is a need for additional training, prevention and protection. Robbins et al. (2008) have used community-based participatory research (CBPR) to study the chromosomal abnormalities in human sperm cells resulting from environmental, occupational and lifestyle exposures. Rogers and her colleagues (2000) have researched the effect of antineoplastic agents on health care workers, informing workplace practices and safeguarding workers at risk for airborne infections. Their group is now examining ethical dilemmas facing OHNs. Lipscomb et al. (2010) have also been engaged in policy development for OHN practice following a series of studies on the complex relationships between work and health disparities. Other researchers have studied the relationships between structural and process factors in the workplace (Salazar et al. 2003), self-care among ageing workers (Dickson et al. 2008), workplace screening and treatment for women victims of domestic violence (Felblinger & Gates 2008), as well as other women's health issues in the workplace (McGovern et al. 2007).

EVIDENCE FOR PRACTICE

What research questions would help you, as a new OHN develop the evidence for your practice strategies?

All of these studies have illuminated the role of the OHN in primary, secondary and tertiary prevention for the working population, most in partnership with other disciplines. What remains to be researched includes the role of PHC in the workplace, effective health promotion strategies, factors that influence workers' return to work, the health effects of ageing in the workforce, ergonomic and hazardous issues in the workplace, strategies for influencing workers to use protective devices as well as emergency preparedness of organisations (McCauley 2012). These issues are somewhat different from those identified by Safe Work Australia (SWA, Online. Available: www .safeworkaustralia.gov.au/sites/SWA [accessed 21 March 2013]), all of which are concerned with regulation, compliance and reporting. The nursing research agenda is aimed more closely at the complexities of human and structural factors with a view toward highlighting the important role played by nurses in maintaining the health and safety of this substantial portion of the population. It is now up to the profession to take further steps to advance the knowledge base for this role and its impact on the health of workers.

TABLE 5.5 Attributes of a health-literate organisation

1. Leadership that makes health literacy integral to mission, structure and operations
2. Integrates health literacy into planning, evaluation, safety and quality improvement
3. Prepares health literate workforce and monitors their progress
4. Adopts partnership approach to design, implement, evaluate health information and services
5. Meets population needs with range of skills, avoiding stigmatisation
6. Uses health literacy strategies in communications, confirming understanding at all points of contact
7. Provides easy access to health information and services, including navigation assistance
8. Designs and distributes print, audiovisual and social media content that is understandable and easy to act on
9. Addresses health literacy high-risk situations such as care transitions, communication about medicines
10. Communicates policies and service costs

(Adapted from Wong 2012:366)

ENTREPRENEURIAL NURSING ROLES

As nursing has grown as a profession in its own right, many nurses have explored opportunities beyond the traditional employee/employer relationship that has long been the hallmark of nursing practice. The community is an ideal setting for nurses to expand services into areas where needs are not being met, or into roles traditionally filled by other practitioners. There are numerous examples in the US and the UK where nurse practitioners and advanced practice nurses have taken an entrepreneurial approach to practice, establishing their own businesses and often providing access to populations underserved by other health practitioners. Their practice model is typically independent, directly accountable to the client, and established either as a profitable business, or for the purpose of consulting on health care, education or research (Wilson et al. 2012). The largest majority of nurse entrepreneurs are in the UK, and these nurses, like many nurse entrepreneurs in the US, manage their own health centres that provide a safety net for uninsured or underinsured people (Hansen-Turton et al. 2010; Wilson et al. 2012). These nurses are among the most well-known entrepreneurs in the profession and, like others, they are connected through a network that provides mutual support and advice on legal, marketing and professional issues (Online. Available: www.nurse-entrepreneur-network.com [accessed 2 May 2013). There are also a number of nurse entrepreneurs in Australia and New Zealand, some of whom are semi-retired academics who consult on nursing curricula, staff development or regulation, and others who provide research consultancies to clinicians, educators or health agencies.

Some of the changes in legislation and/or funding arrangements mentioned earlier in the chapter have led to a number of nurses in Australia and New Zealand establishing their own practice or business. Often though, it is simply the nurse seeing or creating an opportunity and being bold enough to take the first steps, often with very successful outcomes for both themselves as practitioners and for the communities with whom they work. In 1989, Annette Milligan was one of the first nurses in New Zealand to set up her own business, contracting directly with the Ministry of Health to provide sexual health services to the community (originally called Independent Nursing Practice, it is now called INP Medical to reflect the fact that Annette also employs doctors as well as nurses). Traditionally, sexual health services were provided by large non-governmental organisations such as the Family Planning Association or by District Health Boards. Annette broke down many of the barriers that had limited nurses from contracting directly with government to provide services. She has subsequently gone on to establish an occupational health service (Ramazzini), Health Click Ltd, which produces sexuality education resources with specialty resources available for people with learning disabilities, and is also founding trustee of the Safeguarding Children initiative established in 2011 aimed at preventing child abuse (INP, Online. Available: www.inp.co.nz/annette.html [accessed 28 April 2013).

Kim Carter is another nurse moving beyond the traditional boundaries of nursing practice in New Zealand. Frustrated by the lack of influence on her practice due to funding streams and employers that had more control over how she practised than she did, Kim formed a business partnership with a general practitioner in rural practice. She is an equal business director with the GP partner and both make financial and business decisions equally. The governance and clinical roles are separate with both Kim and the GP employed by the business to provide clinical services. Remuneration for clinical work is separate from any dividends or directors' fees. Both Kim and the GP had particular and compatible goals for the working environment they wanted to create and after two years in partnership, they believe they have developed a model that may work well for other nurse/GP partnerships (Carter 2012/13). Additionally, the rural community in which they work has benefited by the retention of primary care services that otherwise may have been lost as practitioners have retired or moved out of the area.

Wilson et al.'s (2012:3) research has found that these innovative approaches come from nurses with strong leadership skills, those with personal vision and passion, 'self-confidence, courage, integrity, self-disciplines, and the ability to take risks, deal with failure and articulate their goals', which are typically to improve health. Although some work in a 'for-profit' mode, many are social entrepreneurs, striving for social rather than financial gain. Australian nurse/psychologist/personal trainer Sue Vaughn is one such person, who began a company on the Gold Coast called 'Health Ventures' (www.healthventures.com.au). Sue has had a long-term commitment to promoting fitness among older people. The program combines cardiovascular exercise, strength, flexibility, agility and coordination training as part of the Gold Coast City Council's 'Get Active' initiative. Subsidised by the council, participants pay a nominal fee which helps cover the rental and equipment used. The program has been so successful Sue has undertaken a study with women 65–75 years of age which shows substantial improvements in mental abilities as well as physical fitness and balance (see Chapter 11).

Some Australian nurse entrepreneurs have collaborated with general practitioners to provide new models of practice to enhance patient access to timely, efficient care. However, other entrepreneurial nurse practitioners have had a mixed reception by GPs. In Western Australia, the 'Revive Clinics' have had an interesting history since 2008 when they first began offering out of hours services in local pharmacies to help deal with GP shortages and long waiting lists at emergency departments (www.reviveclinic.com.au). Services are funded by Medicare, and evaluation data indicate that patients are very satisfied with the services and their location, which allows access to pharmacist advice as well as that of the nurses. After seeing 20 000 patients, the business is about to expand Australia wide. However the nurses have attracted a backlash from members of the medical profession, who have instituted a media campaign to warn GPs that they stand to lose up to 50% of their business in treating minor ailments (*Medical Observer*, Online. Available: www.medicalobserver.com.au [accessed 2 May 2013]). Undaunted, the nurses continue to focus on the patient, convinced that their combination of social and economical entrepreneurship is the essential element that motivates their practice. As UK medical practitioners have concluded, the major value in acknowledging nurse entrepreneurs accrues to the patient, through greater efficiency and effectiveness of the system, which negates the 'Turf Wars' that arise from monolithic provider models of care (Traynor et al. 2008). We revisit this issue in Chapter 14, in discussing the future of health care systems.

CASE STUDY: Occupational health for the Smiths and Masons

The occupational health nurses employed by the mining company that employs Jason and Colin, have developed several employee programs to support healthy lifestyles. They are experienced nurses who understand the social and geographic problems faced by the mining community and who work closely with safety personnel to deal with injuries and risks to wellbeing. Jason and Colin have been fortunate in not requiring any primary care services, but both are feeling the effects of isolation, after one year of employment in the mine. Both are connected to their families via the internet and have had relatively stable internet access with only few disruptions. Colin attended one of the sessions put on by the OHN for stress management but didn't attend a second. He and Jason tend to go to the pub when they have a break, but otherwise stay in the men's quarters instead of socialising with the others.

The Maddington child and school health nurses are familiar with the difficulties of FIFO families and run a number of support groups to help enhance their capacity to cope with the lifestyle. Practice nurses in the area are also aware of the issues faced by the FIFO families in the communities, and the PN attached to Rebecca's GP practice had a discussion with her about her lifestyle the last time they met, which was at her exercise group, where both are trying to lose weight.

As FIFO families are uncommon in the Papakura community the nurses are not familiar with the issues faced by Jason and Huia; however, the local practice nurse has been able to help Huia to manage Jake's asthma. In addition the exercise group that Huia volunteers with at the local Marae has been developed by a new Māori nurse practitioner in the area. She has identified access issues for the local Māori community and has been contracted with the local primary health organisation to provide services for local Māori.

REFLECTING ON THE BIG ISSUES

- There is considerable overlap in nurses' roles in the community, with the need for population and place-based interactions that incorporate physical, mental and social needs.

- Primary, secondary and tertiary prevention activities are integral to all community nursing roles.

- Many aspects of the roles are related to the practice setting and the regulatory environment that determines their scope of practice.

- Population ageing and increasing rates of chronic illnesses have a significant impact on the roles of nurses in all community settings.

- All nursing specialties in the community suffer from a lack of research evidence that would advance the knowledge base and help provide role clarity.

- Models of interdisciplinary collaboration in practice and research can provide better health outcomes in communities.

- Nurses' professional activities could be enhanced by standardising titles and expectations, and developing evaluation studies of the impact of their practice on community health and wellness.

REFLECTIVE QUESTIONS: How would I use this knowledge in practice?

1 What elements of primary health care are transferable across the range of nursing roles?

2 As a practice nurse what would be your role in working with Rebecca to help her, the children and Colin deal with his occupational situation?

3 What would be the most important implications of Jason and Huia residing in a New Zealand community as the only FIFO family in the neighbourhood?

4 As the school nurse, what would be your approach to assessing John's developmental progress?

5 What four major elements would Emily's school nurse be planning to help her become more engaged in her studies?

6 As the occupational health nurse how could you help Jason keep his blood pressure under control?

7 As the child health nurse, to what resources would you refer Huia to manage Jake's asthma?

8 How would you research the impact of the OHN role on worker health in the mining community?

References

Abramowitz, S., Flattery, D., Franses, K., et al., 2010. Linking a motivational interviewing curriculum to the chronic care model. J. Gen. Intern. Med. 25 (Suppl. 4), 620–626.

Allan, J., Annells, M., Clark, E., et al., 2012. Mixed methods evaluation research for a mental health screening and referral clinical pathway. Worldviews Evid. Based Nurs. doi:10.1111/j.1741-6787.2011.00226.x.

Australian Government Department of Health and Ageing, 2010. Building a 21st century primary health care system. Australia's first national primary health care strategy. AGPS, Canberra.

Australian Government Department of Health and Ageing, 2011. Practice Nurse Incentive Payments Guidelines. AGPS, Canberra.

Australian Government Department of Education, Employment and Workplace Relations, 2011. Early Childhood Policy Agenda. AGPS, Canberra.

Australian Government Productivity Commission, 2011. Early childhood development workforce. AGPS, Canberra.

Australian Health Ministers, 2009. National Mental Health Policy 2008. AGPS, Canberra.

Australian Institute of Health and Welfare, 2010. About chronic disease. Online. Available <www.aihw.gov.au/chronic-disease-publications/> 30 March 2013

Aziz, B., 2009. Making more of nurses. Occup. Health (Auckl) 61 (5), 22–23.

Bagshaw, S., 2011. Sexually healthy young people. In: Gluckman, P. (Ed.), Improving the transition: Reducing social and psychological morbidity during adolescence. Office of the Prime Minister's Advisory Committee, Wellington, pp. 133–144.

Baisch, M., Lundeen, S., Murphy, K., 2011. Evidence-based research on the value of school nurses in an urban school system. J. Sch. Health 81 (2), 74–80.

Basch, C., 2011. Healthier students are better learners: A missing link in school reforms to close the achievement gap. J. Sch. Health 81 (1), 593–598.

Baker Laughlin, C., Beisel, M., 2010. Evolution of the chronic care role of the registered nurse in primary care. Nurs. Econ. 28 (6), 409–414.

Barnes, M., Courtney, M., Pratt, J., et al., 2004a. School-based youth health nurses: Roles, responsibilities, challenges, and rewards. Public Health Nurs. 21 (4), 316–322.

Barnes, M., Walsh, A., Courtney, M., et al., 2004b. School based youth health nurses' role in assisting young people access health services in provincial, rural and remote areas of Queensland, Australia. Rural Remote Health 4, 279. Online. Available: <http://rrh.deakin.edu.au/> 22 August 2009.

Belle, M., Willis, K., 2013. Professional practice in contested territory: Child health nurses and maternal sadness. Contemp. Nurse 43 (2), 152–161.

Benkert, R., Templin, T., Myers Schim, S., et al., 2011. Testing a multi-group model of culturally competent behaviors among underrepresented nurse practitioners. Res. Nurs. Health. 34, 327–341.

Bidmead, C., Davis, H., Day, C., 2002. Partnership working: What does it really mean? Community Pract. 75 (7), 256–259.

Bloomer, M., Cross, W., 2011. An exploration of the role and scope of the Clinical nurse consultant (CNC) in a metropolitan health service. Collegian 18, 61–69.

Borrow, S., Munns, A., Henderson, S., 2011. Community-based child health nurses: An exploration of current practice. Contemp. Nurse 40 (1), 71–86.

Boyle, F., Mutch, A., Dean, J., et al., 2011. Increasing access to consumer health organisations among patients with chronic disease—a randomised trial of a print-based intervention. Prim. Health Care Res. Dev. 12 (3), 245–254.

Brennan, W., 2010. Safer lone working: assessing the risk for health professionals. Br. J. Nurs. 19 (22), 428–430.

Brooks, F., Kendall, S., Bunn, F., et al., 2007. The school nurse as navigator of the school health journey: developing the theory and evidence for policy. Prim. Health Care Res. Dev. 8, 226–234.

Brown, S., Nobiling, B., Teufel, J., et al., 2011. Are kids too busy? Early adolescents' perceptions of discretionary activities, overscheduling, and stress. J. Sch. Health 81 (9), 574–580.

Bruce, E., Klein, F., Keleher, H., 2012. Parliamentary inquiry into health promoting schools in Victoria: Analysis of stakeholder views. J. Sch. Health 82 (9), 441–447.

Buckley, S., Gerring, Z., Cumming, J., et al., 2012. School nursing in New Zealand: A study of services. Policy Polit. Nurs. Pract. 13 (1), 45–53.

Burgel, B., Childre, F., 2012. The occupational health nurse as the trusted clinician in the 21st century. Workplace Health Saf. 60 (4), 143150.

Bushy, A., 2000. Orientation to nursing in the rural community. Sage, Thousand Oaks.

Buss, J., 2012. Associations between obesity and stress and shift work among nurses. Workplace Health Saf. 60 (10), 453–458.

Callander, R., Ning, L., Crowley, A., et al., 2011. Consumers and carers as partners in mental health research: Reflections on the experience of two project teams in Victoria, Australia. Int. J. Ment. Health Nurs. 20, 263–273.

Cant, R., Birks, M., Porter, J., et al., 2011. Developing advanced rural nursing practice: A whole new scope of responsibility. Collegian 18, 177–182.

Carryer, J., Boddy, J., Budge, C., 2011. Rural nurse to nurse practitioner: an ad hoc process. J. Prim. Health Care 3 (1), 23–28.

Carryer, J., 2012. An area of workforce development: catch 22. Te Puawai August, 4.

Carter, K., 2012/13. To boldly go ... some thoughts on buying a general practice. Nurs. Rev. 13 (2), 8–9.

Chamberlain-Salaun, J., Mills, J., Park, T., 2011. Mental health nurses employed in Australian general practice: Dimensions of time and space. Int. J. Ment. Health Nurs. 20, 112–118.

Chiarella, M., Salvage, J., McInnes, E., 2010. Celebrating connecting with communities: coproduction in global primary health care. Prim. Health Care Res. Dev. 11, 108–122.

Clancy, A., Svensson, T., 2010. Perceptions of public health nursing consultations: tacit understanding of the importance of relationships. Prim. Health Care Res. Dev. 11 (4), 363–373.

Clendon, J., 2004/5. Demonstrating outcomes in a nurse-led clinic: How primary health care nurses make a difference to children and their families. Contemp. Nurse 18 (1/2), 164–176.

Clendon, J., 2009. Motherhood and the Plunket book: a social history. Unpublished doctoral thesis. Massey University, New Zealand.

Clendon, J., 2010. Government policies open up new roles for primary mental health nurses. Kai Tiaki Nursing New Zealand 16 (8), 20–22.

Clendon, J., Dignam, D., 2010. Child health and development record book: tool for relationship building between nurse and mother. J. Adv. Nurs. 66 (5), 968–977.

Clendon, J., Carryer, J., Walker, L., et al., 2013. Nurse perceptions of the Diabetes Get Checked Programme. Nurs. Prax. N. Z. 29 (3), 18–30.

Clendon, J., Walker, L., 2011. Characteristics of younger nurses in New Zealand: implications for retention. Kai Tiaki Nursing Research 2 (1), 4–11.

Clendon, J., Walker, L., 2013. Nurses aged over 50 and their experiences of shiftwork. J. Nurs. Manag. doi:10.1111/jonm.12157.

Comino, E., Harris, E., 2003. Maternal and infant services: examination of access in a culturally diverse community. J. Paediatr. Child Health 39, 95–99.

Commonwealth of Australia, 2009. Capabilities for supporting prevention and chronic condition self-management. DOHA and Flinders University, Canberra.

Connor, M., Nelson, K., Maisey, J., 2009. The impact of funding on a rural health nursing service: the Reporoa experience. Nurs. Prax. N. Z. 25 (2), 4–14.

Coombs, T., Curtis, J., Crookes, P., 2012. What is the process of comprehensive mental health nursing assessment? Results from a qualitative study. Int. Nurs. Rev. 60, 96–102.

Coyle, M., Al-Motlaq, M., Mills, J., et al., 2010. An integrative review of the role of registered nurses in remote and isolated practice. Aust. Health Rev. 34 (2), 239–245.

CRANA Council of Remote Area Nurses of Australia, 2003. Aust. J. Rural Health 11, 107.

Crawford, P., Brown, B., Majomi, P., 2007. Professional identity in community mental health nursing: a thematic analysis. Int. J. Nurs. Stud. 45, 1055–1063.

Crollard, A., de Castro, A., Tsai, H., 2012. Occupational trajectories and immigrant worker health. Workplace Health Saf. 60 (11), 497–502.

Dawson, A., 2011. Home based nursing service aims to reduce health inequalities. Profile 2011 Kai Tiaki Nursing New Zealand 17 (3), 12–13.

DeBell, D., 2006. School nurse practice: a decade of change. Community Pract. 79 (10), 324–327.

Dickson, V., McCauley, L., Riegel, B., 2008. Work-heart balance: The influence of biobehavioral variables on self-care among employees with heart failure. AAOHN J. 56 (2), 63–73.

Dowell, A., Garrett, S., Collings, S., et al., 2009. Evaluation of the primary mental health initiatives : Summary report 2008. University of Otago and Ministry of Health, Wellington.

Downie, J., Chapman, R., Orb, A., et al., 2002. The everyday realities of the multi-dimensional role of the high school community nurse. Aust.J. Adv. Nurs. 19 (3), 15–24.

Downie, J., Clark, K., Clementson, K., 2004-5. Volunteerism: Community mothers in action. Contemp. Nurse 18 (1/2), 188–198.

Driscoll, A., Harvey, C., Green, A., et al., 2012. National nursing registration in Australia: A way forward for nurse practitioner endorsement. J. Acad. Nurse Pract. 24, 143–148.

Duffield, C., Gardner, G., Chang, A., et al., 2011. National regulation in Australia: A time for standardization in roles and titles. Collegian 18, 45–49.

Duke, M., Street, A., 2003. Hospital in the home: constructions of the nursing role—a literature review. J. Clin. Nurs. 12, 852–859.

Edwards, N., MacLean Davison, C., 2008. Social justice and core competencies for public health. Can. J. Public Health 99 (2), 130–132.

Elsom, S., Happell, B., Manias, E., 2009. Informal role expansion in Australian mental health nursing. Perspect. Psychiatr. Care 45 (1), 45–53.

Expert Advisory Group on Primary Health Care Nursing, 2003. Investing in health: Whakatohutia te Oranga Tangata A Framework for activating primary health care nursing in New Zealand. Ministry of Health, New Zealand, Wellington.

Felblinger, D., Gates, D., 2008. Domestic violence screening and treatment in the workplace. AAOHN J. 56 (4), 143–150.

Ferriolo, A., Acree Conlon, H., 2012. Pain management in occupational health. Workplace Health Saf. 60 (12), 525–530.

Finlayson, M., Sheridan, N., Cumming, J., 2009. Nursing developments in primary health care 2001-2007. Victoria University of Wellington, Wellington. Online. Available: <http://www.vuw.ac.nz> 10 August 2009.

Flinders University, 2013. The Flinders Program, School of Medicine. Online. Available <www.flinders.edu.au/medicine/sites/fhbhru/self-management.cfm> March 30 2013.

Foster, K., O'Brien, L., Korhonen, T., 2012. Developing resilient children and families when parents have mental illness: A family-focused approach. Int. J. Ment. Health Nurs. 21, 3–11.

Francis, K., Mills, J., 2011. Sustaining and growing the rural nursing and midwifery workforce: Understanding the issues and isolating directions for the future. Collegian 18, 55–60.

Gagan, M., Maybee, P., 2011. Patient satisfaction with nurse practitioner care in primary care settings. Aust.J. Adv. Nurs. 28 (4), 12–19.

Gardner, K., Bailie, R., Si, D., et al., 2011. Reorienting primary health care for addressing chronic conditions in remote Australia and the South Pacific: Review of evidence and lessons from an innovative quality improvement process. Aust. J. Rural Health 19, 111–117.

Ghaddar, S., Valerio, M., Garcia, C., et al., 2012. Adolescent health literacy: The importance of credible sources for online health information. J. Sch. Health 82 (1), 28–36.

Graham, E., Duffield, C., 2010. An ageing nursing workforce. Aust. Health Rev. 34, 44–48.

Green, C., Kler, P., Leeves, G., 2007. Immigrant overeducation: Evidence from recent arrivals to Australia. Econ. Educ. Rev. 26, 420–432.

Green, R., Reffel, J., 2009. Comparison of administrators' and school nurses' perceptions of the school nurse role. J. Sch. Nurs. 25 (1), 62–71.

Grootjans, J., Newman, S., 2013. The relevance of globalization to nursing: a concept analysis. Int. Nurs. Rev. 60, 78–85.

Guzys, D., Kenny, A., Bish, M., 2013. Sustaining secondary school nursing practice in Australia: A qualitative study. Nurs. Health Sci. doi:10.1111/nhs.12039.

Haag, A., 2013. Writing a successful business plan. Workplace Health Saf. 61 (1), 19–29.

Halcomb, E., Hickman, L., 2010. Development of a clinician-led research agenda for general practice nurses. Aust.J. Adv. Nurs. 27 (3), 4–11.

Halcomb, E., Davidson, P., Brown, N., 2010. Uptake of Medicare chronic disease items in Australia by general practice nurses and Aboriginal health workers. Collegian 17, 57–61.

Hallett, C., Pateman, B., 2000. The 'invisible assessment': the role of the staff nurse in the community setting. J. Clin. Nurs. 9, 751–762.

Hamden, A., Newton, R., McCauley-Elsom, K., et al., 2011. Is deinstitutionalization working in our community? Int. J. Ment. Health Nurs. 20, 274–283.

Hanson-Turton, T., Bailey, D., Torres, N., et al., 2010. Nurse-managed health centers: Key to a healthy future. Am. J. Nurs. 110 (9), 23–26.

Happell, B., Hoey, W., Gaskin, C., 2012a. Community mental health nurses, caseloads, and practices: A literature review. Int. J. Ment. Health Nurs. 21, 131–137.

Happell, B., Scott, D., Nankivell, J., et al., 2012b. Nurses' views on training needs to increase provision of primary care for consumers with serious mental illness. Perspect. Psychiatr. Care ISSN 0031-5990.

Hardy, S., 2012. Training practice nurses to improve the physical health of patients with severe mental illness: Effects on beliefs and attitudes. Int. J. Ment. Health Nurs. 21, 259–265.

Hart, C., Parker, R., Patterson, E., et al., 2012. Potential roles for practice nurses in preventive care for young people. A qualitative study. Aust. Fam. Physician 41 (8), 618–621.

Harvey, C., Driscoll, A., Keyzer, D., 2011. The discursive practices of nurse practitioner legislation in Australia. J. Adv. Nurs. 67 (11), 2478–2487.

Harvey, S., Fisher, L., Green, V., 2012. Evaluating the clinical efficacy of a primary care-focused, nurse-led, consultation liaison model for perinatal mental health. Int. J. Ment. Health Nurs. 21, 75–81.

Hatem, M., Sandall, J., Devane, D., et al., 2008. Midwife-led versus other models of care for childbearing women. Cochrane Database Syst. Rev. (4), CD004667.

Hedley, C., Thompson, S., Morris Matthews, K., et al., 2012. The B4 school check behaviour measures: findings from the Hawke's Bay evaluation. Nurs. Prax. N. Z. 28 (3), 13–23.

Henderson, J., Willis, E., Walter, B., et al., 2008. Community mental health nursing: keeping pace with care delivery? Int. J. Ment. Health Nurs. 17, 162–170.

Henwood, T., Eley, R., Parker, D., et al., 2009. Regional differences among employed nurses: A Queensland study. Aust. J. Rural Health 17, 201–207.

Hogg, R., Kennedy, C., Gray, C., et al., 2012. Supporting the case for 'progressive universalism' in health visiting: Scottish mothers and health visitors' perspectives on targeting and rationing health visiting services, with a focus on the Lothian Child Concern Model. J. Clin. Nurs. 22, 240–250.

Holden, L., Williams, I., Patterson, E., et al., 2012. Uptake of Medicare chronic disease management incentives. A study into service providers' perspectives. Aust. Fam. Physician 41 (12), 973–977.

Holm, A., Severinsson, E., 2012. Chronic care model for the management of depression: Synthesis of barriers to, and facilitators of, success. Int. J. Ment. Health Nurs. 21, 512–523.

Holt, H., 2010. Health and labour force participation. New Zealand Treasury Working Paper 10/03. New Zealand Treasury, Wellington New Zealand.

Humphreys, J., Gregory, G., 2012. Celebrating another decade of progress in rural health: What is the current state of play? Aust. J. Rural Health 20, 156–163.

Hurley, J., Linsley, P., 2007. Expanding roles within mental health legislation: an opportunity for professional growth or a missed opportunity? J. Psychiatr. Ment. Health Nurs. 14, 535–541.

International Council of Nurses: International Nurse practitioner-advanced nursing network, research sub-group, 2001. Online. Available <http://icn-apnetwork.org> March 26 2013.

International Council of Nurses, International Nurse-Practitioner-Advanced Practice Nursing Network, 2005. Scope of practice, standards and competencies of the advanced practice nurse. Online. Available: <http://icn.aanp.org> 27 March 2013.

Jackson, D., Saltman, D., 2011. Recognising the impact of social exclusion: The need for advocacy and activism in health care. Editorial. Contemp. Nurse 40 (1), 57–59.

Jacobs, S., 2007. The pivotal role of politics in advancing nursing practice. Kai Tiaki Nursing New Zealand 13 (11), 14–16.

Johnston, S., Liddy, C., Mill, K., et al., 2012. Building the evidence base for chronic disease self-management support interventions across Canada. Can. J. Public Health 103 (60), 462–467.

Jones Warren, B., 2011. Two sides of the story: The bully and the bullied. J. Psychosoc. Nurs. 49 (10), 22–29.

Journal of School Nursing, 2008. The American Academy of Pediatrics Policy Statement. The role of the school nurse in providing school health services. J. Sch. Nurs. 24 (5), 269–274.

Joyce, C., Piterman, L., 2011. The work of nurses in Australian general practice: A national survey. Int. J. Nurs. Stud. 48, 70–80.

Kawi, J., 2012. Self-management support in chronic illness care: A concept analysis. Research and Theory for Nursing Practice. Int. J. 26 (3), 108–125.

Keatinge, D., Fowler, C., Briggs, C., 2007. Evaluating the Family Partnership Model (FPM) program and implementation in practice in New South Wales, Australia. Aust.J. Adv. Nurs. 25 (2), 28–35.

Keleher, H., Joyce, C., Parker, R., et al., 2007. Practice nurses in Australia: current issues and future directions. Med. J. Aust. 187 (2), 108–166.

Keleher, H., Parker, R., Abdulwadud, O., et al., 2009. Systematic review of the effectiveness of primary care nursing. Int. J. Nurs. Pract. 15, 16–24.

Kilpatrick, S., Cheers, B., Gilles, M., et al., 2009. Boundary crossers, communities, and health: Exploring the role of rural health professionals. Health Place 15, 284–290.

King, A., Boyd, M., Carver, P., et al., 2011. Evaluation of a gerontology nurse specialist in primary health care: case finding, care co-ordination and service integration for at-risk older people. Workforce New Zealand Innovation Projects Funding, Waitemata PHO, Waitemata DHB, University of Auckland, Auckland New Zealand.

Kitson, A., Conroy, T., Wengstrom, Y., et al., 2010. Defining the fundamentals of care. Int. J. Nurs. Pract. 16, 423–434.

Kitzman, H., Olds, D., Cole, R., et al., 2010. Enduring effects of prenatal and infancy home visiting by nurses on children: Follow-up of a randomized trial among children at age 12 years. Arch. Pediatr. Adolesc. Med. 164 (5), 412–418.

Knight, T., 2012. Heart health programme making big difference. Short Takes Newsletter of the New Zealand Occupational Health Nurses Association. Available: <http://www.nzohna.org.nz/uploaded/file/Short%20 Takes%20Feb%202012.pdf> 27 April 2013.

Kool, B., Thomas, D., Moore, D., et al., 2008. Innovation and effectiveness: Changing the scope of school nurses in New Zealand secondary schools. Aust. N. Z. J. Public Health 32 (2), 177–180.

Krothe, J., Clendon, J., 2006. Perceptions of nurse-managed clinics: A cross-cultural study. Public Health Nurs. 23 (3), 242–249.

Kruske, S., Barclay, L., Schmied, V., 2006. Primary health care, partnership and polemic: Child and family health nursing support in early parenting. Aust. J. Prim. Health 12 (2), 57–65.

Kruske, S., Grant, J., 2012. Educational preparation for maternal, child and family health nurses in Australia. Int. Nurs. Rev. 59, 200–207.

Laurant, M., Reeves, D., Hermens, R., et al., 2004. Substitution of doctors by nurses in primary care. Cochrane Database Syst. Rev. 4, doi:10.1002/14651858.CD001271.pub2.

Lenthall, S., Wakerman, J., Opie, T., et al., 2009. What stresses remote area nurses? Current knowledge and future action. Aust. J. Rural Health 17, 208–213.

Lenthall, S., Wakerman, J., Opie, T., et al., 2011. Nursing workforce in very remote Australia, characteristics and key issues. Aust. J. Rural Health 19, 32–37.

Litchfield, M., 2004. Achieving health in a rural community: A case study of nurse-community partnership. Central Publishing Bureau, Hastings New Zealand.

Litmus Ltd, 2013. Implementation and formative evaluation of the rheumatic fever prevention programme—final report. Litmus Ltd, Wellington.

Lipscomb, J., Sokas, R., McPhuL, K., et al., 2009. Occupational blood exposure among unlicensed home care and home care registered nurses: Are they protected? Am. J. Ind. Med. 52 (7), 563–570.

Lipscomb, J., Schoenfisch, A., Shishlov, K., et al., 2010. Nonfatal tool—or equipment-related injuries treated in US emergency departments among workers in the construction industry 1998-2005. Am. J. Ind. Med. 53 (6), 581–587.

Lobaton Cabrera, S., Beaton, R., 2009. The role of occupational health nurses in terrorist attacks employing radiological dispersal devices. AAOHN J. 57 (3), 112–119.

Long, K., Weinert, C., 1989. Rural nursing: Developing the theory base. In: Lee, H., Winters, C. (Eds.), Rural nursing: concepts, theory and practice, second ed. Springer, New York, pp. 3–16.

Lusk, S., Hagerty, B., Gillespie, B., et al., 2004. Acute effects of workplace noise on blood pressure and heart rate. Arch. Environ. Health 59 (8), 392–399.

Machado, R., Tomlinson, V., 2011. Bridging the gap between primary care and mental health. J. Psychosoc. Nurs. 49 (11), 25–29.

Maloney-Moni, J., 2006. Kia mana: A synergy of well-being. Copy Press, Nelson New Zealand.

Marinescu, L., 2007. Integrated approach for managing health risks at work—the role of occupational health nurses. AAOHN J. 55 (2), 75–87.

Maslow, G., Haydon, A., McRee, A., et al., 2012. Protective connections and educational attainment among young adults with childhood-onset chronic illness. J. Sch. Health 82 (8), 364–370.

Mazza, D., Shand, L., Warren, N., et al., 2011. General practice and preventive health care: a view through the eyes of community members. Med. J. Aust. 195 (40), 180–183.

McCarver, P., 2011. Success of a diabetes health management program in employer-based health care centers. AAOHN J. 59 (12), 513–518.

McCauley, L., 2012. Research to practice in occupational health nursing. Workplace Health Saf. 60 (40), 183–189.

McCoy, C., 2009. Professional development in rural nursing: challenges and opportunities. J. Contin. Educ. Nurs. 40 (3), 128–131.

McGovern, P., Dowd, B., Gjerdingen, D., et al., 2007. Mothers' health and work related factors as 11 weeks post-partum. Ann. Fam. Med. 5 (6), 519–527.

McKinlay, E., Clendon, J., O'Reilly, S., 2012. Is our focus right? Workforce development for primary health care nursing. J. Prim. Health Care 4 (2), 141–149.

McKinlay, E., Garrett, S., McBain, L., et al., 2011. New Zealand general practice nurses' roles in mental health care. Int. Nurs. Rev. 58 (2), 225–233.

McCloughen, A., Gillies, D., O'Brien, L., 2011. Collaboration between mental health consumers and nurses: Shared understandings, dissimilar experiences. Int. J. Ment. Health Nurs. 20, 47–55.

McMurray, A., 2013. Healthy communities: the evolving roles of nursing. In: Daly, J., Speedy, S., Jackson, D. (Eds.), Contexts of Nursing, fourth ed. Elsevier, Sydney, pp. 305–323.

Mehta, S., Cornell, D., Fan, X., et al., 2013. Bullying climate and school engagement in ninth grade students. J. Sch. Health 83 (1), 45–52.

Mellor, G., St John, W., 2009. Managers' perceptions of the current and future role of occupational health nurses in Australia. AAOHN J. 57 (2), 79–87.

Merrick, E., Duffield, C., Baldwin, R., et al., 2012. Expanding the role of practice nurses in Australia. Contemp. Nurse 41 (1), 133–140.

Miller, C., 2011. An integrated approach to worker self-management and health outcomes. Chronic conditions, evidence-based practice, and health coaching. AAOHN J. 59 (11), 491–501.

Mills, C., Reid, P., Vaithianathan, R., 2012. The cost of child health inequalities in Aotearoa New Zealand: A preliminary scoping study. BMC Public Health 12, 384. doi:10.1186/1471-2458-12-384.

Mills, J., Birks, M., Hegney, D., 2010. The status of rural nursing in Australia: 12 years on. Collegian 17, 30–37.

Mills, J., Lindsay, D., Gardner, A., 2011. Nurse practitioners for rural and remote Australia: Creating opportunities for better health in the bush. Aust. J. Rural Health 19, 54.

Milne, R., Lennon, D., Stewart, J., et al., 2012. Incidence of acute rheumatic fever in New Zealand children and youth. J. Paediatr. Child Health 48 (8), 685–691.

Mitchell, C., Ellis, I., 2011. Promoting family and child health. In: Kralik, D., van Loon, A. (Eds.), Community Nursing in Australia, second ed. John Wiley & Sons, Milton, Qld, pp. 314–351.

Moses, K., Keneally, J., Bibby, H., et al., 2008. Beyond bandaids: Understanding the role of school nurses in NSW—Project summary report. Online. Available: <http://www/caah.chw.edu.au/projects/summary_report.pdf> 24 August 2009.

Nardi, D., 2011. Integrated physical and mental health care at a nurse-managed clinic. J. Psychosoc. Nurs. 49 (7), 28–34.

National Nursing and Nursing Education Taskforce, 2006. Final Report. Online. Available: <www.nnnet.gov.au> 30 March 2013.

National Party, 2012. Prime Minister's youth mental health initiative. National Party New Zealand, Wellington.

Nelson, K., Christensen, S., Aspros, B., et al., 2011. Adding value to stretched communities through nursing actions: The Wellington South Nursing Initiative. Contemp. Nurse 40 (1), 87–102.

Newhouse, R., Stanik-hutt, J., White, K., et al., 2011. Advanced practice nurse outcomes 1990-2008: A systematic review. Nurs. Econ. 29 (5), 230–250.

New Zealand Guidelines Group, 2012. New Zealand Primary Care Handbook 2012, second ed. New Zealand Guidelines Group, Wellington.

New Zealand Health Workforce Information Programme, 2009. Health workforce projections modeling: rural nursing workforce. Health Workforce New Zealand, Wellington New Zealand.

New Zealand Ministry of Health (NZMOH), 2001. The Primary Health Care Strategy. MOHNZ, Wellington.

New Zealand Ministry of Health (NZMOH), 2002. Primary mental health: A review of the opportunities. MOHNZ, Wellington.

New Zealand Ministry of Health (NZMOH), 2006. Te Kokiri: The Mental Health and Addiction Action Plan 2006-2015. MOHNZ, Wellington.

New Zealand Ministry of Health (NZMOH), 2008. The B4 school check: a handbook for practitioners. MOHNZ, Wellington.

New Zealand Ministry of Health (NZMOH), 2010. Changes to the well child/tamariki ora framework. MOHNZ, Wellington.

New Zealand Ministry of Health (NZMOH), 2012. Mātātuhi Tuawhenua: Health of Rural Māori 2012. MOHNZ, Wellington.

New Zealand Ministry of Health, Nursing Council of New Zealand, DHBNZ, NPAC-NZ, 2009. Nurse Practitioners: A healthy future for New Zealand. MOHNZ, Wellington.

New Zealand National Health Committee, 2007. Meeting the needs of people with chronic conditions. National Advisory on Health and Disability, Wellington.

New Zealand Nurses Organisation & The College of Nurses Aotearoa (NZ) Inc, 2007. Investing in health 2007: An update to the recommendations of Investing in health: A framework for activating primary health care nursing (2003, Ministry of Health). New Zealand Nurses Organisation & the College of Nurses Aotearoa (NZ) Inc, Wellington.

Nugus, P., Greenfield, D., Travaglia, J., et al., 2010. How and where clinicians exercise power: Interprofessional relations in health care. Soc. Sci. Med. 71, 898–909.

Nursing Council of New Zealand, 2008 Nurse Practitioner Scope of Practice Online. Available <www.nursingcouncil.org.nz/index.cfm/1,41,htm/Nurse-Practitioner> April 15 2013.

Nursing Council of New Zealand, 2012a. The New Zealand nursing workforce. Nursing Council of New Zealand, Wellington.

Nursing Council of New Zealand, 2012b. Annual report. Nursing Council of New Zealand, Wellington.

Nursing Council of New Zealand, 2013. Consultation on two proposals for registered nurse prescribing. Nursing Council of New Zealand, Wellington.

Nursing Review, 2012. NPs push the boundaries. RCNA, Canberra. August.

O'Brien, A., Hughes, F., Kidd, J., 2006. Mental health nursing in New Zealand primary health care. Contemp. Nurse 21 (1), 142–152.

O'Connor, M., Alde, P., 2011. Older persons' health and end-of-life care. In: Kralik, D., van Loon, A. (Eds.), Community Nursing in Australia, second ed. John Wiley & Sons, Milton, Qld, pp. 354–386.

Olavarria, M., Beaulac, J., Belanger, A., et al., 2009. Organizational cultural competence in community health and social care. J. Cult. Divers. 16 (4), 140–149.

Olszewski, K., Parks, C., Chikotas, N., 2007. Occupational safety and health objectives of Healthy People 2010 A systematic approach for occupational health nurses—Part 11. AAOHN J. 55 (3), 115–123.

Parker, R., Forrest, L., Ward, N., et al., 2013. How acceptable are primary health care nurse practitioners to Australian consumers? Collegian 20, 35–41.

Parker, D., Clifton, K., Shams, R., et al., 2012. The effectiveness of nurse-led care in general practice on clinical outcomes in adults with type 2 diabetes. Joanna Briggs Library of Systematic Reviews JBL 000242 10 (38), 2514–2558.

Paton, L., Grant, J., Tsourtos, G., 2013. Exploring mothers' perspectives of an intensive home visiting program in Australia: A qualitative study. Contemp. Nurse 43 (2), 191–200.

Phillips, C., Pearce, C., Hall, S., et al., 2009. Enhancing care, improving quality: the six roles of the general practice nurse. Med. J. Aust. 191 (2), 92–97.

Pope, W., 2011. Another face of health care disparity. Stigma of mental illness. J. Psychosoc. Nurs. 49 (9), 27–31.

Pulcini, J., Jelic, M., Gul, R., et al., 2010. An international survey on advanced practice nursing education, practice, and regulation. J. Nurs. Scholarsh. 42 (1), 31–39.

Randolph, S., 2012a. Strategic thinking. Workplace Health Saf. 60 (2), 52.

Randolph, S., 2012b. Living well with chronic disease. Workplace Health Saf. 60 (7), 244.

Reineholm, C., Gustavsson, M., Ekberg, K., 2011. Evaluation of job stress models for predicting health at work. Work 40 (2), 229–237.

Ridgway, L., Mitchell, C., Sheean, F., 2011. Information and communication technology (ICT) use in child and family nursing: What do we know and where to now? Contemp. Nurse 40 (1), 11–129.

Robbins, W., Wei, F., Elashoff, D., et al., 2008. Y:X sperm ratio in boron-exposed men. J. Androl. 29 (1), 115–121.

Roberts, J., Floyd, S., Thompson, S., 2011. The clinical nurse specialist in New Zealand: How is the role defined? Nurs. Prax. N. Z. 27 (20), 24–35.

Rogers, B., Goodno, L., 2000. Evaluation of interventions to reduce needlestick injuries in health care occupations. Am. J. Prev. Med. 18 (4suppl), 90–98.

Rogers, B., Marshall, J., Garth, K., et al., 2011. Focus on the aging worker. AAOHN J. 59 (10), 447–457.

Ross, J., 2011. Place-based practice: a New Zealand nursing education model. In: Molinari, D., Bushy, A. (Eds.), The rural nurse: transition to practice. Springer Publishing Ltd, New York, pp. 85–94.

Royal College of Nursing Australia (RCNA), 2006. Position Statement Advanced Practice Nursing. Online. Available <www.rcna.org.au> (27 March 2013).

Ryan, K., 2008. Health promotion of faculty and staff: the school nurse's role. J. Sch. Nurs. 24 (4), 183–190.

Salazar, M., Takaro, T., Gochfeld, M., et al., 2003. Occupational health services at ten US Department of Energy weapon sites. Am. J. Ind. Med. 43 (4), 418–428.

Schmied, V., Donovan, J., Kruske, S., et al., 2011. Commonalities and challenges: A review of Australian state and territory maternity and child health policies. Contemp. Nurse 40 (1), 106–117.

Schneiderman, J., 2006. Innovative pediatric nursing role: public health nurses in child welfare. Pediatr. Nurs. 32 (4), 317–323.

Schofield, R., Ganann, R., Brooks, S., et al., 2011. Community health nursing vision for 2020: Shaping the future. West. J. Nurs. Res. 33 (8), 1047–1068.

Schwem, M., 2009. Generalized public health and industrial nurses work together. Public Health Nurs. 26 (4), 380–382.

Searle, J., 2007. Nurse practitioner candidates: shifting professional boundaries. Australasian Emergency Nursing Journal 11, 20–27.

Seigart, D., Dietsch, E., Parent, M., 2013. Barriers to providing school-based health care: International case comparisons. Collegian 20, 43–50.

Sen, A., 2000. Development as freedom. Knopf, New York.

Shepherd, M., 2011. Behind the scales: Child and family health nurses taking care of women's emotional wellbeing. Contemp. Nurse 37 (2), 137–148.

Sheridan, N., Kenealy, T., Connolly, M., et al., 2011. Health equity in the New Zealand health care system: a national survey. Int. J. Equity Health 10, 45–55.

Shi, X., Tubb, L., Fingers, S., et al., 2013. Associations with physical activity and dietary behaviors with children's health and academic problems. J. Sch. Health 83 (1), 1–7.

Signal, L., Walton, M., Ni Mhurchu, N., et al., 2012. Tackling 'wicked' health promotion problems: a New Zealand case study. Health Promot. Int. 28 (1), 84–94.

Smith, S., Firmin, M., 2009. School nurse perspectives of challenges and how they perceive success in their professional nursing roles. J. Sch. Nurs. 25 (2), 152–162.

Spence, D., Garrick, H., McKay, M., 2012. Rebuilding the foundations: Major renovations to the mental health component of an undergraduate nursing curriculum. Int. J. Ment. Health Nurs. 21 (5), 409–418.

Starr, S., Wallace, D., 2011. Client perceptions of cultural competence of community-based nurses. J. Community Health Nurs. 28 (2), 57–69.

St John, W., Fraser, K., Bennett, E., 2007. Home visiting. In: St John, W., Keleher, H. (Eds.), Community Nursing Practice, Theory, Skills and Issues Crows Nest NSW. Allen & Unwin, pp. 230–248.

St Leger, D., Nutbeam, D., 1999. Health promotion in schools, The Evidence of Health Promotion Effectiveness. European Commission, Brussels, pp. 110–122.

Strasser, P., 2011. Scope of practice issues for occupational and environmental health nurses. AAOHN J. 59 (1), 12–14.

Thomas, E., 2011. Implementation of occupational health service improvements through application of total quality management processes. AAOHN J. 59 (6), 267–273.

Thompson, M., Wachs, J., 2012. Occupational health nursing in the United States. Workplace Health Saf. 60 (3), 127–133.

Torp, S., Grimsmo, A., Hagen, S., et al., 2012. Work engagement: a practical measure for workplace health promotion. Health Promot. Int. doi:.10.1093/heapro/das/022.

Traynor, M., Drennan, V., Goodman, C., et al., 2008. 'Nurse entrepreneurs' a case of government rhetoric. J. Health Serv. Res. Policy 13 (1), 13–18.

Tyrell, L., 2013. Mental health professionals are getting together—by many means. NRHA, Partyline, pp. 10–11.

Underwood, J., Mowat, D., Meagher-Stewart, D., et al., 2009. Building community and public health nursing capacity: A synthesis report of the national community health nursing study. Can. J. Public Health 100 (5), 1–10.

van de Bovenkamp, H., Trappenburg, M., 2012. Comparative review of family-professional communication: What mental health care can learn from oncology and nursing home care. Int. J. Ment. Health Nurs. 21, 366–385.

Villegas, W., Allen, P., 2012. Barriers to advanced practice registered nurse scope of practice: Issue analysis. J. Contin. Educ. Nurs. 43 (9), 403–409.

Wallace, M., 2009. Occupational health nurses—the solution to absence management? AAOHN J. 57 (3), 122–127.

Walker, L., Clendon, J., 2013. NZNO biennial employment survey. New Zealand Nurses Organisation, Wellington.

Walker, L., Clendon, J., 2012a. A multi-cultural nursing workforce: views of New Zealand and internationally qualified nurses. Kai Tiaki Nursing Research 3 (1), 4–11.

Walker, L., Clendon, J., 2012b. Ageing in place: retirement intentions of New Zealand nurses aged 50+. Proceedings of the New Zealand Labour and Employment Conference, Wellington.

Wallis, K., Smith, S., 2008. Developmental screening in pediatric primary care: the role of nurses. J. Spec. Pediatr. Nurs. 13 (2), 130–134.

Wand, T., 2013. Positioning mental health nursing practice within a positive health paradigm. Int. J. Ment. Health Nurs. 22, 116–124.

Ward-Griffin, C., McWilliam, C., Oudshoorn, A., 2012. Relational experiences of family caregivers providing home-based end-of-life care. J. Fam. Nurs. 18 (4), 491–516.

Weber, M., 2010. The importance of exercise for individuals with chronic mental illness. J. Psychosoc. Nurs. 48 (10), 35–40.

Weist, M., Mellin, E., Chambers, K., et al., 2012. Challenges to collaboration in school mental health and strategies for overcoming them. J. Sch. Health 82 (2), 97–105.

Weist, M., Paternite, C., Wheatley-Rowe, D., et al., 2009. From thought to action in school mental health promotion. International Journal of Mental Health Promotion 119 (3), 32–41.

Whitehead, D., 2006. The health-promoting school: what role for nursing? J. Clin. Nurs. 15, 264–271.

Wilkinson, J., 2012. Places for nurse practitioners to flourish: Examining third sector primary health care. Aust.J. Adv. Nurs. 29 (4), 36–42.

Wilson, H., Huntington, A., 2009. An exploration of the family partnership model in New Zealand. Blue Skies Report No 27/09. Families Commission, Wellington.

Wilson, A., Whitaker, N., Whitford, D., 2012. Rising to the challenge of health care reform with entrepreneurial and intrapreneurial nursing initiatives. Online J. Issues Nurs. 17 (2), Manuscript 5:1-13.

Wong, B., 2012. Building a health literate workplace. Workplace Health Saf. 60 (8), 363–369.

Wong, S., Regan, S., 2009. Patient perspectives on primary health care in rural communities: effects of geography on access, continuity and efficiency. Rural Remote Health 9 (1142), 1–12.

World Health Organization, 1996. Promoting health through schools. The World Health Organization Global School Health Initiative WHO, Geneva.

World Health Organization, 2007. Workers' health: global plan of action. Sixtieth World Health Assembly. WHO, Geneva.

World Health Organization, 2012. Chronic diseases. Online. <http://www.who.int/topics/chronic_diseases/en> 31 March 2013.

Yarwood, J., 2008. Nurses' views of family nursing in community contexts: an exploratory study. Nurs. Prax. N. Z. 2 (2), 41–51.

Zeller, J., Levin, P., 2013. Mindfulness interventions to reduce stress among nursing personnel. An occupational health perspective. Workplace Health Saf. 61 (2), 85–89.

Zinner, P., 2006. Preparing the work force for retirement—the role of occupational health nurses. AAOHN J. 54 (12), 531–536.

Useful websites

www.ngala.com.au—Early parenting support in Western Australia

www.tresillian.net—Early parenting support in New South Wales

www.plunket.org.nz—Royal New Zealand Plunket Society

www.starship.org.nz—New Zealand telemedicine programs

www.mindnet.org.nz—Vibe—mental health promotion and prevention newsletter

www.mentalhealth.org.nz—New Zealand mental health promotion

www.aifs.gov.au—Australian Institute of Family Studies

www.msd.govt.nz/what-we-can-do/families/index.html—New Zealand Families Today

www.kidshealth.org.nz—New Zealand kids health

www.anu.edu.au/aphcri—Australian Primary Health Care Research Institute

http://nrha.ruralhealth.org.au—Australian National Rural Health Alliance

www.cyh.com/SubContent.aspx?p=102—Australian Parent Helplines

www.australia.gov.au/topics/health-and-safety/occupational-health-and-safety—Australian Government sites for Occupational Health and Safety

www.moh.govt.nz/moh.nsf/indexmh/nursing-initiatives—Nursing initiatives in New Zealand

www.cph.co.nz/About-Us/Education-Settings/Health-Promoting-Schools.asp NZ Canterbury District Health Board site for Health Promoting Schools

www.chnwa.org.au—National Nursing and Nursing Education Taskforce (N3ET) NP standards

www.nzno.org.nz/groups/colleges/college_of_primary_health_care_nurses NZNO College of Primary Health Care Nurses website

www.mhpn.org.au—Mental Health Professionals' Network

Working with groups

CHAPTER 6

Introduction

Practising as an enabler of community health includes individual, community-level and group activities. This chapter focuses on working in groups to help people create and maintain their health, change their health behaviours or enhance their community. As experienced community nurses know, group work can be rewarding, particularly when group members energise and support one another. It can also be challenging, especially where individuals overwhelm the ideas of others by dominating the group, or when group members find the topic difficult to share. People behave in a myriad of ways when they participate in groups, sometimes unpredictably. To meet the goals of the group the leader must accommodate different cultures, attitudes, behaviours, experiences and styles of relating to other people. The markers of successful groups are varied, and linked to the extent to which participants feel they have been acknowledged, participated to the best of their ability, and achieved their goals and those of the group itself. This chapter outlines some of the theoretical foundations for group work, and provides examples of how groups are used by community nurses to help people achieve some of their goals for health and wellbeing. The discussion then moves to the specific strategies nurses are using to help people change and the important role of leadership in facilitating groups. The major outcome of the chapter is to show how group work can be a helpful tool for health promotion, recovery from illness and supportive, sustainable relationships in daily life. As with earlier chapters, we build the foundations for group work on the primary health care (PHC) philosophy and principles. We begin by explaining content and process issues in group work and how these are interrelated.

SUCCESSFUL GROUPS: CONTENT AND PROCESS

The success of group work depends on two main elements: content and process. In some cases, the content of the group is pre-determined by the reason it was constituted, which can be to provide group therapy, mutual support for a common issue or condition, to develop group or community solutions to problems, or a combination of all of these goals. Garcia et al.'s (2011) review of the literature on group work identifies nine different types of groups, with examples of those that may be used by nurses in community roles (see Box 6.1).

Community action groups are almost always formed from the grassroots ideas of people living in a certain community who become 'activated' by something that has been externally imposed on them. The anti-tobacco lobby is, to date, the most successful example of how members of the public in numerous countries banded together against the tobacco companies to help stamp out smoking in

OBJECTIVES

By the end of this chapter you will be able to:

1. identify the most important elements of successful group work
2. explain the differences between therapeutic, self-help, problem-solving and community action groups
3. develop a plan for conducting a therapeutic group for new mothers suffering from postnatal depression (PND) in the community
4. develop strategies for conducting a self-help group for employees with chronic illness in their work setting
5. develop a healthy school initiative that includes student and staff group work
6. identify the most significant principles in helping people change
7. explain the characteristics of effective leaders and their application to practice.

BOX 6.1 **Types of groups**

- Community activism (community development, capacity building)
- Support (peer groups for mutual support)
- Activity therapy (child health and development activities)
- Coaching (health education, promotion)
- Counselling (group therapy)
- Intervention (working with migrant groups)
- Psychoeducational (prevention of developmental risk factors)
- Psychotherapy (age-appropriate behaviour change)
- Therapy (therapies for mental health issues such as cognitive behavioural therapy (CBT), mindfulness, yoga, meditation, resilience training)

public places, eliminate tobacco advertising and educate the public about the hazards of smoking. Another community action that began in the last century became the international environment movement, once people began to see that the shift from an agrarian society to industrialised economies was harming the environment, and there were inadequate safeguards in place to ensure global sustainability for the next generations. These global movements have had numerous spinoff effects, where various communities have found their voice and articulated local needs in relation to global problems; the 'think global, act local' approach. The 'bugga up' campaign associated with the quit smoking campaign began in the 1970s with a group of public health professionals, who were determined to destroy tobacco advertisements, and did so, everywhere they could access them, beginning on the streets of Sydney. Since then, the community activist group 'GetUp!' (www.getup.org.au) has used the internet and social media effectively to make people aware of public policies that disadvantage certain groups in our society. Their objective is to ensure that members of the public have a voice in political decisions. This approach is also visible in the current major worldwide campaign by the 'lock the gate alliance' and other groups to communicate to citizens of the world the risks to the environment, especially rural lands, from explorations for coal seam gas (CSG). With internet communications and social media providing instant messages around the globe, the 'lock the gate alliance'

(www.lockthegate.org.au/groups), and the 'clean water healthy land' community action groups (www.cleanwaterhealthyland.org.au/content/building-community-action-groups) are able to attract an unprecedented number of concerned communities. The 'clean water healthy land' group goes beyond simply disseminating information by providing instructions for community activism, explaining online how to get people involved, to plan and to take action.

On a smaller scale, many local councils make decisions that spawn protests among citizens, who often react by lobbying for cleaner rivers, or more recreational facilities, child care, or police patrolling the streets, or socially responsible laws around issues such as problem gambling (see Box 6.2). Although there may be a group leader who initiates the lobby, in some cases the leadership is shared between smaller groups of people who typically have access to the tools for communicating with others. The role of nurses in this type of group is sometimes that of a knowledgeable participant who can provide advice on health and development matters. In other cases, nurses may decide to instigate a community group where political and policy decisions have compromised their ability to provide equitable, accessible services to the community. This type of action is often warranted by decisions that have created disadvantage or discriminated against the most vulnerable in society. The nurses who do get involved at this level use their advocacy skills to articulate to policymakers the difficulties people experience from discontinued rural health services, reduced child and school health services, or community support systems such as drop-in centres for the homeless or housing for the mentally ill or victims of violence. Leading a community action group is demanding and time-consuming, and although it is an important part of working with community groups, nurses often spend a larger proportion of their professional time in health promotion, support, self-help or therapeutic groups.

GROUP EXERCISE: Groups

In groups of three or four, list the elements that you think need to be present for successful group work—base this list on your own experiences in class or in other groups. As you work through the chapter add other elements to your list that you may uncover from the examples given.

BOX 6.2 **A grassroots community action group: Darci's story**

Darci Goldsworthy of Ngāpuhi descent, tells the story of his instigating a grassroots community action to prevent problem gambling in his New Zealand community. Darci grew up in a family of four brothers and two parents, originally in the North Island and then, when he was 10, rural Nelson in the South Island, where he attended the local school. When Darci was 14, his father was tragically killed in a forestry accident, leaving Darci to grow through his formative years with no father figure in the home. He left school at 16, and, following in his father's footsteps, entered the forestry industry where he worked for eight years. He bought his first home at 18 and became a father at age 20. After the breakdown of his relationship with the mother of his child, he took on full-time solo care of his daughter when she was three and then in 2011 also took on the care of his two nephews and niece. Darci's sense of responsibility extends to caring for his community. Victory is a small, socio-economically deprived community of Nelson—a community that has fought hard to build a sense of pride and ownership and that won the inaugural New Zealand Community of the Year in 2010. But in the same year, the local city council in Nelson changed their gambling policy to allow poker machines into communities where they had previously been banned. The policy change occurred without community consultation. Here Darci takes up the story:

'It all began for me when I read an article in the *Nelson Mail* about how the Nelson City Council had changed their Gambling Policy to allow nine pokie machines to be placed into the heart of our community of Victory, all for one Landlord's economic gain. This sparked outrage in me at how our local government would change a section of our gambling policy that was originally put in place to protect the overall wellbeing of communities from the harmful effects of gambling addictions, all for one man's economic gain!

Originally on my own I spoke with council, and I was then joined by another community member, David Johnston. We spoke with the Mayor, spoke in chambers with council, and finally set up a community meeting in Victory. The purpose of the first community meeting was to provide awareness of the situation and also to gather community support. During the meeting we were very alarmed to find that the majority of those who attended were completely unaware of what had happened, and how the changes to the gambling policy would affect the Victory community.

We held a further two community meetings, gaining increasing community support. It was not long after the third meeting that we formed the Nelson Gambling Task Force Incorporated Society. Once formed, I became Chairperson.'

Although they had no money, the Taskforce made submissions to the council and arranged a protest march. Despite these efforts, the council persisted with the changed policy, arguing that there was nothing the community could do until the policy came up for review again in three years' time. At this point, Darci and the Taskforce approached the local community law centre and with their support and a pro bono legal team, the community was able to challenge the city council in the high court and win. It took over two years, but eventually the efforts of the community paid off and the poker machines were removed.

Darci has since gone on to be a finalist in the Young Māori of the Year Awards in 2012 and has started studying philosophy, politics and economics at university. He is also an avid rapper and DJ, teaching rap classes to children at local primary schools, and DJ'ing and MC'ing at local festivals including running dance competitions and programs for children and youth. Darci has also made his own hip-hop music including a problem-gambling song, and has performed throughout New Zealand. Most recently he has spoken and performed at a rally in Adelaide and is starring in a Canadian documentary about the effects of problem gambling on indigenous people. You can view Darci's Rap about gambling on YouTube: www.youtube.com/watch?v=kIyXgmXBNdIv

Darci says he has grown immensely from the experience of taking on the fight to remove pokie machines from the Victory community—particularly in regard to social awareness, public health, processes of local governance, leadership, parenthood, communication, public speaking and team work. Darci again: 'Underestimate not the power of communities, but the words of those who choose not to understand unity. No matter how much faith we place in local or central government to do what is right for us as a whole, we must NEVER neglect the power we give them to bring about change.'

For more information on problem gambling in New Zealand, see www.choicenotchance.co.nz.

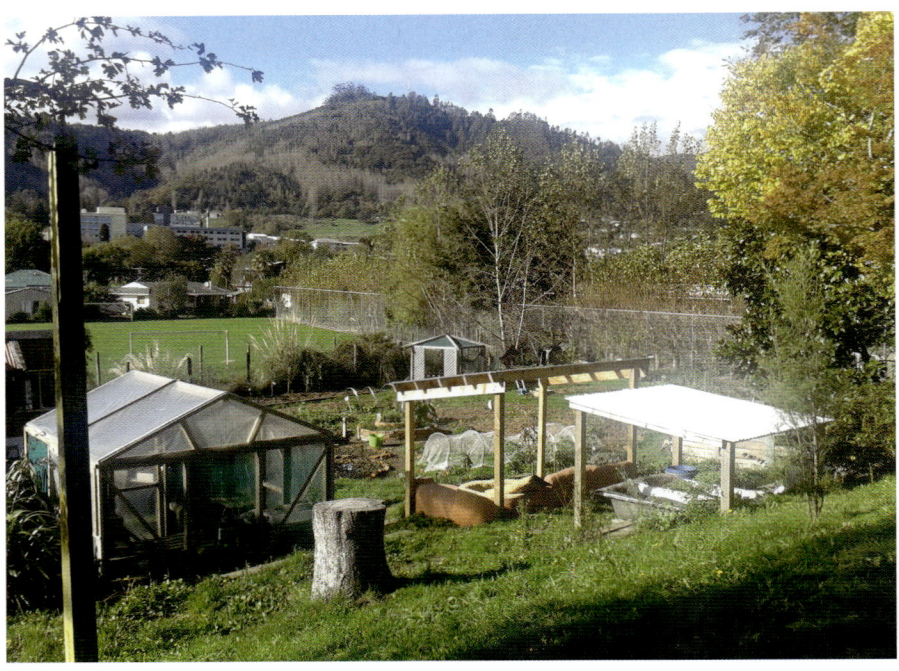

Victory community garden—part of the Victory Community Health Centre community hub (with permission)

REMINDER: PHC principles

- Equity of access to health care
- Appropriate technology
- Intersectoral collaboration
- Cultural sensitivity, safety
- Health promotion
- Community participation

When nurses get involved in community groups, either as a leader, member or support person, the principles of PHC should prevail (see Box 6.3). Some community development groups may be convened by local councils, schools or interest groups to lobby for resources that promote equity or bring about greater public participation. Other community groups are co-operatives of like-minded people who pool their resources to make the community a healthier place for their families or themselves. Examples include groups that build community gardens to improve food security for residents, mothers' groups that provide a social forum for sharing parenting information or neighbourhood exercise groups. These community groups are usually intended to maximise community capacity through access to opportunities or resources for health. Like other groups, community groups create

knowledge and appropriate supports for health through culturally sensitive discussion and interactions.

In the context of PHC our overriding goal is social justice, which is promoted through group empowerment. This means that, despite individual differences, when people work together in a group, the group can create 'bonding' or 'bridging' social capital (Townley et al. 2011). This doesn't mean that everyone in a group is similar, or that the group aims to promote uniformity, but by identifying themselves as a member of a group they can build solidarity and a sense of purpose (Townley et al. 2011). Sometimes, it is simply important to be there for the group. Solidarity can be motivating, inspiring faith in the group's collective wisdom and activism for change (Wiggins 2011). Each person who feels they have participated in the discussion may find the experience empowering in building self-esteem and the self-confidence to continue interacting (Wiggins 2011). Some groups are more similar or homogeneous than others, which has positives and negatives. The positives are evident in developing mutual support, such as occurs in cultural groups who are able to overcome racism or other oppressive circumstances by pulling together and developing a sense of physical and emotional safety. This is a type of 'bonding' social capital. A negative aspect of belonging to a homogeneous group may be in-group biases that create less favourable attitudes towards

BOX 6.3 Post-disaster groups for social justice

A classic example of the PHC approach in group work is reported by two of the counsellors who worked with victims of Hurricane Katrina and the San Diego Wildfires in the US, the earthquakes in Haiti and Costa Rica, Cyclone Nargis in Burma and the Thailand Tsunami (Bemak & Chung 2011). Using a social justice framework they facilitated groups to help people recover from these situations, and to help protect them against trauma and despair following the disasters. Using a group, rather than individual approach, they tried to help people work out ways to overcome the loss of their communities as well as the personal trauma, to build a sense of the future through hope, purpose and mastery. Groups were facilitated following a planned Disaster Cross-Cultural Counselling (DCCC) model. Cultural considerations were pre-eminent in all the groups, as the facilitators were sensitive to the fact that many people had lost friends and family members who helped sustain their cultural identity. They established a group ethos aimed at eliminating any cultural domination, so that participants could feel they had equal access to all interactions and group dynamics. Group process began by exploring people's existing coping strategies, gradually working to convey a sense of psychological safety. Next, the facilitators helped participants develop new coping skills through the formation of surrogate families, new communities, and new healing rituals that would help build social connections. This was particularly important in helping them overcome their existing sense of disenfranchisement and oppression that

was compounded by the disaster. The counsellors felt that many people who are victims of disasters are those who are already vulnerable because of a lack of access to resources, safe housing or other supports that impinge on their ability to recover from this type of major trauma. Their ongoing focus on social justice reminded people that they had equity of access to whatever measures would help them gain empowerment and recovery. The third step in the group process was aimed at groups exploring a combination of new and old coping strategies that could help foster hope, through group empowerment, and a sense of purpose and stability, by joining with others in forging the future and developing mastery over the small things that would help recovery. The fourth phase was aimed at psychological stability through discussions of meaning, purpose and realistic goals for the future; finding culturally appropriate solutions to any barriers that prevented them from developing the skills to move forward (Bemak & Chung 2011).

What aspects of this model could you apply in working as a community nurse or a volunteer following the natural disasters such as floods, bushfires and earthquakes that have occurred in Australia and New Zealand? How would you go about persuading others to use this type of approach?

? What research does this example suggest for working with groups in the context of your community?

other groups (Townley et al. 2011). The paradox of this type of situation is that a group may come together as a collective voice against those who discriminate against them, and without strong leadership, may actually become discriminatory towards others. One of the solutions is 'bridging' social capital, interacting across different social or demographic groups.

REMINDER

Bonding social capital—trusting and cooperative relationships between groups who have similar demographic or social characteristics

Bridging social capital—relations between individuals who are dissimilar with respect to social identity and power

Group process

Many groups are facilitated by interdisciplinary teams, which adds an extra dimension to group processes, and a number of advantages. Groups that incorporate the perspectives of other disciplines can enhance problem resolution, promote holistic views, and sometimes lead to collaboration for other problems (Clark 2003). Leadership development for group work, especially group counselling, is typically interdisciplinary, and this promotes collaborative problem-solving in the context of conducting groups. Some courses, such as the Diploma of Counselling provided by the Australian Institute of Professional Counsellors, are provided online, and others have a mix of online and face-to-face learning (Online, www.aipc.net.au/adwords.adw_diploma/?gclid=CKz _wcGL67sCFYHqpAod8gOAGg, www.group -counseling.com/index.html [accessed 8 January 2014]). In working with other disciplines, leadership that promotes good communication is critical to success. In some cases, co-facilitators or facilitators from different disciplines take turns leading the group, while in others, the leadership role is assigned to one individual who is able to provide a bridge between disciplines. Interprofessional input into the discussions and deliberations can promote efficiency and effectiveness in setting realistic goals and ensure the feasibility of plans, especially when the group is small, communication is clear, and the leader encourages a diversity of opinions (Xyrichis & Lowton 2008). Interdisciplinary groups also tend to attract organisational support, as they are seen as cost effective. They tend to encourage innovation and implementation of change through the synergies created between disciplines, which can strengthen partnerships that may be readily sustained (Cramm et al. 2013; Fatchett & Taylor 2013; Xyrichis & Lowton 2008).

PRACTICE STRATEGY

How do you think group dynamics change when the group is interdisciplinary?

What strategies would you use to ensure that everyone's opinion was heard and valued?

A similar dynamic occurs when groups combine professionals and volunteers from the communities, like the approach taken in the Community Mothers (CM) program, which began as a partnership between the Department of Health Western Australia, child health nurses, teaching staff from the School of Nursing and Midwifery at Curtin University, new parents and volunteer mothers from the Perth community (Downie et al. 2004–05). The volunteer mothers were recruited to visit first time parents during their first year of parenting, providing role support and helping them access local resources with maternal and child health nurses and teaching staff overseeing the program. The CM program included groups of volunteers who received professional guidance to help new mothers with parenting skills and support in several communities in Perth and nearby towns. The model was successful; however, with reductions in funding for local programs, CM has now been reframed as an Indigenous parenting initiative funded by the Commonwealth Better Health Initiative (CBHI) to provide parenting support in five regional communities with high needs (Munns 2010) (see Chapter 13).

Some groups are led by maternal and child health nurses or midwives, where nurses encounter group members through maternity care or child

health clinics. One such parenting group in Sydney, the Foundations for Young Parents program (FFYP) combines home visiting with a parenting program for younger parents in a socio-economically disadvantaged area of Sydney (Mills et al. 2012). The Sydney program connects expectant mothers by encouraging them to attend antenatal classes tailored to the needs of young mothers. A range of strategies are used to foster mutual support, including social networking and focusing on relationships as well as activities. Nurses involved in the program report that they use a partnership approach, balancing educational components about child care and developmental issues with topics that emerge from the participants. They described this aspect of the groups as being 'in the moment' with the young women, sharing their stories, building trust, role modelling and acknowledging their concerns (Mills et al. 2012:668). Like the Community Mothers program, the FFYP helps new mothers identify their assets and build on their strengths while they are connecting with others and developing parenting skills. Some groups adopt particular learning frameworks, while others are relatively pragmatic. One Australian group teaches parents the basic safety skills and works with participants in a relatively structured way using instruction, modelling, role-play, feedback and various exercises to ensure they are fully engaged in the process (AIFS, Online. Available www.aifs.giv.au/cfca/pubs/practice/a144434/index.html [accessed 6 May 2013]).

These groups represent a few select examples of parenting groups, which are part of a widespread movement by governments to assist parents. An important element of the parenting support agenda is a new Australian Parenting Research Centre (2012) that acts as a clearinghouse for research into the effectiveness of parenting programs internationally, and we discuss these further in Chapter 8. Although each group is different in its own way, it is always important to be receptive to the diversity of group participants, their opinions and behaviours, and group dynamics. When the group seems to need a more structured approach, facilitators often use a staged approach. Clark's (2003) model follows Tuckman's (1965) stages of 'forming', 'storming', 'norming' and 'performing', which she has adapted to reflect the components of the nursing process. The stages of group development are listed in Box 6.4 below.

Problem-solving groups

Although groups are formed for many reasons, many come together to address a common problem. To find solutions, these groups tend to use a relatively structured approach. In the first stage of the group, both the group and the problem are assessed,

BOX 6.4 **Stages and tasks of group development**

Stage	Tasks
1 Orientation (forming)	Selecting group members
(Assessment)	Training for group participation
	Identifying goals and purposes
2 Accommodation (storming, norming)	Establishing modes of decision-making
(Planning)	Developing mechanisms for conflict resolution
	Developing a communication network
	Developing a climate conducive to collaboration
Negotiating	Negotiating roles
	Developing methods for task assignment
3 Operation (performing)	Assigning specific tasks to accomplish goals
(Implementation)	Performing actions to accomplish goals
4 Dissolution (leaving)	Planning evaluation of outcomes
(Evaluation)	Assigning member roles and tasks in evaluation
	Data collection
	Analysis of evaluation data
	Possible group dissolution

(Source: Clark 2003:282)

reflecting content and process. Whether the group is intended for assessment, therapy, problem-solving, knowledge development, self-help, empowerment or lifestyle change, the group requires clarity of purpose. From the outset it is important to establish a constitution for the group, including the number of members, the timing and location of group meetings and what inclusion criteria were used to invite members. For problem-solving groups Clark (2003) recommends using her assessment tool to identify the dimensions of the problem (see Chapter 3). Based on these assessment data the nurse can then identify the strengths and weaknesses of the group, and any opportunities and threats to group process. The leader then helps clarify the goals of the group and encourages members to brainstorm ('storming') ideas for decision-making, including strategies for conflict resolution, communication and negotiating their respective roles in the group processes. We like to call these the rules of engagement. In groups that are focused on collaborative decision-making or community support groups, tasks and responsibilities can often be democratically decided, negotiated in the spirit of trust, respect and collaboration, with the leader 'on tap' rather than 'on top'.

GROUP GOALS

- Needs assessment
- Therapeutic interventions
- Problem-solving
- Knowledge development
- Self-help
- Community empowerment
- Lifestyle change

Communication strategies are crucial to problem-solving. Good communication skills include launching the discussion in a way that is informative but doesn't preclude others' ideas, controlling the fairness and flow of the discussions, ensuring that familiar language is used and that there is a balance between guided discussion and self-direction. These measures are intended to promote group cohesion. A skilful leader will be able to interpret the 'words' and 'music'; what is being said as well as what is not being said (Puskar et al. 2012). Again, where decisions are expected by the group it is often up to the leader to guide the group in selecting a decision-making strategy. Clark (2003) suggests that decisions can be made in one of six ways: by default, by the leader, by a subgroup, by majority vote, consensus or unanimous consent. In the process of assessing the group and establishing group processes and goals some of the questions that may arise include whether or not the 'problem' needs to be solved within the group or whether the group is simply establishing the foundation for problem-solving; the capacity to which the group seems to be able to work together; the expertise of members relative to the task, decision or roles; and whether there are any organisational constraints that may affect group process (Clark 2003).

ACTION POINT

The example provided by Garcia et al. addresses the explicit needs of girls. Can you think of some differences in group dynamics that should be anticipated in an adolescent boys' group?

Garcia et al. (2011) explain how all of these factors come together in the context of school health. They explain that groups can be the most appropriate strategy for connecting adolescents, especially girls, as their identity is often formed through relationships and verbal engagement. A well-facilitated group can help to enhance girls' psychological health, addressing issues of gender identity, self-confidence, authenticity in relationships and judgement skills. A good facilitator for such a group is 'respectful and patient, trustworthy and caring, engaging and relevant, and flexible. S/he must also be a role model and maintain self-awareness' (Garcia et al. 2011:430). The facilitator must also be knowledgeable about female adolescent development, the influences on their lives, particularly from school, and have a working knowledge of local resources that may be needed by the group. Risks and benefits of this type of group need to be addressed in a balanced way, discussing issues of confidentiality and privacy as well as rules for mandatory reporting of any threatening circumstances. Effective group facilitators understand the importance of group processes, and the need to develop a sense of shared purpose. They are also able to monitor group progress while maintaining personal boundaries, understanding what is appropriate in terms of self-disclosure, particularly when drawing on personal experiences. They create a safe space for conversation, maintaining a non-judgemental attitude, and consistency in the way they approach conflict

resolution. In these groups the facilitator also acts as the role model for good communication skills. Communication skills include simultaneously concentrating on one person's comments while observing others' reactions and addressing these appropriately. With this type of approach the group dynamics are more likely to elicit positive outcomes from all members.

GROUP PLANNING, MANAGEMENT

- Establish purpose, goals, leadership
- Set tone for communication
- Discuss organisational issues
- Decide tasks, responsibilities
- Monitoring and evaluation strategies
- Progress markers
- Conflict resolution

Bringing nurses together in a group can also be useful for problem solving. Poor retention in the profession and a lack of support for young nurses were identified as issues by researchers examining the experiences of young nurses in the workplace (Clendon & Walker 2011; Clendon & Walker 2012). As a result, the researchers recruited a group of young nurses interested in addressing these issues to work together to identify strategies for supporting young nurses at work. Although living in different parts of the country, the nurses met monthly via video conference and held email and Facebook discussions to develop their plans. Although facilitated by one of the researchers, the group selected a leader from within the group and each member took on responsibility for different aspects of the two projects developed. The first project was to develop a website aimed at young nurses—a website that provides content on how to manage the challenges of nursing as well as a forum and a place to share the lighter moments of nursing (www.nznursesstation.org). The second project was to develop the Young Nurse of the Year Awards as a means of providing a way of recognising the work of young nurses and provide an incentive to keep them both in New Zealand and in nursing. Allowing the group to lead and develop the projects themselves was key to the group's success.

Therapeutic groups

Group therapy is one of the most effective tools used to help people deal with or overcome mental illnesses. Community mental health nurses (CMHNs) often conduct groups to help people deal with depression, anxiety, substance abuse or other behaviours that may be preventing them from leading satisfying, confident lives (Puskar et al. 2012; Wand 2013). This type of group can be powerful in helping people identify with others in a similar situation and gain from their experiences and insights throughout recovery and beyond (Puskar et al. 2012). Group therapy is also used by midwives and child and family nurses to help women with postnatal depression or other conditions that may affect their parenting ability as well as their own mental health (Scope et al. 2012). Other types of groups do not follow a strictly therapeutic model, but are designed to provide a forum for education, sharing and support (Puskar et al. 2012). Examples of these groups are self-help groups to help people deal with illness, such as cancer or chronic conditions, bereavement, or to develop and strengthen their coping skills following a disaster (Bemak & Chung 2011; Wand 2013). Regardless of the specific goals of the group, most therapeutic and self-help groups are solution-focused, emphasising individual and group strengths and assets to promote recovery from a condition or situation, and build capacity for the future (McAllister 2010; Wand 2013).

In terms of group process, the leader initially sets the tone of the group, focusing on communication, ensuring transparency by first explaining structural and organisational issues such as whether the group will have rotating leaders, whether they can be joined by others once they begin, how meeting information will be disseminated (verbally, in writing or electronically), any strategies that will be used to ensure integrity of communication, and how progress will be monitored and evaluated. In some cases, these issues will have been decided prior to the group meeting, at the time of invitation, but when it is possible to involve group members in making these organisational decisions, there is a greater likelihood that participants will feel a sense of belonging and ownership, which promotes group cohesion. In therapeutic groups, tasks and responsibilities may be assigned by the leader, including evaluation responsibilities (Clark 2003). Evaluation data should analyse the extent to which group goals were met, whether communication was effective, conflicts resolved and any other information that may be helpful in subsequent meetings (Clark 2003). In addition to these summative measures, other measures of group success should indicate clear progress markers and how these reflect the goals of the group (formative assessment data).

> ### Formative assessment
> - Progress markers
>
> ### Summative assessment
> - Goals met?
> - Communication effective?
> - Conflicts resolved?

In all groups, content and process are closely linked, and the group leader must be sufficiently knowledgeable to assess the group dynamics and determine the best processes to achieve their goals (Puskar et al. 2012). Group processes include interactions between group members and the leader, including emotions, responses and outcomes (Puskar et al. 2012). For example, in working with cancer support groups it is important that leaders have the necessary educational background to understand group members' medical conditions as well as the personal qualities and facilitation skills to interpret group interactions and the solutions that emerge from group discussions (Puskar et al. 2012). Cancer support groups may also need to be sensitive to group members' need for anonymity, and this can present a dilemma when designing a group process for peer and professional support. Wiljer et al. (2011) have found that for women experiencing sexual distress because of gynecologic cancers, the internet can be an ideal format for group work. Women in this situation, like others experiencing psychosexual difficulties, tend to have negative feelings about body image and sexuality, with difficulty sharing ideas and strategies. To overcome their hesitancy to come together as a group, a multidisciplinary group of clinicians/researchers developed an online bulletin board or forum using two platforms to host weekly private forums and live chats (Online. Available: www.CaringVoices.ca, www.womenshealthmatters.ca [accessed 23 April 2013]). In this process, group members could participate to the extent that they were comfortable, spontaneously raising topics of importance, or simply reading what others were discussing (Wiljer et al. 2011). Feedback from the women after 12 weeks indicated that they were able to gain courage, feel less lonely and become more confident in their own recovery through a very private means of mutual validation and support (Wiljer et al. 2011). This example shows the interrelatedness of content and process. The lesson for planning groups is that it is always important to determine which structure will be most effective for the particular participants the group is intending to attract, and to consider their views on the duration, frequency of sessions and optimal group size (Scope et al. 2012). The internet group was an ideal solution for this group of women, but other cancer support groups tend to meet in person. However, for these groups it is also important to work out the best place, time and duration of group meetings in relation to participant preferences, treatments and other schedules affecting participation.

Leg ulcer clubs are a further example of a therapeutic group environment that supports people with a health condition. Leg ulcers can frequently result in people (usually older) becoming isolated in their communities due to pain, exudate, immobility and odour (Lindsay 2013; Green & Jester 2010). Leg ulcer clubs were established as a means of bringing together people with ulcers into a community-based social environment that encourages social interaction and provides individual care for people's specific physical needs. Volunteers provide transportation to the club where required, and nurses facilitate the group and provide any care that is required. Research into the outcomes among members of the clubs has found previously house-bound, non-concordant patients have taken on responsibility for self-managing their condition, healing rates have improved, recurrence has been low, quality of life has improved and costs have been low (Lindsay 2013). Key elements to survival of such groups are having nurses committed to the model and responsive to the needs of the community, interested volunteers, and funders with an understanding of the value of such groups. In a primary health care context this type of partnership approach enhances the effectiveness of the group. It is also essential to provide culturally safe groups which resonate with participants' worldviews.

Culturally embedded groups

For many cultures, successful outcomes are most likely when the foundations for a desired change are built on cultural mores and values. For cultures that have strong connections to a group culture—group work may be an effective way to elicit and sustain change. Many indigenous cultures, for example, are founded on the collective. For Māori, a collective or group approach that includes whānau (family), hapu (sub-tribe) and iwi (tribe)—the groups that make up the collective—has been proven to be more successful than simply adopting an individual approach. For example, project REPLACE (part of a government funded healthy eating, healthy action program [HEHA]) was developed to support Māori living in the Bay of Plenty area lose weight, increase exercise, eat healthily, reduce smoking and reduce alcohol consumption (Mercer et al. 2013). Evaluation of the project identified that one of the most successful

elements was the 'Māori ways of doing'—in particular the group aspect (in this case whānau) activities that resulted in greater accountability and incentive to participate (Mercer et al. 2013). Unanticipated benefits included a reduction in social isolation, greater social participation and intergenerational learning (Mercer et al. 2013). A similar approach is used with Australian Indigenous parenting programs which are based on drawing parents together within the security of a cultural group (AIHW 2012b). Although all of these share the similarities of fostering good parenting in a culturally safe context the groups are focused according to slightly different needs; some to promote parental attachment (The Boomerangs Aboriginal Circle of Security Parenting); discussion of caregiving behaviours (Group Triple P Positive Parenting Program adapted for Indigenous families); and preventing serious social problems (Exploring Together) (AIHW 2012b). Although they have not been introduced widely there are strong indicators that groups have greater viability when they are culturally embedded. This principle of group work has also been illustrated in evaluating the Community Mothers program that began in Perth but is now offered in remote Aboriginal communities in Western Australia (Munns 2010; Walker 2010). The program's strength is that it is delivered in the local language with input from community mothers (Walker 2010). The evidence has shown how embedding cultural meanings, just like the 'Māori ways of knowing' (Mercer et al. 2013), can be helpful in promoting family engagement and mothers' knowledge of postnatal and maternal health, assets and risk factors for parents and their children (Walker 2010).

> ### CULTURALLY EMBEDDED GROUPS
> - Embedding cultural meanings, ways of knowing, values, worldview, language
> - Culturally responsive by challenging cultural oppression, power structures
> - Promote family engagement, knowledge of risks and assets

Extensive work in New Zealand on Kaupapa Māori approaches to research and participation and 'by Māori for Māori' initiatives, as well as group work developments in North America, are starting to provide a strong basis for the development of more appropriate models and theories that support behaviour change among these groups (Chino & DeBruyn 2006; Dyall et al. 2013; Kerr et al. 2010).

Kaupapa Māori knowledge validates a Māori world view that incorporates the validity and legitimacy of Māori language, culture, values and knowledge, and challenges and engages with existing power structures that have perpetuated colonial oppression (Kaupapa, Online. Available: www.kaupapamaori.com/theory/6/ [accessed 5 May 2013]; Kerr et al. 2010). While Kaupapa Māori approaches exclude non-indigenous practitioners to a certain extent, partnerships with indigenous practitioners enable non-indigenous practitioners to engage with communities in a Māori-centred way that can draw on the learning obtained from Kaupapa Māori knowledge and theory. Understanding the way in which differing cultures understand the world enables practitioners to engage in group work that facilitates behaviour change in culturally responsive ways, with greater likelihood of success.

HELPING PEOPLE CHANGE: FROM THEORY TO PRACTICE

WHAT'S THE POINT?

How do you think knowledge, motivation, group support and behaviour are linked?

In many practice settings, community nurses will lead groups that are working towards healthy lifestyle changes. Working within a PHC focus, the overarching focus is on working in partnership with the group to plan and make changes according to their own needs and motivations, and at their own pace. The role of the nurse in these groups is to provide health education and support, and to act as a facilitator/manager to document and evaluate goals and progress. When groups are encouraged to manage change in systematic steps with adequate evaluation and communication throughout the process, it is more likely to result in successful outcomes. A good facilitator will encourage group members to identify and reflect on personal attitudes and concerns that may affect their motivation or ability to change, which, in turn, will promote understanding by all those involved in the change, and garner support for the change (Critchley et al. 2012). A wide-ranging review of health promotion studies of behaviour change has found that the most effective strategies are self-monitoring of behaviour, risk communication and social support (Van Achterberg et al. 2010). This suggests that simply providing knowledge, materials and professional support is inadequate in helping people change (Van Achterberg et al. 2010). Yet many

health professionals provide advice on *why* change is necessary, without following through and monitoring progress or providing other types of support.

EVIDENCE-BASED TAXONOMY OF BEHAVIOUR CHANGE

- Knowledge
- Awareness
- Social influence
- Attitude
- Self-efficacy
- Intention
- Action control
- Maintenance
- Facilitation

Advice is important, but it should be part of an ongoing multi-component approach. The evidence supporting this contention is very strong, particularly in research findings from studies addressing the management of chronic conditions such as diabetes and heart disease and factors such as poor nutrition, obesity and smoking that precipitate such conditions (AIHW 2012a; Critchley et al. 2012; Stead & Lancaster 2005). With the increased prevalence of obesity and diabetes in the population, health promotion experts and researchers are now focusing on group-based programs, especially for weight control. Analysis of diabetes prevention programs reveals that when people are ready to make lifestyle changes, a combination of psychosocial, educational and motivational support can be most effective (Critchley et al. 2012). However, there is still so much about human behaviour in groups that is not well understood, which creates a dilemma for health promotion, particularly in helping people quit smoking. Stead and Lancaster (2005) conducted a Cochrane review to evaluate the effectiveness of group behaviour therapy programs for smoking cessation. They compared 53 clinical trials and found only limited evidence that adding group therapy to other forms of interventions, such as advice from a health professional or nicotine replacement, can produce extra benefits. The reviewers did conclude that multi-component processes are likely the best option for smoking cessation, but there are considerable differences in effectiveness, with some smokers preferring quit smoking groups, and others preferring individual strategies (Stead & Lancaster

2005). As these researchers argue, this type of research needs to be extended to analyse the relative contribution of different components of the interventions. It is interesting that after many years of research there remains a lack of conclusive evidence for what works best, for which groups of people, in specific circumstances.

The wider body of lifestyle research also points to the need to understand the theory behind health behaviour change, to develop strategies based on the best evidence of how knowledge, awareness, social influence, attitudes, self-efficacy, intention, action control, maintenance and facilitation can be used in various contexts to support individuals and groups as they begin the change toward healthier lifestyles (Van Achterberg et al. 2010). These nine components form a taxonomy of behaviour change which emerged from Van Achterberg et al.'s (2010) review of the health promotion literature. In some cases, it is the combination of these factors at the right place and time that will influence a person's ability to change; but in others, there may be one or more factors that are more significant than the others. For example, groups can provide social support in times when a person is feeling socially or emotionally isolated, as occurs in many women following pregnancy and childbirth. Sometimes, the problem is a lack of knowledge, but in other cases, despite knowledge and motivation to take control of behaviour, these women have a feeling that there is no one who can identify with their feelings and experiences.

REMINDER: Social marketing

Using business marketing techniques such as mass advertising to achieve behavioural goals for the social good.

Researchers have been studying antenatal and postnatal care for many years, still without conclusions that would provide definitive pathways to positive experiences. However, they have made progress in systematically studying the effect of groups in the context of antenatal care. A Cochrane review of midwifery studies, comparing outcomes for women who had individual or group antenatal care, found no differences between the two models of care on the basis of childbirth outcomes (Ickovics et al. 2007; Kennedy et al. 2011), but women who participated in group antenatal care found the experience positive (Homer et al. 2012). Other studies cited in the review conclude that antenatal care in groups can lead to greater social support,

which could potentially lead to better knowledge and skills, more health-promoting behaviours, and fewer behaviours that might create health risks for the mother and baby (Homer et al. 2012). Again, there is much to learn about the interactions between various factors and a person's inclination to change. An interesting study in Western Sydney found that a group-based model of antenatal care for overweight and obese women provides better support than individual guidance. Davis et al. (2011) convened a multidisciplinary group that combined education, motivation and peer support for this group of women in Western Sydney who were addressing both weight and childbirth issues. The program was highly regarded by participants, which poses a question of whether or not, when people are satisfied with their guidance, they will actually follow through with behaviour changes. Behavioural theorists have varying perspectives on how their responses or intentions might predict whether or not they decide to make changes.

Theories of behaviour change

A number of theories and models for behaviour change (compared in Box 6.6) have been developed to inform how we work with groups. Most of these are familiar to health educators, and they range from theories about social marketing, to those that inform campaigns to create fear of unhealthy behaviours, and cognitive behaviour theories (Edgar & Volkman 2012).

Cognitive behaviour change: the Theory of Reasoned Action

Cognitive behaviour theories tend to be the more widely used theoretical approaches in health. Ajzen and Fishbein's (1980) model has been used extensively by researchers and practitioners, as it provides a set of discrete steps that can be used to promote change. The model was used to test out Ajzen and Fishbein's hypothesis that attitudes can predict behaviour. Following several research studies they developed the Theory of Planned Behavior, also called the Theory of Reasoned Action or the Theory of Planned Change (Ajzen 1991; Ajzen & Fishbein 1980). The theory basically posits that people have three sets of beliefs that affect their intention to change. The first involves behavioural beliefs, which create attitudes toward the behaviour. The second is a set of normative beliefs that may be shaped by their group or community membership or other social factors such as cultural influences. The third set of beliefs involves self-perceptions about the extent to which they have control over their behaviours (control beliefs). The three types of beliefs all affect intention to change, which, in turn, affects behaviours (Ajzen 1991).

PRACTICE STRATEGY

How could an adolescent sexual health group use the 'action, target, time and context' strategy as a model for mutual support?

As the leader, what group dynamics would you have to consider?

BOX 6.5 **Resilence training for Project SafeCare**

1. Describe the target behaviour or skill.
2. Explain the rationale for teaching the skill.
3. Model each behaviour.
4. Ask parents to practise the behaviours.
5. Provide positive feedback on various aspects of performance.
6. Provide constructive feedback, including where people need to improve.
7. Review parents' performance, establishing homework to consolidate their skills, recording progress and repeating teaching until skills are mastered.

(Source: Iannos & Antcliff 2013)

According to Ajzen and Fishbein's (1980) model, to help people develop a foundation for change, behaviours should be defined in terms of four components: action, target, time and context (Sutton 2011). Sutton (2011) elaborates these steps in encouraging a young person to eat a healthy diet, beginning with breakfast. The action is 'eat'; the target is 'breakfast', the time component is 'tomorrow'. The context, which in this case is unspecified, is presumed to be the home. An example of where the context would be more important is in supporting a young person's attempt to change sexual behaviours. The intention might be 'using a condom the next time I have sex with a new sexual partner'. By making the context explicit the person's intentions are clearer, and there is a greater likelihood that their specific intention will predict healthy behaviour (Sutton 2011). Although these theoretical approaches address individual behaviours, they are also used to frame group work, where knowledge of individual behaviour helps inform expectations of how people will behave in groups, including the influence of the group on their health-related behaviours. It is also important for people trying to change to become aware of the various influences on their behaviours, as these factors can help them make informed decisions about making changes.

Social learning theory: resilience-led approach

The Resilience-Led Approach (Daniel et al. 2011) is a program to help families at risk for abuse and/or neglect based on social learning theory (SLT) (Iannos & Antcliff 2013). The program focuses on behaviours, using active learning strategies and role-modelling as well as extensive feedback. Box 6.5 outlines the seven steps.

Box 6.5 outlines what can only be described as a prescriptive approach to teaching parenting. As helpful as this approach can be in some cases, it is also an example of how the application of Western models and theories of behaviour change could be problematic for indigenous cultures as there is no emphasis on the cultural conditions that would influence either the motivation or behaviours involved in the change (Chino & DeBruyn 2006).

The Health Belief Model

Another theory that focuses on people's beliefs about behaviour is the Health Belief Model (HBM) (Becker 1974). Like Ajzen & Fishbein's model, the HBM has also been used in many situations to help guide health behaviour change, particularly those where people are encouraged to take precautions against illness or injury (Becker 1974). The theory is based on the notion that if people have sufficient motivation, and feel they are susceptible or vulnerable to ill health, there is a greater likelihood that they will take positive actions, especially if there are cues available in their social context to inspire those actions. Their decision to change would also be influenced by modifying factors such as personality, demographic (age, stage), or social and cultural factors, and the extent to which they believe they can reduce the perceived threat at a subjectively acceptable cost (Becker 1974). This theory has been adapted for nursing by Pender (2006), who has used it to guide numerous studies of health promotion change, where the nurse helps articulate the perceived threats, motivating factors and cues to action to help the group move forward with their changes.

The HBM is based on social learning theory (SLT), also called social cognitive theory (SCT), which holds that behaviour is determined by two main factors: expectancies and incentives (Rosenstock et al. 1988). Expectancies refer to environmental cues; how things are connected; in other words, what leads to what. Other expectancies are the consequences expected from actions, and self-efficacy; that is, how competent a person feels in performing a certain behaviour that would create better health. These expectancies can be shaped by members of a group, particularly in peer support groups. For example, in working with young people to discourage social media bullying the discussion might revolve around personal experiences of low self-esteem as a result of receiving personal insults or some other form of incivility. Having low self-esteem, the individual might decide to withdraw from recreational or sporting achievements, which can soon become a destructive cycle of declining self-esteem that has lasting effects on all aspects of the person's life. The group leader addressing this type of situation would guide the group toward recognising that everything is connected to everything else (the social ecology of human behaviour). Ideally, acknowledging the 'connected' effect of destructive behaviours will resonate with members of the group, who would then be encouraged to identify alternative behaviours that can have a positive effect on self-esteem. The positive behaviours may act as incentives or reinforcing factors such as approval from others (in this example), or in the case of lifestyle behaviour change, improved health status, physical appearance, economic gain or other consequences (Rosenstock et al. 1988). Thinking about behaviour change this way is closely related to the HBM model, as both are cognitive theories, based on motivating factors and self-perceptions about the chances of success in changing behaviour. The two theoretical approaches are also extensions of the work of Kurt Lewin (Rosenstock et al. 1988).

SCT TO OVERCOME BULLYING

Expectancies: the connections between environmental cues to action; consequences of the action; self-efficacy.

Incentives to change: approval from others, self-esteem.

Lewin's Unfreezing, Changing, Refreezing model

Lewin's (1951) model of unfreezing, changing and refreezing was one of the original guides to help people change health behaviours. In this model the first step is to identify the driving and restraining forces that may be influencing group complacency or unwillingness to change, as well as environmental conditions that may present barriers to change. 'Unfreezing' is a process of ensuring that there is accurate communication of the goals and expectations of the change, and what strategies are being suggested for improvement. The next stage, 'moving', creates awareness of shared understandings that people have

about the change and its outcomes, identification of the key people who will take ownership of the change, and what information will be communicated throughout the implementation to ensure that the change is sustainable. Following implementation, the 'refreezing' stage is focused on communicating the impact of the change and how it will be evaluated and sustained over time (Lewin 1951).

LEWIN'S MODEL FOR POLICY CHANGE

The major challenge for rural people is access to health services, which is related to the distribution of health professionals. If policymakers were motivated to 'unfreeze' the mindset that dictates the need for financial 'return on investment' from the costs of health professionals, develop strategies to create a fairer distribution of these people on the basis of social justice, and 'refreeze' notions of social investment for community development they would be acting on the principles of PHC.

Rogers's Diffusion of Innovations model

Rogers's (2003) Theory of the Diffusion of Innovations advances Lewin's ideas in arguing that innovations or changes are more easily diffused or accepted among those who seek to change if they can see the relative advantage of the change, and its compatibility with their approach or goals. Change will also be more readily accepted if people can see its potential in meeting their needs, if they have a chance to try it out prior to full implementation, and if it can be customised to their environment or circumstances so that it is compatible with their social and cultural perspectives (Rogers 2003). These theoretical concepts also provide a foundation for the trend towards translational research in nursing and other health disciplines. Knowledge translation research, as we explain in Chapter 15, outlines the importance of structuring our knowledge of barriers and facilitating factors in encouraging people to use research evidence for practice improvements (Cane et al. 2012), or for policy changes. If we understand why people are hesitant to change or what structural barriers to change exist in the context of care, it will be easier to address ways of encouraging evidence-based practice.

Another widely used model of change is Prochaska and Velicer's (1997) transtheoretical model, often called the Stages of Change model. This model differs from the theoretical approaches above in that it is focused on the temporal stages of change that explain *when* shifts in attitudes, intentions and behaviours occur, rather than the social cognitive aspects of *why* changes are made. The model is comprised of five stages: precontemplation, contemplation, preparation for change, action and maintenance (Prochaska et al. 1992). In the precontemplation stage there may be resistance to change, which is then reconsidered in the contemplation stage. Once people are convinced of the need for change they begin to make preparations for change, followed by action and activities to sustain the change. They outline the various processes that tend to occur during the five stages of change, where people can be helped to link emotional and cognitive elements through helping relationships and reinforcement for personal control over the behaviour. Numerous studies have reported using the Stages of Change as a guideline to help groups work through cycles of change, especially when they have tried unsuccessfully to make changes such as quitting smoking or reducing stress. Cassidy (1997) outlines the way she has used the model to guide her work as an OHN, in dealing with a highly stressed workforce who were constantly asked to do more with less, and often reacted with unhealthy behaviours such as smoking and overeating. She began the process by creating awareness of the quit smoking message among all employees, to encourage those in the pre-contemplation stage to think about the possibility of change, communicating the fact that she was there to help. She used consciousness raising and dramatic relief techniques (role-playing) to increase understanding and emotional awareness of their plight, while helping people re-evaluate the need to quit smoking. During the action stage she used individual contracts to help workers set goals and meet these successfully, adding relaxation techniques, assertiveness training and positive self-talk to her strategy. She convened groups to provide mutual support for smokers who have tried to quit, and worked with the groups to create awareness of how people could reduce the cues in their environment in the longer term that reinforce the unhealthy behaviours substituting these with healthy behaviours such as exercises or self-rewards (Cassidy 1997).

STAGES OF CHANGE MODEL

- Precontemplation
- Contemplation
- Preparation for change
- Action
- Maintenance

Besides safety surveillance and treating occupational illnesses and injuries occupational health nurses have been involved in healthy lifestyle programs for many years. Their focus on health and wellness in the workplace has become a high priority in the past decade, with worldwide increases in the incidence of diabetes, obesity and other chronic diseases and ageing of the workforce (Miller 2011). Some OHNs are using a health coaching approach in corporate wellness programs, based on evidence-based guidelines for best practice in the occupational setting. Miller's (2011) program involves establishing standards of care that maintain equity of access to all employees in any given industry, and disseminating standardised approaches to reduce practice variation among OHNs. She uses motivational interviewing as an evidence-based health coaching approach to help individuals by monitoring and reinforcing their healthy behaviours.

Motivational interviewing for change

As we outlined in Chapter 4, motivational interviewing is based on client-centred guided interviews that are intended to help individuals and groups create and maintain healthy lifestyles. The objectives are to help people discover their ambivalence toward changing behaviours, reveal their real concerns, and work towards self-discovery and self-management on the basis of the best available evidence to support their choices (Miller 2011). In group work, the nurse is there to activate participants' motivation for change through empathy and compassion. Members of the group are seen as partners, accountable and transparent in sharing beliefs, values, concerns and their agenda for change (Miller 2011). The dialogue for a group dealing with obesity begins with questions such as:

- 'What is the greatest concern about your condition/weight/general health'?
- 'What concerns you the most?'
- 'What concerns you the most about the plan we discussed'?
- 'What would you like to change the most about your condition? The plan?'

Once the group has begun sharing their concerns (self-discovery) the role of the nurse is to help them continue to work towards self-management through goal setting and mutual support. Community mental health nurses use a similar approach, based on social cognitive theories, in helping people through self-discovery of existing states to where they are able to value positive elements in their lives and work from strength to strength. Working with mental health groups has the dual challenge of overcoming the negative labelling to which many have been exposed, and helping them develop aspirations and solutions for positive health (Wand 2013). This can pose a problem in groups where there are different diagnoses, age groups or other factors such as interpersonal difficulties that interfere with promoting group cohesion. Identifying group assets rather than differences can be helpful to keep the group on track. For these and other groups there needs to be a process for ensuring that client psychological safety is the priority.

Using motivational interviewing techniques the nurse begins with a set of broad questions such as those above. Wand (2013) suggests that questions are aimed at prompting people to disclose how they see the problems, then explain how they have coped in the past. This is followed by questioning how they would imagine the situation improving in future, strategies that have been helpful for them and their next steps. In the context of this dialogue the leader tries to elicit responses that reflect people's resources, capacities, strengths and qualities, interspersed with 'problem-free talk' about their lives rather than their problems (Wand 2013). Some of the communication techniques in this type of approach include helping people see their problems as ordinary rather than monumental difficulties, not to minimise their situation, but to help them understand that others share similar experiences. At the same time, using their language to paraphrase comments evokes feelings of sincerity and genuineness, which can be helpful to those who feel overwhelmed by their situation or their lives (Wand 2013).

A similar approach is being used by nurses conducting group cognitive behavioural therapy (CBT) for women suffering from postnatal depression (PND), which can be effective in some, but not all cases. CBT is a combination of techniques from cognitive and behavioural therapies that are widely used with people suffering from moderate levels of depression (Scope et al. 2012). An integrative review of studies of CBT found that group interactions can help normalise the feelings of sadness, emptiness, fatigue, and inability to care for their child that many women have after childbirth, and help with social support (Scope et al. 2012). Some of the studies reviewed by Scope et al. (2012) found that although group CBT is helpful for some women, others experienced adverse or negative effects from the group context, especially women feeling the group was making social comparisons between them (Scope et al. 2012).

Barriers to change

Among the biggest obstacles to change in groups or in entire organisations is failure to articulate the change, its rationale, time frame and individual implementation steps. Clearly, communication is pivotal to successful change in any context. Kotter (1995), one of the most influential leadership advocates from the Harvard Business School, also advocates the need to establish a sense of urgency—motivating people to get outside their comfort zones and helping them become empowered through participation in a powerful guiding coalition to oversee the change. The change agent then develops and communicates a vision for what the change will bring, encourages risk-taking and creative ideas, establishes plans for creating short-term wins, helps them create reward structures for those involved in implementing change, and ensures that victory is declared at the appropriate time and celebrated. This last stage should be accompanied by new ideas or projects that could extend the change and reinvigorate the process, anchoring the change in the local culture (Kotter 1995) (see Figure 6.1).

KOTTER'S GUIDE TO CHANGE

- Establish a sense of urgency
- Create a powerful guiding coalition
- Share the vision for change
- Communicate to energise renewal
- Remove obstacles, encourage risk-taking and creativity
- Plan for short-term wins and rewards
- Ensure sustainability
- Anchor changes in the work culture

THINK ABOUT IT

Theories of behaviour change tend to be grounded in Western philosophical approaches. With growing emphasis on Indigenous self-determination, how much emphasis do you think this will have on the next phase of change theory development?

LEADING, FOLLOWING AND BEING THERE FOR THE GROUP

As we have mentioned previously, each group is different, and the style of leadership can vary depending on the purpose of the group, its progress in meeting goals and expectations, and the leader's personal characteristics. Leadership style is often

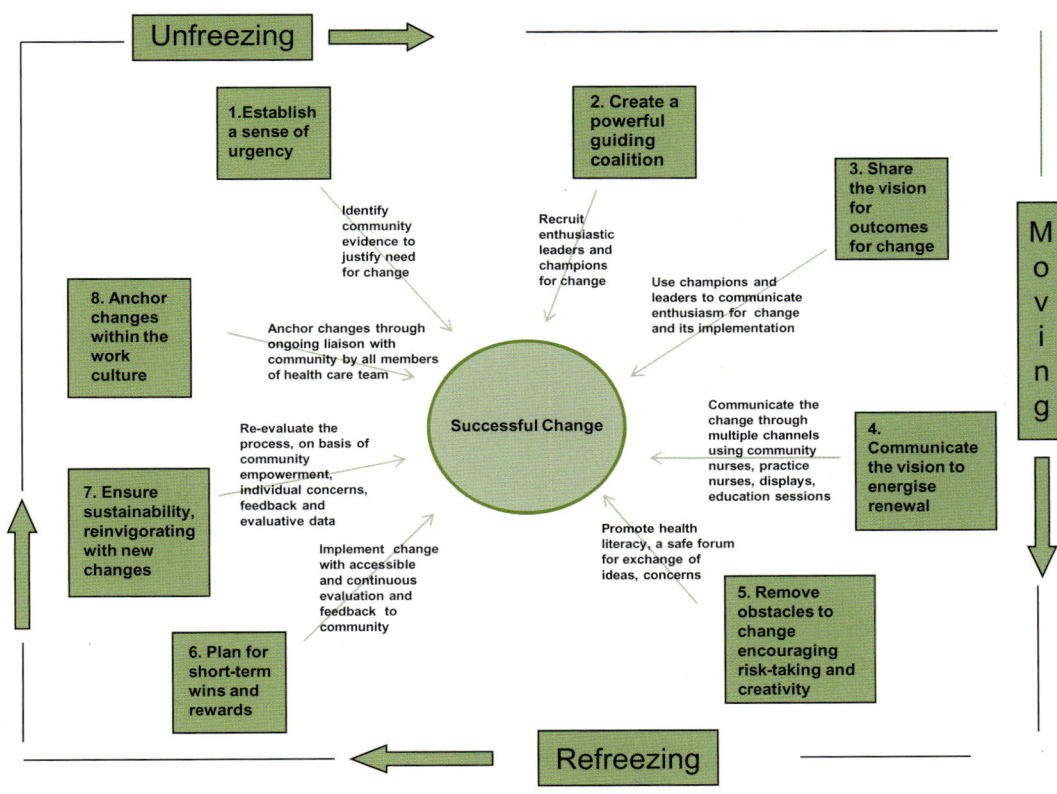

FIGURE 6.1
Helping people change

shaped by a combination of personality, prior experience in group work and expertise in the area under discussion. As people begin to air their differences, or work towards agreement, the leader may alternate between being somewhat directive to being a reflective participant in the group's deliberations. These levels of leader participation tend to vary as the group finds a level of balance and becomes more or less harmonious over successive meetings. In some groups, especially those convened for decision-making, conflicts can present barriers to discussion. Barriers can arise from unclear expectations, communication problems, different values or attitudes, previous conflicts among group members, or competition for resources (Clark 2003). Where this occurs the strengths of the group leader are critical to conflict resolution. To minimise barriers the leader needs to create an open climate for discussion where people's views are not dismissed, and where group members can explore how to proceed in a non-judgemental atmosphere. Good leaders give people permission to have divergent views, acknowledging to the rest of the group that all perspectives will be valued, which communicates an atmosphere of safety.

In some cases, the group leader begins a group by conveying a group philosophy. The leader seeks to encourage health behaviour change based on the principles outlined in Box 6.7 below.

What is a good leader?

Leadership has been described as 'the capacity of a human community to shape its future' (Senge 2002:13). Accepting the mantle of leadership can help nurses create an avenue for influencing groups to develop and sustain their common goals. Good leaders help develop this capacity by combining their innate skills and abilities with deliberate efforts to challenge, inspire, empower and act as a role model for others. For some, this is embellished with artistic flair and charisma. For others it is a deliberate, conscientious and committed progression towards excellence, achieved through careful assessment and rational planning. The best leaders are able to balance both sides of the coin (or the brain) sometimes simultaneously, sometimes sequentially. A charismatic personality, which draws on personal charm, can be helpful, but it must be accompanied by the substance of strategic thinking, change management skills, personal strength,

BOX 6.6 Behaviour change theories: a comparison

Theory	Principles
Theory of Planned Behaviour (Reasoned Action) Attitudes can predict behaviour (Ajzen & Fishbein)	behavioural beliefs + normative beliefs + control beliefs influence intention to change which affects behaviour
Health Belief Model (Becker, Pender)	motivation + beliefs about susceptibility+ environmental cues, lead to likelihood of positive action, modified by personality, demographics, socio-cultural, personal beliefs
Social Cognitive Theory (Rosenstock et al.)	expectancies (consequences, self-efficacy) + incentives (reinforcements) lead to behaviour
Unfreezing, Changing, Refreezing (Lewin)	unfreeze barriers (driving and restraining forces, environmental conditions), create shared understandings for change, implement and sustain change by refreezing
Diffusion of Innovations (Rogers)	understanding relative advantage of change, compatibility with goals, needs, try it out, customise to circumstances to be compatible with socio-cultural perspectives
Transtheoretical model (Stages of Change. When changes occur—Prochaska, Velicer)	precontemplation, contemplation, preparation for change, action, maintenance

BOX 6.7 Philosophical principles for group behaviour change

1 Believe that change is possible.

2 Create an atmosphere of trust for sharing ideas and experiences.

3 Start with what people know.

4 Value experiential knowledge as highly as formal knowledge.

5 Proceed from action to reflection to action (the cycle of praxis).

6 Knowledge is constructed in interactions between people.

7 People are active participants in acquiring knowledge.

8 Acknowledge educational influences from many sources.

9 Decision-making should be democratic.

10 Each member shares life experiences.

11 We learn with our heads, our hearts, and our bodies.

12 The arts are important tools for teaching and organising.

13 Critical thinking should be extended to developing critical consciousness to take action for change.

(Source: Wiggins 2011:359)

confidence, negotiation skills, knowledge management and willingness to form strategic alliances (Jooste 2004).

The ideal image of a good leader epitomises courage. Courageous leaders practise with their eye and their intellect on the big picture, however they also create cycles of personal and professional affirmation and confidence among group members that are fuelled by small, incremental successes. This is where professionalism is paramount. In group work the leader must become adept at articulating the contribution of all participants. This requires not only good communication skills, but an attitude of reflective humility. Being attentive and receptive to the range and breadth of voices around the table creates a meaningful understanding of how culture is captured in the language used by others (Gray 2009). When the group has clear communication it is easier to collaborate with one another, sharing information and engaging in planning processes without dissent. Successful collaborations make visible their acceptance of the leadership role, attract support from those around them, and inspire others to become leaders. The most widely cited description of good leaders comes from Kouzes and Posner (1988). Good leaders:

- challenge process, learning from the past but living in the present

- inspire a shared vision, creating a force that invents the future

- enable others to act, by mentoring, turning followers into leaders

- model the way by example, living the values and planning for their successors, and
- encourage the heart by celebrating the achievements of themselves and others.

Leadership and followership

Good leaders also design opportunities for ideas to flourish with good timing and good judgement. This creates mutual respect and an environment wherein difference, diversity and ambiguity are not just tolerated; they are celebrated (Porter-O'Grady & Malloch 2003). These leadership characteristics are most evident and often most appreciated in working with interdisciplinary groups. The theory of Transformational Leadership (Burns 1978) captures the ideal aspirations of multidisciplinary work because it is inclusive and focused as much on followership as leadership. The theory focuses on capacity development and building circles of trust within the group to advance the agenda and build mutual accountability (Porter-O'Grady & Malloch 2003). Members of the group tend to gravitate to transformational leaders because they are committed to followers, and enable group capacity by understanding not only the followers, but themselves and their place in the scheme of things. They maintain consistency between values, beliefs and actions, and are able to articulate what they stand for (Malloch & Porter-O'Grady 2005). These leadership characteristics are described as emotional competence. The emotionally competent leader understands that:

- leadership is all about relationships
- leadership requires emotional balance
- conflict is present in all relationships
- communication skills are not leadership optional
- the leader never owns others' issues or resolves others' problems
- accountability means that the leader sees that defined outcomes are attained
- friendship is not a component of the role, and
- the leader keeps no secrets, in fact, favours disclosure (Malloch & Porter-O'Grady 2005).

The theory of Transformational Leadership is similar to 'Servant Leadership'. Servant leadership focuses on all levels of service, on valuing and developing people to build capacity and support innovation (Jackson 2008). Both theoretical approaches are based on influence, rather than coercion, and foster personal and professional growth through authenticity, trust and humility. This type of leadership encourages participation and empowerment rather than creating a culture of disempowerment and intimidation, the latter of which can lead to bullying and various forms of incivility.

Being there for the group

As we have mentioned previously, conducting groups is integral to community nursing roles. However, when nurses are isolated from one another, such as occurs in the community, there are few opportunities to learn from the examples of others who might be ideal role models for group work. The alternative is to have a mentor who can provide guidance and support from their own experience. A mentor can be invaluable in helping to clarify the ambiguities and contradictions that sometimes arise when a nurse is isolated, such as in rural practice (Mills et al. 2006). Mentorship programs can be formalised or simply be the spontaneous bonding that occurs informally between mentors and mentees. Mentoring programs vary to some degree, but there is widespread agreement on the fundamental characteristics of a mentor. These include the following:

- trust
- openness to new ideas
- valuing knowledge
- compassion
- presence—being able to 'walk' the journey
- mindfulness
- passionate optimism
- resilience
- balance
- impulse control
- accessibility
- emotional competence (Porter-O'Grady & Malloch 2003; Sambunjak et al. 2009).

MENTORING IN PRACTICE

An example of effective mentoring in the context of group work is the tripartite partnership between a New Zealand Community Trust, Massey University School of Nursing and a local high school. This innovative model of collaboration enabled nursing students to develop skills in group work while promoting health among school students. They worked with the school over the period of their program, providing interactive classroom sessions and collaborating with senior students to facilitate small group workshops for junior students on health issues. The mentoring process in the group context was empowering for both levels of school students as well as the nursing students, all of whom had a chance to develop negotiation skills and shared decision through their unique partnership (Scott 2011).

Being a mentor helps novice practitioners build the toolkit for group work in understanding the vulnerabilities we all have as learners. The mentor then provides the impetus for mentees to stretch their capacity while preserving egos that are porous and receptive, not ones that become a casualty of the process. The opposite of this is toxic mentoring, where the mentor tries to transfer knowledge rather than building capacity. In this case, the mentor sets up a situation where they try to shape the mentee's development to mirror their own. This leads to failure to thrive. If people are being mentored toward emotional competence, they will embrace the *next* step in the journey, rather than the last, and rather than mimic the characteristics of the mentor, they will develop their own career strategies openly and decisively (Porter-O'Grady & Malloch 2003). Of course, mentorship is also reciprocal: as a person fosters another's development they also build their own capacity, which has benefits for individuals, groups and the community. Being a mentor can result in feelings of increased job satisfaction, greater feelings of value, improved interpersonal skills, improved job performance and increased learning for the mentor (Donner & Wheeler 2007; Canadian Nurses Association 2004). For mentees, the benefits can include increased feelings of competence and confidence in practice, decreased stress, increased job satisfaction, expanded networks and leadership development (Dorion 2011; Canadian Nurses Association 2004).

Mentor relationships that foster leadership skills also help strengthen the profession. Goleman (2002) suggests that becoming a good leader requires 'soul'; that is, using the emotion, identity and character that we all have in us, and using it to maximise our leadership potential (Goleman 2002; Shaw 2007). In Goleman's view, professions need a 'tribal feel', where we develop sensitivity to our own and others' capabilities and tendencies by fostering a culture of self-reflection and a place for the safe exchange of ideas and feedback. This type of approach is empowering. Empowerment, even the perception of empowerment, is contagious. Where the leadership is fair and inclusive, and there is organisational support, others become empowered by association and everybody's satisfaction increases.

REFLECTIVE PRACTICE: NURSING TRIBALISM

Think of a time in practice when you've felt the 'tribalism' Goleman describes. To what extent was this shaped by external events? By your own ideas?

What reflections in practice have led you to act as a leader rather than a follower?

Being there for one another involves first, a professional commitment to making nursing work visible. Demonstrating leadership skills in the context of practice may be difficult at times, depending on the level of support from managers or decision-makers at arms-length from practice. In most cases team meetings can dissolve barriers to empowerment, but in other cases the road to successful and rewarding practice can be challenging. Knowing and communicating the things that matter, how *you* are making a difference, and how this fits into the bigger picture can help empower the group. Leadership at all levels can help reinforce your ideas and approaches to practice, which, in turn, can be justified as strategies for another occasion. The second step involves our obligation to work through professional organisations to create a collective voice, share knowledge and skills, and inspire successive generations of nurses by role-modelling and mentoring. As a mentor, enabling 'ordinary people to produce extraordinary things in the face of challenge and change' creates inner leadership that can make a difference to people's lives, and the work of the team or the practice (Jooste 2004:217). It is circumscribed within the simple act of generosity, celebrating yours and others' assets, strengths and challenges. It begins with a clear vision, a willingness to share and a commitment to the work of the health care and practice team, its actions and outcomes. This builds capacity from within and without, perpetrating understanding and shared solutions to the breadth of problems that often seem insurmountable. With strong leadership these can be resolved one step at a time.

CASE STUDY: Group work for the Smiths and Masons

A men's group has been established by the occupational health nurse in the mining community where Jason and Colin are employed, with a focus on mental, physical and social issues. This has proven popular with some of the younger miners but presents challenges for some of the older ones. The nurse is persevering using a range of strategies to include all members of the mining community, including some of the local Indigenous men.

Rebecca has joined a weight management group and is enjoying the social side of the process as well as seeing the effects of exercise and nutritional advice.

In Papakura the local practice nurse has established a support group for mothers and children who have asthma but because she works, Huia struggles to get to the group. The nurse is currently trying to develop a special after-hours group for working parents.

REFLECTING ON THE BIG ISSUES

- The most effective groups are those that have a clear sense of purpose, with identified goals, participative structures, appropriate communication processes, and a leader who is knowledgeable and inclusive.
- Content and process are interrelated in all groups.
- Different agendas are established for different groups, depending on whether they are supportive, therapeutic, self-help, problem-solving or aimed at behaviour change.

- Behaviour change is underpinned by theory.
- Change includes knowledge, awareness, social influences, attitudes, self-efficacy, intention, action control, maintenance, facilitation.
- Barriers to change include failure to articulate the change, its rationale, time frame and implementation steps.
- Good leaders are courageous, articulate, professionally committed role models and mentors who create an open, non-judgemental climate for discussion.

REFLECTIVE QUESTIONS: How would I use this knowledge in practice?

1. What would be the most important characteristics the OHN would bring to the men's group attended by Jason and Colin?
2. What strategies would s/he use to be inclusive and encourage communication in the men's group?
3. Would the Maddington nurses working with the Mason family participate in Rebecca's weight management in any way? Which ones? How would they be part of her goals?
4. How would you explain the differences in the evidence showing that many men do not want to quit smoking in groups, yet many obese pregnant women prefer weight control groups to individual intervention strategies? What is the implication of this information for practice? For research?
5. What behavioural principles would the group leader be using to conduct the asthma support group in Papakura?
6. How could the children's asthma support group be linked to a healthy school initiative?
7. Outline a multidimensional plan for an evidence-based University student healthy lifestyle group that includes goals and objectives, a time line and leadership principles.

References

Ajzen, I., 1991. The theory of planned behaviour. Organ. Behav. Hum. Decis. Process. 50, 179–211.

Ajzen, I., Fishbein, M., 1980. Understanding attitudes and predicting social behavior, Prentice-Hall, Engelwood Cliffs, NJ.

Australian Government AIHW, AIFS, 2012a. Healthy lifestyle programs for physical activity and nutrition. Closing the Gap Clearinghouse Resource sheet no. 9, AIHW, Canberra.

Australian Government AIHW, AIFS, 2012b. Parenting in the early years: effectiveness of parenting support programs for Indigenous families. Closing the Gap Clearinghouse Resource sheet no. 16, AIHW, Canberra.

Becker, M., 1974. The health belief model and personal health behavior. Health Educ. Monogr. 2, 234–335.

Bemak, F., Chung, R., 2011. Post-disaster social justice group work and group supervision. J. Spec. Group Work 36 (1), 3–21.

Burns, J., 1978. Leadership Harper & Row, New York.

Canadian Nurses Association, 2004. Achieving excellence in clinical practice: a guide to preceptorship and mentoring, Canadian Nurses Association, Ottawa.

Cane, J., O'Connor, D., Michie, S., 2012. Validation of the theoretical domains framework for use in behaviour change and implementation research. Implement. Sci. 7, 37–54.

Cassidy, C., 1997. Facilitating behavior change. Use of the transtheoretical model in the occupational health setting. AAOHN J. 45 (5), 239–246.

Chino, M., DeBruyn, L., 2006. Building true capacity: Indigenous models for indigenous communities. Am. J. Public Health 96 (4), 596–599.

Clark, M., 2003. Community Health Nursing, fourth ed. Prentice-Hall, Upper Saddle River, New Jersey.

Clendon, J., Walker, L., 2011. Characteristics of younger nurses in New Zealand: Implications for retention. Kai Tiaki Nurs. Res. 2 (1), 4–11.

Clendon, J., Walker, L., 2012. 'Being young': younger nurses' experiences in the workplace. Int. Nurs. Rev. 59 (4), 555–561.

Cramm, J., Phaff, S., Nieboer, A., 2013. The role of partnership functioning and synergy in achieving sustainability of innovative programmes in community care. Health Soc. Care Community 21 (2), 209–215.

Critchley, C., Hardie, E., Moore, S., 2012. Examining the psychological pathways to behavior change in a group-based lifestyle program to prevent Type 2 diabetes. Diabetes Care 35 (4), 699–705.

Daniel, B., Burgess, C., Antcliff, G., 2011. Resilience practice framework, The Benevolent Society, Paddington, Sydney.

Davis, D., Raymond, J., Clements, V., et al., 2011. Addressing obesity in pregnancy: The design and feasibility of an innovative intervention in NSW, Australia. Women Birth 24 (1 Suppl.), doi:10.1016/j.wombi.2011.08.008.

Donner, G., Wheeler, M., 2007. A guide to coaching and mentoring in nursing, International Council of Nurses, Geneva.

Dorion, N., 2011. Nursing mentorship programs: Creating a culture of mentorship. SRNA News Bull. 13 (1), 27.

Downie, J., Clark, K., Clementson, K., 2004-5. Volunteerism: Community mothers in action. Contemp. Nurse 18 (1/2), 188–198.

Dyall, L., Kepa, M., Hayman, K., et al., 2013. Engagement and recruitment of Māori and non-Māori people of advanced age to LiLACS NZ. Aust. N. Z. J. Public Health 37, 124–131.

Edgar, T., Volkman, J., 2012. Using communication theory for health promotion: Practical guidance on message design and strategy. Health Promot. Pract. 13 (5), 587–590.

Fatchett, A., Taylor, D., 2013. Multidisciplinary workshops: learning to work together. Community Pract. 86 (3), 21–23.

Garcia, C., Lindgren, S., Kemmick Pintor, J., 2011. Knowledge, skills, and qualities for effectively facilitating an adolescent girls' group. J. Sch. Nurs. 27 (6), 424–433.

Goleman, D., 2002. The new leaders, Little Brown, London.

Gray, M., 2009. Public health leadership: creating the culture for the twenty-first century. J. Public Health (Bangkok) 31 (2), 208–209.

Green, J., Jester, R., 2010. Health-related quality of life and chronic venous leg ulceration: part 2. Br. J. Community Nurs. 15 (3), S4–S4-6, S8, S10.

Homer, C., Ryan, C., Leap, N., et al., 2012. Group verses conventional antenatal care for women. Cochrane Database Syst. Rev. 2012, Issue 11. Art. No. CD007622, doi:10.1002/14651858.CD007622.pub2.

Iannos, M., Antcliff, G., 2013. Parent-skills training in intensive home-based family support programs, Australian Institute of Family Studies, Child and Family Australia, Melbourne.

Ickovics, J., Kershaw, T., Westdahl, C., et al., 2007. Group prenatal care and perinatal outcomes: A randomized controlled trial. Obstet. Gynecol. 110 (2), 330–339.

Jackson, D., 2008. Servant leadership in nursing: A framework for developing sustainable research capacity in nursing. Collegian 15 (1), 27–33.

Jooste, K., 2004. Leadership: a new perspective. J. Nurs. Manag. 12, 217–223.

Kennedy, H., Farrell, T., Paden, R., et al., 2011. A randomized clinical trial of group prenatal care in two military settings. Mil. Med. 176 (10), 1169–1177.

Kerr, S., Penney, L., Moewaka Barnes, H., et al., 2010. Kaupapa Māori action research to improve health disease services in Aotearoa, New Zealand. Ethn. Health 15 (1), 15–31.

Kotter, J., 1995. Leading change: why transformation efforts fail. Harv. Bus. Rev. 73 (2), 59–67.

Kouzes, J., Posner, B., 1988. The leadership challenge, Jossey-Bass, San Francisco.

Lewin, K., 1951. Field theory in social science, Harper & Row, New York.

Lindsay, E., 2013. Lindsay Leg Clubs: clinically effective, cost effective. J. Community Nurs. 27 (1), 5–8.

Malloch, K., Porter-O'Grady, T., 2005. The quantum leader: applications for the new world of work, Jones and Bartlett, New York.

McAllister, M., 2010. Solution focused nursing: A fitting model for mental health nurses working in a public health paradigm. Contemp. Nurse 34, 149–157.

Mercer, C., Riini, D., Hammerton, H., et al., 2013. Evaluating a healthy eating healthy action program in small Māori communities in Aotearoa, New Zealand. Aust. J. Prim. Health 19, 74–80.

Miller, C., 2011. An integrated approach to worker self-management and health outcomes. Chronic conditions, evidence-based practice, and health coaching. AAOHN J. 59 (11), 491–501.

Mills, J., Lennon, D., Francis, K., 2006. Mentoring matters: developing rural nurses knowledge and skills. Collegian 13 (3), 33–36.

Mills, A., Schmied, V., Taylor, C., et al., 2012. Connecting, learning, leaving: supporting young parents in the community. Health Soc. Care Community 20 (6), 663–672.

Munns, A., 2010. Yanan Ngurra-ngu Walalja, Halls Creek Community Families Programme. Neonatal Paediatr. Child Health Nurs. 13 (1), 18–21.

Parenting Research Centre, 2012. Evidence review: An analysis of the evidence for parenting interventions in Australia, Parenting Research Centre, Melbourne.

Pender, N., 2006. Health promotion in nursing practice, fifth ed. Prentice Hall, Upper Saddle River, NJ.

Porter-O'Grady, T., Malloch, K., 2003. Quantum leadership: a textbook of new leadership, Jones and Bartlett, Mississauga.

Prochaska, J., DiClemente, C., Norcross, J., 1992. In search of how people change. Applications to addictive behaviours. Am. Psychol. 47, 1102–1114.

Prochaska, J., Velicer, W., 1997. The transtheoretical model of health behavior change. Am. J. Health Promot. 12, 38–48.

Puskar, K., Mazza, G., Slivka, C., et al., 2012. Understanding content and process: Guidelines for group leaders. Perspect. Psychiatr. Care 48, 225–229.

Rogers, E., 2003. Diffusion of Innovations, fifth ed. The Free Press, New York.

Rosenstock, I., Strecher, V., Becker, M., 1988. Social learning theory and the health belief model. Health Educ. Q. 15 (2), 175–183.

Sambunjak, D., Straus, S., Marusic, A., 2009. A systematic review of qualitative research on the meaning and characteristics of mentoring in academic medicine. J. Gen. Intern. Med. 25 (1), 72–78.

Scope, A., Booth, A., Sutcliffe, P., 2012. Women's perceptions and experiences of group cognitive behaviour therapy and other group interventions for postnatal depression: a qualitative synthesis. J. Adv. Nurs. 68 (9), 1909–1919.

Scott, S., 2011. A tripartite learning partnership in health promotion. Nurs. Prax. N. Z. 27 (2), 16–23.

Senge, J., 2002. Servant leadership: afterword. In: Spears, L. (Ed.), Servant Leadership, a Journey into the Nature of Legitimate Power and Greatness, twenty-fifth anniversary ed. Paulist Press, New York, pp. 343–360.

Shaw, S., 2007. Nursing leadership, International Council of Nurses and Blackwell Publishing, Oxford.

Stead, L., Lancaster, T., 2005. Group behaviour therapy programmes for smoking cessation. Cochrane Database Syst. Rev. 2005, Issue 2. Art No. CD001007, doi:10.1002/14651858.CD001007.pub2.

Sutton, S., 2011. The contribution of behavioural science to primary care research: development and evaluation of behaviour change interventions. Prim. Health Care Res. Dev. 12 (4), 284–292.

Townley, G., Kloos, B., Green, E., et al., 2011. Reconcilable differences? Human diversity, cultural relativity, and sense of community. Am. J. Community Psychol. 47, 69–85.

Tuckman, V., 1965. Developmental sequence in small groups. Psychol. Bull. 63 (6), 384–399.

Van Achterberg, T., Huisman-de-Waal, G., Ketelaar, N., et al., 2010. How to promote healthy behaviours in patients? An overview of evidence for behaviour change techniques. Health Promot. Int. 26 (2), 148–162.

Walker, R., 2010. An evaluation of Ynan Ngurra-ngu Walalja: Halls Creek Community Families Program, Telethon Institute for Child Health Research, Perth.

Wand, T., 2013. Positioning mental health nuring practice within a positive health paradigm. Int. J. Ment. Health Nurs. 22, 116–124.

Wiggins, M., 2011. Popular education for health promotion and community empowerment: a review of the literature. Health Promot. Int. 27 (30), 356–371.

Wiljer, D., Urowitz, S., Barbera, L., et al., 2011. A qualitative study of an internet-based support group for women with sexual distress due to gynecologic cancer. J. Cancer Educ. 26, 451–458.

Xyrichis, A., Lowton, K., 2008. What fosters or prevents interprofessional teamworking in primary and community care? A literature review. Int. J. Nurs. Stud. 45, 140–153.

Useful websites

www.nznursesstation.org—Website for young nurses

www.womenshealthmatters.ca—Women's chatroom for gynecologic issues

www.getup.org.au

www.lockthegate.org.au/groups

www.cleanwaterhealthyland.org.au/content/building-community-action-groups

—Social activist groups

www.choicenotchance.co.nz—Problem gambling help

SECTION 2

Sustainable Health for the Family and the Individual

Introduction to the Section

This section reflects the importance of promoting health and wellness at each stage along the life course from birth to death. Chapter 7 focuses on the contemporary family. Because the family is so important to both individual and community health, we provide an extensive chapter to guide your learning in four distinct parts. Part 1 addresses the family in society. In this 21st century, families are increasingly diverse and exposed to a number of contemporary changes. Some of the most significant issues for families in this era revolve around rapid social, technological and workplace changes, including those influenced by global events. The global economy has reshaped the work environment as well as communication systems and various technologies, which have also brought families from one community into contact with many others throughout the world, and these are discussed in depth. In Part 2 we examine couple relationships and family life across the transitions of partnering, marriage and, in some cases, marital separation. In this section we address the new family forms such as same-sex marriage, now entrenched in legislation in many countries, as well as the impact of family separation, divorce and the violence that can disrupt family stability. Part 3 outlines the unique circumstances of some families living in our communities, including migrant and refugee families, families coping with illness or disability, and rural families. The final part of Chapter 7 describes the goals, policies and practices for promoting healthy family life using the framework of the Ottawa Charter for Health Promotion.

Child health is commonly understood as the most significant indicator of how families, neighbourhoods, communities and nations are able to provide health-enhancing conditions for

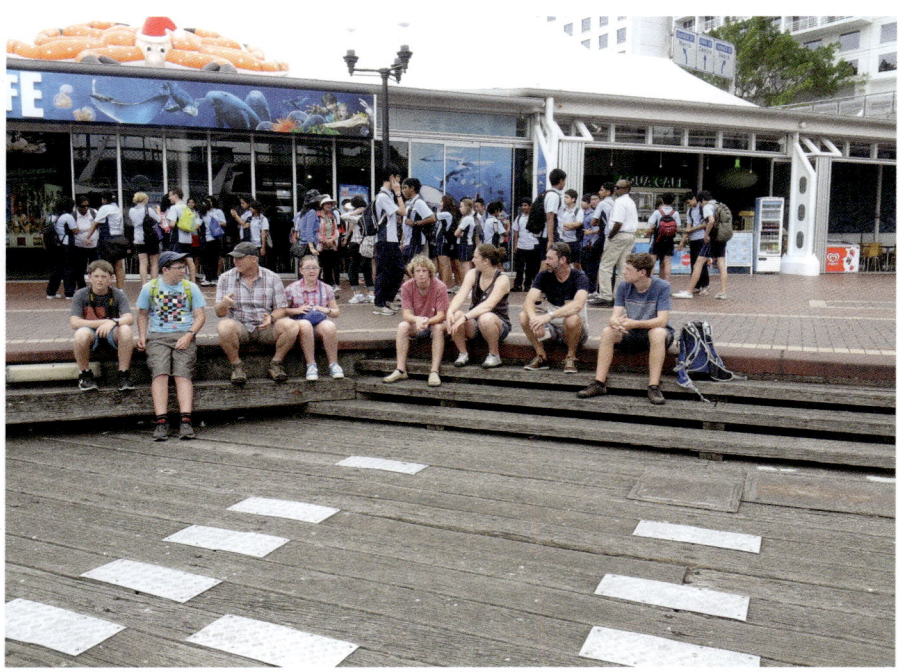

Extended family time (photo: Jill Clendon)

daily living. Chapter 8 places the child at the centre of interest so we can consider the burgeoning body of research into biological embeddedness, the role of environmental stimuli and the social determinants of child health.

The health status of adolescents in any community provides a barometer of a community's progress in creating and supporting a healthy start to life, and creating a template for the future. At this crucial stage, a large segment of the population is launched from childhood to adulthood, from dependence to independence. How adolescents deal with the various challenges and negotiate the many transitions of a few delicate years often heralds how well they will cope with the transitions of adult life; this is addressed in Chapter 9 by exploring the concept of the adolescent 'at promise' rather than 'at risk', in the expectation that there are some ways nurses and other health care professionals can bring the promise of adolescence to fruition.

Healthy adulthood reflects the culmination of socially and environmentally supported choices for health and wellness made by individuals at earlier stages of their development. Adulthood is also the time when many chronic diseases emerge and when the risks of ill health or injury are acute. For younger adults, particularly parents, social and occupational pressures loom large and the discussion in Chapter 10 extends to issues related to formal and informal work and family life that were introduced in Chapter 7. In Chapter 10, the major risk factors and lifestyle determinants of healthy adulthood are discussed in a way that acknowledges the influence of the environment and social structures on personal choices for health. The chapter also reinforces the need for intergenerational consideration of the continuum

of health and illness and primary, secondary and tertiary strategies to help people reach their potential.

Chapter 11 provides an examination of the features of healthy ageing. Managing chronic conditions is of major concern in this part of life's pathway, and we revisit some of the main strategies for helping people shape their lifestyles and their communities to promote healthy ageing. A social perspective of ageing is outlined, including the need to attend to older people's numerous transitions; those related to family members joining or leaving the family home, retirement, loss and the adjustments of widowhood. Our role in assisting older people to expect—and then to achieve—health and wellness is paramount at this time of life. We are encouraged to adopt measures to counter ageism, to procure high-quality lifestyles, and to strengthen older people's voices in the policy arena, particularly now when we are all pondering longer lives.

Throughout these chapters in Section 2, we use the Ottawa Charter for Health Promotion as a guide to working with each of the population groups. After 50 years, the charter represents a timeless approach to managing community health, situating practice within the goals of healthy public policy, creating supportive environments, strengthening community action, developing personal skills and reorienting health services. Our two families, the Smiths and the Masons, also feature in each chapter, as the case study unfolds with a different focus for each, ranging from the family, to the children, adolescents, adults and older persons. As you read through the chapters, we encourage you again to think about the big issues, some of which we mention at the end of each chapter, and reflect on practice and its evidence base.

Healthy families

Introduction

Few people would challenge the notion that the family is the most important influence on the health of a society. The family is where individuals are nurtured and guided to adopt and adapt beliefs, behaviours, values and attitudes that will help their members become healthy and competent citizens of wider worlds. As mentioned in Section 1, there are many influences on health and development that arise from the interactions between families and communities. Some of the most important of these are habits of mind and action that emerge from a child's early experience in the family. Daily interactions between family members create opportunities for inherent traits and predispositions to be shaped into positive or negative behaviours in relation to health and wellbeing. These become habitual and refined as they are reinforced and nurtured, and as family members interact with others external to the family. Families with children play an important role in nurturing their children along their developmental pathways. This has a reciprocal effect on parents or caregivers as each interaction provides not only an opportunity for parental dialogue, but also renewed consideration of the way adult family members are relating to one another. For families without children, regardless of their configuration, interactions are also major opportunities for mutual nurturing and the development of adult competence to deal with the world outside the family. In this era of increasing cross-border migration, there are many lessons to be learned about the distinctiveness of these family interactions in families with different cultural traditions.

Adult family members make lifestyle choices, and this can be crucial to a child's decision-making in relation to healthy lifestyles. Children's choices are cultivated by what is observed and modelled within the family, and how family health is entrenched in the social conditions and relationships beyond the family. In this respect, families play a significant gatekeeping role as the main link between individuals and their environments. Because families themselves are dynamic, their roles change in various ways and this has implications for family health and wellbeing. As individual family members change and develop in the encounters of daily life, the family as an entity also changes to adapt to the outside world, which affects its ability to provide a supportive environment for its members. Each opportunity to adapt and change can be used to share strengths and challenges, and to teach younger family members the skills to be self-regulating and competent, to create and sustain health and wellbeing as they negotiate the critical stages along the pathways to adulthood.

In a contemporary world where change is both rapid and constant, the way family members transact and adapt to the precariousness of their environments determines the extent to which the family can provide solace and refuge, comfort, succour and direction to each of its members. Families that are able to provide a firm grounding for their members to deal with outside stressors can vitalise the community in ways that cultivate understanding, tolerance and social cohesion. Alternatively, a lack of strong family bonds to shelter or protect family members from the outside world can have harmful effects on its members and cast a shadow over the community. Our socio-ecological perspective addresses the multiple, reciprocal, positive and negative influences on family life and how these change over time (Barakat 2012). Toward that end, this chapter examines the family in the context of today's societies, how families change and are being changed by contemporary life, and the role of nurses and other health professionals in helping them achieve health.

POINT TO PONDER

Family is the most important influence on the health of a society.

Part 1: The family and society

When we think of family, some of us think of the protective envelope that provides a refuge from the stresses and strains of contemporary society. Others see family as a combat zone, a kind of repository for the collective problems of both the inside and outside world. Most people hold a view of family that lies somewhere between these two extremes. The family is the filter or mediating structure that functions as a gatekeeper between individuals, their culture and the wider society. It is a conduit through which society transmits to individuals its social and cultural norms, roles and responsibilities. The family also acts as a communicative structure from within, providing a scaffold for interactions, with the goal of bonding individuals into a cohesive whole with shared attitudes, values and opinions. When this goal is achieved, the family is able to give voice to needs and preferences, which should, in turn, inform societal policies and processes that can vitalise the community.

> ### WHAT IS ... THE FAMILY?
>
> A protective gatekeeper between individual family members and their culture, and the wider society.

Most communities situate the family at the centre of social life. From the seeds sown and nurtured in the family, members make decisions affecting access to health care and social services, prevention of illness, preservation of the natural and built environment, the cultivation of knowledge and strategies to manage the social determinants of their health and wellbeing. These are the essential elements of a healthy society. However, family life can also exert a negative influence on these

decisions, subduing or constraining individuals and circumstances, precipitating illness, failing to protect its members from harm, or endangering their physical, social or cultural environments. Families are therefore the pivot point around which societies revolve. As the foundational human institution, the family has been described as:

a cooperative economic and protective powerhouse delivering mutual care and goods and services to its members; a source of succour, nursing and welfare when needed; and a social organization in miniature providing education, ethical instruction, recreation, entertainment, companionship, and love.

(Maley 2009:1)

GROUP EXERCISE: Family

In groups of three or four, discuss what family means to you. Does everyone in the group have a similar understanding or are there differing opinions? What about the wider group? Why is it important that we understand what family means to people? How is this important in the context of a home visit, or in a child health clinic, in the school setting or in an older adult residential facility? Is 'family' more or less relevant in any of these settings?

FAMILY FUNCTIONS

Although there is considerable diversity among families, in most cases, family roles tend to revolve around goal setting, using internal and external resources for the advantage of family members, and the nurturing and socialisation of children (Friedman et al. 2003). Duvall and Miller (1985) describe the family's general functions as the following:

- Affection—an affectionate family environment provides the conditions within which family members can learn to trust one another and those external to the family.

- Security and acceptance—having basic physical and emotional needs nurtured within the family instils a sense of safety and security that will promote the ability to be accepting of others.

- Identity and a sense of worth—reflecting on family interactions allows family members to develop a sense of who they are and how their unique characteristics are linked to those of others.

- Affiliation and companionship—throughout the lifespan the family creates a sense of belonging among members, which establishes a template for bonding together and with others.

- Socialisation—the family transmits a cultural and social identity that will embody the family's history and values and thus contribute to the community's collective identity, particularly in multicultural communities. This influences community cohesion.

- Controls—within the family all members come to recognise the rules and boundaries that provide realistic standards for public behaviour (Duvall & Miller 1985).

The family functions listed above represent an ideal. When families are able to provide these nurturing, protective functions there is a greater likelihood of promoting social cohesion and achieving mutually beneficial goals and bonds of trust, which are the cornerstones of social capital (Putnam 2005). Thinking of the family in terms of social capital ultimately means that family members are part of the system of reciprocal capacity development in the wider society. Societal norms and standards are not imposed from outside the family, but take shape through the way families interact with a range of institutions and processes. This is a 'relational' view, where the family is seen as integrally connecting and shaping one another's lives and the situations, contexts and processes of their external environments (Hartrick Doane & Varcoe 2005).

Families have changed dramatically in the 21st century in form, function and relationships. In this era of globalisation and mass migration, most societies, especially in the wealthy countries, are composed of more culturally and linguistically diverse (CALD) families than in the past. Interactions within and between different cultural groups are influenced by this diversity, adding to the richness,

potential and sometimes risks that pervade our societies. The world of work has also transformed family roles considerably, as have changing attitudes and policies affecting child care and schooling. In the context of these changes the challenge for health professionals is to explore ways of promoting and supporting family choices, enabling and enhancing health for all family members (Nyirati et al. 2012). Promoting family health is, at times, a daunting challenge, given that it occurs in the face of constant change, but it is also fascinating, providing us with constantly evolving understandings of how families define themselves and how they manage their lives and their health across a variety of situations.

DEFINING THE FAMILY

Defining the family is important for several reasons. These include some of the most important social and structural determinants of health, such as the socio-legal family environment. Socio-legal arrangements dictate who is included in insurance policies, which members have access to children's school records, who can be a part of a joint tax return or bank account, and who is eligible for reproductive assistance, sick leave, death benefits, child support, superannuation or other means of income security. Some definitions of family are more traditional; for example, explaining the family on the basis of a common place of residence. The Australian Bureau of Statistics (ABS) (2011) defines the family as:

two or more people that are related by blood, marriage (registered or de facto), adoption, step or fostering, and who usually live together in the same household. This includes newlyweds without children, gay partners, couples with dependants, single mums or dads with children, siblings living together, and many other variations. At least one person in the family has to be over 15.

FAMILY THEORETICAL TRADITIONS
- Structural Functional Theory
- Developmental Theory
- Systems Theory

Family nursing scholars have tended to define the family according to three basic theoretical perspectives. The first is Structural Functional Theory, where families are identified by how they are organised and what they do to maintain and promote family health (Friedman et al. 2003). Another approach to defining the family is within Developmental Theory, which views families in terms of a sequence of lifecycle stages, each with developmental tasks, such as establishing the marriage, childrearing, children leaving home and retirement. The third and most influential theoretical tradition is seen within the rubric of Family Systems Theory, where the family is seen as an entity in itself, consisting of subsystems (of siblings, for example). The family system may be defined by location, blood ties, marriage, legal adoption or residence, or by cultural affiliation, bonds of reciprocal affection and mutual responsibility (Wright & Leahey 2009). Interactions between subsystems (family members) and interactions between members and the family's surrounding environment affect the family as a whole (Doane Hartrick & Varcoe 2005).

'RELATIONAL' VIEW OF FAMILY

Families connect and shape one another's lives and the situations, contexts and processes of their external environments.

All of these theoretical approaches can be used to define the family as a basis for assessing and categorising family needs; however, each carries a presumption of understanding that may not be congruent with the PHC philosophy. The various theories and the assessment tools that accompany them have been criticised on the basis that they tend to purvey a Western dominant view of how family life is lived without considering how the family sees itself (Doane Hartrick & Varcoe 2005). These authors caution against defining the family as a particular configuration of people, which may lead to stereotypical, and therefore limiting, notions of family needs (Doane Hartrick & Varcoe 2006). Families are a microcosm of adaptive interactions that are determined by historical events, cultural mores, preferences for spiritual or lifestyle activities, continuity or discontinuity of relationships, and connections to their neighbourhood and community. Family forms such as single parent or blended households, same-sex couples or intergenerational families often have unique structures, roles and challenges. Because of this variability, the relational view of families is more appropriate in a PHC context. The family as a relational entity is inclusive of the family's perspectives, choices, internal interactions and interactions with the external world in the face of changes and challenges.

Assessing a family on the basis of a set of guidelines or behavioural norms also sends a message that there are normative criteria and expectations for interactions and behaviours. This can be disempowering for families who experience historical or situational disadvantage. A more authentic approach to working with families is first, to discover how the family sees itself, and then encourage their participation in identifying any changes they seek to make or reinforce their strategies for maintaining health and preventing illness or injury. Wright and Leahey's (1987) explanation that family is 'whoever the family says it is' remains the most enduring and practical way of defining the family. It is also a more collaborative, partnership approach to begin helping families meet their needs.

THE FAMILY IS ...

'whoever the family says it is'.

In Australian and New Zealand Indigenous groups, 'family' is pre-eminent. Australian Indigenous groups have variable languages with which to describe their families and the notion of family connectedness, however, government agencies describe all Australian families as 'family' using common terminology. In Australia, working with Aboriginal family groups is always inclusive of Aboriginal people, either child and family health workers who are from the same group as the group they work with, or those who are known to be accepted by the families. The Aboriginal health workers may be part of mainstream services, but they are educated in family therapy, research and policy development as well as having local cultural knowledge. Examples of these services include the Bouverie Centre in Victoria and the Yorgum Aboriginal Family Counselling Service in Western Australia. The Bouverie Centre works in conjunction with participating Aboriginal Community Cooperatives, Child and Family Services and Latrobe University (Online. Available: www.bouverie.org.au/research/family-therapy-training-consultation-aboriginal-child-family-workers-community [accessed 8 January 2014]). The Yorgum Aboriginal Family Counselling Service is an Aboriginal community-controlled family counselling service that provides specialist assessment and counselling and links family members, including Aboriginal grandmother groups, to those who require their services (Online. Available: www.snaic.au/projects.dsp-default.cfm?loadref=84org [accessed 8 January 2014]).

In New Zealand, Māori families are known as whānau. Whānau is an extended family group comprising three to four generations. Traditionally whānau were made up of 20 to 30 people and were generally self-sufficient in everything except for matters of defence where they called on hapū (sub-tribe) and iwi (tribe) for support. Whānau cared for their older members (kaumatua and kuia) and their tamariki (children) collectively; where a child lost a parent or the family was too large to support a child, the child became known as whāngai and was cared for by the larger whānau—this is still common practice today (NZ Government, Online. Available: www.teara.govt.nz/en/tribal-organisation/page-4 [accessed 18 June 2013]). For Māori, whānau is what they say it is. The collective nature of whānau is important to understand in relation to family policy in New Zealand and will be discussed later in the chapter.

FAMILY DEVELOPMENTAL PATHWAYS

Developmental theorists suggest that families and their members go through various stages with some degree of consistency, each of which is quantitatively and qualitatively different from adjacent stages. The stages work through a set of transitions from beginning a partnership or marriage, to parenthood, to having children, seeing them off to school and ultimately to leaving home, to when the couple enters retirement. These stages may reflect the pathway of a traditional nuclear family, but they do not capture the multiple transitions and role changes of contemporary families in today's society. In many cases, children attend child care from very early after birth, and both partners are in some form of employment outside the home. Older children leave and return home. Single adults living together as a family of friends experience stages in their development that are not dependent on children's developmental stages. Same-sex couples may take turns enacting caregiver roles, and older, even retired people re-enter the workforce several times and often re-partner in old age. In addition, the beginning of family life may vary according to the couple's lifestyle choices, for example, at the stage of cohabiting. Cohabitation either prior to or instead of marriage is one of the most predominant trends for couples in the 21st century. It can be a normative stage where a couple lays the foundation for the future, including marriage and children (premarital cohabitation), or it may be an exploratory relationship between the partners to see whether or not they are sufficiently compatible to make a commitment to one another (Lichter & Qian 2008; Tach & Halpern-Meekin 2009; Thornton 2009).

FAMILY EVENTS
- Children's developmental milestones
- Educational transitions
- Leaving the family home
- Forming an intimate live-in relationship
- Changes in housing
- Unsettling events (injury, illnesses, deaths)
- Relationship changes
- Financial changes

(Baxter et al. 2012)

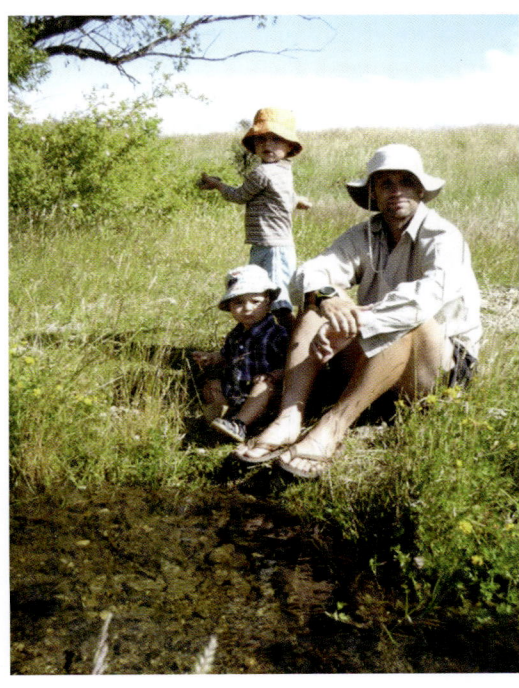

Family time (photo: Penny and Dan Smale)

Many families live in transient groupings with the intermittent involvement of non-resident members. When family members are separated or divorced there are often many new transitions, such as establishing various boundaries, dealing with children's access to parents, consolidating new relationships, reconstituting the family unit and planning for step-parenting. In the case of migrant or refugee families, children may be parented by members of several families, or in some cases, spend periods of time in detention or refugee camps without formal schooling. Family developmental stages with traditional expectations for certain roles at each stage may therefore not be as relevant in today's society as in the past. However, there are some rather predictable events that have an impact on family health and wellbeing. These events symbolise the dynamic nature of families as they respond to various situations, structures and processes. For example, a nuclear family constituting two parents and a child may have fewer, but equally meaningful, interactions than a separated family where the child is nurtured across two households. As the child grows the number and type of interactions s/he experiences may depend on the degree to which each familial household experiences a stable structure or periods of relative stability. The event of additional children joining either or both families affects interactions between all members in both households, as do the various milestones in their development. Children's transitions to school and beyond are also remarkable events in family life. In addition, a range of factors create changes affecting adult family members' relationships with one another, including economic, employment, environmental, social, cultural, relationship or health changes, and the adults' ages and stage in life. Intergenerational families, often described as extended families, may also have unique interactions to accommodate various members' stage in life. These changes and transitions tend to affect family members differentially, affecting psychosocial health, individuals' sense of isolation, stress and general wellbeing (Baxter et al. 2012). Clearly, the role of nurses in working with families in a community context needs to be focused on promoting inclusiveness, family cohesion and the transmission of strengths, needs and preferences along these variable developmental pathways and transitions.

CHANGING FAMILIES, CHANGING PARTNERS, CHANGING ROLES

As mentioned previously, family roles are usually dynamic, adapting to meet family goals and the ebb and flow of developmental and circumstantial events in family members' lives. A century ago when many families lived as an economic unit predominantly on properties, roles were relatively predictable. Nuclear families of husband, wife and several children were the norm. The husband was considered the head of the family, the wife was its heart. Children and parents worked together towards the major goal of productivity and economic survival. Few children were born to unmarried mothers, and some who did have children outside marriage were coerced into having them adopted to two-parent 'traditional' families. As a clear recognition of the perverse nature of this practice, in 2013 the Australian Government formally apologised to women for its

previous forced adoption policies that deprived those women of raising their children (FAHCSIA, Online. Available: www.fahcsia.gov.au/our-responsibilitiews/families-and-children/programs-services/past-forced-adoption-practices [accessed 9 May 2013]).

> ### WHAT'S YOUR OPINION?
>
> What are the key changes that have occurred in family life since the turn of the century?
>
> How would these affect your practice in the community today?

Since the industrial revolution that followed World War II, all Western societies have dramatically changed. The women's movement of the 1970s promoted the idea of women having choices in life rather than predetermined roles as wives and mothers. In recent times there has been a relaxation of sexual morality, reinforced by accessible contraception and a lack of social censure for marriage alternatives such as cohabitation (Maley 2009). In general, but with some exceptions, women have greater opportunities in the workplace, and better financial security than in the last century. Today there is a diverse array of jobs and more flexibility in the workplace for both men and women, who, in some cases, are now able to work from home. Abundant employment opportunities also inspired many women to undertake further education which they may have previously foregone to establish a family. These vast social changes have had profound effects, including declining birthrates, increases in the rate of family separation and divorce, and a dramatic increase in child care outside the family home.

> ## PRACTICE CHALLENGE
>
> How would you help a refugee family identify their assets and needs in relation to preparing their child to enter school after they had spent two years in detention?

In theory, these changes should have improved family life, but there remain some issues yet to be resolved. Five decades on from the women's movement the majority of women receive little assistance from partners in relation to the family's domestic responsibilities (AIFS, Online. Available:

www.aifs.gov.au/insititue/pubs/factssheets/2011 [accessed 9 May 2013]). In the workplace, they have yet to achieve parity with men in wages or executive opportunities. Women also experience greater job insecurity, partly because of family-related absences from the workplace. On the surface it seems that women have become emancipated from the pre-determined roles of their mothers. Yet, for many, the new freedom created by the women's movement has meant additional—rather than substitute—roles. As a result, many women continue to return home from work to complete a 'second shift' of child care and housework. This burden of dual roles often disrupts harmony in the home, creating a dual source of stress.

Globalisation has also had a major impact on the female workforce, with many women being relegated to lower paid casual jobs at the end of large commodity chains. It has exacerbated job insecurity for women, many of whom work in low-wage service industries, which is a particular burden for immigrant women who are disadvantaged in numerous other ways. Concurrently, the increased competitiveness of globalised industries has also created work intensification for men. Like their female co-workers, they have had to adapt to rapidly changing employment environments without the job security of past decades, where rewards flowed from persistence and loyalty rather than rapid transitions to a series of new workplaces. The challenges of the 21st century are multiplied many times over for migrant families. The mass migration of families across porous borders has affected family social and cultural life in their country of origin as well as in the host countries. Opening up national borders to migrants and refugees, and increasing the diversity and range of opportunities for women, has provided greater financial and social independence for those previously excluded from these opportunities, and created the impression of a fairer society in countries of the West.

POPULATION TRENDS, FERTILITY AND CHILD BEARING

Sweeping changes in society have irrevocably changed family life everywhere, including Australia and New Zealand. Australia's population has grown to nearly 23 million people, 19% of whom are children under age 15. The proportion of children is slightly greater in New Zealand, where 21% of the 4.5 million population is under age 15 (NZ Government, Online. Available: www.stats.govt.nz/browse_for_stats/people_and_communities [accessed 10 May 2013]). In both countries the population is ageing, with those over age 65 representing nearly

10% of New Zealanders and 14% of Australians, reflecting successes in preventing maternal and infant mortality and improvements in health. As a result, healthy life expectancy in both countries is among the highest in the world (ABS, AIFS, NZ Government, Online. Available: www.abs.gov.au/ausstats/abs@.nsf, www.aifs.gov.au/institute/pubs/factssheets/2011, www.stats.govt.nz/browse_for_stats/people_and_communities [accessed 10 May 2013]). Another trend shows increasing numbers of adults living alone, particularly older people, but including those who are younger and choose to live alone or are in transition because of relationship breakdown (Qu & De Vaus 2011). However, the majority of families are couples; 84% in Australia, about 40% of whom have dependent children, and 82% in New Zealand, approximately 42% of whom have dependent children. Around 33 000 people live as same-sex couples in Australia (Qu & De Vaus 2011) and approximately 11 800 in New Zealand (Statistics New Zealand 2010). Trends in all OECD countries show that many couples cohabit prior to marriage. In Australia these couples represent 8.9% of the population and in New Zealand 9.3% of the population (OECD Family Database, Online. Available: www.oecd.org/els/social/family/database [accessed 10 May 2013]).

QUICK FAMILY STATS

In both Australia and New Zealand, the marriage rate is declining, more couples are cohabiting and the divorce rate is around 12–12.5% per 1000 marriages.

The dramatic changes to family life since the social revolution of the 1960s and 1970s have had a pronounced effect on fertility, child bearing and projections for the future of the population. Marital instability and the decision of many women to delay child bearing until they have established their careers have conspired against fertility rates, so there are fewer children being born, most to older (>30) first-time parents, although New Zealand continues to have a higher birth rate than Australia. The average age of first-time mothers in Australia is 28, and the overall average age for all mothers is 30 (AIHW 2012). The birth rate in Australia has declined from 3.5 children in 1961 to 1.92 in 2011, and in New Zealand from 4.3 in 1961 to 2.1 in 2012 (AIFS, Statistics NZ, Online. Available: www.aifs.gov.au/institute/pubs/factssheets/2011, www.stats.govt.nz/browse_for_stats/people_and_communities [accessed 10 May 2013]). These rates differ according to socio-economic advantage, with those from low socio-economic advantage (migrants, those with lower education, Indigenous women) having the most births. For example, the Indigenous fertility rate is 2.74 babies per mother in Australia, 2.8 babies per mother for Māori and 2.9 babies per mother for Pacific women in New Zealand (ABS, NZ Government, Online. Available: www.abs.gov.au/ ausstats/abs@nsf, www.socialreport.msd.govt.nz/ people/fertility.html [accessed 10 May 2013]). Because infertility is a growing problem, especially for non-Indigenous women who tend to be older when they marry and begin their families, the rate of assisted reproduction technologies (ART) has increased markedly in many countries, averaging 4% of all Australian births (AIHW 2012).

Government incentives such as child care subsidies, increasing the baby bonus or paid parental leave, have been developed to address the decline in fertility, but there is a broader constellation of factors responsible for low birth rates that should be addressed. These include the need for equitable availability of child care centres, culturally appropriate family and community support, gender relations at home and at work, family-friendly workplace policies, and parity of wages for women and men. Many countries, including Australia and New Zealand, have begun to rely on immigration to sustain the population in the wake of falling fertility rates. New Zealand welcomed 1200 migrants and Australia 55 500 migrants in 2013 and 2012 respectively (ABS, NZ Government, Online. Available: www.abs.gov.ausstats/abs@nsf, www.stats.govt.nz/ browse_for_stats/population/Migration [accessed 10 May 2013]). Migrant families not only help supplement the workforce, but they lend vibrancy to the community, especially when there are 'family reunion programs' that allow a migrant to bring other family members to the host country. The migrant population is only part of the solution to sustaining the population, and policymakers argue that it is also important for a society to replace itself to provide a sufficient workforce and thus a tax base to sustain the ageing population.

A lower tax base places those living alone, with disabilities or the vulnerability of ageing at risk for a lower quality of life. If the trend toward living alone continues, it could also create a shortage of housing, and drive prices upward to where they are not affordable for either young families or older people. This is already a significant problem in large cities such as Melbourne, Sydney and Auckland where high house prices and government policies around lending have made first-home buying extremely difficult for young families. More importantly, when individuals work long hours and live isolated lives

there is a risk to family life and, ultimately, community cohesion.

EVIDENCE FOR PRACTICE

What research should we be conducting now to ensure that community health services are adequate and sustainable for the population in future?

What intervention studies could be undertaken to help older people remain healthy and fit?

Smaller family size is also a concern to demographers and child health specialists. One effect of small families is the number of children growing up without siblings, and the impact of this will likely not be fully realised until the children are adults. Another important consideration is the potential for families with young children to become the minority in the population. This could have implications for the way communities are developed or transformed if they become oriented toward meeting the needs of the older population rather than children. Although it is possible that in future, families will be caring for more adults than children, the impact of an adult-oriented community would be the lack of an influential voice for young families in the public arena. For some time the built environment has been showing the signs of demographic change, with some housing developments being tailored to older singles and child-free couples. With children pushed to the margins of public consciousness it is difficult to imagine who will champion the causes of family-friendly environments, including schools, workplaces, leisure and health services, or the need for communities to be actively involved in children's development (Stanley et al. 2005).

FAMILIES AND WORK PATTERNS

Since late last century, family life has been dramatically transformed by changes in the workplace. Unemployment has always had the most significant impact on the family, straining relationships, financial resources and inhibiting family members' capacity to make the kind of social connections that often occur in the workplace. For those employed, there have also been major changes that affect family life. With shrinking economies, many countries have seen an incremental casualisation of the workforce, which creates problems for some families financially, and in trying to balance career development, fertility, child care and family social time.

TRENDING NOW: Family life and work

- Most parents are both employed, often working long hours.
- Maternal employment is at all-time high.
- Fathers take 1–4 weeks' leave after birth.
- Many jobs have been casualised, leaving parents with job insecurity.
- Some parents work from home.
- Women tend to work part-time, increasing as their children grow.
- Single mothers have low employment rates.
- Most children are in child care by the first year of life.
- Grandparents are undertaking considerable child care.

Casualisation, part-time work and parental leave

A remarkable change that began in the last century is the significant increase in maternal employment for families with very young children, which has also had a profound change on family life (AIFS 2013). The typical work pattern for couples with children is for one person to have a full-time job and the other to work part-time, however many couples work according to different schedules depending on the age of the children. In most Australian families with children (87%) the male partner was engaged in paid employment in 2013, while 68% of couple mothers and 57% of single mothers were employed (AIFS 2013). Predictably, the proportion of single mothers' participation in paid work is lower because of the difficulties of having sole responsibility for child care. In 2011 19% of women and 12% of men worked part-time jobs (31% for single mothers), but the proportion who move into full-time work shows a steady increase as the children grow older. Australian and New Zealand policy changes have meant that workers have the right to negotiate flexible working arrangements, especially after the birth of a child or when other caregiving responsibilities are required. The Paid Parental Leave Scheme is designed to help parents provide a good start to their children's lives, with financial support for up to 18 weeks (14 weeks in New Zealand—see below) to take time off to parent a newborn or recently adopted child. In 2013 the Australian scheme was expanded to include a new two-week payment for working dads or partners (Dad and Partner Pay) to encourage fathers to help with child care (Government of Australia, Online. Available: www.humanservices.gov.au/customer/services/centrelink/parental-leave-pay [available 9 May 2013]). Many Australian fathers (80%) combine parental leave, holiday leave and other opportunities for flexible employment options after a child's birth (AIFS 2013). Mothers tend to take advantage of parental leave for longer periods of time than fathers, who typically take leave for 1–4 weeks, but most return to work earlier after childbirth than in the past, many returning to jobs within the first year (AIFS 2013). With so many parents in the workforce children's involvement in formal child care has risen exponentially over the past 30 years. Parents with children under age two continue to use informal care where possible, but from around age three most Australian children (61%) are in child care (AIFS 2013).

In New Zealand, most adults in families with dependent children work at least some hours per week with 66% of mothers in work and 90% of fathers (Families Commission 2012a). Over the past decade, a range of family-friendly policies have been introduced to support them. These include 14 weeks' paid parental leave (under the *Parental Leave and Employment Protection [Paid Parental Leave] Act 2002* and its amendment in 2004), and 20 free hours of teacher-led care and education for three- and four-year-olds. The 'working for families' tax credit also supports families with parents in work providing a sliding scale of tax credit based on income. Despite these policies, attaining the right mix of working hours and equitable distribution of work and child care responsibilities remains challenging for families (Colmar Brunton 2006). Over 29% of families with dependent children work 80 or more combined hours per week (Families Commission 2009a). Such long working hours bring multiple challenges for families and many call on extended family members to assist with child care responsibilities.

In both Australia and New Zealand grandparents, usually grandmothers, are called upon to provide child care, often at great personal cost, given that many are themselves engaged in part-time employment, and some have carer responsibilities for a spouse or older family member. In these cases, child care is not only physically demanding but may cause a conflict between the flexibility of grandparenting and disciplinary responsibility associated with the parenting role (Lange & Greif 2011). Most grandparents readily accept the responsibility and reciprocity with their grandchildren, recognising the importance and value of the role, but they may also have few opportunities for social support for themselves (Lange & Greif 2011). Despite the pressures, the pleasures and rewards of maintaining connections with grandchildren are great (Hendricks 2010). Many grandparents have adopted technology to support them in maintaining these connections, with mobile phones, texting, Facebook and Skype enabling grandparents and grandchildren to maintain relationships within the global context. However, child care and the many ways it affects contemporary family life, work choices and family planning remains a major issue for social policy planners.

For grandparents raising grandchildren full-time, the stresses and strains associated with this often unexpected role can be great (Hendricks 2010). New Zealand legislation passed in 1989 (*Children, Young Persons and their Families Act*) mandated the extended family as the preferred placement for children requiring care and protection. Based around traditional Māori concepts of whānau responsibility and decision-making, there is now some doubt over how well the model works for European families (Worrall 2009). Financial support for ageing grandparents is also inequitable when compared with the support provided for non-related foster caregivers, contributing to the challenges associated with raising sometimes troubled or disabled children and young people.

Work and stress

The workplace of the 21st century is the source of stress for many workers, in some cases because of long working hours, in others because of job insecurity or the dynamics of workplace interactions. Globalisation has precipitated some of the changes to today's workplaces, which include constant downsizing, restructuring to meet global demands, outsourcing work and relocating industries to gain economies of scale. These changes are a result of the need for companies to respond quickly and competitively to global markets. As a result, men in Australia and New Zealand work extremely long hours compared to men in other countries, with Australian men working the fifth highest hours in the world and 20% of New Zealand men working very long hours (OECD, Online. Available: www.oecdbetterlifeindex.org/countries/new-zealand/ [accessed 28 June 2013]; Patulny 2012). These extended work hours have an impact on the entire family. Some workers caught in the competitive ethos of transglobal companies have been forced to seek alternative employment, relocate to other regions, accept FIFO work patterns or move into other countries for various lengths of times. In many workplaces the 'structure, pace and experience of work has intensified at a time when family structures have weakened their ability to buffer

workers from the stress of the economy' (Palladino Schultheiss 2006:334). This is challenging as people try to reconcile equally important aspirations for a happy family and worklife. Researchers in the US report that nearly half of all workers experience difficulty balancing home and work, in some cases because of long and inflexible work hours and a lack of affordable, quality child care or family leave to spend quality time with their children (Milkie et al. 2010). Many workers lament that they would like to work fewer hours and spend more time with their children, a view that is also shared by their children (Johnson et al. 2013). Their work satisfaction is also affected when they are uneasy about family time. Many workers aspire to experience a sense of embeddedness or social connection with their work culture and workmates, which links them to a work-defined community. For others, work brings a sense of alienation and disconnection, or the impact of intersecting tensions between work and home (Losoncz & Bortolotto 2009; Palladino Schultheiss 2006). Because both types of responses reflect the social worlds within which people interact, the boundaries between work and personal life are somewhat artificial and fluid.

'Spillover' between family and work spheres can have a positive or negative effect, depending on whether a person has a supportive partner who can act as a buffer to difficult workdays and with whom one can share positive workplace experiences (Fincham & Beach 2010). New Zealand researchers found that high job satisfaction can improve home life quality, and has a positive effect on children's attitudes and values related to paid work (Colmar Brunton 2006). Parents in their study reported that working makes them better parents, and helps them deal with personal and practical issues. They also reported making friends at work, developing new interests and appreciating the financial capability to provide their family and children with extra benefits, such as holidays and gifts (Colmar Brunton 2006). However, other researchers have found that spillover of stress in either the work or personal context can leak across the boundaries, creating difficulties, particularly where work is undertaken in highly competitive surroundings or where long or non-standard shifts create a poor fit between workers' actual and preferred hours (Losoncz & Bortolotto 2009). Some of the factors that contribute to negative spillover in the workplace are the quality, complexity and skill level of the job, the amount and pace of work, flexibility, job security and control over the work schedule (Losoncz & Bortolotto 2009). The advent of smart phones that enable instant access to employees at all times of the night and day through email, texting and phone calls is a further contributing factor to spillover. Sometimes these factors are less intense for those working part-time, but part-time work can be stressful if hours are extended and there is little support from a partner. The effects are multiplied for those with child care or elder care needs as well as coping with workplace demands (Losoncz & Bortolotto 2009). Negative 'spillover' is more likely for those with inadequate coping skills, and it can erode a person's self-concept, making both their personal and work role difficult (Michel et al. 2009; Palladino Schultheiss 2006). The challenges are more difficult for immigrant workers, especially if they experience stereotyping, restricted opportunities for advancement, bias or discrimination (Palladino Schultheiss 2006).

EVIDENCE-BASED PRACTICE

What would be an important research question to study work-life balance?

Conflicts in either work or family relationships can either stimulate or inhibit career progress, work-related tasks and family functioning. Both sides of the work-home boundary require clear navigation, and this begins with the opportunity to reflect on the goals of each (Palladino Schultheiss 2006). Palladino Schultheiss (2006) explains that the discourse of 'work-life' balance or 'work-family' balance may have created the misunderstanding that balance, in terms of time, involvement and satisfaction, is attainable. For many people, successful work-family balance is often precarious. Like many men, women's careers are central to their identities. They have high demands in the workplace, often having to outperform expectations, with their careers costing them more in their private lives than men's (Ezzedeen & Ritchey 2008). Some women find they must breach workplace standards that require masculine behaviours, but they also have a parallel problem in breaching social norms of caregiving, often having to relegate child care to outsiders (Ezzedeen & Ritchey 2008). However, researchers have found that support from co-workers and family members, especially partners, can provide a significant buffer for feelings of unease or conflicts about work and family (Coulson et al. 2012). It is important to recognise that obtaining the right work balance is different for everybody depending on their stage of life, family circumstances, and personal desires. Morrison and Thurnell (2012) recommend employers offer a range of work-life benefits that employees can choose from as their circumstances change. Fujimoto et al. (2013) identify significant

gender differences in perceptions of work-life balance among Australian workers and suggest that employers need to move away from the 'ideal worker norm' (where one spouse works—usually the male—and the other spouse stays home to look after the children) to encompassing more gender-sensitive management and work-life balance policies.

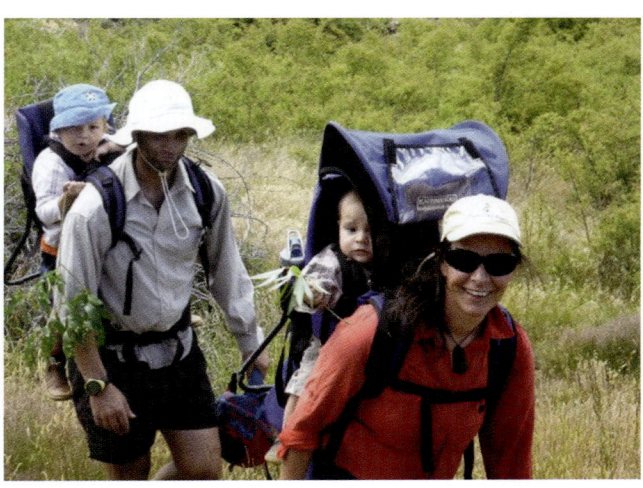

Family work-life balance (photo: Penny and Dan Smale)

Gender and work

Conversations about the elusive (and some would say mythical) 'work-family balance' tend to focus on either single parents or dual-earner couples. The most evident gender issue discussed in the media is the wage gap between male and female workers, but other issues include the challenges faced by single parents, especially women, because of their responsibility for parenting-related absences. In the workplace there are broad benefits from women's employment, including improvements to their mental and physical health, financial resources and often social supports (Coulson et al. 2012). Employers understand these issues, and tend to work towards retaining workers, especially when the costs of replacing and training employees are high. What often occurs with new mothers is that they re-enter the workplace to find the enormity of coping with family and workplace acts as a deterrent to staying in the job, especially where their child's temperament is such that they find it difficult to cope with non-maternal care or have ongoing illnesses (Coulson et al. 2012). In these cases, some women become anxious, depressed or ill. The antidote to these reactions is to provide consistent, accessible and reliable social support to help them feel they have the capability to weave their roles together in a way that sustains them in both home and workplace. To provide a buffer of support for such women, workplaces should help pregnant women plan for their maternity leave, making them feel emotionally supported as well as 'in the loop' and cared for once they return to work (Coulson et al. 2012:40).

Other gender issues are often hidden in workplace relationships, and fail to take account of the level of family diversity in today's society (Habib 2012). The workplace difficulties of lesbian, gay and bisexual families, or unmarried partners with and without children can be exacerbated by stigma, isolation and invisibility (Palladino Schultheiss 2006). In the context of reproductive technologies such as donor insemination and gestational surrogacy, new fathering identities have emerged, particularly in relation to gay fatherhood, which has been embraced widely in Australia (Dempsey & Hewitt 2012). Gay fathers include those who may have fathered children in previously heterosexual families, foster carers, donor dads and gay adoptive parents (Dempsey & Hewitt 2012). The language used in the workplace can also create gender issues; for example, the 'working mother' term, which is usually used in reporting women's stress, and has no parallel 'working father' term. This maintains the stereotype that family responsibilities belong exclusively to mothers (Palladino Schultheiss 2006).

Single employees without family responsibilities also have a unique set of issues, including the risk of having unequal access to benefits, a lack of respect for non-work life, occasional work expectations that exceed those with family responsibilities and social exclusion (Casper et al. 2007). This set of discriminatory influences represents a backlash to the family-friendly workplace where more desirable assignments may be given to employees who are perceived to have greater needs because of parental responsibilities. Research indicates that this type of discrimination may be more problematic for those in low-status, lower income jobs than those in a more privileged position (Casper et al. 2007). Clearly, the goals of a family-friendly workplace should be inclusive and equitable working expectations and the provision of equal opportunities for all employees.

A further workforce pressure in contemporary society lies in the growing number of older workers. Many older workers, especially older women, are seeking to delay retirement to respond to government policies that have reduced the affordability of living on a pension, and this applies to nurses as well as other female-dominated professions. As noted in Chapter 5, a study of nurses aged over 50 in New Zealand found that the

financial crisis in 2008–09, and changes in life circumstances such as divorce were substantial contributors to delayed retirement (Walker & Clendon 2012). Other changes affecting older workers flow from greater use of retrenchment and job redundancies for those unable to keep up with a highly competitive marketplace. On the other hand, some older workers stay in the workplace longer because of robust health, made possible by new medical technologies, or for other personal or professional reasons.

Transient families: FIFO and military families

Although each style of employment poses challenges to family life, the increase in the fly-in fly-out (FIFO) employment pattern described in Chapter 2 has had a major impact on many families. For parents, the FIFO arrangement presents constraints to family life that are similar to those of separated or military families. The experiences of FIFO parents and defence force personnel who are deployed overseas for periods of time are often similar to those of non-residential separated parents in terms of having to make constant adjustments to the multiple entries and exits into family life. For these parents, missing children's significant events or developmental milestones is a source of stress and anxiety. In the case of military families, helping family members adjust to unfamiliar environments is another challenge (Lowe et al. 2012). In preparation for deployment, numerous issues have to be arranged, which adds to the stress and worry about the partner who may be imperilled by having to confront combat (Lowe et al. 2012). The emotional issues are difficult, as the partner left behind assumes the role of managing the family, and then needs to renegotiate roles when the other partner returns. Some deal with this by concealing their fears or pressures, and others by withdrawing for periods of time during the reunion periods (Lowe et al. 2012). Some veterans report that their marriages are stronger after deployment, whereas others are weakened by the long absences and stress, especially where it is the woman who has been away (Fincham & Beach 2010). The children of these military families also suffer from the stress of separation and may have difficulty verbalising their feelings, with young children treating their parent like a stranger, and older children tending to express anger and fear (Lowe et al. 2012). Military nurses understand these issues, but in many communities where the families seek help and guidance from child and school health nurses, there is a challenge for the nurses to become familiar with the disruptions and pressures on this type of family. Similarly, helping FIFO families requires the depth of understanding to see where their greatest needs are during periods when they are together as well as when they are separated by distance. For the workers, moving from a partnered life to a single person's accommodation creates a plethora of stressors. These can include feelings of separation from family and support systems, exacerbated by a lack of telephone and internet access, and having little access to recreational facilities or time for relaxation. Some cope with the isolation in unhealthy ways, with alcohol or illicit substances. For the partner left behind, they can often experience a sense of abandonment and isolation akin to being a sole parent. The parent at home, usually the mother, may have to adjust to having previously enjoyed the closeness of a partner relationship, while being forced by the work schedule to assume total responsibility for child care and the logistics of raising a family, as well as helping the children cope with their father's absences. Although there is wide variation in the way individuals cope with these multiple transitions the accumulation of stress can lead to family disruption, depression and relationship breakdown. Some families adapt to this lifestyle by resettling in communities with a large number of FIFO families who provide an informal support system with a strong social network of families with a similar family situation.

Australian and New Zealand research into the unique challenges of military families is sparse. Although the research agenda for FIFO families is slowly evolving, few studies have been conducted by nurses. A small study of young men's views on the FIFO lifestyle indicated that having a positive attitude and effective coping mechanisms helps with psychological functioning and relationships while they are away, and adjustments when they make the transition to home (Carter & Kaczmarek 2009). Gallegos's (2006) in-depth interviews with FIFO family members in Western Australia found communication crucial to their adjustment, which concurs with the findings of other research (Taylor & Simmonds 2009). Gallegos's (2006) study revealed that family identity issues, child development and attachment concerns, decision-making and communication challenges related to parenting, and dealing with emotional responses of all family members to the father's work schedule were the major issues. Suggestions from both workers and their partners included the need to improve the flow of information from support agencies about the realities of parenting in this type of lifestyle, and ensuring that information from the industry is clear on work schedules, travel requirements and entitlements (Gallegos 2006).

CARING FOR MILITARY FAMILIES

Support for military and FIFO families remains scarce, with few agencies yet to provide appropriate services to meet their needs. Nurses in their home communities and in occupational and child health settings have a growing role in supporting their unique needs.

WHAT'S YOUR OPINION?

Nurses and other health workers have not traditionally used the FIFO model for their own work, yet calls for this as a model for employment of health care workers in remote locations is growing (Margolis 2012). How do you think nurses and other health care workers would cope with a FIFO lifestyle?

FIFO or military employment can add to the strain on marital relationships, or it can help build resilience. An Australian study of postings on a website forum supporting FIFO families found that women who had been in FIFO relationships for extended periods of time self-identified as strong and independent whereas those new to the FIFO lifestyle found the lifestyle emotionally challenging and were worried about becoming 'too independent' from their partners (Pini & Mays 2012). For cohabiting couples with a partner working away, there can also be difficulties in consolidating the partnership because of the intermittent nature of their relationships. In these cases, parenting and/or marriage is often

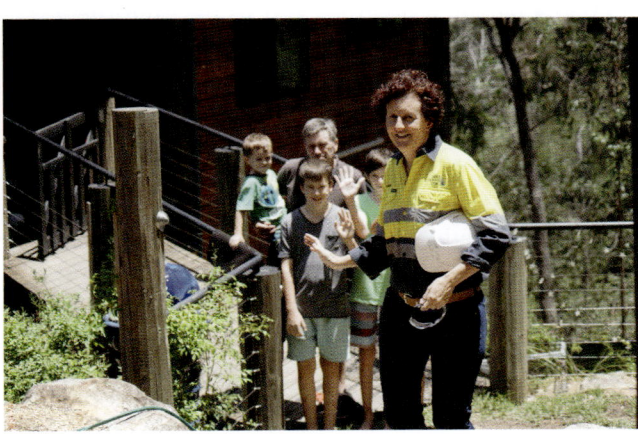

Alison Bourke, Queensland mining company nurse, saying goodbye to the family again (photo: Alison Bourke with permission)

delayed indefinitely until the couple can visualise a predictable future together. These couples spend the majority of their time as single adults, which can be socially awkward, leading to feelings of relationship insecurity. Like married couples, they transition frequently from the freedom of making their own decisions and organising their lifestyle according to personal needs to accommodating their part-time partner's needs when he/she arrives home. This can create a power imbalance in the couple relationship, and erode social relationships because of the tentativeness of their social life.

Part 2: Couple relationships and family life

Although today's families assume various forms and styles, the intimate couple relationship remains central to family members' health and wellbeing, for gay as well as heterosexual couples (Carr & Springer 2010). A strong, intimate couple relationship with warmth and open communication provides family members with a model for other relationships both within and external to the family. The type of partner an individual chooses to share her/his life with depends on personality traits, personal attitudes, values, norms of behaviour, identity and prior experience. All of these influences can be shaped in the family of origin or events in a person's life (Ongaro & Mazzuco 2009). During the pre-marriage courtship period successful couples develop a shared, well-grounded understanding of one another and their mutual expectations for married life (Wilson & Huston 2013). This shared reality reflects concordance, agreement about the relationship, perceptual congruence and a similar depth of love. The way they communicate during this time should set the tone for their relationship, ideally in providing mutual understanding of one another's personal qualities and values, and the ability to cross-check the accuracy of their impressions (Wilson & Huston 2013). On the other hand, couples who idealise one another, embellishing or overselling their enthusiasm for the other partner, minimising or discounting their differences, may create a mismatch between expectations and reality, which often leads to disappointment and a failed relationship (Wilson & Huston 2013). The dating relationship is therefore crucial to the long-term potential of a relationship, as it prefigures the emotional climate within which couples feel free to disclose their feelings, experiences and plans (Wilson & Huston 2013). Couples who set the stage for marriage or a long-term relationship in this way are better able to withstand the pressures of changes over the life course.

SOCIAL INFLUENCES ON COUPLE RELATIONSHIPS

Societal changes also exert an influence on young adults' relationships. Couples are influenced by the general tolerance for divorce and cohabitation that exists in most societies (Thornton 2009). In past times, traditional patterns of union formation saw many couples make companionate decisions about partnering, where a mate was chosen on the basis of compatibility. Today, there is a greater focus on individualised decisions, where a person seeks a partner who will support their personal goals and development. Couples still make choices on the need for companionship and having similar interests such as how they spend their leisure time (Claxton & Perry-Jenkins 2008). What is important is that couples understand each other's needs at the outset and throughout their relationship, and have a commitment to mutual self-development. Gender roles have always played a part in partner formation. Since the beginning of the feminist movement, women's preferences have changed, and women in the 21st century, compared to their mothers, place less importance on signs that a man is a good provider. Men, on the other hand, tend to value women's earning power, which has not historically been an influence in choosing a partner (Goldscheider et al. 2009).

> ## TRENDING NOW
>
> Many couples prior to or just after marriage attend couples relationship education (CRE), which helps them develop communication skills, shared expectations and positive mutual commitment. These programs are available for home study and have been found to be an effective investment in their future (see Halford et al. 2010).

Social policies also affect couples' propensity to make decisions about marriage or cohabitation. In conservative areas such as exist in many rural areas, particularly in the US, there is greater pressure on couples to marry (Heath 2009), particularly among those with a strong religious commitment. Religious commitment has been identified as having a positive effect on relationship quality, through enhancing problem resolution, or adding meaning and structure to support the relationship (Fincham & Beach 2010). Certain other social environments have a more laissez faire attitude, where young people are left to make up their own mind about partnering and marriage. Parental marital history is another important influence on the choice of a partner and the style of partnership. Those who have been previously exposed to marital disruption tend to choose partners with similar experiences and often defer marriage until after a period of cohabitation (Goldscheider et al. 2009). The timing of partnering or marriage also tends to be variable, sometimes influenced by socio-demographic factors such as neighbourhood characteristics (Fincham & Beach 2010).

Another social issue related to marital relationships is the trend towards same-sex marriage, which in some cases has evoked discriminatory responses. Since the turn of the century, liberalisation of marital laws in some countries (Canada, the United Kingdom, South Africa and some states in the United States) have resulted in a trend over the past decade or so toward greater acceptance of marriage between homosexual couples (Kluwer 2000; LeBourdais & Lapierre-Adamcyk 2004). This is also a social trend in Australia and New Zealand. Civil union became legal for same-sex couples in New Zealand in 2004 (*Civil Union Act 2004*, Online. Available: www.legislation.govt.nz/act/public/2004/0102/latest/whole.html [accessed 20 October 2009]), and in 2013, New Zealand legalised same-sex marriage with the passing of the Marriage (Definition of Marriage) Amendment Bill into law. The new Act has resulted in a number of gay and lesbian Australian couples travelling to New Zealand to marry. In Australia, groups lobbying for equal rights in marriage have attempted to secure similar legislation, but as yet there has been little political support for this type of change.

THINK ABOUT IT …

Why do you think it's important to consider same-sex marriage in society?

RELATIONSHIP SATISFACTION

Because of the growing number of couple separations worldwide, researchers have devoted an inordinate amount of time to studying partnership satisfaction (Amato 2010; Claxton & Perry-Jenkins 2008). Australian married couples report that they are highly satisfied with their relationship, while those who are divorced, especially non-resident parents, report low levels of satisfaction (Commonwealth of Australia 2008). Contextual factors play an important role in relationship satisfaction, particularly the

affective climate of the couple wherein they relate to others as well as themselves. Their history, workplace satisfaction and perceived support from one another helps moderate the effects of external forces in their lives (Fincham & Beach 2010). This is important for married couples because marital satisfaction has been identified as a strong predictor of life satisfaction, health and wellbeing (Carr & Springer 2010; Fincham & Beach 2010). On the other hand, infidelity has continued to be a source of dissatisfaction for young men and women (18–25), and a growing problem among older (65–90) men, presumably because Viagra and other accessible treatments for erectile dysfunction have provided new avenues for older men's extramarital sexual encounters (Fincham & Beach 2010).

RELATIONSHIP SATISFACTION

- Internal factors include history, warmth, love, security, trust and mutual support.
- External factors include workplace satisfaction and socio-economic environment.

Cohabitation can provide marriage-like benefits, including intimacy, economic cooperation and sharing (Carr & Springer 2010). The health benefits of cohabiting often depend on gender, life course stage, reasons for cohabiting, events during the cohabitation and the relationship satisfaction of each partner. Some cohabitors who subsequently marry report lower marital quality and less satisfaction with their relationship than married couples (Lichter & Qian 2008). Reasons for this may be related to the tentativeness of living together, which feeds unrealistic expectations of their future as a couple. Cohabiting couples are less likely to pool resources and they must negotiate a number of decisions that may lead to conflict; for example, purchasing a home, having children, or dealing with relatives and friends. When a person has experienced multiple transitions from one union to another a stable relationship is less likely. This may be due to the fact that many serial cohabitors are from low socio-economic groups, some of whom have few resources for a successful marriage (Lichter & Qian 2008). However, it can also reflect an individual's lack of marriage commitment or their unconventionality, or it can be a function of the ease at which successive breakups have been completed. For those who do marry, the odds of divorce have been found to be double of those who have only ever lived with the one person they married (Lichter & Qian 2008).

Research has also shown that marital quality tends to be poor among couples who have had a child during cohabitation (Amato 2010). Others argue that cohabitation prior to marriage creates inertia, and couples tend to marry because they have accumulated possessions and drift towards marriage (Amato 2010).

A HEALTHY COUPLE RELATIONSHIP ...

promotes 'the individual wellbeing of each partner and their offspring, assists each partner to adapt to life stresses, engenders a conjoint sense of emotional and sexual intimacy and ... promotes the long-term sustainment of a mutually satisfying relationship within the cultural context in which the partners live' Halford (2000:14).

Marital commitment involves personal, social, interpersonal, structural and legal elements. Personal reasons include an individual's preference to stay married, which may be an orientation towards sharing with a compatible other, the mutual benefit gained and personal fulfilment. Moral reasons for committing to another relate to feelings of obligation towards the marriage. Structural aspects reflect the constraints or barriers to not being married, which can include children's disadvantage and financial considerations (Byrd 2009). Despite encountering difficulties such as financial strains, the arrival of children or challenging events, a strong relationship is multidimensional, the product of what is valued, shared goals, responses to experiences and the potential of maintaining self-identity within the partnership.

HEALTHY COUPLES, HEALTHY FAMILIES

A committed, well-functioning and stable relationship is associated with greater resilience to stressful events, better physical and mental health, greater work productivity and effective parenting (Black & Lobo 2008). Conversely, there are a number of static and dynamic risks for poor couple relationships (Amato 2010). Static risk factors that predict breakdown include separation, divorce or violence in the family of origin, serial cohabitation, marrying young, being poor and/or unemployed, bringing children into a new marriage, marrying someone from a different race or having a history of depression or anxiety (Amato 2010). Dynamic or changeable risk factors include unrealistic expectations of the relationship, inadequate mutual partner support, lack of balance between individual and shared activities, inequitable division of household responsibilities and poor communication and conflict management (Amato 2010).

The importance of family communication cannot be overstated. Family values, behaviours and relationships are encompassed in the way members communicate with one another and value one another's sense of self. The main characteristics of successful family communication include clarity, open emotional expression, and collaborative problem solving (Black & Lobo 2008). Family members need opportunities to express their feelings, thoughts and concerns; to receive active encouragement of spontaneity and authenticity; to have honest, constructive resolution of conflicts; and to receive clear, consistent and unambiguous messages that convey love, affection, trust, support and acceptance (Amato 2010; Friedman et al. 2003).

COMMUNICATION, POWER, CHANGE AND RESILIENCE

Healthy power structures in the family have a more egalitarian structure where there are flexible opportunities for sharing power, and for complementing rather than subordinating one another. In a healthy family, individual members understand their respective roles in the family hierarchy and the extent to which they have authority over family decisions. This requires clear, predictable understanding of family role expectations and a commitment to sharing authority. Positive patterns of communication are essential, and are the key to family harmony during all periods of family change, including child bearing. Ongoing dysfunctional communication and interparental discord can cause an accumulation of harmful effects for children, particularly if parents also suffer from depression. Together, the co-existence of parental depression and marital conflict creates a multiplier effect, increasing children's risk for emotional insecurity (Kouros et al. 2008).

RESILIENT FAMILIES

- Communicate
- Are mutually committed, supportive
- Balance personal, family needs
- Are flexible, adapt to change
- Have a positive outlook
- Are tolerant, spiritual
- Spend time together; have similar interests, but personal space
- Plan for financial matters

Contemporary families have less predictability in their lifestyles than in previous times, more transitions and different configurations. Culture, experience, personal and contextual factors conspire to create numerous permutations in the way family members adapt to change. Parents with disabilities, for example, face added challenges at times and will often only receive much-needed support when issues reach crisis point (Families Commission 2012b). For lesbian and gay families, creating a child is often the first hurdle to be passed as family configurations change (Gunn & Surtees 2009). Some families are able to accommodate variety and change without too many problems, allowing members their own pathways and styles of coping with change, while others hold fast to a level of protectiveness that may not be helpful to individual members. Most families interact along a continuum of responses, which change over time. To some extent, the family's responses to change depend on the degree to which their boundaries are more or less porous; the extent to which they tend to allow the external world in, and, in turn, open themselves to the outside world. This may also change as members adapt to different circumstances. For example, a tightly woven family with relatively closed boundaries may be temporarily helpful in times of grief and bereavement, which usually occur following a death in the family, or when family members depart the family home to begin their own lifestyle. However, if the family is overly protective in the event of this type of change, family members may not develop the skills they need to personally adapt to the situation or to other changing circumstances. If the family is able to maintain itself as a unit, to balance personal grief and individual needs while allowing compassion and help from others, there is a greater likelihood that family members will develop a more balanced and harmonious perspective.

The key to successful adaptation to change revolves around self-knowledge and being able to access the type and timing of support as it is needed, being flexible and committed to others. These help build resilience in the face of change and adversity, and tolerance for others' needs, strengths and patterns of adjustment. Family resilience is developed in the context of developing a repertoire of positive coping behaviours and attributes. These include a positive outlook, spirituality, family member accord, flexibility, communication, financial management, time together, mutual recreational interests, routines and rituals, and social support (Black & Lobo 2008). Families who have a high level of resilience tend to survive the most difficult times, including the traumas of separation and divorce.

MARRIAGE, SEPARATION, DIVORCE AND PARENTING

The trend towards separation and divorce that began in response to changes in Australia's *Family Law Act* of 1975 and New Zealand's 1981 *Family Proceedings Act*, both of which introduced divorce on the grounds of irreconcilable differences, has continued, although at a slower rate than in the past (AIFS, Statistics NZ, Online. Available: www.aifs.gov.au/institute/pubs/factssheets/2011, www.stats.govt.nz/browse_for_stats/people_and_communities [accessed 10 May 2013]). Current trends indicate that around one in three marriages will end in divorce, and the incidence is greater in previously divorced families. In Australia, just under half of these divorces occur among couples with children, which means that approximately 50 000 children experience their parents' divorce, most of whom will live in lone-parent households. For New Zealand children, nearly one in four lives in a single-parent family, the third highest in the world (AIFS, NZ stuff, Online. Available: www.aifs.gov.au/institute/pubs/factssheets/2011, www.stuff.co.nz/national, www.mydivorce.com.au [accessed 10 May 2013]).

> ### POINT TO PONDER
>
> Research demonstrates that marriage has beneficial effects but that these are not experienced consistently across time or different contexts.

The trend towards cohabitation rather than marriage has left some relationships more fragile than where there has been a formal marriage commitment, especially when there are children born outside of a formal marital relationship (Baxter et al. 2011). OECD figures show 48% of births are outside of marriage in New Zealand and 34% in Australia (Families Commission 2012a). As mentioned above, marriage has beneficial effects, including companionship, everyday assistance and emotional support, and mutual support for healthy behaviours (Amato 2010; Carr & Springer 2010). On the other hand, divorced individuals suffer from more symptoms of depression and anxiety, stress, general health problems, substance use and a greater risk of mortality than married people (Amato 2010). Divorce is a complex and long-lasting event that diverts a person's life course and requires new roles and relationship patterns as well as integration of events and emotions (Eldar-Avidan et al. 2009). In some cases the event of a high-conflict divorce causes symptoms of ill health, but in other cases divorce resolves a difficult situation and the person initiating the divorce may find improved health over time.

POINT TO PONDER

Separation and divorce have significant effects on the family. Successful coping and adaptation can be maximised if the divorce is harmonious and if stress is minimised.

Amato (2004) divides the scholarly debates on marriage into two camps: the marital decline perspective and the marital resilience perspective. The former group sees the retreat from marriage and the spread of single-parent households as a sign of individualistic norms that contribute to numerous social problems, including poverty, delinquency, violence, substance abuse, declining educational standards and the erosion of neighbourhoods and communities. In contrast, the latter group argues that separation and divorce provides a second chance for happiness and an escape from dysfunctional families. This side argues that poverty, unemployment, poorly funded schools, discrimination and the lack of health and other public services represent a more serious threat to the health of society than does the decline in married, heterosexual, two-parent families (Amato 2004). Some theorists contend that the effects of divorce are experienced differentially by men and women, to men's advantage. However, the nature, desirability, selectivity and relative rewards of marriage shift over time and scholars are now equivocal about the gender differences in the experience of divorce (Carr & Springer 2010). What has been identified is that women tend to be more satisfied with marriage in younger age groups, but become more dissatisfied as they get older, which is reflected in the fact that many women initiate separations after several decades of marriage. For some family members, divorce creates new ways of coping and can be capacity building.

WHAT'S YOUR OPINION?

- Divorce as a second chance?
- Divorce as a failure?
- How would you guide someone from a hopeless to a resilient perspective?

Divorce and parenting

Divorce is clearly a major concern for the health and wellbeing of children over time. Many children of divorce have lived with cohabiting parents and partners, dividing their time and emotional energy between stepfamilies and a variety of step siblings. Because the dissolution of marriage is now intergenerational some of these children may be facing the prospect of experiencing divorce themselves, which has implications for their mental health. The anxieties and adjustments that children make during the transitions of parental separation vary by age, temperament and previous experiences, but few go through the experience without some degree of stress. Researchers indicate that children raised by both biological parents score higher on measures of psychological adjustment, self-esteem and academic success (Baxter et al. 2011; Sassler et al. 2009). On the other hand, children of divorce have been described as having poorer health and educational outcomes, experience more behavioural and emotional problems, have a higher propensity to fall into delinquency and crime, are more often in danger of being abused and neglected, and experience more unstable and unsatisfying relationships themselves (Maley 2009; Sassler et al. 2009). Yet there are differences in these outcomes for children who are being removed from a hostile or deteriorating relationship between their parents, and those who are surprised to find their seemingly happy family being dissolved. Children's emotional wellbeing is also dependent on whether they have inherited any of their parents' psychosocial traits or mental health problems, whether or not they are deprived financially or disrupted in terms of school, housing, diminished quality of parenting or loss of contact with one or another parent, and the type of emotional responses and coping being role-modelled to them in the context of the divorce (Baxter et al. 2011).

POINT TO PONDER

The impact of divorce on children and adolescents is significant. Although some demonstrate resilience, distress, apprehension, confusion, anger and destructive behaviours are more common.

Numerous studies have shown that children raised by two happily and continuously married parents have the best chance of developing into competent and successful adults (AIFS 2012; Hetherington & Kelly 2002). Couples who maintain a satisfying relationship have been found to have skills, attitudes and behaviours that translate into higher levels of parental warmth towards their children (Zubrick et al. 2008). Early studies on the effect of divorce on children focused on studying why some children become resilient and well adjusted, while others experience negative and pervasive effects (Amato & Rivera 1999; Kouros et al. 2008). Some of this research sought to allay the fears of separating parents that their actions would have adverse effects on their children by showing that it is better for the children when parents separate rather than remaining in a home with high marital conflict (Hetherington 1999; Wallerstein et al. 2000). However, after 25 years of studying the effects of divorce on children, researchers have concluded that many children do not do as well as was expected (Hetherington 1999). Some children of divorce may be disadvantaged by poverty or the cumulative effects of a parent who may have existing mental health problems, which can contribute to their stress as much as the process of family separation (Hunter & Price-Robertson 2012).

WHAT'S YOUR OPINION?

- Is it helpful to aggregate information on children of divorce, or would it be better to just look at individual cases of resilience in responding to family changes?

- Are the statistics useful in improving family health?

Although some children show resilient behaviours, more often than not they experience distress, apprehension, confusion and anger in response to marital conflict and divorce (Amato 2004; Hetherington 1999; Kouros et al. 2008; Wallerstein et al. 2000). As adults, children of divorce also experience higher marital instability themselves and tend to have a reduced belief in marriage as a long-lasting institution (Ongaro & Mazzuco 2009, Teachman 2002). Young children and adolescents have the highest rates of difficulty adjusting to marital separation and stepfamily life (AIFS 2012). For adolescents, adjusting to the transitions that follow separation and divorce presents an enormous personal challenge, with studies showing that they have lower verbal ability, school test scores, school and university completion rates, and higher rates of behavioural and mental health problems, delinquency, teenage pregnancy and early parenthood (AIFS 2012). Some of these

negative impacts are related to a lack of consistency. Many children of divorce experience transient family groupings and a number of stressful challenges as the family establishes various boundaries, deals with children's access to parents, consolidates new relationships, reconstitutes the family unit and plans for step-parenting.

Divorce and the blended family

The blending of two families can be a difficult situation with many ups and downs as some or all of the members of both families become part of the core family for indeterminate lengths of time. Parental conflict, distress and the adjustments of divorce place children at risk for emotional difficulties and a sense of loss. In some cases, their difficulties occur because parents are too preoccupied with their own adjustment to adequately meet their emotional needs. Inadequate role-modelling or a lack of support can create lasting difficulties for children in developing intimate relationships as adults (Eldar-Avidan et al. 2009). On the other hand, when both parents are sensitive, responsive, nurturing and able to stimulate their children, there is a greater likelihood of favourable outcomes for children (Berlyn et al. 2008). Blended families can also result in increased parental supervision of children, which may have been lacking in a single-parent household, and have a positive effect in cases where the mother has an enhanced sense of wellbeing from the new partnership (AIFS 2012).

GROUP EXERCISE: Parenting

Parenting has a considerable influence on the health of children. Working in pairs, make a list of determinants that influence caregivers' ability for positive parenting. Make some notes on how you think nurses can support families in parenting. Consider the differing settings that nurses practise in, such as schools, clinics and in the home. Share your notes with the wider group.

The impact of divorce on parenting

As Parkinson (2012:2) argues, 'marriage may be dissoluble but parenthood is not'. For divorcing couples without children there are often major emotional sequelae that may last for a finite length of time, but for parents the trauma of divorce tends to have protracted and sometimes severe emotional and financial impacts. Diminished financial resources can create dramatic changes to their lifestyles, especially for women left with the responsibility for children. Single mothers have also been found to have poorer physical and mental health than mothers who are part of a couple (AIFS 2012). Mothers' economic disadvantage is a result of systemic inequities where women tend to have lower earning capacity than men, yet are left with the greatest proportion of child care expenses. The poverty of mothers raising children alone, called the 'feminisation of poverty' or the 'pauperisation of motherhood', has been documented throughout the world. It is not only an issue for the women themselves but a significant predictor of child outcomes (Keating & Hertzman 1999; Stanley et al. 2005; UNFPA 2000). However, with the trend toward shared parenting rather than one parent having 'custody' of the children, there is a greater likelihood of joint responsibility for parenting and a more equitable distribution of the financial costs associated with this (Parkinson 2012). The policy of shared parenting as a first consideration in Australian divorce cases was developed 'in the best interests of the child' so that each parent would have both rights and responsibilities; the opportunity to continue a close and supportive relationship with their children and the obligation to protect them from harm (Parkinson 2012:2). Since its inception in 2006 the policy has had mixed outcomes, working well in some cases, but the majority of divorces continue to result in one parent living with the children and the other being a non-resident parent (AIFS 2012).

Non-resident parenting

Being the parent in the home has the advantage of being accessible to children at times of their greatest need, and being part of significant moments in their lives. Despite a growing proportion of single-father families, it is still mostly men who become non-resident parents following divorce (Goldscheider et al. 2009). These fathers typically experience a deterioration of their lifestyle related to shrinking finances, but a more serious problem for non-resident fathers is their difficulty in maintaining a warm and enduring father–child relationship with their children. The typical pattern of non-resident parenting sees the father spending alternate weekends and an evening midweek with the children (AIFS 2012). However, around 19–28% of Australian men do not follow this pattern, seeing their children only intermittently (AIFS 2012). A number of factors affect the quality of the father–child relationship from this pattern of involvement. These factors include the father's pre-divorce parenting practices and relationships, financial resources, his satisfaction with access arrangements, his relationship with the children's mother in terms

of parenting, the closeness of his residence to the children, their age, stage and gender, whether he is fathering children from a new family, and any difficulties caused by the children having to adjust to multiple family transitions (AIFS 2012; Baxter 2012). However, non-resident fathers are not a homogeneous group and men react to the situation in a variety of ways (AIFS 2012). Some live in close proximity to their children, while others may be at a distance, reflecting a diversity of child–father arrangements. In addition, the presence of another man acting as the social parent to his children, whether from a live-in or external relationship, can not only change the context within which children are raised but also affect a non-resident father's relationship with his children (AIFS 2012). Studies of fathering comparing 'biological fathers' and 'social fathers' have shown mixed results, with some indications that social fathers engage in higher cooperative parenting styles and accept more shared responsibilities for parenting than married fathers. However, this may be due to the mother's selection of this type of husband, or because the new social father may be working to ensure quality and stability in the new relationship (Berger et al. 2008).

NON-RESIDENT PARENT FACTORS

- Pre-divorce parenting
- Financial resources
- Access arrangements
- Parental relationship
- Proximity to children
- Children's age, stage, gender, number of transitions

The importance of fathers remaining involved with their children is widely acknowledged, as fathering plays a significant role in children's health and wellbeing as well as fathers' satisfaction as parents (Gillies 2009; Halle et al. 2008). Where legal arrangements dictate access and child support, there are sometimes lower levels of contact between fathers and their children, often because of financial difficulties, which has a reciprocal effect on both fathers and their children. Some fathers suffer from Parental Alienation Syndrome (PAS), where embattled parents conduct an unrelenting campaign of denigration, criticism and sometimes hatred against each other (Farkas 2011). Deliberate and malicious strategies place the child at the centre of parents' anger rather than their support, with the child used as a pawn in their conflict, which is a form of emotional abuse (Farkas 2011). As a result, not only does the child suffer from confusion or ambivalence about the parents, but the non-resident target of abuse may become so alienated from the family that he withdraws from the father–child relationship. This type of situation decries the large body of research that has shown an association between the quantity and quality of father involvement and improved cognitive outcomes for their children (Amato & Rivera 1999).

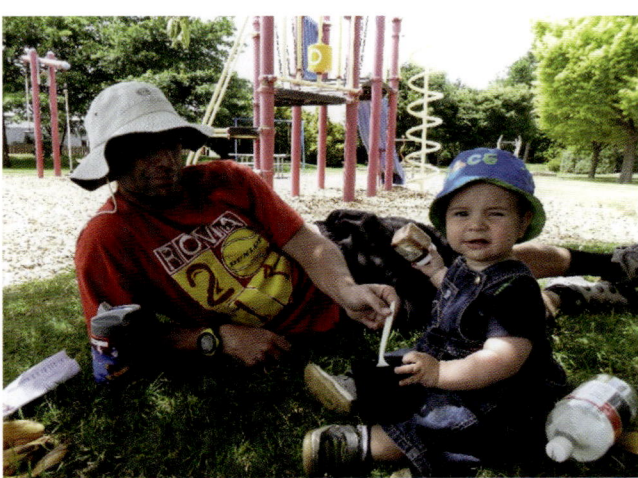

Dad time (photo: Penny and Dan Smale)

In addition to the children's adjustment to separation and divorce, the father's health and wellbeing is a major consideration. Leaving the family home can be devastating and have long-lasting effects. Even without PAS the loss of a partner is often accompanied by loss of other social networks, including those related to child care and family friendships (Patulny 2012). Australian fathers also face a loss of social contact time because of work intensification and long hours on the job, yet they manage to spend more time caring for children than men in any other country (Patulny 2012). They also experience deeper and less supported loneliness than women (Patulny 2012). Research has shown that fathers' education, mental health and perceived parental relationship quality or self-efficacy can play a role in helping them maintain confidence in their role (AIFS 2012). Another issue for fathers is the feeling of ongoing social isolation, which has been known to last into older age (Patulny 2012). Without the civilising influence of the family, many divorced fathers are at risk of being the population most in need of support during ageing (Gillies 2009; Lin 2008).

Parenting, child support and the rights of the child

EVIDENCE FOR PRACTICE

Family diversity can create controversy among those who take a narrow view of what constitutes a family.

What research studies would help reframe these debates?

Most non-resident parents in Australia and New Zealand provide financial support for their children through formal child support laws. In Australia around 90% of non-resident fathers have signed formal child support agreements, many of whom also add informal support when their children need 'extras' for sports or other events (AIFS 2012). These arrangements generally work well, but there are also cases where, despite the formality, the non-resident parent fails to provide child support. In some cases, this is because child support laws can disadvantage low socio-economic fathers by requiring a greater proportion of their finances than wealthier men (Swiss & Le Bourdais 2009). Low-earning fathers may be further disadvantaged by having to work variable shifts or during weekends when their children are available to see them. Swiss and Le Bourdais (2009) suggest that these difficulties faced by fathers are not well understood in the legal justice system, and practical factors should therefore be taken into account by those determining fathers' access to their children. In many cases, when financial barriers or the multiple responsibilities of two families arise, fathers tend to distance themselves, which reduces children's opportunities to have the advantage of both parents' support.

TRENDING NOW

- Shared parenting
- Parenting plans
- Best interests of the child

In many countries, new approaches to divorce laws have followed the lead set by the *British Family Law Act* of 1992, which mandated a parenting plan to be devised at the time of divorce. This ensures that the rights of children supersede the rights of either parent. Parenting plans represent one of the most important initiatives in helping families adjust to divorce. They are designed to document both parents' negotiated goals and intentions to ensure safety, physical and emotional care, education and legal responsibilities throughout their children's childhood. Parenting plans consist of detailed information on children's living arrangements and contact schedules, financial support, parents' decision-making responsibilities and dispute-resolution processes (Smyth 2004). Development of a parenting plan also helps to separate the processes of resolving money and property disputes from those involving the children. The plan is based on a humanising approach to providing for the children's wellbeing after parental separation to help counter the effect of emotionally intense legal negotiations that often interfere with rational decision-making.

The focus of contemporary research into divorcing families is not so much on laying blame as it is in emphasising the importance of parental support in ensuring love, security and support to achieve healthy social and cognitive development in children (Eldar-Avidan et al. 2009; Kouros et al. 2008; Swiss & Le Bourdais 2009; Wallerstein et al. 2000). New legislation in many countries has seen the language of separation and divorce changed to reflect the fact that custody of children is no longer the most important issue. Instead, the emphasis is on allowing children access to parents, rather than the other way around. This elevates the role of the non-residential parent to a more equal status than previously, when the emphasis was on survival of the single-parent headed household.

In situations where a resident parent chooses to move to another location, it is often the non-resident parent who suffers further separation and alienation from their child or children. Attempts to identify the best outcomes for children in situations where a parent wishes to move to another location have identified more dilemmas than solutions. Taylor et al. (2010) interviewed children and parents about their experiences in the aftermath of a relocation decision which either allowed the children to move with their resident parent or required them to remain living in close proximity to their non-resident or shared care parent. The intention of the study was to assist lawyers and the Family Court identify which issues ought to be examined most carefully in determining what is likely to be in the welfare and best interests of children affected by their parent's relocation dispute. Taylor et al. (2010) note that while in many cases decision are clear cut, for others the issues are complex and frequently there is no simple solution.

Today, it is expected that both parents will create opportunities to contribute to their children's development not only financially, but emotionally and socially as well. Widespread public debate about marriage, fertility, reproductive technologies and adoption have also drawn areas of discrimination into sharp focus. As a result, there is greater visibility of diverse family forms and a family's rights to raise children, regardless of the family composition. However, when the subject of family diversity is aired publicly, it tends to attract heated criticism from those who believe that alternative family forms erode family values. The people on this side of the argument tend to favour the neoliberal, moral right wing of politics, which is often argued on the basis of a narrow religious view of what constitutes a legitimate family (Heath 2009).

Coltrane (2001) argues that confining the debate to what constitutes a 'legitimate family' encourages rigid social mores such as premarital sexual abstinence, male family headship, females having to identify with the family, and resistance to feminism, homosexuality, cohabitation, abortion and related issues. Instead, the discourse of family issues should recognise the gendered and generational power dynamics that disadvantage both mothers and fathers when the children are not at the centre of policies and practices (Fletcher 2008; Gillies 2009). Clearly, there is a need in society for consideration of how parents can be supported in doing the best they can for their children. Polarised arguments to the right or the left side of politics do the family a disservice by focusing attention on morality and historical family structures, rather than jobs, poverty, equity, diversity, safe neighbourhoods, parenting, child care and health care; in other words, the SDH that make families strong.

VIOLENCE IN THE FAMILY

One of the greatest risks to the health and wellbeing of families is violence among family members, the infliction of abuse by one family member against another. This can include child-to-parent violence, elder abuse, intrafamilial abuse or intimate partner violence, the latter of which is the most frequent form of violence in the family (Schofield & Walker 2008; Thornton et al. 2008). Abusive intimate relationships can be categorised in terms of legal, fear-based or injury-based definitions (Sheehan & Smyth 2000). The legal definition includes the occurrence, attempt or threat of violence. Fear-based violence includes any act or threat to a person, causing fear for their wellbeing and safety. Injury-based violence refers to the severity of the act, as one that requires clinical intervention (Sheehan & Smyth 2000).

GENERATING THE EVIDENCE

How can we promote assessment of family violence in the nurse–family encounter?

What research questions remain unanswered to guide community nurses in helping families who have suffered family violence?

In the 1990s a declaration by the United Nations (UN) identifying violence against women as a human rights violation attracted global attention and outrage (Campbell 2001). At the same time, the WHO declared domestic violence a public health problem, and in 1995 the World Conference for Women in Beijing incorporated women's right to live without violence into a set of recommendations to the 23rd special session of the UN General Assembly (UNFPA 2000). In 2002, in response to continuing rates of violence around the world, WHO commissioned a first World Report on Violence and Health (Heise & Garcia-Moreno 2002). In 2008 Ellsberg et al. published the results of another WHO study across 10 countries, which showed that 15–71% of ever-partnered women had experienced physical or sexual violence or both by a former partner. These reports by the WHO and UN drew international attention to what is now considered a major public health problem affecting families and communities.

Intimate partner violence

The most common form of violence in the family, intimate partner violence (IPV), is linked to gendered relations of power and control (Parkinson 2012; Vincent & Eveline 2008), and usually follows marital conflict (Fincham & Beach 2010). IPV includes many types of abuse ranging from humiliation, belittling insults, property damage, threats of harm and actual physical abuse (Parkinson 2012). In the context of marriage IPV may be instigated by a man believing that he has the right to control his wife and the family resources. It can also be an aggressive response to acute negative events when he is under chronic stress (Fincham & Beach 2010). In some cases, the woman may escalate family conflict through aggression, which, in turn, disinhibits her partner's use of physical aggression (Fincham & Beach 2010). In the context of separation and divorce the abuser may be reacting to the spouse gaining exclusive access to family resources, including children. Where children are involved parental stress and conflict can create a lethal cocktail of reactions that have long-lasting effects on everyone involved. Without personal resources many women tend to stay in abusive families to ensure their children have a home. However, this leaves the situation unchanged, and the woman typically becomes more disempowered over time, causing poor mental and physical health, anxiety, low self-esteem and often post-traumatic stress symptoms and/or suicidal ideation, all of which can hamper her capacity for effective parenting (Letourneau et al. 2011). For many women the cycle of daily disempowering conditions becomes the norm for their lives in the ordinary interactions of marriage or partnership. Liang et al. (2005:75) explain that the 'fluid, liberal, and intimate nature of these interactions may make subtle violations and abuses difficult to detect and harder still to understand or define'.

PRACTICE STRATEGY

What factors could mediate the relationship between family structure and IPV?

How could you use this knowledge in planning strategies to help women and their children?

The prevalence of IPV is difficult to judge due to under-reporting and concealment of the problem, particularly in the case of psychological abuse. In many cases, women are hesitant to disclose their abuse even to emergency nurses, feeling that exposure and a loss of control will further disrupt their lives or result in incarceration of their partner (Catallo et al. 2012). Some researchers indicate that 8–66% of women are victims of violence at some time in their life (Letourneau et al. 2011). Many women suffer psychological abuse from partners who control their activities, their friendships and their access to support systems. One third of Australian women with a current or former partner report having experienced at least one form of violence, with 40% experiencing at least one incident of physical or sexual violence since age 15 (Murray & Powell 2009). In New Zealand, the figures are even higher with 55% of ever-partnered women having experienced any form of IPV in their lifetime (Fanslow & Robinson 2011). The accuracy of figures on violence against Indigenous women is nearly impossible to estimate, as many Indigenous women conceal their injuries not only from health care staff but from their friends and neighbours, because of their cultural obligation to protect family and kinship culture at any cost, even their personal wellbeing. It is estimated that Indigenous women may be up to 45 times more likely to be victims of IPV and ten times more likely than non-Indigenous women to be murdered (Vincent & Eveline 2008). For Māori, family violence is considered to be at epidemic levels (Te Puni Kokiri 2010). However, as we discuss in Chapter 13, the experience of Indigenous women is complex and includes a combination of factors related to colonisation history, racism and marginalisation as well as their social and economic vulnerability (Cripps & McGlade 2008).

PRACTICE STRATEGY

What visible behaviours might you see in a child health clinic in encountering a mother and child who had been previous victims of partner abuse?

Societal factors also have an impact on violence in the home. IPV, like rape and other forms of sexual coercion, occurs in a microcosm of societal conditions fuelled by economic exclusion and patriarchal attitudes of entitlement (McMurray 2006; Moloney 2008). When this becomes entrenched in society, it sends a signal to women that they are not worthy of participating in certain aspects of social life. IPV is therefore a public health problem that compromises the capacity of women and children who are its victims to live safe, dignified, empowered lives (McMurray 2006). Victims of IPV are often subjected to multiple forms of abuse, with many women experiencing a combination of physically threatening acts, verbal abuse and sexual violence, all of which violate societal norms of behaviour in a civilised society and have destructive effects on other family members.

IPV and the children

Witnessing IPV has a profound effect on children's emotional, social, behavioural and cognitive development (Letourneau et al. 2011). In some families, there is a co-occurrence of IPV and child abuse (Terrance et al. 2008; Wilson et al. 2004/5). It is estimated that 12 114 New Zealand children witnessed IPV in 2011/2012 (Bennett 2012a). Witnessing violence can cause children to experience the same psychological and behaviour problems as having been abused themselves (Johnson & Sullivan 2008), and it has also been associated with an increased likelihood of becoming a perpetrator

(Families Commission 2009b). This is a serious threat to child health and wellbeing. In some cases, mothers tend to become overly enmeshed with their child or children, drawing comfort from them rather than providing comfort for their distress. Others have been described as distancing themselves from their children, creating problems for the children who have no boundaries or guidance (Letourneau et al. 2011). Young children especially tend to react by externalising behaviours in anger, aggression and punitive treatment of their mothers. As we mentioned in the previous chapter, social learning theory (Bandura 1977) suggests that when children are exposed to violence they may acquire similar aggressive behaviour patterns, developing the perception that violence and aggression are normal and acceptable. In this way observing and experiencing violence creates a 'cradle of violence' for anti-social adulthood (Strauss 2001: 187).

Marital separation is a well-known time of risk for violence, but prevalence rates are difficult to estimate, as many couples experience unprecedented levels of conflict during and for some time after separation and divorce. In those cases that reach the family court, no separate statistics on family violence are kept as distinct from undifferentiated parenting disputes, and the relationships are complex, and prone to be misunderstood (Parkinson 2012). A woman's decision to end her marriage is often a precipitating factor for violence and this may be exacerbated by the injustice felt by male partners in an era of heightened awareness of men's roles in parenting. Heightened awareness of issues around fathering and the protracted grief experienced by many men often precipitates violence, even among men who have not previously been violent. In terms of the law and the family court system, the issue is about safety for the children as well as the woman, ensuring that interparental conflict, especially coercive controlling violence, is considered in decisions about sole or shared parenting orders (Parkinson 2012). The special issues of migrant couples are also a consideration in the courts and in social services. In some cultures, a woman's decision to separate from her husband may be a trigger to violence that would have been tolerated in their home culture. Sometimes migration instigates a change in power relations, and at the time when a migrant wife first enters the workplace she may envision a life without being controlled. This type of event can precipitate violence, often with dire outcomes, especially for women without extended family support (Naeem et al. 2008).

Part 3: Families with special needs

MIGRATION AND FAMILY LIFE

Migrant families have created indelible changes to the evolving national character of Australian and New Zealand community life (AIFS 2011a). In both countries, the last few decades have seen a steady growth of migrants from Asian countries and the subcontinent, the UK and other European countries, as well as cross-migration between the two countries. Refugee families also contribute to the multicultural vibrancy of the family and society in both countries in spite of the difficulties many of these groups experience in the maze of resettlement processes. At a societal level migration from poor to wealthy countries can create tensions, particularly if public opinion debates focus on the strain on the host country's resources from waves of migration. At the same time, there is widespread discussion over how to meet skill shortages. Obviously, the two issues need to be resolved in the same arena, but the challenge remains for health and social service planners to identify how migrant people can be educated and employed in the areas of greatest need without disempowering them, or denigrating their lifestyles.

> **POINT TO PONDER**
>
> Migration to a new country can create new opportunities for families but can also be one of the most stressful periods in a family's life course.

The transition to a new country is complex for all family members and affects family interrelationships in both subtle and overt ways. Many migrant workers suffer from having left behind family members, coping with family separation until their spouse or children can join them through family reunification processes (Glick 2010). Some families experience a conflict of competing cultures and new family structures, as young family members straddle old and new ways of thinking about such things as child care, being working parents, separation and divorce, and the need for space and solitude in their frenetic lives (Glick 2010). Their experiences can be more intense where they are treated with discrimination,

prejudice and feelings of isolation, even when they are broad-brushed as part of a homogeneous cultural group rather than having a distinctive ethnic identity with diverse views in relation to their country of origin (Glick 2010). These situations can evoke intense emotions as they waiver between creating family stability and acculturating to their new lifestyle and opportunities for prosperity. Many immigrant and refugee families migrate to countries with better opportunities than they have previously experienced because of poverty, dangerous or destructive living conditions, political or individual freedom, or to provide better opportunities for their children (Chuang & Gielen 2009). Leaving their homes, friends and relatives is stressful, as is the need to make adjustments to completely new lifestyles, social, education and employment systems. Successful adaptation to the new culture during the migration experience depends on multiple spheres of influence in the community context of the new home and family environment, and the family's orientations and attitudes (Glick 2010).

The timing of migration is also important to family life, especially in the child-bearing years, as negotiating parenting and family life in a new culture and within different social structures can present major challenges (Glick 2010; Renzaho & Vignejevic 2011). In many cases, young families make the transition to both parenthood and a new country at the same time, which increases their level of transitional stress. Their culturally bounded view of parenting may be challenged by their children's assimilation into the new culture, transforming family dynamics and values across the generations (Chuang & Gielen 2009). Searching for adequate employment after resettlement can also place multiple strains on family members, especially if they experience multiple moves to gain employment. Where these families are able to maintain old and new family ties and bonds in their new country, there is a greater likelihood of building a successful new life (Glick 2010). Community support at this time can be a major influence on subsequent patterns of family development and the family's ability to connect with networks in the wider community.

Migration stress and coping

Economic deprivation or traumatic pre-migration experiences can also have profound effects on the family's adaptation to the new environment. In many cases, highly educated migrants arrive in their new country to learn that they must retrain or work at lower level jobs. Adolescents can also experience problems when they are required to help support the

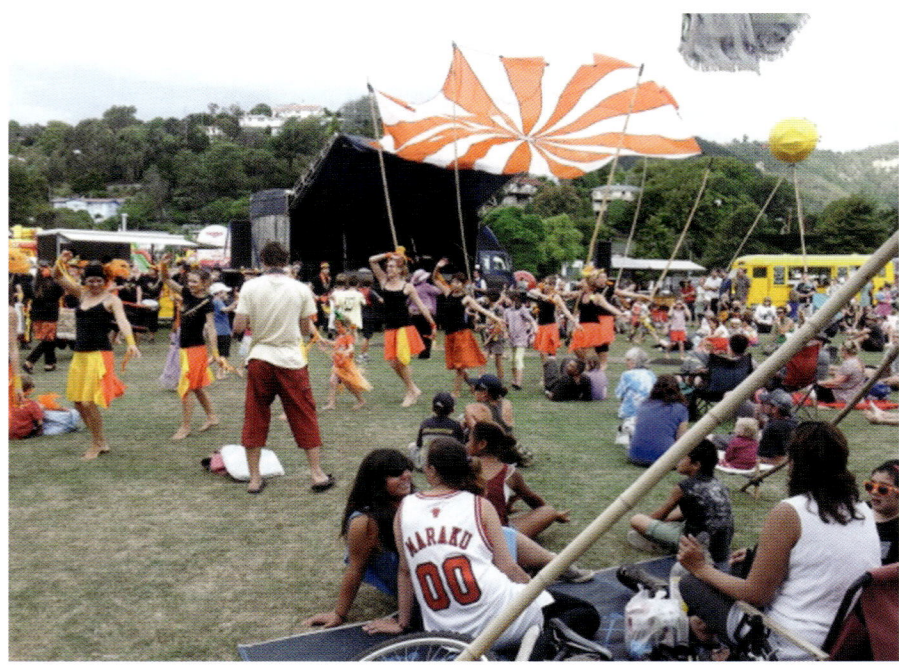

Race Unity Day festival (photo: Jill Clendon)

family instead of pursuing an education (Glick 2010). Sometimes they are the family member who leads migration, by travelling to the host country to attend school in advance of other family members (Glick 2010). These young people often find themselves in situations of conflicted values and mores, attempting to fit in to the wider community while maintaining cultural ties to their parents and ethnic group, often acting as language brokers for their parents (Glick 2010). Sometimes the transition of migration is made easier by resettlement in a place where there is an enclave of people sharing the same ethnic identity, but this is not always possible, especially if employment dictates otherwise.

Refugee families often endure long periods of adjustment when family members have experienced torture and trauma, changing roles, separation or death of family members, language difficulties or cultural behaviours that conflict with their country of origin (Lewig et al. 2009). These difficulties can be eased if support systems are provided by health and social professionals who have a good understanding of their unique experiences and expectations (Lewig et al. 2009). Lewig et al.'s (2009) research into refugee families' parenting challenges in South Australia found that the major challenges were linked to tensions between Australian laws and cultural norms and traditional cultural parenting beliefs and practices. Disciplining children was a particular area of difference in parenting. Refugee families found the

inappropriateness of physical discipline in Australia challenging, as they had been used to stronger control over children's behaviour (Lewig et al. 2009). Parents also believed that child care should be done in the family, often by older siblings. They were also concerned about the lack of structured activities in the community where mothers could meet one another and share parenting skills, as well as activities for adolescents after school to encourage their engagement with the community (Lewig et al. 2009).

A longitudinal study that traced the resettlement of a group of Bhutanese refugees in New Zealand found that initial expectations sometimes differed from the reality of resettlement. For example, despite not having worked in some cases for nearly 18 years, refugees believed that being able to find work would be easy once settled in their new country (Krishnan et al. 2011). The reality was quite different with some taking over a year to find work and others still to find a job despite their strong desire to work. Other challenges included the cooler climate and housing differences such as cold and large houses (Krishnan et al. 2011). Despite the Bhutanese group being identified as a strong and cohesive community with good links despite geographical separation within New Zealand, greater support in up-skilling and access to vocational opportunities are still required by many refugee groups, including those with strong community connections (Krishnan et al. 2011).

PRACTICE STRATEGIES

Working with refugee and migrant families can be challenging. Nurses must ensure the care they provide for these families is non-judgemental and based on the various needs and preferences of family members.

The migrant experience is an extended process rather than a discrete event that affects family life for many years after physical relocation (Lassetter & Callister 2009). Even for voluntary migrants the processes of adaptation create health effects linked to 'stress of the move, climate differences, racism, separation from family members and modifications in their physical environment, lifestyle and cultural milieu' (Lassetter & Callister 2009:94). These effects can interfere with acculturation or cause deteriorating health. Although adjustment to a new country can be confronting, marital stability and family reunion programs can help protect the family's integrity. Supportive factors in the host community include the presence of cultural and religious supports, accessible education and health care resources, social support services and a political environment in their resettlement country that is amenable to peace and stability.

GROUP EXERCISE: Refugee families

Refugee families face significant challenges settling into their new communities due to the traumatic circumstances of their past. Working in groups of three to four, make a list of the various issues nurses may need to support refugee families to address as they settle in their new country. Present this to the larger group as a mind map with the refugee family in the centre. On one side, make a list of the particular skills you think a nurse may need to have when working with refugee families.

FAMILIES CARING FOR MEMBERS WITH ILLNESS OR DISABILITY

For many families, the capacity to live the life they would choose is influenced by the need to care for a member with an illness or disability. Many families cope with a situation of illness with modest adjustments, especially if it is a transient situation that can be resolved over time, as is the case with many childhood illnesses. For others, the chronic

illness or disability of a family member can bring dramatic changes to family life (see Box 7.1). Relative to other countries, Australia and New Zealand have low rates of disability, yet around 15% of middle aged people and 10% of seniors in Australia care for elderly or disabled adult relatives (AIFS 2011a). For Indigenous families, even though they represent only 2.3% of the Australian population (AIFS 2011b) and 15.3% of the population of New Zealand (NZ Government, Online. Available: www.stats.govt.nz/browse_for_stats/population/estimates_and_projections/historical-population-tables.aspx [accessed 5 July 2013]) the problems of disability are severe, as they have greater rates of disability than non-Indigenous people, creating multiple stressors on those families who are among the most disadvantaged in society.

Of major significance to family life, around 7% of Australian children aged 0–14 live with a disability, ranging from mild or moderate limitations (43%) to those who have severe limitations on their lives (57%) (ABS, Online. Available:

BOX 7.1 Parents with disabilities

Many adults with disabilities go on to have children themselves. Being a parent with a disability brings a range of added challenges and rewards to family life. Many parents with disabilities struggle to gain employment and are often in situations of economic hardship. A study of 20 New Zealand families that included a parent with a disability found families demonstrated great resilience through shared family belief systems, maintaining an optimistic outlook and persevering in the face of challenge. Adaptability, flexibility and support from extended families and friends were also essential support mechanisms (Raffensperger et al. 2012). Despite these strengths, connectedness to community and financial resources were low and many remained in situations of financial difficulty that were compounded by the costs of their disability. Raffensperger et al. (2012) suggest five principles to bear in mind when working with families that include a parent with a disability:

1. Every family is unique.
2. Disabilities co-exist with abilities and strengths.
3. Spending time together having fun helps to build family resilience.
4. Families function as a unit.
5. Poverty and social isolation are challenges in themselves.

www.ausstats@abs.nsf [accessed 12 June 2013]). Approximately 11% of New Zealand children live with a disability (Bascand 2007). Disabilities include young children's sensory and speech limitations, chronic asthma, and intellectual, mental or behavioural disorders such as autism spectrum disorders (ABS, Online. Available: www.ausstats@abs.nsf [accessed 12 June 2013]; Bascand 2007). In many families, children's disabilities are compounded by the health problems that affect all young people today, especially obesity, which has a significantly higher worldwide prevalence among children with physical and cognitive disabilities (Rimmer 2011). In all cases, the onus is on the family to help them become part of the community and society, whether they live in the family home or in assisted care, so that they can live as normal a life as possible.

The financial costs associated with family care are substantial, and it is estimated that supporting a child with an illness or disability in this part of the world is 29–37% higher than supporting a well child (WHO & the World Bank 2011). In addition to the financial burden there are also significant opportunity costs when parents or other family members are unable to maintain their employment or usual lifestyle (UNICEF 2013). Many caregivers are also disadvantaged by having to forego predictability and long-term planning for their own lives as they become trapped in a situation where they are unable to make career changes, relocate or implement retirement plans (Donelan et al. 2001). Some find they are no longer able to participate in community life, either through lack of time, mobility, or social exclusion and discrimination, the latter of which are often more severe for families from vulnerable and minority groups (Vargas et al. 2012). The emotional costs are substantial, and the strain of caregiving can create undue pressure on family relationships, sometimes creating disorganisation of family functioning and compromising the health of all family members (Simpson & Jones 2012). The sense of social isolation experienced by caregivers can also be severe. In some cases, the family becomes isolated either by the desire of the ill person to remain out of public view, or by the altruistic desire to manage the situation as well as possible (Tsai & Wang 2009). Often, the caregiver gets caught up in a cycle of caring without respite, becoming exhausted to the point of emotional breakdown. Whether this occurs because of a lack of available resources, a situation that prevents accessing help or an unwillingness to seek assistance, it is a dysfunctional state for both the caregiver and the rest of the family. After long periods of time, some caregivers find that the burden of care

precipitates a much faster deterioration in their physical and mental health than they had anticipated and they may withdraw from social interactions and be at risk of developing clinical depression. This can also occur where they experience gradually diminishing support from others.

PRACTICE STRATEGY

Family caregiving is an issue affecting multiple social determinants of health. How would you systematically address these in practice?

The emotional effects can change profoundly over the trajectory of the illness or disability, as, for example, parents try to adjust to an unexpected event at birth and then endure the ups and downs of caring for a child with precarious health issues. In cases such as the birth of a pre-term baby, parents become hypervigilant This style of parenting may be resolved over time with psychosocial support, parenting education and therapeutic developmental support for the infant (Benzies et al. 2013). However, in other cases, family life is forever changed by the need for caregiving, especially in caring for a child with an intellectual disability. Many parents caring for children with even mild disabilities live stressful lives of trying to cope with the combination of their child's physical, emotional and behavioural problems while dealing with their own adjustments (Brookman-Frazee et al. 2010; Daire et al. 2011).

Caring for a chronically disabled child poses a number of crises over time, and for parents it can lead to feelings of guilt, separation from society, depression, marital problems and anxiety about their child's future (Daire et al. 2011; Tsai & Wang 2009). The practical aspects of caregiving often create uncertainty about their other relationships, and many couples have to work at organising sufficient time out from caregiving to maintain the partner relationship as well as deal with the needs of other children (Daire et al. 2011). This is easier when disability services provide respite care and when the family has a strong family support network. It is estimated that 420 000 New Zealanders care for ill, elderly, disabled or seriously injured loved ones over the age of 18 at home (Carers NZ, Online. Available: www.carers.net.nz/news_and_events/media_releases/6 [accessed 5 July 2013]). Family members who care for a disabled adult child in New Zealand have traditionally received no financial support from the government to provide this care, despite non-family members providing equivalent care getting paid through government agencies. Court action by family members incensed by this inequity resulted in the government setting aside $23 million a year (equating to the minimum wage) to support family carers from 2013 (NZ Carers, Online. Available: www.carers.net.nz/news_and_events/media_releases/7 [accessed 5 July 2013]).

The burden of caring for others is predominant among middle-aged women, who are often 'sandwich carers', acting as the primary caregiver for children as well as older persons with disabilities or ageing parents. Older carers often have chronic illnesses of their own, and this can create considerable personal stress, especially for those who live in the same home as the person requiring assistance. With population ageing the future burden of caregiving in the family will be significant, as many older people require some form of assistance, ranging from help with hearing devices to the constant help needed for those who develop dementia (Commonwealth of Australia 2008). Deinstitutionalisation of the mentally ill and policies that have eliminated many disability and aged care services in the past have also placed increased burden of care on family caregiving. Other pressures on informal caregivers are related to increased rates of family breakdown, leaving even fewer family members available for caregiving, especially for their elders. However, new models of disability care in New Zealand and the National Disability Insurance scheme planned for Australia are aimed at greater support for families with a disabled member, expanding choices for the type of care to be provided, and tailoring disability services to local and cultural needs (Online. Available: www.health.govt.nz/our-work/disability-services, www.ndis.gov.au [accessed 13 June 2013]).

All disabled persons, carers and families need cooperation and support from others as well as a sense of control over decisions and support services. Participation in planning and implementing care strategies is empowering and must take into account the context in which families and those they care for interact (Pullmann et al. 2010; Wilcox & Woods 2011). The challenge for health advocates is to recognise the bi-directional impact of family caregiving and to help families in this situation become empowered to make these choices. Although health professionals attempt to provide sufficient information and support to family caregivers, research studies have revealed that they often overestimate family members' health-related knowledge, underestimate the ill person's functional status, have poor understanding of the family's cultural needs and are sometimes insensitive to the family's intergenerational needs (Donelan et al. 2001; Kinrade et al. 2009; Teel & Carson 2003). As a result, family members may be left to deal with medical crises, symptom management and other maintenance issues with less than adequate professional backup, relying primarily on their own judgement, wisdom and resourcefulness. This is a major challenge for disability care in rural families.

RURAL FAMILY CAREGIVERS

Compared with families in urban environments, rural families throughout the world have higher rates of illness, disability and mortality, all of which are exacerbated by poor access to care and caregivers (AIFS 2011b; Pullmann et al. 2010). The proportion of rural families in Australia and New Zealand is relatively stable, at approximately 31% of the Australian population and 13% of New Zealanders (AIFS 2011b; NZ Government, Online. Available: www.tradingeconomics.com/new-zealand [accessed 13 June 2013]). Their disproportionate health status increases with the distance from metropolitan health services, and it is not clear how much of the difference is a result of biological factors, structural determinants of health or the rural lifestyle (Bourke et al. 2009). Rural and remote communities also contain disproportionately large numbers of Indigenous people, whose health is compromised by factors other than geography (AIFS 2011b). Rural life can have advantages, especially when families pull together in the face of difficulty, but these are usually outweighed by the disadvantages of a lack of access to services and support systems. The burden of family caregiving is therefore often pronounced for families living in rural areas, where resources are extremely scarce. In addition to the financial and emotional stressors mentioned in the previous sections, families caring for children with health problems away from urban centres face the additional stress of inadequate transportation, isolation, poverty, a lack of respite and fewer social networks than in urban areas. In the case of psychiatric or emotional problems these issues are often exacerbated by stigma, gossip and public surveillance of everyday life (Pullmann et al. 2010).

POINT TO PONDER

Rurality impacts on people's access to health services. Few options for accessing care limit rural family's choice of health care provider, in some cases, meaning a family does not seek care and does their best to 'manage'.

As mentioned in Chapter 2, rural families have less financial security than in past times, especially when they have experienced years of drought and more competitive markets for their goods due to the global economy. This has eroded the health status of many families, which is often compromised by exposure to harsh environments, occupational hazards associated with rural work and long working hours. The convergence of culture, gender, isolation, illness, ageing and a lack of service access can create multiple pressures on rural families, reflecting the intensity of the SDH for these populations. Other lifestyle pressures exist in the more remote settlements, which are disadvantaged by unreliable and expensive communications, continually rising fuel costs and a lack of access to fresh food, safe housing, adequate education and health services. As a result, young children and their families in remote and rural communities lack the advantages of having access to the internet and other educational tools for developing health literacy and skills for a changing workplace. Because of the lack of educational opportunities many adolescents leave home early to study in cities. When the family business is farming, their departure can create additional work pressures for those left behind. It can also be difficult for parents, especially for farming families who often spend more time with their children than urban families. For young people, the isolation and loneliness of being separated from the family can cause stress and difficulties associated with dislocation at a time when they most need family support.

Another difference between urban and rural people lies in the way rural people use health services. Most people make greater use of hospital emergency departments for primary care (AIHW 2012). This can be a problem for family members seeking the personalised care and privacy of a general practitioner, as there are few alternatives for care. Interventions for mental illness, family conflicts or other issues may rely heavily on friendship networks rather than professionals, as rural families seek to pull together, and give back to the community as a mutual support system (Sampson et al. 2011). But even this type of reciprocity can pose difficulties in a small community. In particular, rural women who experience violence may have unique needs that are not acknowledged by either police or health care professionals, and geographic isolation can amplify their perpetrator's control over them and their subsequent loneliness and isolation. In some cases, the prominence of firearms in a traditional, patriarchal rural home can heighten women's vulnerability by creating fear and intimidation (Wendt 2009). Some rural women

in this situation become trapped in violent relationships through 'financial insecurity, dependency, and stress; a perceived lack of confidentiality and anonymity; and stigma attached to the public disclosure of violence' (Wendt 2009:175). These situations and other aspects of family life therefore require sensitivity by health professionals and community planners to ensure that services are tailored to the needs of the population. Most community nurses in rural areas carry cards with emergency numbers that can be quietly provided to women at risk of violence, including the telephone numbers available in both Australia (1800 737 732) and New Zealand (0800 456 450).

Part 4: Goals, policies and practices for family health

Regardless of location, the family unit is today diverse and dynamic in its composition, perceptions and performance. What it means to belong to a family is defined in many ways, depending on the meanings held by family members and the ways they are bound together. The family itself is a metaphor for belonging and this should have a positive connotation for quality of life and life satisfaction. But despite the strength in connectedness, the family is also the most fragile of all human institutions; the place where we hold our deepest tensions, fears and hatreds, and sometimes violence, madness and despair (Curthoys 1999). For some families, having a wider range of choices has enhanced the quality of members' lives, while in others, the result has been dissatisfaction and disharmony. In the wealthy nations, the casualisation of workers and the intrusion of social media into family life has played havoc with family expectations. In the developing world, death, disease and civil strife continue to re-shape the family and create the impetus for migration. In the face of unremitting change, families will need the support of societal structures and policies and the commitment and guidance of health professionals to ensure sustainability throughout the precariousness of this century.

GOALS FOR FAMILY HEALTH

The goals listed below are relative to all families, and aimed at creating societies that will provide:
- physical, emotional and culturally inclusive support for all families
- access to a family-friendly means for economic sustainability

- a common bond from which to relate to the outside world
- opportunities for self-development for each of its members
- a connection to other families
- sense of place, heritage and continuity.

To achieve these goals, strategies for assisting families must be linked to the wider social and cultural context of their lives.

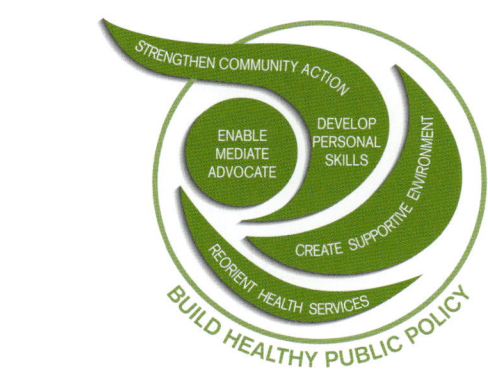

Building healthy public policy

The term 'family-friendly policy' has become increasingly distorted with political usage. A family-friendly policy is designed in collaboration with families who will be not only recipients, but co-creators of strategies that enhance health and wellbeing. Yet often, governments devise family-friendly policies on the basis of economic gains and without genuine collaboration with those who would enrich policies with practical wisdom. For example, parents should be involved in planning child care policies and other policies to deal with education, child health services, transportation, women and men's health, disability services and a range of other areas that affect family life. Family-friendly policies must be inclusive, which means they gather input from people in a variety of cultures and lifestyles. Such policies need to be based on in-depth knowledge of the various permutations of family life and the actual experiences of families. This means, for example, that policymakers should understand the SDH and support policies that promote reproductive choices for mothers, services that maintain health for family members across the developmental continuum and throughout health and illness, pregnancy and child care. Flexible

workplace policies that protect parental health and support parenting are also family-friendly policy goals. These need to include fathers' work schedules and organisational practices that do not discriminate against any type of parent. Father involvement in child care can be promoted by greater intersectoral collaboration, including cross-service discussions of how workplace policies affect social service policies and child access as determined by legal orders. Closer collaboration would provide an opportunity to solve some of the challenges faced by both men and women who have intermittent or variable work patterns affecting family life, such as occurs with FIFO families or those who must travel for work.

> **FAMILY**
>
> One of the most important but most vulnerable structures in society. Family-friendly policies are necessary for their long-term sustainability.

Another policy area requiring attention revolves around ensuring that the legal system supports parenting and families. Family law is a major concern for family advocates because current Australian and New Zealand law, like that of some other countries, allows unilateral divorce, which can be imposed upon an unwilling and possibly exploited spouse with legal impunity. This creates a disincentive to work towards partnership stability and responsibility (Maley 2009). The trend toward shared parenting has both strengths and weaknesses, and requires monitoring on the basis of individual cases, to ensure that the best interests of the child are served, and that children are protected from potential violence (Parkinson 2012).

Policies protecting human rights and non-violence

> **FAMILY LAW**
>
> Policies that assist parents to discuss all issues associated with children in a supportive manner are essential.

Violence in the home and community has become a more visible policy issue since the activism of the feminist movement in the 1970s (Murray & Powell 2009). A positive step in developing government policies to address the true nature of violence against women has been to reframe 'family violence' within a human rights discourse (Murray & Powell 2009). This means that each of us has a right to be safe and to have equality of opportunity. For women, unequal status in many areas compromises their human rights. Indigenous women, for example, are marginalised by gender, culture, economic and historical factors such as colonisation. This intersection of factors impinges on their human rights. Yet policies are developed on the basis of 'family violence', a term that tends to overlook the gendered issues of economic and social inequality inherent in violence against women. Therefore, situating responses to domestic violence within women's right to have control over their lives should be the foundation for policy development as advocated by the United Nations Declaration on the Elimination of Violence Against Women (UN 1993). There also remains a need for appropriate discussion of Indigenous women's violence and all forms of discrimination against Indigenous people, also enshrined in the UN Declaration on the Rights of Indigenous People (2007) (UN, Online. Available: www.un.org/esa/socdev/unpfii/documents/DRIPS_en.pdfg [accessed 13 June 2013]), to overcome 'the combined effects of racism, colonisation, and the socio-economic disadvantages of unemployment, poverty, and social isolation' (Murray & Powell 2009:542). Such an inclusive, culturally embedded policy response to the issue of violence against Indigenous women would be more appropriate in drawing attention to the social and structural determinants of their health and wellbeing. For all members of the community, policies for policing and emergency services should promote safety and a peaceful environment for family life, including emergency accommodation for those made vulnerable by violence when women and their children have to leave their home. Family services policies should continue to focus on housing strategies for the homeless and modifications to the built environment for families trying to provide care for members with a disability or impairment so that they are not excluded from social participation (Rimmer 2011). These policies should be developed in close collaboration with families to recognise the family's decision-making capacity in the context of the community environments that will promote wellbeing (Woods et al. 2011).

PRACTICE STRATEGY

Advocate for the rights of any group in the community who may be disadvantaged or vulnerable.

Inclusive policies

Public policies represent the shared values of society, which can reflect a moment in time or a vision for the future (Murray & Powell 2009). Implementation of policies is likely to be more equitable when they are developed from a deep understanding of the people affected by them. Inclusiveness should therefore be a major concern for all family policies. The way a family is defined sets boundaries for inclusion and exclusion when funding allocations are made. Government policies should therefore be developed in consultation with the community and the families who reside there, rather than be instigated above the grassroots level. For example, government agencies that fund programs for ageing families on the basis of such criteria as age and frailty fail to recognise that in doing so, they may sever a vital relationship between ageing couples or siblings who may need to remain together as a first priority. Older families with caregiving needs, and families with children suffering disabling conditions, can find the maze of social service policies difficult to understand or access, particularly when they change with each new government. This brings the role of advocating for families in clearer focus, and provides the impetus for all nurses, midwives and health professionals to have a working knowledge of policies and how they affect various families.

ACTION POINT

Collaborate with families to ensure cultural and environmental appropriateness.

Policies for vulnerable families

The special needs of rural and migrant families, those with extended family households, Indigenous people and those whose family of definition is based on sexual preference need also be addressed within a family-friendly context. Migrants and refugees are among the most vulnerable families in our communities whose lives are being imperilled by unhealthy policies. Detaining those who have sought asylum from global conflict, for example, without preserving family integrity, contradicts the human rights principles of actively engaging with people to encourage participation in decision-making and self-help. Everyone should have a right to social participation through employment and a happy family life (AIFS 2011a). Policies governing migrant and all other workers therefore need to be carefully conceived to maintain the rights of current and future residents. A family policy introduced in New

Zealand in 2010 entitled 'Whānau Ora' is designed to reduce health and social wellbeing disparities among vulnerable families. Underpinned by Māori values, although not exclusive to Māori families, the family-centred approach seeks to achieve the goal of 'Whānau Ora' (wellbeing of the extended family). The policy requires health services to work across traditional sector boundaries to improve individual, family and community health (Boulton et al. 2013). The policy has the potential to radically transform health service delivery to vulnerable families in New Zealand and will be evaluated carefully.

Policies protecting the community

In many of our large cities, we are surrounded by open, public debate on how to create cohesive, vibrant, trusting, family-friendly environments that promote social capital. At the local council level, interdisciplinary teams are developing policies for clean air, water conservation, more green spaces for recreation and better opportunities for education. This acknowledges the important role of communities in health and acceptance of the SDH. In Australia, the state of Victoria now mandates city council-level health and wellbeing policies, with many other states following its lead. This is one of the most important policy developments of recent times, as it entrenches the notion that it takes a whole community to raise a family. Numerous policies have also been developed around safety and quality of life. These include food security policies, public awareness of nutrition and food safety, new standards of food packaging, labelling and marketing, pricing sanctions and elimination of junk food advertising to deter families from overconsumption of high cholesterol and fatty foods, alcohol and tobacco.

It takes a village ...

It takes a community ...

At the global level, we have seen the policies of the most powerful governments move further away from social programs by severely limiting budget allocations to programs that would ensure health and safety for families raising children. This is ironic at a time of declining rates of childbirth and widespread knowledge of the inequities between rich and poor. At the national level, government policies protect markets abroad, yet there is no policy support to ensure local markets are able to compete with their goods, or that local community services are available for those most in need of them. New

Zealand, which has the advantage of national policy development, has been better able to facilitate policies for families across both Islands. With the fragmentation of policies in Australian states and territories this has not yet been achievable with the concordance of all. Policies for rural communities are virtually non-existent, despite the need to revitalise rural areas in order to leave a safe, cohesive and vibrant environment for the next generation. Rural families have relatively high rates of social capital, which they draw upon in times of need, but they also need support and infrastructure to ensure families have the right to make choices for health and wellbeing.

Creating supportive environments

In the rush of today's busy lifestyles, the need for community and societal support has never been greater. Supportive communities can develop ways of providing safety for families where abuse or other types of trauma are interfering with their health and wellbeing. Caregiving families, rural families, Indigenous families and those suffering family disruption need sensitive, resourceful health professionals to understand their needs. One of the most important elements of helping families is to convey a sense of non-judgemental support to help promote family resilience (Simpson & Jones 2012). This support can be embedded in the language we use. Being supportive means ensuring inclusiveness in all aspects of describing family life, being supportive of people's rights to what is enshrined in law, including single and gay parenting, same-sex marriage and a range of other family changes that have transformed the family in contemporary society. Those dealing with domestic abuse need equally sensitive treatment, and when they present to hospitals, and other health and community services, professionals working in these environments should be aware of the signs indicating that the person is living under threat. Where a family member is victimised by family violence, the individual's safety is paramount. Timely and appropriate assessment is crucial, which requires that all health professionals are provided with advanced training in family assessment, particularly in relation to family violence. A culturally safe approach begins with reflecting on one's own family, then seeking to engage safely with family members as appropriate. Critical skills include the ability to make decisions about who should be present at the assessment and to judge when the priority is to protect the victim rather than the family. Box 7.2 provides links to resources that will assist health practitioners assess people at risk of family violence. It is also important that the physical environment in health centres and hospitals provides safe places for discussion with those who are under threat of violence, including support for the nurse who may also be vulnerable to psychological risk in helping family members.

PARENT AND FAMILY ADVOCACY
Non-judgemental support for family choices.

Family parenting groups

First-time mothers gain enormous benefit from parent groups. Some groups are organised informally, from neighbourhoods or churches or individuals, as we mentioned in Chapter 6, but where these are not available, health professionals have an important role to play in bringing new and experienced mothers together, particularly those vulnerable families at risk for child neglect because of a lack of knowledge or experience. The benefit of these types of groups is well documented, especially when this type of teaching and support is accompanied by home visiting to reinforce parenting skills. The Community Mothers program that began in Perth has now evolved to a culturally embedded program as part of the Halls Creek Healthy Lifestyle Project for Indigenous mothers in Western Australia (Walker 2010). The program, which was developed in the local language for local mothers, has shown how understanding cultural meanings can be helpful in promoting family engagement and mothers' knowledge of postnatal and maternal depression, child neglect, alcohol and substance abuse, suicide and self-harm, domestic violence, transgenerational grief and loss, and worries about a new stolen generation as well as high levels of illness and incarceration (Walker 2010). The success of this program also demonstrates what constitutes a supportive environment, one that deals with issues from community-based participation in the language of local families. It also shows how focusing on early parenting can have far-reaching effects across all areas of family life and throughout the lifespan.

Programs focusing on fathers' needs are often overlooked and many provide supportive environments such as men's outreach services, or father and son camps, father-friendly places where they can pick up and drop off their children if necessary. Man-friendly services, with materials written in male-oriented language, are especially important for migrant and/or Indigenous men, and those living in rural areas who may be isolated from others (O'Brien & Rich 2002). Men's networks have also been developed for men who are unable to meet in person for mutual support. The Australian Fatherhood Research Network connects many of these men's initiatives through their bulletin from the University of Newcastle reporting on a wide range of men's issues (www.aracy.org.au/networks/australian-fatherhood-research-network) which can be downloaded without a subscription. Support for families experiencing separation and divorce is also essential. A number of organisations offer programs and information including the Family Justice in New Zealand who provide a free 'Parenting through Separation' program that supplies information and resources to support parents through separation and divorce, focusing on practical support for helping children through the process (www.justice.govt.nz/family-justice/about-children/making-decisions-about-children/getting-help-outside-the-court/parenting-through-separation) and Relationships Australia, who also provide a variety of support options for parents (www.relationships.org.au/relationship-advice/relationship-advice-topics/managing-separation-and-divorce).

Supportive environments must be tailored to the family's need to balance the conventions of their culture with the circumstances of their lives (see the 'Research in practice' box). For example, it is unacceptable in some communities to be divorced, yet violence against women and children is tolerated because it is embedded in people's culture and social mores. Similarly, some families are adamant about retaining child rearing practices, and their preferences must be respected while acting sensitively to promote healthy environments within which their children will flourish. We can all assist families by becoming knowledgeable about other cultures, being aware of how our stereotypes can influence our understandings of family life as we help them bridge old and new cultural influences in a culturally safe way.

RESEARCH TO PRACTICE: The African migrant parenting study

Australian researchers conducted a parenting program with 39 migrant and refugee parents (21 mothers, 18 fathers) from four African countries to help them negotiate the change in parental expectations of children, attitudes towards corporal punishment and restriction of children's access to food. The sessions, which were delivered by bilingual assistants, included eight culturally competent parenting skills including child development, children's self-confidence, communication and language, family relations, education pathways, legal issues, managing family stress, and parenting children and teenagers in a new culture. The researchers measured parenting attitudes and child-rearing practices using a validated tool before and after the program. The program produced positive change in terms of parents' expectations for their children, increased empathy, diminished belief in corporal punishment and a reduced tendency to reverse parent–child role. However, parental attitudes to children's independence were resistant to change, suggesting that participants retained their traditional views about children needing to submit to parental authority (Renzaho & Vignjevic 2011).

? Do the results of this study suggest any cultural issues that need to be resolved before the program is repeated? How would you go about providing such a program for parenting?

Supportive environments are those that respond to the combination of SDH affecting various families. For many women who are members of traditional cultures, the road to empowerment has been long and arduous as they have attempted to change patriarchal systems of marriage. Social structures and services need to be based on understandings of the tensions between individual and family transformations. This begins with the way conflict, especially IPV, is dealt with in Emergency Departments, where the healing environment should minimise intrusion while allowing a woman the time and space to relate her unique, multi-layered story in her way in a caring, supportive environment (Catallo et al. 2012; Davis & Taylor 2006). Some commonalities exist for all women in these situations, including social and institutional failures to hold the perpetrators responsible for their actions. These system-level failures create a situation of entrapment, where

women and often their children cannot escape a violent home because of economic reasons and fears for their safety (Johnson & Sullivan 2008). To change the situation requires more than immediate treatment and ongoing support for women's personal resilience. Our role as nurses also focuses on providing structural supports for gender-based empowerment through social activism, advocating for equitable circumstances for all members of society and strengthening community action.

Strengthening community action

The key to strengthening community action is family participation in identifying and resolving issues that may be constraining their health and wellbeing (see Box 7.3). This begins by helping them recognise the contextual influences that can be rearranged to support their health and development capacity. A genogram and ecomap produced in collaboration with family members can help illustrate their different connections and networks and the external influences that affect them (see Appendixes A, K). From this information a family-centred approach involves assessing their shared beliefs, relationships and interactions (Nyirati et al. 2012), strengths, weaknesses, threats and opportunities.

PRACTICE STRATEGY

Community action begins from a base of knowledge of family structures, processes and connections to the community and to one another.

A more detailed family assessment model is seen in Appendix H. The Australian Family Strengths Nursing Assessment Guide was developed and refined by Lindsay Smith (Smith & Ford 2013) on the basis of the resources of the Family Action Centre and St Luke's Innovative Resources. The model is based on the language Australian families use when talking about their own family. The uniqueness of the model lies in identifying each family's strengths in relation to Togetherness, Sharing activities, Affection, Support, Communication, Acceptance, Commitment, Resilience and Spiritual Wellbeing. Under each of these areas the nurse notes areas of strength and those that may be earmarked for growth.

As nurses and other health professionals working with families, our role is to allow family members to 'own' their own problems, rather than telling them what to do. Working in partnership with families to assess their needs can help ascertain

BOX 7.3 A family assessment tool

Holtslander et al. (2013) have developed an evidence-based, three-step, 15-minute family interview based on the Calgary Family Assessment Model (CFAM) and the Calgary Family Intervention Model (CFIM) (Wright & Leahey 2009, 2013). The objective of the exercise is to establish a therapeutic conversation, listen to families and understand their needs. In addition to good listening skills this assessment approach requires compassion and a willingness to make a connection with the family. The first step is to engage with the family in the process of compiling a genogram and an ecomap (see Appendices A, K). The next step involves developing three therapeutic questions for family members that elicit information on family information or other needs, which is typical of other types of assessment strategies. The final step is to offer commendations on family strengths and resources, which helps family members identify solutions based on personalised information in the context for change. This brief assessment strategy is considered by the authors as a good way to learn the skills of involvement with challenging problems and issues, and develop the confidence to interact with families and help them develop resilience and plan their preferred future.

? What do you think are the strengths and weaknesses of this brief approach to family assessment?

Do you think three questions are sufficient to establish a baseline of information?

To what extent is a prescribed approach such as the 15-minute interview helpful for assessing all types of families?

Are there any alternative learning approaches that might be helpful for family assessment?

Where do you think nurses could access advanced training in family assessment?

how family members experience the structural influences of their communities. Families should also be aware of early education opportunities their children are able to access, and this requires intersectoral planning between educators, health professionals and others involved in the health and social development of children. A family-inclusive approach helps them make informed, appropriate and acceptable choices. Working with families this way can maximise social action, addressing the influences in society which affect the structures and services that promote enhanced caregiving capacity among families supporting a member with a disability, for example (Brookman-Frazee et al. 2010; Daire et al. 2011). For rural people, collaborating with families can help draw attention to their need to overcome systemic barriers such as human resources, policy and funding issues that inhibit appropriate service delivery (Pullmann et al. 2010). At a societal level, participating in decision-making for effective solutions to family challenges is more desirable than trying to engineer families' strategies for change or critical decisions.

ACTION POINT

Get involved with what is happening in your community.

In the workplace, one target for social action is in lobbying for changes in organisational culture that will create supportive family opportunities. Companies need to recognise that worker loyalty will be multiplied many times over by systems of work that allow people to fulfil the obligations of both family and work. Good managers recognise the value added to their productivity from supporting family members with greater flexibility and attention to their emotional needs. This means helping people understand the value of developing emotionally intelligent ways of interacting rather than tolerate anti-social behaviours such as bullying in the workplace (Goleman 2000). This approach is foundational to the development of health literacy and helps promote people's self-confidence in their decision-making abilities. For FIFO families there is an additional need to include and support their views in community development debates about their working conditions. A relatively new initiative has seen the development of a FIFO newsletter and online chat forum (www.fifofamilies.com.au), which can be disseminated to all families involved. FIFO families can also be supported using research data focusing on the health impact assessment of FIFO employment at the individual, family and community levels (Australian Centre of Excellence by Local Government 2012). This type of information can help families work towards a more family-sensitive, empowering approach than simply complying with existing workforce constraints.

A PHC partnership approach to social action dictates the need for ongoing communication. The communications media has awakened us to the large number of hidden facets of family issues and sparked a debate over the public versus private nature of the family, including issues of collective morality. As health professionals, it is important that we stay involved in community dialogue, to provide the opportunities for family members to weigh in to debates that affect their health and wellbeing, and to transmit helpful information to them. To be of real assistance to families, we must keep issues of concern to them at the centre of public focus.

Developing personal skills

We hear much today about skills shortages, and, as mentioned above, policies should be developed carefully and inclusively, to create employment for successive generations of young people. This is particularly important with declining fertility and an ageing society that will require care and economic support for many years to come. In countries such as Australia with low unemployment, it is easy to overlook the need for building both personal and community skills, but it is important to have both. For countries with higher unemployment such as New Zealand (NZ Government, Online. Available: www.stats.govt.nz/browse_for_stats/snapshots-of-nz/top-statistics.aspx [accessed 6 July 2013]), ensuring re-training is available where needed and providing opportunities for community engagement are important for supporting families facing unemployment.

For many families, their day-to-day lives are stressful, for a variety of reasons. Many people require strategies for building resilience that can transfer across the work to home boundaries. These strategies can be discussed during health encounters in the context of promoting an ecological perspective where people work towards harmony in all of the settings of their lives. This is a capacity development approach, wherein the relational aspects of family life can be explored and validated as major steps on the pathway to community cohesion, trust and capacity for change.

Supporting personal skill development also contributes to civic participation. The rise of the voluntary sector over the past decade has shown the improved sense of wellbeing that occurs in communities where volunteering and participation in community life has become the norm, which makes a significant contribution to social capital. The contribution of volunteers should be recognised and their needs considered, especially those caring for family members with illness. The volunteer sector also includes parents' groups and self-help groups who provide invaluable assistance to families in helping them prepare for the future, especially those who are vulnerable or disadvantaged in

society. These groups should also attract ongoing recognition as their activities can make the difference between confident parenting and caregiving, or experiencing social isolation (Robinson et al. 2012).

Supporting family relationship skills

Although family life is coloured by the normal ups and downs of daily life, satisfaction is both the entry and end-point of the couple relationship. It is an ideal to which most young people aspire and a source of consternation among those who either find it elusive, do not understand it when they find it, or have found it and lost it. One of the most important things we, as health professionals can do to assist families is to understand at least the foundation of family relationship skills, so that our guidance and referrals are appropriate. Couples often need guidance from health professionals at the 'teachable moment', such as child health visits or school health encounters. In some cases these include aspects of their intimate relationship, such as resuming sexual activity following childbirth to try to promote closeness at this time (Williamson et al. 2008), or maintaining couple strengths when they are caring for a disabled child (Daire et al. 2011). In addition, becoming informed about parenting plans can help ease the strain on separated parents. When families in the community are encouraged to participate in designing services such as family post-separation services there is a positive impact on the wellbeing of children and their families, especially for marginalised families (Family & Community Relationship Services Australia 2012). As family health practitioners, if we can help family members develop self-esteem by feeling competent as parents and as partners, they have a better opportunity to build healthy communities. From a human rights or social justice perspective, there is a moral imperative for all children to have access to a home setting where their needs can be met (UNICEF 2013). Support for kinship care, including care provided by relatives and non-relatives such as family friends, is a significant aspect of maintaining children's potential for a satisfying life (O'Neill 2011). Our guidance for parents and caregivers often lies in helping them teach their children effective ways of coping with family stress, not only in the short term, but as a long-term strategy for living (Kouros et al. 2008). This is crucial in so many families who are undergoing marital disruption, particularly with the prospect of long-term effects on the children. It involves ensuring that intervention programs for children of divorce are both proactive and reactive, helping parents respond according to children's ages and developmental stage, as well as including culturally appropriate support for the family unit and sibling subsystems (Eldar-Avidan et al. 2009).

Reorienting health services

A family-sensitive, family-focused approach to health services means that the family and its issues lie at the centre of models of care. Community engagement maximises the opportunities for families to identify priorities and take ownership of problems, improving service access, delivery and better family and community relationships (Family & Community Relationship Services Australia 2012). In those cases where families experience ongoing crises, such as occurs in caring for children with special needs, it is important to be aware of resources where the family can access both emergency and ongoing support to meet what are often specialised needs (Daire et al. 2011). These parents also need ongoing financial, emotional and relationship support, as well as respite care. Families in the various stages of separating also may have a need for crisis care, but in most cases, visits to child health services reveal the need for an empathetic ear. Some health professionals shy away from dealing with difficult issues such as divorce or intimate partner violence because of a fear of opening 'Pandora's box' and being unsure of what to do to help. In many cases, working in partnership with victims of violence or other types of family issues can provide reciprocal knowledge of viable solutions. Women themselves have indicated that what they need from service providers is ongoing validation as women and as mothers, and non-judgemental health professionals who can help them work through their problems and solutions (Letourneau et al. 2011).

In New Zealand, all District Health Boards (DHBs) have established violence intervention programs. The aim of these programs is to reduce and prevent the health impacts of violence and abuse through early identification, assessment and referral of victims presenting to DHBs. These programs often employ a nurse to coordinate screening and intervention activities for people identified as at risk for family violence. While there is still significant work to do, an audit of all 20 DHBs found that approximately 30% (n = 6) are screening at least half of all eligible women (Koziol-McLain & Gear 2012). Plunket nurses (child health nurses) have been screening for family violence with all families who come into contact with the service for the past five years. While nurses found this challenging at first, it is now considered a normal part of the assessment process (Vallant et al. 2007).

Support for rural families requires services that are philosophically aligned with rural life, community-based, culturally competent, integrated, comprehensive and provided in the least restrictive environment and with the full participation of family members (Pullmann et al. 2010). Services planned for rural residents must be cognisant of the inequities between urban and rural populations and the disparity in service providers among the two types of communities. American researchers describe the solution to rural family needs as a system of 'wraparound services', which is a process of organising and coordinating service delivery for family members that may need multiple services such as therapies, special education, medication, employment services and transportation. This type of approach requires team work to ensure that the priority is 'family voice and choice' and support systems welcome friends, extended family and neighbours as partners in care (Pullmann et al. 2010:212).

Health promotion services are also sparse in rural areas. The lack of health professionals and programs for rural families indicate that there needs to be a concerted effort to connect the needs of families in the community with best practice in the cities, the rural areas and the wider global agenda. Developing and publicising a collective social consciousness may be one way to advocate for the equitable rationalisation of resources. As partners in service provision, rural community members have strong insights into the major economic and demographic changes affecting their communities from fertility rates, ageing, migration and wars, to employment and development patterns. Regional needs are therefore dependent on encouraging their input and intersectoral, community collaboration.

In implementing PHC for all families, it is important that links be made between the policy arena and people's access to health services. This involves making sure that links between policy and practice address not only health status and demographic information, but education, social protection, child care, housing, land use, the preservation of cultural and societal values, and adequate investment in health professionals. The latter includes the distribution of personnel across rural and urban areas, as well as permeable services that promote access for vulnerable people to move in and out of the system with ease (Beckfield & Krieger 2009; Peiris et al. 2008).

EVIDENCE-BASED FAMILY CENTRED PRACTICE

In working with families, new combinations of skills and services need to be developed from a base of research evidence to inform accessible, adequate and appropriate care. The evidence base for family nursing begins with a quest for understanding families, rather than searching for certainty, then examining ways of working with them from practice-derived knowledge (Doane Hartrick & Varcoe 2005). To date, there is a serious shortage of studies on the separating or divorcing family, and a dearth of investigations on appropriate ways of assisting couples undergoing marital separation. We need to redress these deficiencies and also reorient our research strategies from focusing on problems, to case studies of what works, to provide exemplars of good and best practice in family care. To this body of evidence we should add our practice-based arguments for preventive care, which is visionary, culturally and regionally relevant, and inventive. Caring, as the fundamental essence of professional practice, mandates our involvement in social and political processes. This guides us toward extending our role into society in order to work intersectorally at optimal capacity as community partners to secure access, equity and empowerment for better health and wellbeing.

CASE STUDY: Family life for the Smiths and Masons

Returning to our families, we see that Rebecca and Huia attended child health clinics in their respective communities for their children's annual check-up. As the parents outlined relatively minor child health issues, the nurses conducted an in-depth assessment of some of the special family issues, including those related to FIFO work, the father–child relationships, father role identity, the marital relationship, couples counselling, the need for extended family support or appropriate substitute support systems. These are sensitive issues, so communication strategies were foremost in their respective approaches to working with the two mothers during the family interviews.

In the mining community the occupational health nurse conducted a company-endorsed interactive family training session for all workers, where she addressed issues related to housing, transportation, community support for transient families and mining management support for families.

Both families have been struggling with the fly-in fly-out nature of Colin and Jason's work. Huia in particular has been struggling with managing their 12-year-old son John's behaviour alone for most of the time and Jason is not sure how he can support her. The Plunket nurse performing Jake's four-year-old before school check had some helpful suggestions for parenting strategies and Huia has shared these with Jason. The couple plan to implement some of these strategies, work together as a team and be consistent in their parenting.

REFLECTING ON THE BIG ISSUES

- Family life is multidimensional and consists of the family system, sibling subsystems and extended kinship networks.
- Family health and wellbeing is a product of individual and family interactions and the way family members interact with the external world, including the immediate community and society.

- The primary goal for empowering family members is to work in partnership with them to undertake collaborative planning to help them develop individual, family and community capacity and choices for family health and wellbeing.
- It is important for nurses and other health professionals to be aware of family issues such

as marital separation, family violence, family caregiving, work-life issues and the intersection of gender, culture and family histories in affecting family change.

- The environments within which families interact influence their health and wellbeing, with urban and rural families experiencing differential levels of vulnerability.

- Nursing interventions should be based on research evidence as well as careful assessment of the family and the circumstances and events surrounding them.

REFLECTIVE QUESTIONS: How would I use this knowledge in practice?

1 Prepare a genogram and ecomap of the Smith and Mason families.

2 What family goals would you establish for each family to ensure health and wellbeing for all family members?

3 How would you approach family assessment if you were conducting a home visit?

4 Would you alert the school nurse of any problems with the family? Why or Why not?

5 What actions would you take if family violence was disclosed during the family interview with either of the mothers?

6 During the interactive sessions with the miners how would you address family relationship issues and conflict resolution?

7 What resources would you use to ensure you had access to current research evidence for your actions?

References

Amato, P., Rivera, F., 1999. Paternal involvement and children's behavior problems. J. Marriage Fam. 61, 375–384.

Amato, P., 2004. Tension between institutional and individual views of marriage. J. Marriage Fam. 66 (4), 959–965.

Amato, P., 2010. Research on divorce: Continuing trends and new developments. J. Marriage Fam. 72, 650–666.

Australian Bureau of Statistics, 2011. Labour Force, Australia: Labour Force Status and Other Characteristics of Families, June 2011. Online Available: <www.abs.gov.au/ausstats/abs@nsf> 5 May 2013.

Australian Centre of Excellence for Local Government, 2012. Impact of fly-in-fly-out/drive-in-drive-out work practices on local government, ACELG, Sydney.

Australian Institute of Family Studies, 2011a. Families in Australia: Sticking together in food and tough times, AIFS, Melbourne.

Australian Institute of Family Studies, 2011b. Families in regional, rural and remote Australia, AIFS, Melbourne.

Australian Institute of Family Studies, 2012. New father figures and fathers who live elsewhere. Occasional Paper No. 42, Australian Government, Department of Families, Housing, Community Services and Indigenous Affairs, Canberra.

Australian Institute of Family Studies, 2013. Parents working out work, AIFS, Canberra.

Australian Institute of Health and Welfare, 2012. Australia's mothers and babies 2010, AIHW, Canberra.

Bandura, A., 1977. Social learning theory, Prentice-Hall, Englewood Cliffs, NJ.

Barakat, L., 2012. Advancing the family management style framework: Incorporating social ecology. Editorial. J. Fam. Nurs. 18 (1), 5–10.

Bascand, G., 2007. Hot off the press: 2006 disability survey, Statistics New Zealand, Wellington, New Zealand.

Baxter, J., 2012. Fathering across families: How father involvement varies for children when their father has children living elsewhere. J. Fam. Stud. 18 (2–3), 187–201.

Baxter, J., Weston, R., Qu, L., 2011. Family structure, co-parental relationship quality, post-separation paternal involvement and children's emotional wellbeing. J. Fam. Stud. 17, 86–109.

Baxter, K., Qu, L., Weston, R., et al., 2012. Experiences and effects of life events: Evidence from two Australian longitudinal studies. Aust. Inst. Fam. Stud. Fam. Matters 90, 6–16.

Beckfield, J., Krieger, N., 2009. Epi+ demos + cracy: Linking political systems and priorities to the magnitude of health inequities—evidence, gaps and a research agenda. Epidemiol. Rev. 31, 152–177.

Bennett, P., 2012a. The White Paper for Vulnerable Children, Ministry of Social Development, Wellington.

Benzies, K., Magill-Evans, J., Hayden, K., et al., 2013. Key components of early intervention programs for preterm infants and their parents: A systematic review and meta-analysis. Pregnancy Childbirth 13 (Suppl. 1), S10–S25.

Berger, L., Carlson, M., Bzostek, S., et al., 2008. Parenting practices of resident fathers: the role of marital and biological ties. J. Marriage Fam. 70, 625–639.

Berlyn, C., Wise, S., Soriano, G., 2008. Engaging fathers in child and family services. Occasional Paper No. 22, Australian Government Department of Families, Housing, Community Services and Indigenous Affairs, Canberra.

Black, K., Lobo, M., 2008. A conceptual review of family resilience factors. J. Fam. Nurs. 14 (1), 33–55.

Boulton, A., Tamehana, J., Brannelly, T., 2013. Whānau-centred health and social service delivery in New Zealand. Mai J. 2 (1), 18–32.

Bourke, L., Humphreys, J., Lukaitis, F., 2009. Health behaviours of young, rural residents: a case study. Aust. J. Rural Health 17, 86–91.

Brookman-Frazee, L., Taylor, R., Garland, A., 2010. Characterizing community-based mental health services for children with Autism Spectrum Disorders and disruptive behavior problems. J. Autism Dev. Disord. 40, 1188–1201.

Byrd, S., 2009. The social construction of marital commitment. J. Marriage Fam. 71, 318–336.

Campbell, J., 2001. Global perspectives on wife beating and health care. In: Martinez, M. (Ed.), Prevention and Control of Aggression and the Impact on Its Victims, Kluwer Academic/Plenum Publishers, New York, pp. 215–227.

Carr, D., Springer, K., 2010. Advances in families and health: Research in the 21st century. J. Marriage Fam. 72, 743–761.

Carter, T., Kaczmarek, E., 2009. An exploration of generation Y's experience of offshore fly-in/fly-out employment. Aust. Community Psychol. 21 (2), 52–66.

Casper, W., Weltman, D., Kwesiga, E., 2007. Beyond family-friendly: The construct and measurement of singles-friendly work culture. J. Vocat. Behav. 70, 478–501.

Catallo, C., Jack, S., Ciliska, D., et al., 2012. Minimizing the risk of intrusion: a grounded theory of intimate partner violence disclosure in emergency departments. J. Adv. Nurs. 69 (6), 1366–1376.

Chuang, S., Gielen, U., 2009. Understanding immigrant families from around the world: Introduction to the special issue. J. Fam. Psychol. 23 (3), 273–278.

Claxton, A., Perry-Jenkins, M., 2008. No fun anymore: Leisure and marital quality across the transition to parenthood. J. Marriage Fam. 70, 28–43.

Colmar Brunton, 2006. Work, family and parenting study: research findings, Ministry of Social Development, New Zealand, Wellington.

Coltrane, S., 2001. Marketing the marriage 'solution': misplaced simplicity in the politics of fatherhood. Sociol. Perspect. 44 (4), 387–418.

Commonwealth of Australia, 2008. Families in Australia: 2008, Department of the Prime Minister and Cabinet, Canberra.

Coulson, M., Skouteris, H., Dissanayake, C., 2012. The role of planning, support, and maternal and infant factors in women's return to work after maternity leave. Fam. Matters 90, 13–44.

Cripps, K., McGlade, H., 2008. Indigenous family violence and sexual abuse: Considering pathways forward. J. Fam. Stud. 14 (2–3), 240–253.

Curthoys, A., 1999. Family fortress: Chronicles of the future, The Australian, Sydney. 13 November.

Daire, A., Munyon, A., Carlson, M., et al., 2011. Examining distress of parents of children with and without special needs. J. Ment. Health Couns. 22 (2), 177–188.

Davis, K., Taylor, B., 2006. Stories of resistance and healing in the process of leaving abusive relationships. Contemp. Nurse 21, 199–208.

Dempsey, D., Hewitt, B., 2012. Fatherhood in the 21st century, Editorial. J. Fam. Stud. 18 (2–3), 98–102.

Doane Hartrick, G., Varcoe, C., 2005. Family nursing as relational inquiry, Lippincott Williams & Wilkins, Philadelphia.

Doane Hartrick, G., Varcoe, C., 2006. The 'hard spots' of family nursing: connecting across difference and diversity, Plenary Address, 7th International Family Nursing Conference. J. Fam. Nurs. 12 (1), 7–21.

Donelan, K., Falik, M., DesRoches, C., 2001. Caregiving: Challenges and implications for women's health. Womens Health Issues 11 (3), 185–200.

Duvall, E., Miller, B., 1985. Marriage and family development, sixth ed. Harper & Row, New York.

Eldar-Avidan, D., Haj-Yahia, M., Greenbaum, C., 2009. Divorce is a part of my life … resilience, survival, and vulnerability: Young adults' perception of the implications of parental divorce. J. Marital Fam. Ther. 24 (1), 30–46.

Ellsberg, M., Jansen, H., Heise, L., et al., 2008. Intimate partner violence and women's physical and mental health in the WHO multi-country study on women's health and domestic violence: An observational study. Lancet 371, 1165–1172.

Ezzedeen, S., Ritchey, K., 2008. The man behind the woman. A qualitative study of the spousal support received and valued by executive women. J. Fam. Issues 29 (9), 1107–1135.

Families Commission, 2009a. Finding time: parents' long working hours and time impact on family life, Families Commission, Wellington New Zealand. Online. Available: <http://www.familiescommission.govt.nz/research/work-life-balance/finding-time> 28 June 2013.

Families Commission, 2009b. Family violence statistics report, Families Commission, Wellington, New Zealand. Online. Available: <http://www.familiescommission.govt.nz/research/family-violence/family-violence-statistics-report> 26 February 2010.

Families Commission, 2012a. New Zealand families today: a brief demographic profile, Families Commission, Wellington, New Zealand. Online. Available : <http://www.familiescommission.org.nz/publications/briefs-and-statistics/fact-sheet-01-%E2%80%93-new-zealand-families-today> 20 June 2013.

Families Commission, 2012b. Disabled parents: diversity, experiences and support needs, Families Commission, Wellington, New Zealand. Online. Available: <http://www.familiescommission.org.nz/sites/default/files/downloads/disabled-parents.pdf> 29 June 2013.

Family & Community Relationships Services Australia, 2012. Community engagement in post-separation services: An exploratory study, Australian Government, Attorney-General's Department, Canberra.

Fanslow, J., Robinson, E., 2011. Sticks, stones or words? Counting the prevalence of different types of intimate partner violence reported by New Zealand women. J. Aggress. Maltreat. Trauma 20 (7), 741–759.

Farkas, M., 2011. An introduction to parental alienation syndrome. J. Psychosoc. Nurs. 49 (4), 20–26.

Fincham, F., Beach, S., 2010. Marriage in the new millennium: A decade in review. J. Marriage Fam. 72, 630–649.

Fletcher, R., 2008. Father-inclusive practice and associated professional competencies. Aust. Fam. Relat. Clgh Brief. 9, 1–10.

Friedman, M., Bowden, V., Jones, E., 2003. Family Nursing: research, theory & practice, Prentice Hall, Upper Saddle River, NJ.

Fujimoto, Y., Azmat, F., Hartel, C., 2013. Gender perceptions of work-life balance: management implications for full-time employees in Australia. Aust. J. Manag. 38 (1), 147–170.

Gallegos, D., 2006. Fly-in-fly-out employment: managing the parenting transitions, Centre for Social and Community Research, Murdoch University, Perth.

Gillies, V., 2009. Understandings and experiences of involved fathering in the United Kingdom: Exploring classed dimensions, Annals of the American Academy of Paediatric Social Services, 624. doi:10.1177/0002716209334295.

Glick, J., 2010. Connecting complex processes: A decade of research on immigrant families. J. Marriage Fam. 72, 498–515.

Goldscheider, F., Hofferth, S., Spearin, C., et al., 2009. Fatherhood across two generations. Factors affecting early family roles. J. Fam. Issues 30 (5), 586–604.

Goleman, D., 2000. Emotional Intelligence, Bantam Books, New York.

Gunn, A., Surtees, N., 2009. We're a family: How lesbians and gay men are creating and maintaining family in New Zealand, Families Commission, Wellington, New Zealand. Online. Available: <http://www.familiescommission.org.nz/sites/default/files/downloads/BS-were-a-family.pdf> 29 June 2013.

Habib, C., 2012. The transition to fatherhood: A literature review exploring paternal involvement with identity theory. J. Fam. Stud. 18 (2–3), 103–120.

Halford, K., 2000. Australian Couples in Millennium Three, Commonwealth of Australia, Canberra.

Halford, W., Wilson, K., Watson, B., et al., 2010. Couple relationship education at home: Does skill training enhance relationship assessment and feedback? J. Fam. Psychol. 24 (2), 188–196.

Halle, C., Fowler, C., Dowd, T., et al., 2008. Supporting fathers in the transition to parenthood. Contemp. Nurse 31, 57–70.

Hartrick Doane, G., Varcoe, C., 2005. Family nursing as relational inquiry: Developing health-promoting practice, Lippincott Williams & Wilkins, Philadelphia.

Heath, M., 2009. State of our unions. Marriage promotion and the contested power of heterosexuality. Gend. Soc. 23 (1), 27–48.

Heise, L., Garcia-Moreno, C. (Eds.), 2002. World report on violence and health, WHO, Geneva.

Hendricks, A., 2010. Changing roles: the pleasures and pressures of being a grandparent in New Zealand, The Families Commission, Wellington, New Zealand.

Hetherington, E., 1999. Should we stay together for the sake of the children? In: Hetherington, E. (Ed.), Coping With Divorce, Single Parenting, and Remarriage, Lawrence Erlbaum Associates, New York, pp. 93–116.

Hetherington, E., Kelly, J., 2002. For Better or For Worse: Divorce Reconsidered, Norton, New York.

Holtslander, L., Solar, J., Smith, N., 2013. The 15 minute family interview as a learning strategy for senior undergraduate nursing students. J. Fam. Nurs. 19 (2), 230–248.

Hunter, C., Price-Robertson, R., 2012. Family structure and child maltreatment, Child Family Community Australia Information Exchange, CFCA Paper No. 10.2012.

Johnson, S., Sullivan, C., 2008. How child protection workers support or further victimize battered mothers. J. Women Soc. Work 23 (3), 242–258.

Johnson, S., Li, J., Kendall, G., et al., 2013. Mothers' and fathers' work hours, child gender, and behavior in middle childhood. J. Marriage Fam. 75, 56–74.

Keating, D., Hertzman, C., 1999. Developmental Health and the Wealth of Nations, The Guilford Press, New York.

Kinrade, T., Jackson, A., Tomnay, J., 2009. The psychosocial needs of families during critical illness: comparison of nurses' and family members' perspectives. Aust. J. Adv. Nurs. 27 (2), 82–88.

Kluwer, E., 2000. Marital quality. In: Milardo, R., Duck, S. (Eds.), 2000 Families as Relationships, John Wiley, Chichester, pp. 59–78.

Kouros, C., Merrilees, C., Cummings, E., 2008. Marital conflict and children's emotional security in the context of parental depression. J. Marriage Fam. 70, 586–697.

Koziol-McLain, J., Gear, C., 2012. Hospital responsiveness to family violence: 96 month follow-up evaluation, Interdisciplinary Trauma Research Centre AUT, Auckland, New Zealand.

Krishnan, V., Plumridge, E., Ferguson, B., 2011. The Bhutanese refugee resettlement experience, The Labour Department, Wellington, New Zealand.

Lange, B., Greif, S., 2011. An emic view of caring for self: Grandmothers who care for children of mothers with substance use disorders. Contemp. Nurse 40 (1), 15–26.

Lassetter, J., Callister, L., 2009. The impact of migration on the health of voluntary migrants in Western societies. J. Transcult. Nurs. 20 (1), 93–104.

LeBourdais, C., Lapierre-Adamcyk, E., 2004. Changes in conjugal life in Canada: Is cohabitation progressively replacing marriage? J. Marriage Fam. 66 (4), 929–942.

Letourneau, N., Young, C., Secco, L., et al., 2011. Supporting mothering: Service providers' perspectives of mothers and young children affected by Intimate Partner Violence. Res. Nurs. Health 34, 192–203.

Lewig, K., Arney, F., Salveron, M., 2009. Challenges of parenting in a new culture: Implications for child and family welfare. Eval. Program Plann. doi:10.1016/j.evalprogplan.2009.05.002.

Liang, B., Goodman, L., Tummala-Narra, P., et al., 2005. A theoretical framework for understanding help-seeking processes among survivors of intimate partner violence. Am. J. Community Psychol. 36 (1/2), 71–84.

Lichter, D., Qian, Z., 2008. Serial cohabitation and the marital life course. J. Marriage Fam. 70, 861–870.

Lin, I., 2008. Consequences of parental divorce for adult children's support of their frail parents. J. Marriage Fam. 70, 113–128.

Losoncz, I., Bortolotto, N., 2009. Work-life balance: The experiences of Australian working mothers. J. Fam. Stud. 15, 122–138.

Lowe, K., Adams, K., Browne, B., et al., 2012. Impact of military deployment on family relationships. J. Fam. Stud. 18 (1), 17–27.

Maley, B., 2009. Family on the edge: stability and fertility in prosperity and recession. CIS Policy Monograph 101, Centre for Independent Study, Sydney.

Margolis, S., 2012. Is fly in/fly out (FIFO) a viable interim solution to address remote medical workforce shortages? Rural Remote Health 12, 2261 (Online).

McMurray, A., 2006. Peace, love and equality: Nurses, interpersonal violence and social justice. Preface. Contemp. Nurse 21, vii–x.

Michel, J., Mitchelson, J., Pichler, S., et al., 2009. Clarifying relationships among work and family social support, stressors, and work-family conflict. J. Vocat. Behav. doi:10.1016/j.jvb.2009.05.007.

Milkie, M., Kendig, S., Nomaguchi, K., et al., 2010. Time with children, children's well-being, and work-family balance among employed parents. J. Marriage Fam. 72 (5), 1329–1343.

Moloney, L., 2008. Violence allegations in parenting disputes: Reflections on court-based decision-making before and after the 2006 Australian law reforms. J. Fam. Stud. 14 (2–3), 254–270.

Morrison, E., Thurnell, D., 2012. Employee preferences for work-life benefits in a large New Zealand construction company. Aust. J. Constr. Econ. Build. 12 (1), 12–25.

Murray, S., Powell, A., 2009. What's the problem? Australian public policy constructions of domestic and family violence. Violence Against Women 15 (5), 532–552.

Naeem, F., Irfan, M., Zaidi, Q., et al., 2008. Angry wives, abusive husbands: relationship between domestic violence and psychosocial variables. Womens Health Issues 18, 453–462.

Nyirati, C., Denham, S., Raffle, H., et al., 2012. Where is the family nurse practitioner program? Results of a US family nurse practitioner program survey. J. Fam. Nurs. 18 (3), 378–408.

O'Brien, C., Rich, K., 2002. Evaluation of the Men and Family Relationships Initiative, Commonwealth Department of Family and Community Services, Canberra.

O'Neill, C., 2011. Support in kith and kin care: The experience of carers. Child. Austr. 36 (2), 88–99.

Ongaro, F., Mazzuco, S., 2009. Parental separation and family formation in early adulthood: Evidence from Italy. Adv. Life Course Res. doi:10.1016/j.alcr.2009.06.002.

Palladino Schultheiss, D., 2006. The interface of work and family life. Prof. Psychol. Res. Pr. 37 (4), 334–341.

Parkinson, P., 2012. When is parenthood dissoluble? Sole parental responsibility and restructions on contact in an era of shared parenting. Presentation to AIFS conference, Melbourne. July 2012.

Patulny, R., 2012. Social contact, efficacy and support amongst Australian fathers. J. Fam. Stud. 18 (2–3), 222–234.

Peiris, D., Brown, A., Cass, A., 2008. Addressing inequities in access to quality health care for indigenous people. Can. Med. Assoc. J. 179 (10), 985–986.

Pini, B., Mayes, R., 2012. Gender, emotions and fly-in fly-out work. Aust. J. Soc. Issues 47 (1), 71–86.

Pullmann, M., VanHooser, S., Hoffman, C., et al., 2010. Barriers to and supports of family participation in a rural system of care for children with serious emotional problems. Community Ment. Health J. 46, 211–220.

Putnam, R., 2005. Civic Renewal and Social Capital, Round Table Discussion, Alcoa Research Centre for Stronger Communities, Curtin University, Perth.

Qu, L., De Vaus, D., 2011. Starting and ending one-person households: A longitudinal analysis. J. Fam. Stud. 17, 126–145.

Raffensperger, M., Morton, M., Gage, J., et al., 2012. From our perspective: exploring the strength and resilience of families that include a parent with a disability, Families Commission, Wellington, New Zealand.

Renzaho, A., Vignjevic, S., 2011. The impact of a parenting intervention in Australia among migrants and refugees from Liberia, Sierra Leone, Congo, and Burundi: Results from the African Migrant Parenting Program. J. Fam. Stud. 17, 71–79.

Rimmer, J., 2011. Promoting inclusive community-based obesity prevention programs for children and adolescents with disabilities: The why and how. Child. Obes. 7 (3), 177–184.

Robinson, E., Scott, D., Meredith, V., et al., 2012. Good and innovative practice in service delivery to vulnerable and disadvantaged families and children, Child Family Community Australia Information Exchange, AIFS, CFCA Paper No. 9: 1–20.

Sampson, K., Goodrich, C., McManus, R., 2011. Rural families, industry change and social capital: Some considerations for policy. Soc. Policy J. N. Z. 37, 1–13.

Sassler, S., Cunningham, A., Lichter, D., 2009. Intergenerational patterns of union formation and relationship quality. J. Fam. Issues 30 (6), 757–786.

Schofield, M., Walker, R., 2008. Innovative approaches to family violence. Editorial. J. Fam. Stud. 14 (2–3), 160–166.

Sheehan, G., Smyth, B., 2000. Spousal violence and post-separation financial outcomes. Aust. J. Fam. Law 14 (2), 102–112.

Simpson, G., Jones, K., 2012. How important is resilience among family members supporting relatives with traumatic brain injury or spinal cord injury? Clin. Rehabil. 27 (4), 367–377.

Smith, L., Ford, K., 2013. Communication with children, young people and families—a family strengths-based approach. In: Barnes, M., Rowe, J. (Eds.), Child, Youth and Family Health: Strengthening Communities, pp. 91–110.

Smyth, B., 2004. Parent-child Contact and Post-separation Parenting Arrangements, Australian Institute of Family Studies, Report No. 9, AIFS, Melbourne.

Stanley, F., Richardson, S., Prior, M., 2005. Children of the Lucky Country, Pan Macmillan, Sydney.

Statistics New Zealand, 2010. Characteristics of same-sex couples in New Zealand, Statistics New Zealand, Wellington New Zealand. Available at: <http://www.stats.govt.nz/browse_for_stats/people_and_communities/marriages-civil-unions-and-divorces/same-sex-couples-in-nz.aspx>.

Strauss, M., 2001. Physical aggression in the family. In: Martinez, M. (Ed.), Prevention and Control of Aggression and the Impact on its Victims, Kluwer Academic/Plenum Publishers, New York, pp. 181–200.

Swiss, L., Le Bourdais, C., 2009. Father-child contact after separation. The influence of living arrangements. J. Fam. Issues 30 (5), 623–652.

Tach, L., Halpern-Meekin, S., 2009. How does premarital cohabitation affect trajectories of marital quality? J. Marriage Fam. 71, 298–317.

Taylor, J., Simmonds, J. G., 2009. Family stress and coping in the fly-in fly-out workforce. Aust. Community Psychol. 21 (2), 23–36.

Taylor, N., Gollop, M., Henaghan, M., 2010. Relocation following parental separation: the welfare and best interests of children, Centre for Research on Children and Families and Faculty of Law University of Otago, Dunedin New Zealand.

Teachman, J., 2002. Childhood living arrangements and the intergenerational transmission of divorce. J. Marriage Fam. 64, 717–729.

Teel, C., Carson, P., 2003. Family experiences in the journey through dementia diagnosis and care. J. Fam. Nurs. 9 (1), 38–58.

Te Puni Kokiri, 2010. Arotake tukino whānau literature review on family violence, Te Puni Kokiri, Wellington, New Zealand.

Terrance, C., Plumm, K., Little, B., 2008. Maternal blame. Battered women and abused children. Violence Against Women 14 (8), 870–885.

Thornton, J., Stevens, G., Grant, J., et al., 2008. Intrafamilial adolescent sex offenders: Family functioning and treatment. J. Fam. Stud. 14 (2–3), 362–375.

Thornton, A., 2009. Framework for interpreting long-term trends in values and beliefs concerning single-parent families. J. Marriage Fam. 71, 230–234.

Tsai, S., Wang, H., 2009. The relationship between caregiver's strain and social support among mothers with intellectually disabled children. J. Clin. Nurs. 18, 539–548.

UNICEF, 2013. The State of the World's Children: Children with Disabilities New York, UNICEF.

United Nations (UN), 1993. Declaration on the Elimination of Violence against Women Online. Available: <www.un.org/documents/ga/res/48/a48r104.htm> (accessed 13 June 2013).

United Nations Family Planning Association, 2000. The State of World Population 2000, United Nations, New York.

Vallant, S., Koziol-McLain, J., Hynes, B., 2007. Plunket family violence intervention project, Interdisciplinary Trauma Research Unit, Auckland University of Technology, Auckland, New Zealand.

Vargas, C., Arauza, C., Folsom, K., et al., 2012. A community engagement process for families with children with disabilities: Lessons in leadership and policy. Matern. Child Health J. 16, 21–30.

Vincent, K., Eveline, J., 2008. The invisibility of gendered power relations in domestic violence policy. J. Fam. Stud. 14, 322–333.

Walker, R., 2010. An evaluation of Ynan Ngurra-ngu Walalja: Halls Creek Community Families Program, Telethon Institute for Child Health Research, Perth.

Walker, L., Clendon, J., 2012. Ageing in place: retirement intentions of New Zealand nurses aged 50+. Proceedings of the Labour, Employment and Work Conference, Wellington New Zealand.

Wallerstein, J., Lewis, J., Blakeslee, S., 2000. The Unexpected Legacy of Divorce: a 25 Year Landmark Study, Hyperion, New York.

Wendt, S., 2009. Constructions of local culture and impacts on domestic violence in an Australian rural community. J. Rural Stud. 25, 175–184.

Wilcox, M. J., Woods, J., 2011. Participation as a basis for developing early intervention outcomes. Lang. Speech Hear. Serv. Sch. 42, 365–378.

Williamson, M., McVeigh, C., Baafi, M., 2008. An Australian perspective of fatherhood and sexuality. Midwifery 24, 99–107.

Wilson, A., Huston, T., 2013. Shared reality and grounded feelings during courtship: Do they matter for marital success? J. Marriage Fam. 75, 681–696.

Wilson, D., McBride-Henry, K., Huntington, A., 2004/5. Family violence: Walking the tight rope between maternal alienation and child safety. Contemp. Nurse 18 (1–2), 85–96.

Woods, J., Wilcox, M., Friedman, M., et al., 2011. Collaborative consultation in natural environments: Strategies to enhance family-centered supports and services. Lang. Speech Hear. Serv. Sch. 42, 379–392.

World Health Organization and the World Bank, 2011. World Report on Disability, WHO, Geneva.

Worrall, J., 2009. Grandparents and whānau/extended families raising kin children in Aotearoa/New Zealand: a view over time, Grandparents Raising Grandchildren Trust New Zealand, Auckland, New Zealand.

Wright, L., Leahey, M., 1987. Nurses and Families: a Guide to Family Assessment and Intervention, second ed. FA Davis, Philadelphia.

Wright, L., Leahey, M., 2009. Nurses and Families: a Guide to Family Assessment and Intervention, fifth ed. FA Davis, Philadelphia.

Wright, L., Leahey, M., 2013. Nurses and families. a Guide to Family Assessment and Intervention, sixth ed. FA Davis, Philadelphia.

Zubrick, S., Smith, G., Nicholson, J., et al., 2008. Parenting and families in Australia, Social Policy Research Paper No. 34, Department of Families, Housing, Community Services and Indigenous Affairs, Australian Government, Canberra.

Useful websites

www.aifs.gov.au/—Australian Institute of Family Studies

www.aracy.org.au—Australian Research Alliance for Children and Youth

www.dss.gov.au/our-responsibilities/families-and-children—Australian Department of Social Services, Families and Children

www.familycourt.gov.au/—Family Court of Australia

www.ruralhealth.org.au—National Rural Health Alliance

http://nccdh.ca/organizations/entry/social-determinants-of-health-listserv—Social determinants of health listserv

www.stats.govt.nz/browse_for_stats/people_and_communities/Families.aspx—New Zealand child and family information

www.australianmarriageequality.org—Australian Marriage Equality

www.familiescommission.govt.nz—New Zealand Families Commission, Kōmihana ā Whānau, research and publications to support the family

www.myfifofamily.com/resources—Resource for FIFO families

www.fifofamilies.com.au—Newsletter and online forum for FIFO families

www.rainbows.org—International support for families experiencing divorce

www.newcastle.edu.au/research-centre/fac/research/fathers/afrn.html
—Family Action Centre

Additional resources

Emergency telephone assistance: Australia 1800 737 732

Women's Infolink—1800 177 577

Family violence—It's Not OK—www.areyouok.org.nz, phone 0800 456 450

CHAPTER 8

Healthy children

Introduction

One of the greatest indicators of health and wellness in a community is the extent to which it invests in and nurtures its children. As we outline in this chapter, our knowledge of the factors that contribute to child health is growing at a rapid rate, and there is widespread understanding that the most important avenue to good health in any community is supporting a healthy start to life. This includes support for parents from the time they begin to plan a family, through conception, childbirth and parenting. Community life is crucial to good parenting, and it requires commitment at all levels of society to develop community structures and processes that will be helpful to parents and others who interact with children.

> ### THE BEST INVESTMENT
> One of the greatest indicators of health and wellness in a community is the extent to which it invests in and nurtures its children.

As we mentioned in Chapter 7, fertility rates in Australia and New Zealand are relatively low with only minor fluctuations in the birth rates over the past few years. Nearly 300 000 Australian mothers gave birth in 2010, 3.9% of whom were Indigenous or Torres Strait Islanders (Li et al. 2012). In New Zealand close to 63 000 mothers gave birth in 2011, nearly 22% of whom were Māori women (NZ Government, Online. Available: www.m.stats.govt.nz [accessed 17 June 2013]). It is a challenge of great magnitude to consider how our communities can support these children and their parents as they grow and develop into healthy members of the population. The children born in these first decades of the 21st century will be raised in families that are substantially smaller than in past generations, and many will attend child care outside the home because both of their parents will be engaged in

formal employment. They will have relatively long and healthy lives because they were born in countries with strong health and social support systems and environments that are comparatively safe and well resourced. Most will have access to bountiful sources of food, clean air and water, recreational spaces for play, safe and stimulating child care, early learning and other developmental opportunities. In many cases, their parents will be supported through policies that protect their health and security in the workplace and the neighbourhood. Compared with children in other OECD countries, these children should thrive. However, like children in other countries, there are health and development issues that continue to require attention; including obesity, intellectual disabilities, behaviour problems, respiratory illnesses, oral health and accident prevention. For some children social exclusion permeates many of these health issues, which directs our professional attention to the most vulnerable and disadvantaged. The challenges for nurses and parents is to maintain the momentum we have established in both countries towards better health for children, promoting early education, safety, healthy eating patterns, outdoor play and other forms of physical exercise, and the socio-emotional supports they require. One of the most widely discussed challenges for children is in pondering the influence of electronic media on their lives, and the extent to which the time they spend in front of a television, computer or mobile electronic device impedes their physical and emotional growth. In addition, there is a need to support parents in promoting healthy lifestyles, harmony in the home, and sustaining sufficient resources to circumvent risks to family life. As nurses, we must also remain vigilant to ensure that families at risk of injury, low socio-economic status, a lack of access to services, or relationship difficulties are brought to the attention of those agencies that can help them. This also includes drawing attention to the education system and those who allocate resources to promote equity of access for rural, remote, migrant and Indigenous children.

OBJECTIVES

By the end of this chapter you will be able to:

1 identify the most important influences on child health in contemporary society

2 describe the major risk and protective factors that influence child health

3 develop a set of community level strategies for promoting positive parenting

4 explain how you would assess the assets and resources related to the SDH in any

given community for supporting child health

5 describe how you would use the principles of primary health care to create a model for child health promotion in the community

6 identify the nursing roles that provide a common base of expertise for child health and parenting across a range of settings (school, clinic, home visiting, support groups).

EQUITY FOR CHILDREN

Our children as a whole are healthy, but disparities exist in both Australia and New Zealand between children of privileged backgrounds and those born to families disadvantaged by low socio-economic position or other vulnerabilities. Our efforts should be directed towards achieving equitable outcomes for all children.

At the community level, there are enormous challenges for parenting and child health from some of the societal changes mentioned in the previous chapter. These include increasing population diversity, the need for work and family harmony, financial constraints, and the need for accessible, affordable child care. Understanding these as global as well as local issues can help us connect knowledge of child health and wellbeing in our communities with that being generated elsewhere. This will help us understand how we are all similar rather than different and how we can learn from one another how to make things better for children. Guided by the principles of primary health care (PHC) we seek common ground as a basis for promoting a socially just world. In the process, we have to ensure that our work continues to create a thirst for the kind of wisdom that will help provide a safe, healthy, equitable, accessible and culturally appropriate pathway from before birth to the end of life. Then, we can use this knowledge as the impetus for change that will sustain our children well into their future.

REMINDER

'Think global, act local'.

THE HEALTHY CHILD: FROM THEORY TO PRACTICE

Healthy children can be defined on the basis of a wide variety of indicators, some of which change throughout childhood. Being born healthy to a family with adequate resources and supports gives a child a head start, whereas coming into an environment of social disadvantage or experiencing ill health or disability compromises a child's chance of achieving health and wellbeing over the life course. After birth, a child's health depends on the combination of biology, family and environments that provide opportunities to lead a healthy, nurtured and well-nourished lifestyle with a minimum of stress. Children's health is a product of receiving warm and consistent parenting, a good education and health services when these are required; and having more protective factors in their environment than risk factors. These determinants of healthy childhood are underpinned by several theories of child health and development. For example, Bronfenbrenner's (1979) theory of social ecology or 'bioecology' addresses four 'systems' or levels of influence on children's development. These include cultural beliefs and values (macrosystem); neighbourhood and community (exosystem); family (microsystem); and individual characteristics and development stage. Bronfenbrenner's theory focuses on interactions between the different systems. Although environmental influences such as peers, school and neighbourhood are important in shaping children's health and development, family is the most significant influence (Lamont & Price-Robertson 2013; Li et al. 2008). The resources a family brings to children's lives include socio-economic position, time, attentiveness, cognitive and emotional support, moral values, expectations and motivation (Hertzman & Boyce 2010; Marmot et al. 2012; Zubrick et al. 2008). Clearly, children's health is closely intertwined with the health of their community (Bronfenbrenner 1979; Edwards & Bromfield 2009).

Another theory, Bandura's *self-efficacy* theory, is based on the expectation that a person can master certain behaviours by engaging in those behaviours to achieve their goals (Bandura 1977). As we mentioned in Chapter 1, behaviours that develop self-efficacy are undertaken in a dynamic, ecological exchange called *reciprocal determinism.* Applying Bandura's theory to parenting means that when parents are provided with both information and trust in their own judgement in the context of their lives, they will be more likely to make decisions that promote better health for their children. As a result, their children are more likely to develop physical, cognitive and self-regulating capabilities that will endure over the life course (Heckman 2012). To some extent, these can be developed in the context of parenting groups (see Chapter 6). Numerous parenting programs have shown positive results in terms of parent self-efficacy and competence in the parenting role, which, in turn, reduces the stress of parenting (Bloomfield & Kendall 2012; Australian Government, FAHCSIA, 2013a). A third theory that demonstrates the primacy of family in children's development is Bowlby's (1969) theory of human attachment. Bowlby's theory posits that newborn infants are predisposed to seek attachment to their caregivers in times of stress, illness or fatigue. Attachment is also important for parents. When parents have had secure attachments in their lives they are more likely to be sensitive, responsive, engaged caregivers for their own children and supportive of one another as partners (Fraley 2010). What all of these theories have in common is reciprocal determinism: children affect and affected by influences in their external world. All of these theories provide insights into how children develop into healthy adults, beginning from their early experiences in the womb and birth, when their earliest predispositions are biologically embedded in their lives. Box 8.1 summarises the theories.

BIOLOGICAL EMBEDDING

Biological embedding is a relatively new science of human development that is rapidly growing among interdisciplinary researchers as a way of explaining health and development across the lifespan (Hertzman 2013). Research that combines genetics, epigenetics and neuroscience has revealed that children begin life with a set of predispositions, biologically embedded to respond to what lies within

BOX 8.1 Theoretical approaches to child health and development

Bronfenbrenner's bioecological theory: child health is a product of reciprocal interactions between:

- macrosystem (cultural beliefs and values)
- exosystem (neighbourhood and community)
- microsystem (family)
- individual characteristics and development stage.

Bandura's self-efficacy theory: children master certain behaviours by engaging in those behaviours to achieve their goals.

Bowlby's theory of attachment: newborn infants are predisposed to seek attachment to their caregivers in times of stress, illness or fatigue.

Biological embedding (gene-environment interactions): Children's interactions with the world around them at 'critical moments' along their developmental pathway determine their endocrine, neurological, cardiovascular and immunological development, and how they learn to modify incoming stressors.

the sphere of their lives. This 'biological embeddedness' provides a template for interactions between children and the array of social and environmental circumstances of their lives as they develop. Children's interactions with the world around them at 'critical moments' (times of heightened sensitivity) along their developmental pathway determine their endocrine, neurological, cardiovascular and immunological development, and how they learn to modify incoming stressors (Hertzman 2001a, b; Hertzman & Boyce 2010). In this way, the environments of their lives that either stress, stimulate, support or nurture them, can 'speak to their genes' through biochemical and physiological mechanisms. When these mechanisms are activated the genes themselves may be transformed in ways that influence the child's health throughout the life course (Hertzman 2013). So children's interactions along the critical pathway from fetal and early childhood literally help 'sculpt' their developing brains to build their coping capacity for later life (Mustard 2007). Their early experiences can create risks to adult health in two ways: by cumulative damage over time, or by biologically embedding adversities during sensitive developmental periods (Leckman & March 2011).

ADVERSE CHILDHOOD EXPERIENCES (ACE)

- Emotional, physical, sexual abuse
- Emotional, physical neglect
- Witnessing domestic violence
- Household with mentally ill or substance abusers
- Losing a parent
- Household member incarcerated

In some cases, children's cultural, spiritual and physical environments allow them to use their biological strengths to greater advantage. In other cases, children fail to reach their potential because of socio-cultural determinants. These can include any of the social determinants of health (SDH). They can be adversely affected by cycles of intractable poverty, exposure to family violence, mental illness or substance abuse, parental neglect, traumatic events in their life such as losing a loved one, a lack of early learning or environmental protection, or failure of the community to provide supportive policies for child health. Instead of enhancing their coping capacity, certain combinations of these social factors

may conspire to stifle a child's ability to be nurtured in the community (Larkin et al. 2012; Shonkoff et al. 2009). Some of these conditions have been identified as *Adverse Childhood Experiences (ACE)* (Larkin et al. 2012). The combined and cumulative effect of multiple adverse experiences can create inequalities for children that persist into adult life by altering their developmental processes and influencing health, wellbeing, learning or behaviour throughout the life course (Hertzman 2012). Stress in the womb or in childhood is therefore extremely important, as it can establish effects that become permanently incorporated into the child's regulatory physiological processes. Childhood stress 'weathers' the body, creating an 'allostatic load', which dysregulates and overuses the pathways that were originally designed for an individual's adaptation to stress. This transforms the brain's management systems from being adaptive to being pathogenic and accelerates the ageing processes (Power et al. 2013; Shonkoff et al. 2009).

Researchers have found that the allostatic load, or cumulative effect of stress from adverse events, can lead to heart disease, cancers, lung disease, skeletal fractures, liver disease, sexually transmitted diseases, a range of mental health disorders, general health and social problems and premature mortality (Larkin et al. 2012). The impacts also include development of a range of risk factors throughout the life course, such as smoking, alcohol abuse, obesity, physical inactivity and other risky behaviours (Larkin et al. 2012). For this reason, interventions to deal with these diseases in adulthood are nowhere near as effective as ensuring a healthy childhood relatively free from stress.

ALLOSTATIC LOAD

The cumulative effect of stress, which dysregulates, overuses and transforms adaptive processes into pathogenic processes, which accelerates ageing.

GROUP EXERCISE: The growth and development of children

Social circumstances, biology, genetics, and parental interaction and attachment can affect the growth and development of children profoundly. In small groups, discuss how each of these can impact on a child and what governments and communities are doing to improve the life circumstances of children. Feed back to the wider group.

SOCIO-ECONOMIC FACTORS AND CHILDHOOD STRESS

One of the greatest sources of pathogenic effects in children is the effect of living in impoverished or low socio-economic families, where children can be exposed to numerous stressors. These stressors include such things as maltreatment, traumatic fear, family conflict and/or chaos, inadequate nutrition, recurrent infections, having mentally unstable or absent parents, punitive parental behaviour, neighbourhood violence, dysfunctional schools and social exclusion (Marmot et al. 2012; Shonkoff et al. 2009; Waldegrave & Waldegrave 2009). Hostility between parents, even in the early postnatal period, can also have an effect on a child, creating anxiety, aggression, attention deficit, insecure attachment, poor self-esteem and poor peer relations (Velders et al. 2011).

Although it may not be possible to completely reverse the effects of these social stressors, sensitive, positive parent–child interactions, exposure to a new vocabulary and stability of parental responsiveness can actually alter a child's physiological responses (Hackman & Farah 2009). Some of the adverse effects of early life conditions may also be partially reversible with lifestyle interventions that improve diet, exercise and stress reduction (Puterman & Epel 2012), especially if these are supported by the family. With this optimistic outlook there has been renewed research and policy interest in examining a child's lifetime socio-economic position (SEP), lifetime growth trajectory, and cognitive and emotional development across the different life stages (Power et al. 2013).

A number of birth cohort studies have tracked children's progress through the pathways of their lives to gain a better understanding of the origins and impacts of social inequalities in health. Most, including the Longitudinal Study of Australian Children (LSAC) (AIFS 2012a), the Longitudinal Study of Indigenous Children (LSIC) (Australian Government 2013a) and the Longitudinal Study of New Zealand Children (LSNZC) (Morton et al. 2013) are finding common links between poorer health in adult life and the socio-economic conditions of children's lives. Other research indicates that the effects of being born into low socio-economic conditions are intergenerational (Power et al. 2013). Yet along the life course, certain influences, such as enhancing cognitive and behavioural capacities during adolescence, can also act as a buffer, especially if there are stable and supportive relationships at the family, community and societal levels (Gluckman 2011; Shonkoff et al. 2009; Zubrick et al. 2008). Investing in 'equity from the start' (Hertzman 2013:4) through supportive environments and programs to develop parenting skills are therefore the most effective ways for communities and global societies to ensure health and wellbeing in the population across the life course. Enabling environments for child health are those that also enhance family life. They nurture connectedness through features of the physical landscape, places and opportunities for community interactions, attitudes of inclusiveness and tolerance, and empowering policies and support services that help build capacity throughout the journey (McMurray 2011) (see Figure 8.1).

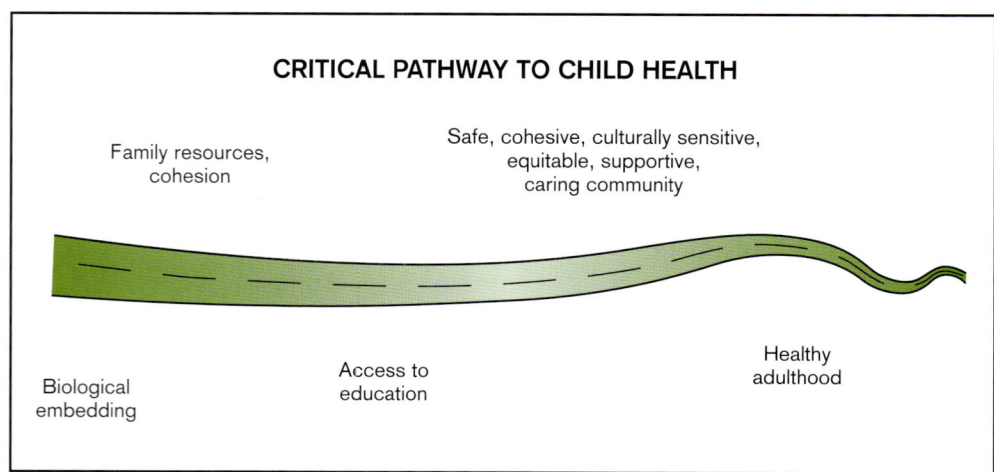

FIGURE 8.1
Critical pathway to child health and wellbeing

EVIDENCE FOR PRACTICE

Why do you think it's important to undertake population cohort studies like the LSAC, LSIC and LSNZC?

How can we use the evidence from cohort studies in practice?

TROUBLING STATS

While most children in the world are cared for and loved, more than 2000 children a day die in the world as the result of an injury, and over 1 billion children under the age of 5 live in the midst of armed conflict.

GLOBAL CHILD HEALTH, DISADVANTAGE AND POVERTY

The health of the world's children is of concern to everyone who claims global citizenship. Most children in the world are cared for and loved, but many other children suffer from violence, exploitation and abuse. UNICEF (2009) considers child wellbeing as comprising six dimensions:

- material wellbeing
- health and safety
- educational wellbeing
- family and peer relationships
- behaviours and risks
- subjective wellbeing.

Globally, many children do not meet these conditions. Although global infant mortality has halved since 1970, the world's population has doubled, so there remains a need to guard against any reversal of the successes of the past decades (Save the Children 2013). In most Western countries, those living in impoverished circumstances with few resources to mitigate risks are most vulnerable to ill health (Marmot et al. 2012). Every day, more than 2000 die from an injury (WHO 2008b). In some regions, children are sexually abused or forced into child marriages, while others may be trafficked into exploitative conditions of work. Just over one billion children under age 5 live in the midst of armed conflict (UNICEF 2009). Many children die on the first day of life, and 3 million a year die in their first month of life due to birth complications, prematurity and infections (Save the Children 2013). Worldwide, nearly 7 million children under age 5 die each year. Most of these deaths occur in developing countries where women and their newborns lack access to basic health care services before, during and after childbirth, underlining the link between poverty and the risk of dying.

Although the Millennium Development Goals (MDGs) have aimed at reducing the under-5 mortality rate, progress has been slow (Save the Children 2013). Extreme poverty has been reduced by half; the number of people with a lack of clean drinkable water has been halved; 200 million people have been removed from slums (double the target); primary school enrolment of girls now equals that of boys, and maternal newborn deaths are steadily declining (UNICEF 2012a). However, even in some Western countries, many children do not stay in education long enough to develop reading, mathematical and science literacy or long enough to transition to employment or training (Heckman 2012). Many children have problematic family and peer relationships, particularly the children of migrant and refugee families and those with disabilities (Heymann et al. 2013; Marmot et al. 2012). Working families do not always have income protection when they become unemployed, and surprisingly, some countries do not provide tuition-free education throughout secondary education (Heymann et all 2013).

The issue of child labour continues to plague many countries, with 215 million child labourers aged 5–17 throughout the world. Some struggle to combine work and education, and some undertake hazardous work for extreme hours in unhealthy or dangerous conditions. They are poorly protected by legal arrangements, and interestingly, Australia and New Zealand are among those countries with no legislated minimum age for full-time employment (Heymann et al. 2013) although there are restrictions around the hours people under the age of 18 can work, the machinery they can operate and where they can work in New Zealand (NZ Govt, Online. Available: www.dol.govt.nz/workplace/knowledgebase/item/1293 [accessed 8 July 2013]). Child marriages are another problem for many women, often marrying older men who tend to restrict their independence. These younger women are the most likely to die in childbirth. Clearly, in all countries of the world the two overarching goals should be to improve health for everyone, and to address inequities by bringing the health of everyone up to the level achieved by the most advantaged (Marmot et al. 2012).

Poverty is rife among children in developing countries, but in the countries of the West, *relative* child poverty continues to be a major problem affecting 15% of the world's children (UNICEF 2012b). Relative poverty refers to those children living in homes receiving less than 50% of the median national income, and this affects approximately 11% of children in Australia and 12% of New Zealand children, which represents a slight improvement in recent years (UNICEF 2012b). Child poverty in New Zealand has become recognised as a particularly significant problem. While poverty has always been an issue for some children, the vast numbers currently living in poverty in New Zealand (some say as many as 25% of all children) are of significant concern (Expert Advisory Group on Solutions to Child Poverty 2012). Unless addressed quickly and effectively, this issue will have long-term consequences for the health and prosperity of New Zealanders. Impoverished childhoods cause food and housing insecurity, inadequate support for illnesses and injuries and impediments to social and emotional development. Poverty adds insult to injury for Indigenous children in both countries, many of whom are already living in conditions of social inequity. Other factors related to poverty that place children at risk of disadvantage include child abuse or neglect, violence, contact with the juvenile justice system, family joblessness and homelessness (AIFS 2012b).

HOMELESSNESS

'living situations where people with no other options to acquire safe and secure housing: are without shelter, in temporary accommodation, sharing accommodation with a household or living in uninhabitable housing.'

(Statistics New Zealand 2009:6)

Homelessness is one of the most serious consequences of relative poverty, and although housing policies in Australia and New Zealand have helped reduce the rate of homelessness in both countries it is a problem with dire consequences.

Every day nearly 1 in 200 Australians are homeless, 23% of whom are children (Homelessness Australia, Online. Available: www.homelessnessAustralia.org.au [accessed 23 June 2013]). The problem of homelessness in Australia has been continually rising over the past decade, which is surprising for an economy that is ranked the 12th or 13th most powerful in the world by the United Nations. In New Zealand, homelessness is well defined by Statistics New Zealand (2009) but figures that tell us how many people in New Zealand are homeless are harder to come by. Overcrowding is problematic— New Zealand has greater overcrowding issues than Australia, the United Kingdom and Canada (Goodyear & Fabian 2012), and crowded living conditions are often a sign that people have lost their homes. However, it is unclear how many live on the streets, live in uninhabitable housing or live in temporary or shared accommodation. Without this information, homelessness remains a hidden problem making it very difficult for policymakers to make decisions regarding resource allocation. Some of the specific effects of living in relative poverty, as summarised in Box 8.2, can impede children's potential for the duration of their lives.

BOX 8.2 Impact of impoverishment in childhood

- High infant mortality
- High unintentional injury rates
- Low birth weight
- Poor overall child wellbeing
- Low immunisation rates
- Juvenile homicide
- Low educational attainment
- Non-participation in higher education
- Dropping out of school
- Aspiring to low-skilled work
- Poor peer relations
- Bullying at school
- Teenage pregnancy
- Physical inactivity and childhood obesity
- Not having breakfast
- Mental health problems, including loneliness
- Living in a cold, damp house
- Missing out on school outings and sports activities

(Source: Emerson 2009; Expert Advisory Group on Child Poverty 2012)

INDICATORS OF CHILD HEALTH IN AUSTRALIA AND NEW ZEALAND

As we mentioned in the previous chapter, children under age 14 comprise 19% of the Australian and 21% of the New Zealand populations respectively. In Australia this represents 4.3 million children, 5% of whom are Indigenous (AIHW 2012a, b). In New Zealand, with a smaller population, there are 891 700 children, 26% of whom were Māori (NZ Govt, Online. Available: www.stats.govt.nz/browse_for_stats/population/estimates_and_projections/NationalPopulationEstimates_HOTPSep12qtr.aspx, www.stats.govt.nz/browse_for_stats/population/estimates_and_projections/maori-population-estimates.aspx [accessed 9 July 2013]). In both countries the proportion of children in relation to the rest of the population is gradually declining because of decreasing fertility and population ageing (AIHW 2012a). A comprehensive report on child health in Australia in 2012 indicates that there has been steady progress in reducing child mortality to comparable rates in OECD countries, and, since 2007, a reduction by half in deaths from injuries (AIHW 2012a). The prevalence of both childhood diabetes and cancer has remained stable, and cases of asthma have decreased, except among Indigenous children. Other indicators of child health show that, in general, their health is improving. Almost three-quarters of young children have stories read or told to them regularly, and most reach the national standard for reading and numeracy. Parental smoking has decreased, and risky behaviours such as drinking and smoking among children have declined. Most children report living in safe neighbourhoods where they can get assistance in times of crisis (AIHW 2012a).

Despite the gains in child health indicators several areas for improvement remain. These include reducing the number of women who smoke in pregnancy (1 in 7) or consume alcohol. Around 90% of mothers initiate breastfeeding but only 2 in 5 (40%) infants are exclusively breastfed at 4 months. Many children (45%) continue to have dental decay, and around a quarter of children enter school with some type of developmental delay. Fifteen per cent of children have parents affected by mental health problems, which can be a risk factor for poor emotional development (AIHW 2012a). Bullying at school is among the most significant difficulties experienced by school-age children and adolescents. Cyber bullying, often through SMS messaging and email, is a particularly serious problem, as we outline in Chapter 9. Some form of bullying has been reported by around half of all Australian children between 5 and 9 years of age, especially boys and those from a different cultural background than the majority of the school population (AIHW 2012a; Jacobs et al. 2012). However, researchers from the Australian Institute of Family Studies (AIFS) have found that the gender divide in bullying is not quite clear, as girls are more devious in the strategies they use, which include nasty note-writing or excluding someone from a friendship group. Children living with a single mother and Indigenous children also reported higher rates of bullying than others (Lodge & Baxter 2012). As we have come to realise in recent years, bullying is insidious throughout the world, and has significant effects on children's social and emotional development, creating low self-esteem, interpersonal difficulties, loneliness and low school achievement (Lodge & Baxter 2012).

Improvements in child health have been slower in New Zealand than Australia, and in 2009 New Zealand was ranked 29th out of 30 OECD countries, based on relatively poor rates of infant mortality, immunisation, deaths in under 5 year olds from accidents and injury, rates of child maltreatment, and hospitalisation for communicable diseases such as pertussis, pneumatic fever and rheumatic fever (Morton et al. 2013). Many New Zealand children live in relative poverty and inequitable conditions, especially the children of Māori and Pacific Island families and, in some cases, these inequalities have worsened rather than improved (NZ Govt, Online. Available: www.growingup.co.nz [accessed 24 June 2013]). The Longitudinal Study of New Zealand children has now surpassed the 9-month mark of the cohort and has found that most babies enrolled in the study are healthy at birth and breastfed to begin their lives. However, like Australian babies, exclusive breastfeeding tends to cease around 4 months of age (NZ Govt, Online. Available: www.growingup.co.nz [accessed 2013]). Among all New Zealand children immunisation rates are mixed, but generally below required standards, particularly for Māori children, with Asian children having the highest rates of immunisation coverage (NZMOH 2012a). New Zealand children are also hospitalised at higher rates than children in Australia, the UK and the US, often for skin and/or respiratory infections, injuries/poisoning, gastroenteritis and asthma (NZMOH 2012a).

WHAT'S THE POINT?

Knowing the indicators and trends helps inform evidence-based practice. It also provides a basis for promoting health literacy and developing collaborative intervention strategies.

The 2011–12 New Zealand Child Health Survey found that 98% of parents believe their children are in good health. Most children are read to at least daily by 9 months, but 1 in 3 are also watching TV by that same month. Some improvements in child care have been evident, including a trend towards later introduction of solid foods, and more general practitioner visits for young children. However, there remains a high prevalence of asthma (14%), overweight (21%) and obesity (11%) among children, especially for Māori (17%) and Pacific (23%) children, and those living in the most deprived areas (19%) (NZMOH 2012a).

The New Zealand survey also found increasing rates of emotional and behavioural problems among children aged 2–14 years, with boys twice as likely to be diagnosed with these issues as girls (NZMOH 2012a). Predictably, the review of children's health found that those in the most deprived areas experienced poorer health habits, including the lack of having breakfast at home. These are also the children who spend more time watching television than other children, although the overall number of children who watch TV more than 2 hours per day has decreased over the past few years (NZMOH 2012a). This is reassuring for several reasons, including the influence of television in portraying sexualised images as well as violence and advertising for non-nutritious food.

THE SOCIAL DETERMINANTS OF CHILDREN'S HEALTH AND LIFESTYLE

As children grow the compound effects of the SDH become more evident, and this is particularly concerning in relation to the global 'obesity epidemic'. Overweight and obesity is as much a problem for Australian and New Zealand children as it is throughout the world, which is a concern, given that obesity is a risk factor for heart disease, type 2 diabetes and some types of cancer (NZMOH 2012a). There is evidence of a social gradient effect, which means that children who are disadvantaged socially, economically and geographically are at increased risk of becoming overweight (AIFS 2012a). To some extent, this may be linked to a lack of available, accessible and affordable fresh fruit and vegetables and opportunities for exercise. Although most children (65%) in New Zealand are normal weight, 21% are overweight and 11% are obese. Māori and Pacific children are also more likely to be obese than other New Zealanders, with Māori children twice as likely to be obese as non-Māori (NZMOH 2012a). Around 23% of Australian children are overweight (AIFS 2012a; AIHW 2012a), and 6% are obese (ABS 2010). Of these children, a large proportion live in

remote areas. A related issue is that remote living children also have more decayed, missing and filled teeth (Australian Indigenous HealthInfoNet, Online. Available: www.healthinfonet.ecu.edu.au/health-facts/ summary [accessed 25 June 2013]). Similarly, in New Zealand Māori children have a disproportionate number of oral health problems, and are more than 1.7 times more likely than non-Māori children to have a tooth removed, especially those who live in deprived neighbourhoods (NZMOH 2012a). Poor oral health can exacerbate dietary problems, especially when parents are attempting to encourage children to eat fresh fruit and vegetables.

To counter the 'obesity epidemic', clinicians and public health researchers have focused on the combination of foetal epigenetic and maternal physiology (Water 2011) as well as lifestyle factors. The cohort studies (LSAC, LSNZC, LSIC) are tracking our children's status in each of these areas to investigate the extent to which children who are overweight, obese, poorly nourished and inactive develop adult conditions such as coronary heart disease, high blood pressure, diabetes and other endocrine disorders, certain cancers, gall bladder disease, osteoarthritis and any other outcomes. These associations, and the prevalence of social and mental health problems, have already been found in research over the past few decades (AIHW 2012a). Researchers have also found that not only is there a greater population prevalence of overweight and obesity, but the BMI (the measurement of individual obesity), of the average child has gradually increased (AIHW 2012a). The effects of overweight and obesity are closely intertwined with children's emotional development, as these children experience discrimination, victimisation, teasing and bullying (AIFS 2013a). As time goes by, obesity becomes entrenched, and by the later years it is less reversible. Parental early intervention is therefore the best option to instil healthy food preferences and dietary habits and patterns of physical activity (AIHW 2012a). Yet some parenting factors have been found to contribute to children's propensity to become obese, including having an overweight or obese father, even when the child's mother is a normal weight, or having a father who is disengaged from the child's life.

In terms of nutrition and physical activity, most Australian and New Zealand children meet the national guidelines of 60 minutes of activity every day, but very few meet the nutrition standard for fruit and vegetable consumption (AIHW 2009; Craig et al. 2007). Studies have found that children may be erratic in their physical activity, but averaged over a period of days, most meet the criterion of one hour per day (AIHW 2012a). Sedentary leisure time also

WHY AN OBESITY EPIDEMIC?

- Genetic predisposition
- Excess maternal weight gain
- Social disadvantage, poverty
- Poor nutrition (high salt, sugar diets)
- Poor oral health
- Fast food outlets in neighbourhoods
- Trend towards 'eating out'
- Unscheduled meal times
- Inadequate physical activity
- No parks, walkable/ safe/ playable spaces
- Poor parental role-modelling
- Education, knowledge, skills
- Too much 'screen time'
- Lack of school support

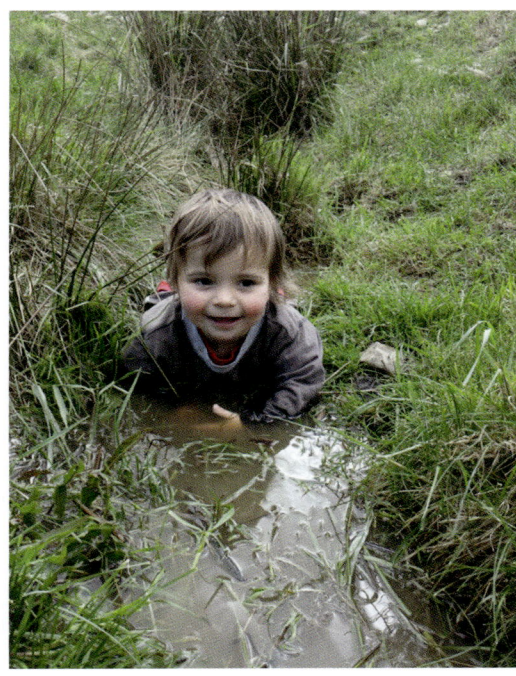

Happy kids are healthy kids (photo: Penny and Dan Smale)

has an influence on physical activity. Few young children conform to the 'screen guidelines', which recommend no more than 2 hours of non-educational screen time (computers, video, TV) per day (AIHW 2012a; NZMOH 2012a). Children who engage in more than 2 hours of screen time per day are more likely to be less physically active; drink more sugary drinks; snack on foods high in sugar, salt and fat; and have fewer social interactions. Because children from disadvantaged backgrounds watch twice as much television as other children, they are doubly disadvantaged in terms of lifestyle risks, given that television 'steals' time from other healthy activities such as physical activities or reading (AIFS 2012a).

Some studies have shown that for each additional hour in front of a screen the odds of being overweight increase by 20%–30% (Steffen et al. 2009). A review of research by the LSAC team demonstrates the links between children's consumption of television and obesity, sleep disruption, delayed language acquisition, poor school performance, aggression and commercialisation of children (AIFS 2012a). Violent and traumatic content affects children's socio-emotional development, because in many cases, they are unable to distinguish between screen action and real life (Cantor 2001). Cantor (2001) suggests that parents can effectively comfort children if they watch these shows with their children, but even with this intervention, there remains the problem of desensitising children to violence. The depiction of aggression is often associated with heroism, and

sends a message that this should be the first response in any situation (Christakis & Zimmerman 2007). Children are also 'commercialised' by watching so many television advertisements, some of which 'groom' children to be consumers, often for unhealthy products (AIFS 2013a). On the other hand, appropriate television can help increase vocabulary, literacy and numeracy, but these desirable outcomes are only achieved when the exposure to learning programs is accompanied by interaction with parents (Saxton 2010). A growing trend is also occurring in the development of video games designed to support the learning needs of children. For example, researchers have found that some children with disabilities are benefiting significantly from video games that enhance memory, coordination and mobility (Bennett et al. 2013; Sandlund et al. 2011; Tanaka et al. 2010).

Although some obesity researchers have created the impression that inappropriate diets are either destiny or unwise choices among those living disadvantaged lives, increased attention has been drawn to obesogenic food environments (Drewnowski 2009). For example, low-income neighbourhoods tend to have many fast food outlets and convenience stores, which encourages consumption of inexpensive foods with refined grains and high sugar and fat content. On the other hand, people living in affluent neighbourhoods have the wealth and access to healthy, low fat foods. In addition, these neighbourhoods often have walkable spaces and parks for child-driven play, which can help them develop confidence and social skills as well as physical wellbeing (Castonguay & Jutras 2009). Food security is a problem for rural families which makes it difficult to maintain a healthy diet. Problems of transporting fresh food are intensified by high fuel prices and, for families living remotely, food storage can be difficult. The neighbourhood is therefore an important factor in determining behaviour. Unless children have safe, adequate transportation, they will be discouraged from walking, playing or riding their bikes to the various places they need to go, which underlines the importance of health and place.

It is tempting to blame parents for the problems, but there is actually a web of social and environmental factors that have created 'obesogenic' environments, many of which affect both parents and children. Solutions therefore have to be aimed at the broader circumstances that create unhealthy lifestyles for the entire family. There is a proliferation of food choices available to busy families these days and the foods marketed to them are often refined and calorie-dense. Many busy families tend to buy foods for convenience and price rather than nutrient value, adding to children's incentives to eat large quantities of fast, easily prepared foods. The growing trend toward more meals consumed outside the home, and a shift to larger portion sizes also play a part (Harnack et al. 2000). Because fast foods are less filling than fresh fruits or vegetables and pleasurable to eat, children tend to eat larger quantities of them. Fresh fruits and vegetables are also more expensive than fast foods, but not as aggressively marketed. It is also ironic that some fast food outlets market 'healthy' options to children, which creates confusion as to what is in fact healthy, and what may be laden with empty calories.

The school environment also plays a role not only in nutrition, but in children's physical activities. Just as family attitudes are conveyed to children in the way mealtimes are structured, and whether other family members engage in physical activities, school environments convey strong messages about how physical exercise and good dietary habits are valued. Opportunities and availability of healthy meals at school have been shown to have an effect on learning and fewer behavioural or academic problems in children (Shi et al. 2013). A number of school-based programs have also found that including structured sessions on weight reduction, physical activity or play, and dietary behaviours can have a significant impact in children's weight loss,

particularly if the parents are involved (Manger et al. 2012; Werner et al. 2012). These results point to the need for multi-level, comprehensive interventions as the way to ensure sustainability of healthy lifestyles over time (Werner et al. 2012).

Many public schools have reduced the physical education component of their curricula. With shrinking education budgets and a virtual explosion of curriculum content, physical education is easy to dispense with, especially where educational managers are not strong advocates of healthy lifestyles. Government regulatory agencies and various education authorities have been moving toward standardised curricula, and their plans often fail to include strong voices for physical education. Like other government agencies today, schools are required to manage risk in a way that reduces the threat of accidents and injuries, and these typically occur during sports and physical activities, making the reduction of sport and activity easy to justify. After-school programs have also changed. Because of the increase in working mothers, a large proportion of children attend after-school care, and these relatively low-funded programs are easier to manage indoors. Where children do attend formal activities after-school, the major focus of these is often oriented towards preparing them to compete in the intellectual rather than lifestyle domain.

From the parents' perspective, it is more convenient to pick children up from school rather than have them ride their bikes. Concerns for children's safety also leave many students taking passive, rather than active transport to and from school. Workplace stressors can also cause parents to be too exhausted to exercise with their children. Together with a reduction in physical education classes at school, these factors create a web of causation for obesity (Salmon et al. 2005). The solutions to the current obesity epidemic thus lie in a combination of healthier family lifestyles, and eliminating obesogenic environments rather than focusing on lifestyle modification programs that create stress by blaming the victims.

Indigenous and ethnic minority child health

Social disadvantage affects many Indigenous people and prevents many of their children from having a healthy start to life. Indigenous mothers are younger than non-Indigenous mothers, and in Australia, Aboriginal and Torres Strait Islander mothers have more births on average than other mothers (2.7 compared with 1.9 births respectively) (Australian Indigenous Health InfoNet, Online. Available: www.healthinfonet.ecu.edu.au/health-facts/summary

EVIDENCE FOR PRACTICE: Physical activity

Numerous studies have examined the combination of psychosocial and environmental supports that would encourage children to increase their physical activity. Researchers conducted a systematic review of the efficacy of physical activity studies to identify those factors that act as mediators of activity (Brown et al. 2013). They found strong effects from studies that used multiple cognitive approaches, including goals setting, problem-solving, relapse prevention, and strong effects from studies that used behavioural reinforcement. The mediators were defined as 'intervening causal variables that are necessary to cause an effect pathway between an intervention and physical activity' (Brown et al. 2013:166). These mediators are identified in behavioural theories such as social cognitive theory and the theory of planned behaviour. The researchers analysing the data explained the challenges of measuring the effects of behavioural interventions in children as being linked to their different rates of maturation and development, their lower cognitive functioning compared to adults, and their sporadic activity patterns. The analysis revealed that self-efficacy, knowledge, intentions, enjoyment and social support are all important in children's participation, but studies should also include the full ecological framework for intervention; the social, physical, cultural, policy and environmental influences on their behaviour (Brown et al. 2013).

? So how will we use this evidence for practice?

If we understand what approaches have been used to encourage physical activity, the degree to which they were successful with different types of children of different ages, in different socio-cultural environments, it may be easier to plan effective interventions and to guide parents on 'what works'.

[accessed 25 June 2013]). Nineteen per cent are teenage mothers, compared with 4% of non-Indigenous mothers. Their babies weigh almost 200 grams less than those born to non-Indigenous mothers, and they are twice as likely as other babies to be of low birth weight (under 2500 grams), which has been linked to the fact that around 50% of Indigenous mothers smoke during pregnancy

(Australian Government 2013b). Indigenous people experience the largest proportion of infant mortality, primarily because of the combination of younger age at birth and social disadvantage. For example, in 2010 the rate of infant mortality for Australian Indigenous women was 11.1 per 1000 births, compared with 7.1 per 100 births for non-Indigenous mothers (AIHW 2012a). There were also differential rates of neonatal deaths, with Indigenous rates at 6.9 per 1000 births and rates for non-Indigenous infants at 2.7 per 1000 births. Perinatal deaths show similar trends with twice as many among Indigenous babies (17.1 per 1000 births) than non-Indigenous babies (8.8 per 1000 births) (AIHW 2012a).

New Zealand Māori families experience similarly disproportionate losses. In 2011, the New Zealand infant mortality rate among Māori was 6.8 per 1000 births, as compared to 5.1 per 1000 births for non-Māori (NZ Govt, Online. Available: www.m.stats.govt.nz/browse_for_stats/population/birthsAndDeaths_HOTPYemar11/commentary.aspx [accessed 24 June 2013]). Migrants in both countries and Pacific people in New Zealand also suffer disproportionate rates of morbidity and mortality because of social disadvantage. Supporting a child with a disability or chronic condition adds another layer of disadvantage for these and other families.

Children with disabilities or chronic illness

Some Australian and New Zealand children have disabilities that interrupt their interactions and effective participation in society. Disabling conditions among children range from moderate impairments for home and school life to those that severely limit core activities of development and require lifelong support. In Australia 7% of young children suffer from a disability, around half of whom have severe or profound core activity limitations (AIHW 2012a). In the 2006 national health survey, 11% of New Zealand children were found to have a disability (Craig et al. 2007).

Indigenous children in Australia have a 30% greater incidence of core disabilities than non-Indigenous children (AIHW 2012a). Many children with disabling conditions are limited in their capacity to overcome or cope with their condition because of barriers that exclude them from social participation, particularly in education (AIFS 2012a). They rely heavily on parents, siblings, other family members and teachers for assistance in the core activities of daily living; mobility, self-care and communication (AIHW 2012a). Their parents are also constrained financially and in the workplace, by having to care for their children for longer periods and sometimes in more intense caregiving than they would with other children. Children with disabilities grow into adults with disabilities and frequently care requirements will continue and are sometimes greater as a child grows and becomes heavier to assist. For family caregivers the grief associated with caring for a disabled child can be compounded when milestones such as leaving home, finding a partner and starting a family are not reached (Clendon 2009). In the LSAC cohort, researchers found that parents of children with disabilities, particularly lone parents, were more likely than other parents to be jobless, which creates additional layers of disadvantage for the child as well as the family (AIFS 2012a). Joblessness in itself is also a risk factor for parental psychological distress, which can have a profound effect on the children living in these families as it often causes a lack of parental warmth (AIFS 2012a). International researchers have also found that caring for a child with a chronic illness or disability can be a barrier to providing preventative care, such as immunisation or medical check-ups, especially for working parents who cannot afford to take time from work (Heymann et al. 2013). Much of their distress is due to financial problems, which, according to LSAC researchers, have caused many families in the cohort to go without meals, to be unable to heat or cool their homes or to pay bills on time, or to access emotional/information or tangible support for their disabled children or maintain positive social interactions themselves (AIFS 2012a). Many parents of children with disabilities are unable to find employment with sufficient flexibility to accommodate their caring responsibilities.

QUICK STATS

Approximately 7% of Australian children and 11% of New Zealand children experience some type of disability that interrupts their ability to participate in society.

Although children who live with chronic diseases are not considered disabled, they and their parents are often subjected to considerable stress from having to monitor and manage their conditions over long periods of time. Chronic conditions can affect children's growth and physical, emotional and social development, either directly or indirectly (AIHW 2012a). In addition to the direct effects of physical pain and discomfort, children with chronic conditions can experience stigma, school absences or inability to participate in age-appropriate activities (AIHW 2012a). These are major problems for New

Zealand children, who have the highest rates of severe asthma in the world, leaving them with a higher risk of developing many common mental health problems from having to cope with the illness (Goodwin et al. 2013). Having a child with behavioural or mental health problems can be traumatic for parents and other family members, who may also end up suffering high levels of distress and depression. For this reason, research continues into the multiple interactions between various factors leading to asthma, with an emphasis on the environment (Sampson 2012). In relation to asthma, New Zealand researchers are examining housing conditions in socially deprived neighbourhoods, on the basis that damp and mould in the home or unflued gas heaters have been associated with the development of asthma and other respiratory conditions. The results have been profound. In a randomised controlled trial of heating intervention in 409 households containing a 6–12-year-old child with asthma, the installation of a more effective heater than was previously in place resulted on average in 21% fewer days of absence from school (Free et al. 2010). The combination of conditions that lead to the disease, including lack of resources, access to care or other factors affecting children living in deprived conditions, will all be investigated further in the Longitudinal Study of New Zealand Children (Morton et al. 2013).

HEALTHY PREGNANCY

Child health begins with a healthy pregnancy. The fruits of a healthy pregnancy are celebrated daily, throughout the world. For some mothers, though, a healthy pregnancy is a conquest of the human spirit over dire social circumstances, made worse by a lack of care and support. In developing countries, the rate of accessing antenatal care steadily increased throughout the 1990s, although progress in some countries like Indonesia and other parts of South-East Asia has been variable (WHO 2005). Save the Children (2013) and the Commission on the Social Determinants of Health (CSDH 2008) recommend a global perspective that will provide mothers and children with a continuum of care from pre-pregnancy through pregnancy and childbirth to the early years of a child's life (CSDH 2008). Their recommendations include support for exclusive breastfeeding initiation within the first hour of life and for the first 6 months, skin-to-skin contact immediately after birth, extended breastfeeding to age 2, and educational support for children and their mothers. Both agencies argue that if these recommendations were adopted worldwide, it would have an intergenerational effect, shaping lifelong trajectories and opportunities for health as well as promoting mothers' educational attainment as a way of countering gender and other inequities (CSDH 2008; Save the Children 2003).

HEALTHY PREGNANCY

A key determinant for a healthy childhood.

Other risks to healthy pregnancy lie in the workplace. Many pregnant women maintain full or part-time employment, exposing them to workplace hazards. Others may be exposed to dangerous conditions in their home, neighbourhood or community. In any of these settings, the availability of sufficient nutritious food is an important influence on healthy pregnancy. Another important goal of pregnancy is to ensure that both parents are in good health and free from infections, harmful drugs or other substances that can interfere with the construction of a healthy child. It is important for expectant parents to understand the multiplier effects of all factors, to gain a clear understanding of how lifestyle factors can interact with biological or genetic factors and environmental circumstances to either enhance or override a child's healthy development.

Antenatal care

Antenatal care by a health professional from the earliest stages of pregnancy can help pregnant women and their partners identify the need for any dietary or lifestyle changes and ways of sustaining those changes throughout the pregnancy and beyond the birth of the child. It also provides an opportunity to help parents create the emotional foundations for the child's life; one of the most important elements of early parenting. Ultrasound examinations and population studies show that from about 10 weeks, an infant moves spontaneously, and by 15 weeks, movements may be felt as a reaction to the mother's laugh or cough, suggesting a response of self-protection or self-assertion (Shonkoff & Phillips 2000). During this stage, a high level of stress in the mother can affect the function of the fetal-placental unit, compromising fetal growth and causing a risk of preterm birth or low birth weight (Hobel et al. 2008). Knowledge of this early neurological development of the fetus, along with our understanding of the effects of stress on neural development during the critical periods, underlines the importance of early and ongoing antenatal care (Hobel et al. 2008; Shonkoff et al. 2009).

ANTENATAL CARE

Provides an opportunity for parents to create the emotional foundations for a child's life.

An additional goal of antenatal preparation is to establish a birth plan, one that empowers parents to make decisions on the place of birth, and the choice of birth attendant or birth companion. Yet another important opportunity afforded by antenatal visits is the chance to discuss the diagnostic approach to the pregnancy, including the choice of vaginal or caesarean birth and whether or not an induction will be indicated. Antenatal preparation also provides an opportunity for parents to talk through their emotional needs in relation to parenting, which is especially important for pregnant adolescents and first-time parents (AIHW 2012b). The antenatal visits can therefore act as a platform for planning and empowerment as a parent through a trusting relationship with a health professional that will help women develop the skills for lifelong decision-making (WHO 2005). Birth preparation includes gathering information about breastfeeding and how to access help with infant problems such as feeding, crying and sleep disruptions, which are typically the most problematic for parents, especially for their first child. Parents often use the antenatal visit to seek guidance on conditions such as Sudden Infant Death Syndrome (SIDS, often called Sudden Unexpected Death of an Infant, or SUDI), which is a major risk in the perinatal period, along with low birth weight, congenital abnormalities and complications of the placenta, cord and membranes (AIHW 2012b). The prevalence of SIDS has shown a dramatic, worldwide reduction, which, to some extent, is directly related to antenatal guidance, and campaigns urging parents to breastfeed and to place their infants in a supine, or back-lying position while sleeping (AIHW 2012b). Sharing a bed with an infant should be avoided; however, for some parents, keeping the infant nearby during sleep is part of their cultural expectations of parenting. Where parents are determined to sleep with their infants, the safest option is to use a sleeping 'pod' that can be brought into the parents' bed, provided the infant is kept inside the pod. In Chapter 15 we describe research into the viability of these sleeping pods, including those such as the wahakura developed by New Zealand Indigenous mothers.

Save the Children's Mothers' Index assesses the wellbeing of mothers and children in 176 countries, many of which show steady improvement. For the first time, Australia has made the top 10 countries,

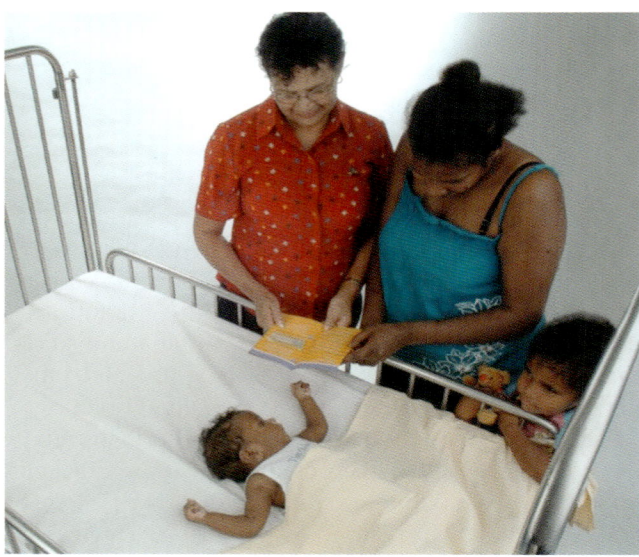

Aboriginal health worker instructing new mother and little sister on safe sleeping (photo courtesy of Professor Jeanine Young, SIDS and Kids Australia and Queensland Health)

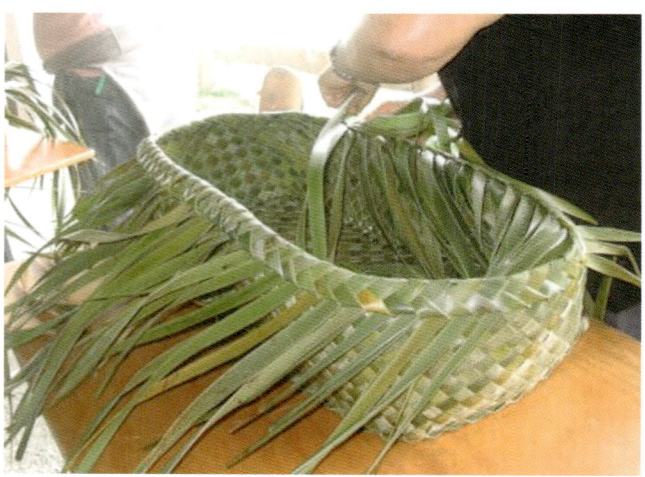

The wahakura (http://whakawhetu.co.nz/)

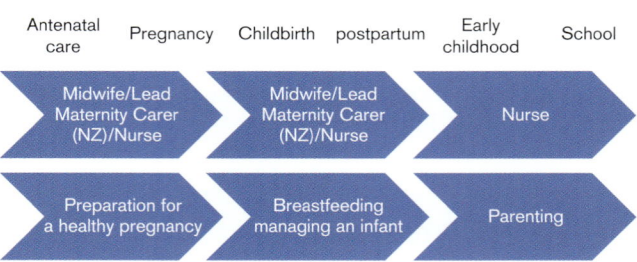

Antenatal care	Pregnancy	Childbirth	postpartum	Early childhood	School

Midwife/Lead Maternity Carer (NZ)/Nurse → Midwife/Lead Maternity Carer (NZ)/Nurse → Nurse

Preparation for a healthy pregnancy → Breastfeeding managing an infant → Parenting

FIGURE 8.2
Continuum of care from pregnancy to child health

programs. Those who did attend antenatal classes did so intermittently and at a later stage in their pregnancy (AIHW 2012a). However, this is gradually changing, perhaps because of increasing attention at all levels of health care to providing culturally appropriate services, and in 2010 around 97% of Indigenous mothers attended at least one antenatal visit (Australian Government 2013b).

Some Indigenous women are disadvantaged by the lack of adequately prepared midwives, especially in rural, regional and remote areas. In many cases it is up to the Maternal, Child and Family Health Nurse (MCAFNA, Online. Available: www.mcafhna.org.au [accessed 20 June 2013]) working in the Australian community or the Public Health Nurse in New Zealand (Morton et al. 2012) to provide culturally appropriate guidance throughout the continuum of care, beginning in the antenatal period. Among the specific issues to be addressed in this period are healthy pregnancy benchmarks, family planning, and parenting issues such as identifying any resources for breastfeeding support if these are required, family and community support during the immediate period after birth, childhood immunisations, plans for child care and managing any stresses related to employment. Figure 8.2 depicts the role of nurses and midwives in helping maintain a continuum of care.

CHILDBIRTH

Skilled care in the birth period and beyond can reduce the health threats to mother and baby, especially during the first month which is the period of highest risk (Save the Children 2013). The first-day mortality rate in countries of the West is highest in the United States, and fifth and sixth highest respectively in Australia and New Zealand (Save the Children 2013). Some people find it surprising that the US has such a dire outcome for so many infants, but this is due to the young average age of the mother, with the US having the highest rate of

with rankings reflecting global standings of mothers' and children's health, educational, economic and political status. New Zealand is not far behind in 17th position (Save the Children 2013). Despite these successes there remains a need for consideration of how we manage the continuum of care for mothers and newborns in our part of the world, especially for Indigenous mothers. For many years Australian Indigenous women have not attended antenatal care because of distance from services, and in some cases, because of cultural inappropriateness of available teenage pregnancy in the industrialised world, predominantly among poor and minority groups (Save the Children 2013). Australian Indigenous women also have a high rate of teenage pregnancy compared to non-Indigenous women, accompanied by the risk of low birth weight or neonatal death (AIHW 2012a). For underweight babies 'Kangaroo Mother Care' is used in many countries as a simple, cost-effective way to keep their newborns warm through skin-to-skin contact on the mother's chest. In some cases, this approach can also circumvent the need for incubators by providing the baby with energy to produce its own body heat. It is also a way for mothers to bond with their babies, and can encourage not only emotional warmth but the baby's ability to breastfeed at will. Researchers estimate that Kangaroo Care could save half a million newborns if it was implemented throughout the world (Save the Children 2013).

For babies who survive the perinatal period there are other threats to life, including exposure to perilous social and environmental conditions, especially for Indigenous children (Jacobs et al. 2012). Those who live in remote areas are often far from health services, and they tend to experience considerable eyesight problems and ear infections, the latter being linked to overcrowding, poor hygiene and exposure to tobacco smoke. The cultural preference of many Indigenous women is to have 'birth on country', which is a cultural rite of passage at childbirth, where women's identity and connections with the land and country are transferred, shared and celebrated (Commonwealth of Australia 2009a). In some cases, state and national health policies prevent birthing on country due to concerns about the risks to mother and baby of being isolated from health services.

PRACTICE STRATEGY

Nurses have an important role in supporting breastfeeding mothers and normalizing the breastfeeding process, given unequivocal evidence for the benefits of breastfeeding for both infant and mother.

For most mothers and their partners, childbirth is a joyous occasion, but there are also risks to health. These can include injuries to the vaginal canal, temporary anaemia due to blood loss and, for some mothers, dramatic changes in their emotional state. Another issue is the risk of infection from a surgical birth. This is a growing problem, with the rates of caesarean section increasing worldwide. The WHO (2005) guideline recommends a maximum proportion of 15% for caesarean sections compared with vaginal births, but the rate of caesarean births in many countries exceeds this proportion (Althabe & Belizan 2006). Most Australian women (68.4%) have vaginal births, with the rate of caesarean births rising to 31.6% in 2010 (AIHW 2010). In New Zealand the rate varies between 11–29% (NZMOH 2012b). These rates are above the 15% considered normal for caesarean rates around the world (WHO 2010). The WHO report argues that overuse of caesarean sections creates a set of financial pressures on the health care system, and in some cases it can lead to morbidity in women and their infants. The rate of inductions at birth has also increased worldwide to 25–30% of births (25.4% in Australia, and 4.9% in New Zealand) with considerable variability across different regions (AIHW 2010; NZMOH 2012b). Unnecessary inductions can also increase risks to the mother related to epidural analgesia, and morbidity such as birth injury and lengthened hospital stay (MacKenzie 2006). At this stage on the childbirth continuum the focus should be on health care systems that develop local evidence for prioritising needs, developing targets for improvement, in-service training for health professionals and others who can assist mothers and babies, including home visiting nurses (Save the Children 2013).

BREASTFEEDING

The WHO has been steadfast in underlining the need for all babies, wherever possible, to be breastfed for the first six months of life (WHO & UNICEF 2003; WHO 2009b). The research evidence supporting the health benefits of breastfeeding for infants and mothers is unequivocal (Heymann et al. 2013). Compelling evidence suggests that breastfeeding protects infants against some chronic diseases, and deaths due to diarrhoea, respiratory tract infections, otitis media, pneumonia and other infectious diseases (Heymann et al. 2013). Breastfeeding also reduces the child's exposure to potentially harmful agents, especially in developing countries where clean water and sanitation facilities may not be available (Heymann et al. 2013). For unknown reasons, breastfeeding seems to reduce the risk of SIDS/SUDI. Breastfed babies have also been found to have better cognitive development, which some attribute to mother–infant bonding and secure attachment (Bryanton et al. 2009; Heymann et al. 2013). Benefits of breastfeeding also extend to the mother, improving recovery after childbirth, assisting with postpartum weight loss, and leading to possible reductions in the risk of breast and ovarian cancers, post-menopausal hip fractures, osteoporosis and maternal depression (Heymann et al. 2013).

Globally there have been many attempts to improve rates of breastfeeding, primarily through UNICEF programs that encourage mothers to initiate breastfeeding at birth. However, many countries, including Australia and New Zealand, have high rates of initiation but low rates of persevering with breastfeeding to six months as recommended in the WHO UNICEF (2003) guidelines (Schmied et al. 2012). Data collected for the LSAC on 5000 Australian families showed that 91% were breastfed at birth, and 46% continued to four months, with 14% continuing to the six-month period as recommended by the WHO (AIHW 2009). New Zealand figures from this same period indicate that 70% of infants were exclusively breastfed at six weeks of age; at three months, just over 50% of infants are exclusively breastfed, and by six months this had dropped to approximately 7.5% (NZMOH 2008). By 2011 this had dropped to 66.3% at six weeks, but increased to 54.9% at three months and 25.2% at six months (Craig et al. 2013). However, in the LSNZC cohort, 97% were breastfed at birth and nearly half of the babies who were living with their mothers were breastfed four times a day at nine months (Morton et al. 2012). It will be interesting in future analyses to see whether these cohorts have better childhood outcomes than those who ceased breastfeeding earlier. For Māori babies, the figures are less encouraging: 60.8% were exclusively breastfed at six weeks, 44.6% at three months and 16% at six months (Craig et al. 2013). Rates for Pacific infants in New Zealand are similar to those of Māori infants (Craig et al. 2013).

The challenges of persevering with breastfeeding pose a question for nurses as to whether or not there are steps that could be taken to encourage women to sustain exclusive breastfeeding for longer periods of time. One innovative program conducted in Perth devised a father-inclusive perinatal education support group with a view toward encouraging fathers to support their partners in breastfeeding. The sessions were conducted by five male educators and included information about their changing role as a man and a father, the importance of communication, and the benefits of breastfeeding for both mother and baby. Evaluation of the program revealed that the men found the 'gender-specific' nature of the program valuable in helping them discuss the issues surrounding birth, including breastfeeding. They also showed an interest in learning more about topics such as postnatal depression (PND), fatigue, sleeplessness and what to expect in the first month after birth. Their feedback

included the suggestion that men would likely find internet or DVD information helpful in terms of childbirth education, which the researchers are planning to explore (Tohotoa et al. 2010).

BREASTFEEDING

Benefits for the infant

- protects against some chronic diseases
- reduces deaths due to diarrhoea
- reduces instances of respiratory tract infections, otitis media, pneumonia and other infectious diseases
- reduces exposure to potentially harmful agents such as waterborne disease in developing countries
- reduces risk of SIDS/SUDI
- increases cognitive development
- promotes bonding and attachment to the mother.

Benefits for the mother

- improved recovery after childbirth
- assists with postpartum weight-loss
- possibly reduces risk of breast and ovarian cancers, post-menopausal hip fractures, osteoporosis, maternal depression.

Both Australia and New Zealand have national strategic plans for breastfeeding. These government-initiated plans are based on the principles of protecting, promoting, supporting and valuing breastfeeding as a biological and social norm for infant and young child feeding (Commonwealth of Australia 2009b; NZMOH 2009). Both plans are aimed at a whole-of-society approach to supporting breastfeeding for all population groups and successive generations across the continuum from pregnancy to child care. Their goals are also congruent with the WHO–UNICEF Baby-Friendly Hospital Initiative, which began in 1991 (UNICEF, Online. Available: www.unicef.org.au/ [accessed 1 July 2013]). The BFI initiative is a structured method of encouraging breastfeeding, which has been adopted by a number of hospitals throughout the world. However, women's busy lives outside the home, an early return to work after childbirth, or the lack of community and peer support can run counter to successful breastfeeding, especially where workplace practices constrain a woman's ability to breastfeed her child.

Nurses and midwives in the UK have been attempting to use the BFI initiative as an incentive for training health visitors and midwives in breastfeeding management, with some recent success. In the UK, rates of initiation are high, but 50% of mothers there cease breastfeeding at 6 weeks, which is among the lowest rate of continuation in the world (Ingram et al. 2011). As in Australia and New Zealand, midwives in the UK have the first level of influence on new mothers, and many are successful in helping them establish breastfeeding, but then the care of mothers is transferred to the health visiting team who conduct child health clinics and home visits. To help enhance their success in encouraging perseverance with breastfeeding, the health service provided a Baby Friendly Initiative (BFI) program for home visiting teams affiliated with one health area. The course was well received by mothers, 85% of whom were breastfeeding at eight weeks. It was also evaluated positively by the nursing staff, who felt they had gained confidence and pride in adopting a consistent approach to counselling mothers about breastfeeding (Ingram et al. 2011). This program is an example of a simple, effective way to achieve consistent breastfeeding advice, which is a key element in persuading mothers that they have the skills to continue breastfeeding. The question remains as to whether or not health policymakers have the commitment to institute and resource such programs.

The other major influence on continuation lies in the workplace situation that either impedes or encourages breastfeeding. Research has shown that when women have access to paid maternity leave and breastfeeding breaks in the workplace, breastfeeding rates increase (Heymann et al. 2013). Heymann et al. (2013) report on two large studies, including one based on 25 years of data from 16 European countries, which found that providing 10 weeks of paid maternity and parental leave was associated with a 1–2% reduction in infant mortality rates, a 3.5% reduction in postnatal mortality and a 3–3.5% reduction in child mortality (Heymann et al. 2013). They attribute some of these outcomes to the fact that when parents are able to take leave they tend to provide better daily care, ensure adequate immunisations, are more

inclined to persevere with breastfeeding and seek both preventative and curative care for their children (Heymann et al. 2013). This evidence illustrates the links between family-friendly workplaces and family-friendly governments. Although most countries have paid leave for new mothers (the US being a notable exception), some mandate paid leave for fathers. Those countries that support fathers to take paid leave after birth have also shown that this type of support increases fathers' involvement with their child during the leave period and after returning to work, indicating better gender equity in child care (Heymann et al. 2013). Australia and New Zealand are among those with modest arrangements for parental leave (18 and 14 weeks respectively) (Government of Australia, Online. Available: www.fahcsia.gov.au/our-responsibilities/families-and-children/programs-services/paid-parental-leave-scheme, www.dol.govt.nz/er/holidaysandleave/parentalleave/ [accessed 1 July 2013]). Paid parental leave has also been shown to increase the likelihood of a woman returning to her previous employment, which has financial benefits not only for the woman but also for employers in improving retention rates, employee stability and reduced training costs (Heymann et al. 2013).

The link between breastfeeding and work schedules confirms the complexity of breastfeeding behaviour in relation to the combination of individual and environmental factors (Commonwealth of Australia 2009b). Studies have found that mothers who returned to work for fewer

EVIDENCE FOR PRACTICE: Migrant women's experiences of breastfeeding in a new country

Australian researchers conducted an extensive review of the published literature to investigate what evidence had been generated on the beliefs and experiences of migrant and refugee women in breastfeeding once they migrate to a new country. The issue is important because migrant and refugee women may initiate breastfeeding in their host country but fail to reach the ideal of six months breastfeeding (WHO UNICEF 2003) as they succumb to the work pressures or cultural mores and practices in the new country. In most countries of the West 20% of women cease breastfeeding before six months (Schmied et al. 2012). The researchers conducting this review were therefore interested in examining how migrant and refugee women could be better supported in the health care system and the community to persist with breastfeeding. The authors conducted a meta-analysis of existing research studies, systematically analysing the evidence using a critical skills appraisal tool. Their analysis revealed that for numerous migrant and refugee women breastfeeding in a new country means facing contradictions and conflicts. From this overarching theme they identified four main subthemes describing women's views:

- Breastmilk is best.
- Producing breastmilk requires energy and good health.
- Female relatives play a dominant role in breastfeeding.
- With no access to traditional postpartum practices, women may cease breastfeeding.

The researchers explained that many women experience tensions between cultures and between family members. They cited studies indicating that sometimes these tensions are exacerbated by a woman's expectations and her material circumstances (McFadden et al. 2012). Stereotypes held by health professionals also play an important role in whether or not a woman persists with breastfeeding, as some hold the belief that most women from other cultures are influenced more by their family members than health professionals. This indicates not only apathy but a view that women migrants and those from ethnic minorities are a homogenous group. The authors concluded that as health professionals, we need to assist these women sensitively, and wherever possible, provide educational opportunities for them and extended family members (Schmied et al. 2012).

? So how will we use this evidence in practice?

Stereotyping impedes our ability to provide culturally appropriate care in many practice contexts. Understanding the perspectives of women requires in-depth assessment of their individual and family needs.

Understanding the factors that will allow women to undertake culturally safe practices while transitioning to their new culture will help professionals encourage breastfeeding for longer periods of time.

than 10 hours per week or were self-employed had the highest rates of breastfeeding (Hector et al. 2005). A number of psychological factors have also been found to predict breastfeeding success (O'Brien et al. 2008). These include the mother's anxiety level, whether or not she had an optimistic disposition towards breastfeeding, self-efficacy, faith in breastmilk for her baby, expectations and planned duration of breastfeeding prior to the birth, and the timing of making the decision to breastfeed (O'Brien et al. 2008). On the other hand, barriers to breastfeeding include the health and risk status of mothers and infants, their socio-economic status, education, knowledge and skills, confidence in their ability to breastfeed, their expectations of the infant's weight gain, separation of mother and infant for non-medical reasons, the availability and media portrayal of supplements to feeding, misdiagnosis or mismanagement of common breastfeeding problems, and support in the hospital, workplace, family, community and policy environment (Commonwealth of Australia 2009b).

POSTNATAL DEPRESSION (PND)

One of the most serious challenges for many women at the time of childbirth and in the first four to six weeks postpartum is related to the emotional aspects of adjusting to parenthood (Hewitt & Gilbody 2009). Postnatally, many women experience being a bit down for various lengths of time, having a depressed mood or tiredness that can begin prior to the birth (Figueiredo et al. 2009; Seimyr et al. 2009). These feelings can intensify for women who are socially isolated, lacking an intimate confidant, friend or extended family available after the birth (Dennis et al. 2009). Migrant, Non-English Speaking Background (NESB) women and those living in rural areas tend to be among those most socially isolated. For some mothers, their emotional state evolves into the more serious problem of postnatal depression (PND), which is characterised by 'feelings of inadequacy and failure, a sense of hopelessness, exhaustion, emptiness, anxiety or panic, decreased energy and motivation, and a general inability to cope with daily routines' (Rush 2012:322). PND is reported to occur in around 12–14% of new mothers in Western societies (Apter et al. 2012; Scope et al. 2012), and affects 15% of Australian mothers (Rush 2012), with many more (35%) experiencing adjustment disorders (Harvey et al. 2012). A 2006 study undertaken to determine the prevalence of postnatal depression in New Zealand women (New Zealand European) found approximately 16% experienced symptoms of depression sufficiently severe enough to warrant intervention (Thio et al. 2006). Of greatest concern, however, was that 75% of these women were not receiving treatment (Thio et al. 2006). Prevalence among Māori and Pacific mothers in New Zealand is also high (Ekeroma et al. 2012; NZMOH 2011). Although the LSNZC cohort remains in the early stages, data from the mothers involved have shown that there is a strong relationship between experiencing depressive symptoms during pregnancy and developing PND after birth (Morton et al. 2012, 2013), a finding that concurs with other studies (Apter et al. 2012). Some researchers have found an association between PND and a history of abuse; however, women who have been abused often have an excess of other stressful events which may compound the risk of PND (LaCoursiere et al. 2012). Box 8.3 lists some of the factors contributing to PND.

A study of maternal, child and family health nurses in Victoria, Australia, found that nurses can be effective in helping women deal with postnatal depressive symptoms, which concurs with international studies showing that MCH nurses have the highest level of awareness of PND. At the four-week child health consultation the nurses engage all mothers in a 'conversation' to assess whether they have a history of anxiety or depression, fatigue or loss of energy, insomnia or changes in appetite. If the mother reveals any of these symptoms, the nurse uses the beyondblue (www.beyondblue.org.au) 'Emotional health during pregnancy and early parenthood' booklet, which also includes use of the Edinburgh Postnatal Depression Scale (EPDS) to identify the extent of the woman's stress, depression, and support and referral options. Where women are identified as at risk of PND, additional consultations

---

BOX 8.3 Factors contributing to postnatal depression

Factors include:

- unwanted or stressful pregnancy
- poor relationship with the child's father or other family members
- criticism or lack of social support, either from family members or peers
- poverty and the social conditions it precipitates, such as crowding, substandard housing or unemployment
- being a migrant mother without a support network
- prior psychiatric problems or a history of depression
- stressful life events
- sleep deprivation or anxiety
- having an infant born with a medical problem or not surviving the birth
- poor physical health or coincidental adverse life events, such as the loss of a partner or abuse
- being depressed prior to birth
- having a depressed partner.

(Source: Dennis et al. 2009; Figueiredo et al. 2009; LaCoursiere et al. 2012; WHO 2005)

---

are provided through home visits or telephone support, and the nurses provide information, advice, counselling and referral to GPs who they know are aware of PND and its treatments. Their screening and assessment strategy establishes rapport that helps provide continuity of care (Rush 2012). In New Zealand, Plunket nurses use the patient health questionnaire (PHQ3) with all mothers they suspect may be experiencing symptoms of postnatal depression. Where mothers are identified as at risk, the nurse provides appropriate support and referral (personal communication, Erin Beatson, 15 July 2013).

For Aboriginal women, PND is assessed as part of family and parenting discussions about how a woman is feeling about the birth. Discussions should take place through Aboriginal women's networks, or through mothering conversations or 'yarning' with other mothers and/or Aboriginal health workers (Our Children Our Future, Online. Available: www.health.gov.au/internet/publications/publishing.nsf [accessed 8 January 2014]). For all families where PND has occurred, the infants and children are particularly vulnerable because of the risk of attachment insecurity, cognitive and developmental delay, social and interaction difficulties (Dennis et al. 2009; Rush 2012). Yet many new mothers are reluctant to seek help for PND, attempting to deal with the condition on their own. This sometimes creates a cycle of despair which can erode self-esteem and potentially damage a mother's relationship with her child (Harvey et al. 2012; Rush 2012). Researchers have found that less than 50% of postnatal depression cases are detected by health care professionals, which indicates the need to screen all new mothers for the condition (Hewitt & Gilbody 2009). Once detected, treatment varies according to the severity of the PND, ranging from clinical and psychological treatment to organising support for the mother, counselling, antidepressants and hospitalisation (Rush 2012). Antidepressants are the least desirable treatment, particularly for breastfeeding mothers (Morrell et al. 2009). As mentioned in Chapter 6, cognitive behavioural therapy (CBT) has been found effective in those with severe PND, especially where partners can also be included (Scope et al. 2012). Where feasible, exercise programs are also helpful in helping women and their partners develop self-efficacy for parenting.

Although exercise programs are sometimes difficult to organise in the early weeks postpartum, women who do participate find they can relieve pregnancy-associated weight gain, reduce symptoms of depression and anxiety, and increase mood states (Cramp & Bray 2011). Several studies, including a Cochrane systematic review, have shown that PND can be treated effectively with psychosocial and psychological techniques. Telephone-based peer support provided by volunteer mothers over 12 weeks postpartum have also been known to reduce the incidence by half among those at risk of PND (Dennis et al. 2009). Telephone support is ideal for this purpose, given that it is flexible, private and non-stigmatising, and it overcomes the problems of accessibility to services, especially for mothers of low socio-economic status or at a distance from services. Support for mothers experiencing maternal mental health issues has been poor in New Zealand (NZMOH 2011), but in 2013 the government allocated a further $18.2 million for maternal mental health service development and it is hoped this will alleviate many of the issues unwell New Zealand mothers have faced.

Men are often inadvertently excluded from discussions of the mental health issues during pregnancy and after the birth of a child (O'Connell-Binns 2009). Yet PND has been estimated as affecting 3–10% of men, even though it manifests differently (Matthey et al. 2000). Some men experience PND as intensely as women, but may hide their vulnerability behind hostility, aggression, work obsession, destructive thoughts or refusing help (O'Connell-Binns 2009). There is some evidence that including fathers in antenatal preparation results in an increased awareness of the maternal experience and it has been suggested that father-specific sessions may be helpful in preparing men for the transition to fatherhood (Habib 2012; Schumacher et al. 2008; Tohotoa et al. 2010).

CHILDREN'S PSYCHOSOCIAL WELLBEING

Measurements of mental health and wellbeing among Australian children are imprecise because of a lack of national data. However, as in other OECD countries, mental illness affects around 20% of the population at some point in their lives, which is important, given the influence of parental mental health on children's mental health (AIHW 2012a). It is estimated that, in general, 17.6% of children under the age of 11 have some type of mental health problem with up to 5% suffering from conduct disorder (WHO 2009a; Craig et al. 2007). Children with these complaints are disadvantaged not only from the disease, but also socially, in terms of stigma, discrimination, functional impairment and the risk of premature death (AIHW 2009). The New Zealand children's health survey (NZMOH 2012a) indicated that only 3.2% of young children have been diagnosed with a mental or emotional health problem but these problems are increasing, especially among boys. Most common diagnoses are anxiety disorder, attention deficit disorder (ADD) or attention deficit and hyperactivity disorder (ADHD) and depression (NZMOH 2012a). Interestingly, the prevalence of these problems was found to be lower for Māori, Pacific and Asian children (NZMOH 2012a). The lower rates of these specific problems may be related to a number of factors, including reliance on family rather than formal help seeking for social and emotional issues, fear or unfamiliarity with treatment options, or a preference for family care rather than external assistance from the health care system.

FIND THE LINK

How do physical activity patterns affect mental health?

The Pacific Islands Families (PIF) study (a longitudinal birth cohort study of 1000 Pacific families which aims to increase our evidence and understanding related to family health and development of Pacific families in New Zealand) provides some evidence around why rates may be lower for Pacific children. Although child behavioural outcomes among the cohort determined a prevalence of externalised behavioural issues (for example, aggression and attention-seeking) of 14.6% at age six across a range of measures, and children whose mothers had experienced symptomatic depression were more likely to exhibit internalised behavioural issues (for example, withdrawal, emotional reaction, anxiety and somatic complaints), a protective factor was found across all dimensions for children whose mothers described themselves as strongly aligned with Pacific traditions such as retaining strong social connectedness with their Pacific community, attending traditional gatherings, and close extended ties (Paterson et al. 2013).

In the Australian LSAC study higher rates of mental health problems were found in the Indigenous families as compared with the non-Indigenous families (AIFS 2012a). However, the actual cause is unclear, as when the prevalence of socio-emotional problems was compared between Indigenous and non-Indigenous children living at the lowest levels of disadvantage, no significant differences were found. This would suggest that, despite the fact that there is often a familial, intergenerational link between child and parental mental illness, in this case, it was disadvantage, rather than family or any cultural factors that led to these problems (AIHW 2012a). Another issue affecting many Indigenous families is the lack of secure housing, and overcrowding. Studies have found that overcrowding is a risk factor for high levels of stress in children and their parents, higher rates of infectious diseases, poorer parenting, increased family conflict and child abuse and neglect (AIHW 2012a). When children live in overcrowded households they tend to withdraw and are less likely to explore and play, which has a negative effect on their learning and cognitive development (AIHW 2012a). A New Zealand study found rates of infectious diseases increased from 20.5% of acute admissions between 1989–93 to 26.6% between 2004–08 (Baker et al. 2012). There was a widening social gradient with Māori and Pacific people at significantly increased risk of infectious disease than non-Māori, non-Pacific people. Increased overcrowding during the 20-year period of the study—particularly for Pacific children—was considered a significant contributor to the increased risk (Baker et al. 2012). Family stability is often compromised when people live in overcrowded conditions, as they lose their sense of autonomy, certainty and control over their environment (AIHW 2012a).

RISKS OF CROWDING

- Low autonomy, control
- High parental stress
- Childhood infections
- Family conflict
- Child abuse, neglect
- Less child play, exploration
- Low cognitive development

Parents with mental illness tend to treat their children with less responsiveness or warmth, and are often irritable, angry and critical, and these parenting traits often have long-lasting effects on their children (AIFS 2012a). Both maternal depression and family conflict have been identified as increasing a child's risk of developing behavioural or emotional problems, including substance misuse, antisocial behaviour or delinquency (Kiernan & Huerta 2008). The risk is greatest where there is protracted conflict and/or clinical depression extending beyond the normal circumstances of having a child. Becoming parents is a major event in the lives of many couples, one that can initially cause difficulties in the couple relationship because of sleep deprivation and, often, a decrease in their intimate or leisure time together (Claxton & Perry-Jenkins 2008). Over time, many parents make the transition to parenting, reigniting their relationship as the pressures of new parenting are alleviated and some parents believe that this stage occurs when the sleep deprivation of new parenthood is resolved and when they are better able to attend to their emotional wellbeing. If parents do not retrieve their emotional wellbeing through support, mutual tolerance and encouragement in their parental roles, their children may be at risk of poor mental health outcomes.

Another layer of influence lies in the way others outside the home respond to the child with emotional or behavioural problems. In some cases, unsociable behaviours or emotional responses can manifest in childhood and attract ridicule, discrimination and disadvantage from other children, which can lead to further behavioural and emotional problems. In other cases the child him/herself may be self-critical and withdraw from social activities. For example, children who are depressed or emotionally distressed tend to disengage from any organised sporting activity, which tends to marginalise them in the social context of neighbourhood or school activities. Their personal reaction and that of others can then prevent their participation in sports or other activities, compromising their socio-emotional wellbeing (AIHW 2012a). Because every child is different, the behaviours and others' responses are unpredictable, but in many cases, their social development can be enhanced with patterns of parenting that are supportive across all situations.

Besides parental influences there are other factors that can tip the emotional balance of a child into mental illness. These include slow academic achievement, physical or psychological trauma, abuse and/or neglect, loss of family, or community and cultural factors, such as having low socio-economic position or being discriminated against (AIHW 2009). Numerous examples of the combination of these factors are seen among refugee children living in Australian detention centres awaiting resolution of their family's applications for settlement (see Chapter 14). In addition to their pre-immigration traumas, inhumane treatment, the lack of predictability in their lives and the fragile emotional status of their parents has a strong negative effect on their emotional development over periods of long internment in the centres. Because of the plethora of factors impacting on these children the relative weight of parental mental health is unclear. As in all families, the transmission of psychosocial health in the family is complex.

Parenting patterns and children's psychosocial health outcomes

To some extent, intergenerational transmission of children's psychosocial health is related to family socio-economic conditions, so it is difficult to gauge the relative effect of social conditions and parenting practices on children's outcomes. In some cases, the effects of family interactions remain hidden. We know that child temperament has a role to play in how family members interact with a child, but these interactions are varied and reciprocal, with a wide range of parental responses to the child's behaviours, and child responses to parental behaviours (Zubrick et al. 2008). This reciprocal impact is intensified in parenting by foster carers, who are typically genuine, warm and well-prepared for parenting, but are challenged by problematic child behaviours and intense scrutiny by agencies external to the family environment (Blythe et al. 2013). Children's emotional and behavioural outcomes in the foster care context are therefore a result of many variable factors: the circumstances, the child's temperament

and history, and parenting. These and other complexities, such as social disadvantage, blur the relationship between cause and consequence in the development of social and emotional problems.

As we reported in Chapter 7, parenting structures are important to children's development, particularly in terms of family patterns that may exacerbate low socio-economic status, such as occurs in some single-parent families. Studies of some other patterns of family life such as gay parenting, while not yet extensive, are revealing that children of same-sex couples are thriving. The Australian Study of Child Health in Same-Sex Families has recently reported on 500 children of these relationships (Crouch et al. 2012, 2013). The researchers found that there was no statistical difference between children of same-sex couples and other children on measures of self-esteem, emotional behaviour, and the amount of time spent with parents. The children also scored higher on measures of general health and family cohesion, yet they experienced discrimination in a variety of contexts.

Parenting style is an important determinant of children's health outcomes. Research in the 1960s and 70s identified the three main styles of parenting as *authoritative*, *authoritarian* and *permissive*. Authoritative, characterised by high warmth and responsiveness, was seen as the most desirable (Baumrind 1966, 1971). Other researchers since that time have conceptualised parenting styles on the two broad dimensions of warmth and control (Chaudhuri et al. 2009). Children of parents who are warm and emotionally available, yet encourage the child's development, have been found to foster self-esteem, social skills and academic achievement (Chaudhuri et al. 2009). This begins in infancy, with parental behaviours that maintain physical and emotional closeness, responding with quick, calming, soothing responses that provide control and security (Bryanton et al. 2009). Parental warmth is expressed in affectionate behaviours, high positive regard, expressing enjoyment in the child's company, taking an interest and being involved in the child's activities, being responsive to his or her moods and feelings, and giving positive expression of approval and support (Zubrick et al. 2008). For new fathers, identity theory contends that the transition to parenting can be a major change in their emotional style of interaction, depending on their own experiences of being parented, their personality, beliefs and their relationship with their partners. Satisfaction with the situation, their decision-making, communication, perceived support and child-centred attitudes have all been found to affect men's identity as a father and therefore their bond with the infant

(Habib 2012). However, one could argue that these influences may be similar for both parents.

PARENTING STYLE

• Authoritative

• Authoritarian

• Permissive

Authoritative parenting is characterised by warmth and responsiveness, and is the most effective parenting style.

Dependable, predictable, warm and consistent interactions are key elements of managing a child's behaviour. Warmth and consistency are the opposite of hostile parenting reactions (McCain & Mustard 2002; AIHW 2009). Hostile parenting is akin to Baumrind's (1966) authoritarian style of parenting, where parents use angry or coercive patterns of parenting with criticism, negativity and emotional reactivity. This is the type of harsh discipline that flows from family conflict or depression, which typically leads to poorer cognitive and social development in children (Kiernan & Huerta 2008; Whiteside-Mansell et al. 2008; Zubrick et al. 2008). Consistent parents are firm, structured, yet sensitive in their interactions with children. They set clear, developmentally appropriate boundaries and expectations for their behaviours, following through with intentions and giving the child a sense of direction and competence (Zubrick et al. 2008). This does not negate the fact that there is a reciprocal response in parenting, as we mentioned above, but in general, warmth, consistency and emotional availability lead to the most positive outcomes for children (Chaudhuri et al. 2009; Zubrick et al. 2008). The goals of good parenting are to help the child 'develop emotional regulation, exploratory behaviour, communication, self-direction, intellectual flexibility, introspection, self-efficacy in meeting life's challenges, moral values, expectations and motivation', all of which can flow to the parent as well as the child (Zubrick et al. 2008:5). Parental commitment to these outcomes helps foster the development of trust, security, self-worth and readiness to learn in the child, as well as a sense of self-efficacy in the parents, wherein they feel confident in their parenting capacity (Zubrick et al. 2008). The LSAC and LSNZC data are also showing that most parents are committed to their children's intellectual development, with most children being read to daily (AIFS 2012b; Morton et al. 2012). Parents in the Australian cohort, whose children are

now in school, report feeling positive about their parenting skills in relation to learning, including their ability to help their child with homework and other school-related activities (AIFS 2012b).

GENDERED PARENTING

Identity theory suggests that men have to develop a 'father identity' in their transition to parenting, which is a product of their developmental history, personality and beliefs about fathering.

How would you differentiate this transition from that of mothers?

Learning readiness and social development

Learning readiness is conceptualised in ecological terms as four interconnected components: ready families, ready communities, ready early childhood services, and ready schools, all of which contribute to ready children (Sayers et al. 2012). Family expectations and support for learning have been identified as strong predictors of educational and behavioural outcomes, especially if families have strong community support (Dockett et al. 2012). When families provide support and reinforcement for their children to succeed educationally through such activities as reading to them, they transmit a type of cultural capital, indicating that intellectual development and opportunities for the future are valued (Dunt et al. 2010). The interaction between the family, community, child service providers and schools, and their cumulative effect determine whether a child is able to take advantage of learning, development and social opportunities (Sayers et al. 2012). Early learning enhances a child's functioning, including language development, literacy acquisition, cognitive processes, emotional development, self-regulation and problem-solving skills (Zubrick et al. 2008). Research has shown that these cognitive and social benefits accrue to children in the context of formal early childhood care (ECC) and education (ECCE) programs, which set the stage for lifelong learning and maximise developmental outcomes (AIFS 2013a; Heymann et al. 2013). Yet half the world's countries lack formal ECCE programs for children under age three (Heymann et al. 2013). These programs are of particular assistance to single parents, children from isolated areas who have had few opportunities for social interaction, children who may have language difficulties because they are NESB children, and families without extended family nearby (Heymann et al. 2013). As children make the all-important transition to preschool in preparation for the transition to primary school, it is important that they begin to feel confident in interacting with others and develop the ability to process feedback from the family, school and peer environment. Throughout this transition family support for their changing identity, through the symbols of school (uniform, language, habits, skills, new peers), project visible signs that the family is connected with their school and external world, which helps children gain both cognitive and social competence (Dockett et al. 2012). These benefits of quality ECCE experiences are now recognised in international policy development as the best investment in the early years (AIFS 2012a; Gluckman 2011).

LEARNING READINESS

Ready families +

Ready communities +

Ready early childhood services +

Ready schools +

= Ready children

From 2013 the Australian Government has provided universal early childhood education of 15 hours per week for all children (AIFS 2013a). However, with vast geographical differences and variability throughout the states and territories some children are not able to access ECE (AIFS 2013a). Predictably, it is the socio-economically disadvantaged children that tend to miss out on ECE, including Indigenous children, especially those in remote areas, NESB children, recent migrant and refugee children and those with disabilities and special care needs (AIFS 2013a). These children are at the mercy of a fragmented and inconsistent provision of ECE. Another layer of differential access lies in the distinction between child care and preschool, which is important for working families. Some families find child care unaffordable, given their socio-economic status. Others find that working non-standard hours impedes access to ECE. Research in New Zealand examining how parents working non-standard hours managed child care arrangements found that a complex mix of family and informal caregiving, combined with formal early childhood either in home-based care or early childhood centres, was common (Families Commission 2008). Some children attended multiple child care centres (up to four) with one child spending 57 and a half hours per week in care. Some parents worked mirrored shifts so that the child

could be largely cared for at home. Working non-standard hours was found to place significant stress on parents which subsequently affected their relationship with their child (Families Commission 2008). Others, particularly some Indigenous parents, prefer to have their children at home in the early years. This may be because of their belief in the importance of home care or their own negative experiences at school, which may have been marred by disrespect for their people and their culture (AIFS 2013b). Children living with single parents can find it particularly difficult when their parents are unable to afford child care that would give them an educational advantage, particularly when the family is more likely than intact families to have financial difficulties. Clearly, these disadvantaged families need linked-up services where collaborative structures across demographic and geographic groups promote equity of access. In the current environment, parents often 'shop around' for affordable child care, the quality of which may be variable. This can leave some young children experiencing the stress of multiple moves instead of a smooth transition to their school years. Understanding the importance of the early learning environment in helping children fit into their community and social environment indicates the need for better coordination of ECE and school to help them make these important transitions (Sayers et al. 2012).

The New Zealand Government has introduced the B4 School Check (see Chapter 5) to detect any behavioural or developmental issues that have not been identified in ECCE, and national standards for education. There is a standard national curriculum called Te Whāriki which all ECCE centres are required to follow. Health and wellbeing are core elements of the curriculum, as are belonging, contribution, communication and exploration. The number of children attending early childhood education in New Zealand is increasing. The introduction of 20 hours of free early childhood education for all three- and four-year-olds in New Zealand in 2007 was an acknowledgement of the importance of early childhood education to child health and wellbeing, particularly for children from lower socio-economic groups and for those from NESB (Mitchell et al. 2008). The policy has had an impact on increasing children's participation in childhood education, and in 2010 53.9% of preschool children attended formal early childhood education (ECE) and care, and 44.1% attended informal care, most provided by a grandparent (Statistics New Zealand, Online. Available: www.stats.govt.nz [accessed 23 June 2013]). These figures were slightly higher for European New Zealand children, but 58%

EVIDENCE FOR PRACTICE: Learning readiness

In recognition of the critical importance of early childhood learning experiences, the Australian Government has developed a National Quality Framework for Early Childhood Education and Care to legislate quality standards and processes associated with early childhood education (Australian Government 2011). The framework is based on research into the key domains of early childhood development called the Australian Early Development Index (AEDI), which was adapted from Canadian evidence-based indicators (Brinkman et al, 2007; Goldfield et al. 2009). The AEDI measures five domains of children's development in the early years: physical health and wellbeing, social competence, emotional maturity, language and cognitive skills, and communication skills and general knowledge (Sayers et al. 2012). Since 2009 the AEDI has been administered to all Australian children in their first year of full-time school. The findings have provided educators and policymakers with evidence of which children are developmentally vulnerable on one or more domains. Predictably, the most vulnerable were Indigenous children and those living in the most socio-economically disadvantaged communities. Although more than 80% of Australian children attend preschool or day care, Indigenous children, those with a disability, and NESB children had the lowest rates of participation. These results from the AEDI and evidence from a follow-up study called 'Outcomes and Indicators of a Positive Start to School' will provide policymakers with knowledge of the impact of early childhood education on all five domains of children's development.

ECE/ECCE

Good quality early childhood education is critical for children to develop the skills for lifelong learning.

? So how will we use this evidence for practice?

It will be interesting to see how these initiatives shape the health and wellbeing of generations of children in the future. In the short term, measures that can be taken to upskill the most vulnerable children will be important in terms of social equity. The legislation governing child care will attempt to ensure that all child care organisations maintain basic health and safety measures, including prevention and management of communicable diseases, especially for infants, and that there is sufficient, appropriately qualified staff to give each child age-appropriate attention and skills. This has implications for training staff and ensuring that standardisation does not prevent child care providers from supporting children and families in their local communities. As nurses we need to promote a commitment to intersectoral collaboration, interacting with teachers, parents, policymakers and other community partners to achieve the goals of PHC for children and their families.

of European/Māori, 53.8% of Māori only, and 44.4% of Asian children also had substantial rates of attendance (Statistics New Zealand, Online. Available: www.stats.gov.nz [accessed 23 June 2013]).

RESILIENCE

Whether children are born to traumatic conditions or to a more gentle life, their development capacity depends on their resilience, which is the key to personal and social competence. Resilience is a concept that captures how children display competent, adaptive functioning despite exposure to high levels of risk or adversity (Hunter 2012). It can be shown by children at different ages and stages, and can change depending on the level of the adversity, and whether the adversity is a single traumatic event, multiple stressful events, or chronic exposure to adversity. Child sexual abuse is among the most stressful, traumatic and chronic events, as the effects create a long-lasting legacy for the child, the family and, in some cases, the community (Martsolf & Burke Draucker 2008). A child can also display resilience or adaptive functioning in one area of their life, such as their emotional responses, yet they can experience significant deficits in another; for example, academic achievement (Hunter 2012). Developing resilience is often the culmination of individual, family, and community risk and protective factors. Individual factors include biological or epigenetic influences that, combined with psychological characteristics, build the child's capacity for emotional self-regulation, self-efficacy and self-determination. Family factors include having a close relationship with at least one caregiver or a strong attachment to a sibling; and community factors include social assets such as schools, groups, sporting or recreation clubs, and a sense of community connectedness (Hunter 2012).

A number of assets or protective factors have been identified as helping children develop resilience. As individuals, children with resilient temperaments demonstrate persistence and emotional regulation, which sees them modify, ameliorate, or change their responses to stressors. They tend to take an active approach to problem-solving, an ability from infancy to get positive attention from others, being alert and autonomous, having a tendency to seek out novel experiences and to maintain an optimistic view, even in the face of distressing experiences (Armstrong et al. 2005). Girls seem to be more resilient than boys, perhaps because they are more inclined to reach out and use social networks, gaining the social support they need (Silburn 2003; Stanley et al. 2005). Others demonstrate verbal and non-verbal abilities which help them adapt to various situations. Environmental features such as education, child care and other sectors that affect the child and family all have major parts to play in helping develop resilience. While some of these factors are protective across different circumstances (for example, good parenting), others are dependent on the context,

such as the education arena (Hunter 2012). These important factors are depicted in Figure 8.3.

KEEPING CHILDREN SAFE

Each day, 2000 children around the world die of unintentional injury, half of whom could be saved (WHO 2008b). The most prevalent childhood injuries are from road crashes, drowning, burns, falls and poisoning. The highest rate (95%) of these injuries occurs in developing countries, especially African nations, where children die at 10 times the rate of Australian and New Zealand children, primarily from road traumas (WHO 2008b). Besides being the greatest cause of child mortality, childhood injuries also place an extraordinary burden on health care systems. For those children who survive accidental injuries, many are seriously disabled, creating a lifelong caregiving burden for families. When the child has been injured in the home, there is an often unrelenting emotional toll on family members. This is a major problem, as the most common injuries occur in or around the home.

One of the things health professionals can do to promote child safety from injury is to consider the SDH that impact on child safety, then lobby for

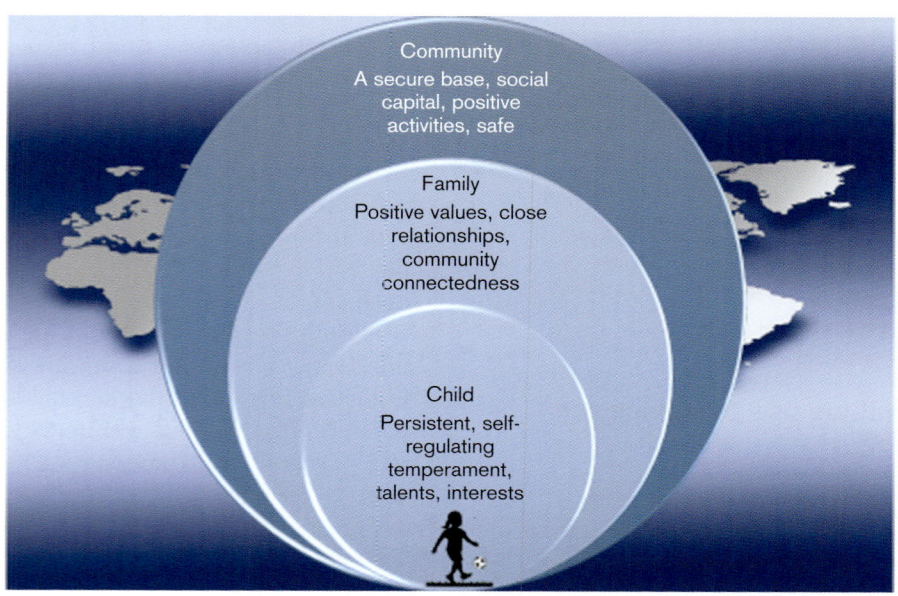

FIGURE 8.3
Child, family and community assets and protective factors

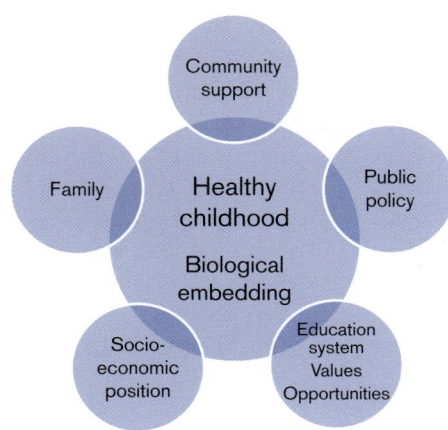

FIGURE 8.4
Interactions between factors involved in healthy childhood

healthy and protective environments within which young children grow, to ensure that the onus is on all of society to help keep children safe from harm (see Figure 8.4). This approach has been effective in advocating for bike helmet use, safer roadways and bicycle paths, and seatbelts on school buses. The whole-of-society approach is also being used to make visible the threats to child health and wellbeing that exist in our society from sexual predators, through groups like Bravehearts (www.bravehearts.org.au). Child and family health nurses also have a major role to play in monitoring safety at the societal level by advocating for vigilance and fostering parental health literacy in relation to threats to their children's health. Strategies include providing parents with information on their child's capacity at each developmental stage, so they will be alert to the precautions needed to ensure their child is safe, or directing parents to the sources of parental advice on child safety, either in print form or on the internet. For new parents there are many websites that provide age-related advice on accident prevention, identifying the behaviours at each stage that create the risks of certain types of accidents. The ability to provide anticipatory guidance for parents and caregivers is a key competency for child and family health nurses, one that Plunket and Tamariki Ora (Māori child health) nurses have integrated into practice since the 1970s (Clendon 2009).

A major source of risk lies in internet safety. Although children are supposed to be age 13 before they engage in social networking, anecdotal information suggests that many young children have the skills and the wilfulness to push the boundaries of internet safety. Most parents are aware of security measures that can help protect their children from accessing inappropriate websites on their home computers, but many children are able to access mobile devices at school or in recreational venues. The popularity of these devices and the rapid growth of sites make it imperative that parents discuss internet safety with their children before they are placed at risk of being exploited or damaged by unsavoury messages or messengers. Family-friendly websites provide a wealth of encouragement for internet safety prevention, and we list some of these at the end of the chapter. UNICEF also has direct advice for accident prevention. Key messages for both the family and community are outlined in Box 8.4.

Many childhood injuries are not caused by children's behaviour, but by the family's social circumstances such as housing and the risk or protective factors in the wider community (AIHW 2012a). As we have mentioned the safety risks for Indigenous children is greater, as many live in housing with few safety features and have poor general health (AIHW 2012a). Safety in young children requires attention to the SDH, beginning with family relationships. From strong family attachments, young people are able to make decisions about the various paths they will take toward independence. These attachments also provide a blueprint for forming subsequent social relationships and a sense of social connectedness. Helping children acquire and refine skills at progressively higher and broader levels sets the stage for later developmental tasks. Refining skills to the level of mastery helps children move from reaching and grasping, to walking, riding a tricycle, playing sport, and developing friendships and intimacies. In mastering lower level skills, children learn confidence, self-esteem and a sense of control over their environment. This attracts recognition from others, a sense of pride, wellbeing and life satisfaction (Stanley et al. 2005). Engaging with the wider community provides opportunities for children to make the most of their own capacities in the context of developing respect for those around them, a sense of integrity, and 'civic friendship' (Stanley et al. 2005:25). As a child grows to adulthood, civic friendship and civic participation can then grow into increasingly wider circles of trust, which helps foster community cohesion and social capital (Putnam 2005).

CRITICAL PATHWAYS TO CHILD HEALTH

From all the research into early parenting and development, we know that the health of children reflects the social determinants that impact on their world; the national policy environment that encourages or discourages the expression of their culture; their genetic make-up, and that of their parents; their ability to access early, high-quality education; the family's socio-economic status, including their place of residence; their access to and preferences for health services; family harmony, the extent to which healthy behaviours are modelled in the family and community; and features of the physical environment.

> **POINT TO PONDER**
>
> Critical step 1 towards healthy children: the health and wellbeing of women.

The first critical step on the pathway to healthy children is to focus on the health and wellbeing of women and this begins with educating women throughout the world (WHO 2005). Women's education and empowerment have significant effects on their socio-economic capability, and that of their children (UNFPA 2000). The pathway to health and wellbeing extends from women's pre-conception health literacy about diet, smoking, exercise and self-esteem, to political decisions aimed at enhancing structural support for families at all stages from birth through maturation to death (McCain & Mustard 2002).

> **POINT TO PONDER**
>
> Critical step 2 towards healthy children: linking child, family and community to build resilience.

A second critical pathway overlaps the first, in that health promotion activities should address the links between individual cognitive development and competence, and the aspects of society and the environment that either provide social buffering, social risk or social enhancement. A socio-ecological view of child health includes attention to the characteristics of the child, family and community, ensuring that a socially just, inclusive society supports the development of resilience along the pathway to maturity. Children also need to be seen from very early in life as learners, right from earliest child care to high school and beyond (Hertzman 2001b; Mustard 2007). Supporting early, high-quality child care and education are therefore important policy initiatives.

> **POINT TO PONDER**
>
> Critical step 3 towards healthy children: early childhood education, high-quality child care.

GOALS FOR CHILD HEALTH

The major health issues for children's health in today's society include adequate societal investment in the early years, supportive communities that protect and enable child and family health, health literacy for parents and their children, and continuing evolution of the evidence base for child and family health. The most optimal circumstance for a healthy child is to be born into a child-friendly, healthy and safe family and community. To support parents in this endeavour nurses need to address key family practices, as outlined in Box 8.5.

To achieve child health in any community, all known risk factors and factors that develop children's resilience and capacity to cope with their environments must be acknowledged and incorporated into a community's goals and target for prevention, protection and health promotion. An intersectoral approach is essential, which is best argued within the strategies of the Ottawa Charter for Health Promotion (WHO, Health and Welfare Canada & CPHA 1986).

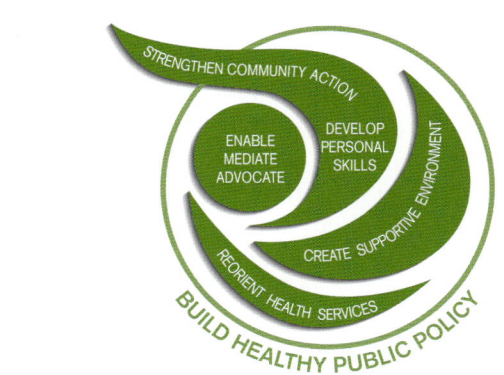

BOX 8.5 Nursing goals for supporting parents

- Maintaining culturally appropriate birthing and social support
- Some resources for Aboriginal and Torres Strait Islander women's birthing services include Congress Alukura in Alice Springs; Nganampa Health Council, Ngua Gundi Mother Child Project in Woorabinda, Qld; Aboriginal Maternal and Infant Health Strategy (AMIHS) NSW; Strong Women, Strong Babies, Strong Culture, NT. For migrant women information can be accessed at: www.migrationinformation.org/Feature/display.cfm?ID=108. Support for Māori women seeking traditional approaches to birthing, including where to find a Māori midwife, can be found through Nga Maia O Aotearoa (www.ngamaia.co.nz). Whakawhetu provides information for Māori whānau on preventing SUDI (www.whakawhetu.co.nz).
- Breastfeeding exclusively for six months and continuing until the child is aged two or more
- Resources for breastfeeding are listed at the end of this chapter and include: www.breastfeeding .asn.au, www.babyfriendly.org.nz, and telephone helplines 1800 686 2 686 (in Australia) and 0800 611 116 (in New Zealand)
- Promoting physical growth and mental and social development, including interactions with others in the household
- Recognising the need for assistance if required for infant settling or feeding
- Resources include: www.plunket.org.nz, www.tresillian.net, www.ngala.com.au; others are listed at the end of this chapter

- Preventing child abuse and neglect
- Accessing health services when required by maintaining sufficient health literacy to recognise needs and seek timely and appropriate care
- Resources include www.healthinfonet.ecu.edu.au, www.health.govt.nz
- Providing access to high-quality child care when required
- Assessing family health in the context of home visits, ensuring the home is peaceful and free from stress, conflict or violence
- Mental/emotional health promotion with the aim of meeting the universal needs of belonging, competence, independence, learning readiness and connectedness to the broader environment
- Keeping children safe from the harm of alcohol, tobacco or other toxic substances
- Immunising children according to the national schedules (www.immunise.health.gov.au, www.health.govt.nz)
- Preventing injuries and accidents
- Accessing helplines, local poison hotline, web safety sites
- Promoting safe, warm housing
- Maintaining food security in all neighbourhoods, promoting safe cooking with good ventilation
- Maintaining health literacy through knowledge of resources for child health

(Source: AIHW 2012a, WHO 2005)

Building healthy public policy

We began the chapter by stating that the greatest investment any society can make for the health of its people is one that facilitates the health of children. This is a global argument, one that directs health policies toward addressing the inseparable relationship between child, family and community health. This relationship is embedded in global, national and local policy declarations. The United Nations Convention on the Rights of the Child, to which Australia and New Zealand are signatories, is a legally binding international instrument to guide the care and protection of children (UNICEF, Online. Available: www.unicef.org.au/ [accessed 4 July 2013]). The Millennium Declaration of 2000 also addresses the explicit need to protect children from conflict, violence, abuse and exploitation (UNICEF 2009). Each of the Millennium Development Goals outlined in Chapter 4 is linked to the needs of children, from poverty reduction to educating children, eliminating gender inequality and reducing child mortality (UNICEF 2009). At the heart of all of these global policies is the need for equity at the start of life, to eliminate disparities and inequitable conditions, and provide a strong foundation for children along their life course (CSDH 2008). This requires policy coherence, commitment and leadership, as well as the integration of health in all government policies (CSDH 2008; WHO 2008a).

In New Zealand, the 2001 Primary Health Care Strategy set in motion a national set of policies to reduce social inequities with a focus on child, family and community health (NZMOH 2001). In 2009, Australia developed its first national Primary Health Care Strategy with a similar intention (Government of Australia, Online. Available: http://www.yourhealth.gov.au/internet/yourhealth/publishing.nsf/Content/nphcs [accessed 4 July 2013]). The National Framework for Protecting Australia's Children 2009–20 and the Communities for Children initiatives embody the commitment to building community capacity to support children and families (Lohoar et al. 2013). A national commitment to children has also been declared in the Australian National Agenda on Human Capital of the Council of Australian Governments (COAG), the Stronger Families and Communities Strategy (2004–09), and the Australian Research Alliance for Children & Youth (ARACY) Declaration and Call to Action to transform Australia for the future of its children (ARACY 2009, see Appendix I) all address the social inclusion agenda of closing the gap on Indigenous disadvantage (AIHW 2009).

Following New Zealand's lead on social inclusion, Australia's National Indigenous Reform agenda has made positive progress in closing the gap in health and longevity between Indigenous and non-Indigenous citizens (Government of Australia, Online. Available: www.fachsia.gov.au/ourresponsibilities/indigenous-australians/program-services/closing-the-gap [accessed 4 July 2013]). One aspect of closing the gap is culturally appropriate policies governing the availability of appropriate early childhood education for Indigenous people, which we discuss further in Chapter 15 (AIFS 2013a). A number of national policies also recognise equal rights to protect all citizens from discrimination on the basis of gender, sexual preference, age or disability (Heymann et al. 2013), many of which affect children in their day-to-day lives.

The most important policy decision governments must make acknowledges the importance of antenatal care in providing and sustaining a good start for improving the health of the entire population. Policies governing antenatal and birth care, immunisation, support for breastfeeding both at home and in the workplace, and early childhood education can be argued on the basis of research into the link between good health and adequate support during pregnancy, the influence of early parenting, and the importance of the nested influences of neighbourhoods and communities in child health. Antenatal care and breastfeeding, in particular, have the capacity to increase lifespan, enhance quality of life and reduce the cost of illness care for the population, making them the most important policy focus in public health. Both Australia and New Zealand have national strategies to promote breastfeeding and the health of breastfeeding mothers as well as national immunisation strategies.

Healthy public policy for children involves ensuring that policies governing illness and injury surveillance, health and fitness promotion, family support systems and sustainable environments are all developed coherently, so that all influences on health are acknowledged by all sectors of society. This type of intersectoral collaboration is advocated in the Australian National Preventative Health Strategy, which sets targets for reducing chronic illnesses through shared partnerships and acting early and throughout life (Government of Australia, Preventative Health Taskforce, Online. Available: www.preventativehealth.org.au/ [accessed 4 July 2013]). At the macro level, there must be coherent action across all sectors to work towards sustainable environments in which families can raise their children in equitable, safe, health promoting circumstances. Taxation and regulation should be part of health promotion policy development, addressing alcohol consumption, smoking and obesity (Marmot et al. 2012). Actions should revolve around knowledge of the SDH embedded into a 'Health in All Policies' agenda, and a strong commitment to social justice, based on everyone's moral right to develop health capacity.

Intersectoral policy collaboration is essential. This includes developing and monitoring manufacturing safety standards, housing standards and advertising codes of conduct, particularly in promoting tobacco products and junk food to children. Collaborative legislation such as that governing seatbelts, bicycle helmets and child care workers is also intended to guide safe behaviour and environments. Other policies affecting children's capacity should address the workplace where wages need to be high enough for people to help families exit poverty and preclude any family having to rely on child labour. Workplace policies should support the ability of working families to balance child care needs, including leave to attend to children's ill health, childhood education or breastfeeding. Laws mandating the licensing of child care workers, accreditation of child care providers and working with children's legislation are a visible signal of society's commitment to protect its most vulnerable citizens. This commitment is embodied in both Australia and New Zealand's paid parental leave schemes, which are also inclusive of a father's right and responsibility to parent his children.

To date, the intersectoral approach has been more widely accepted in New Zealand than in Australia, primarily because of fewer layers of bureaucracy and a stronger commitment to working across sectors (Jacobs 2009). Yet, despite the successes of intersectoral collaboration in New Zealand, there remains much to be done in relation to child health policy development. In 2011, the New Zealand Government published the 'Green Paper for Vulnerable Children' (Bennett 2011). The Green Paper was designed to open up the debate around how New Zealand cares for its vulnerable children. Over 10 000 submissions were received from throughout the country (NZ Govt, Online. Available: www.childrensactionplan.govt.nz/home [accessed 18 July 2013]). As mentioned earlier, up to 25% of New Zealand children live in poverty and many are suffering the effects of this in terms of their health and social development (Expert Advisory Group on Solutions to Child Poverty 2012). There were high expectations that the outcomes from the debate over the Green Paper would provide a future direction for supporting these children through addressing the SDH and, specifically, poverty. Unfortunately, the subsequent White Paper for Vulnerable Children (Bennett 2012a) and Children's Action Plan (Bennett 2012b), while providing useful direction for health

and social care providers, schools, families and communities, have failed to provide any significant plans for addressing child poverty in New Zealand, relying, instead, on a very narrow definition of the term 'vulnerable', limiting the policy to only those children who are at significant risk of abuse and neglect. As a result, although child health is embedded in various policy documents, there has been no specific all-encompassing child health policy since 1998 (NZMOH 1998). Strategic policy direction in this area remains lacking, and there continues to be a need for more inclusive policies that provide a way forward for nurses, midwives, and other health professionals working in the broader field of child and family health.

Healthy public policies should include affordable and accessible high-quality education for all. The poorest children need extra financial support for school costs and transportation and the policies governing school resources should also cover adequately educated teachers—the best teachers for those most in need (Heymann et al. 2013). As a general rule, policies to promote better health among children should respond to children's holistic needs for balance and potential. This means that school boards and education authorities should become aware of the need to accommodate physical education programs as integral to children's development. Schools can also be effective in promoting child health by cultivating health literacy. One example of this is the focus on good nutrition, which is done well by many early child care providers as well as primary schools by eliminating high fat content from school canteens and promoting better nutritional standards. This is an attempt to balance healthy eating policies during the early primary school years with modifications to the environment within which children and their families make healthy choices.

Creating supportive environments

Supportive environments for child health should begin with those conducive to healthy pregnancy. Ideally, services that provide health surveillance and monitoring for pregnant women should be readily available to all and accessible through workplace-based resources. With the current shortage of health care professionals, arrangements should be made to provide new parents with access to alternative sources of information and support to develop adequate levels of health literacy for parenting. This can be accomplished by ensuring appropriate online resources, or distributing information and resources in schools, child care centres or designated family support centres, allowing parents a choice in how and where they access information. The research cited earlier in this chapter is interesting in terms of the impact of maternal, child and family nurses on new mothers' mental health, particularly in relation to PND (Rush 2012; Scope et al. 2012). This evidence should be widely disseminated to highlight the important role of nurses in supporting parents, and in turn, their children, in their neighbourhoods and communities.

Schools are a major context for achieving the Millennium Development Goals (MDGs) worldwide (Godson et al. 2011). Yet in many parts of the world schools are facing considerable environmental problems with inadequate space, air and water quality, teaching resources and many other difficulties. In our part of the world, schools in remote and sometimes regional areas are also finding difficulties in maintaining safe environments within which children can learn and develop. A supportive school environment should be one where both the physical and intellectual environments support health in a sustainable way (Sampson 2012). Schools can also redress inequities; for example, in enrolling children with disabilities in schools with their non-disabled counterparts (Heymann et al. 2013). Another way the school can address the social equity agenda is in the context of the school health literacy agenda, providing information that is both culturally appropriate and family-friendly. This strategy extends to the combination of actions to promote healthy lifestyles. School-based obesity prevention programs have been shown as a cost-effective way to reduce overweight and help with parental health literacy, especially in relation to dietary behaviour (Manger et al. 2012; Werner et al. 2012). Initiatives to promote gender equality should begin at school, in engaging boys to think about health, wellbeing and help seeking, given that their hesitancy often demonstrates the 'inverse care law': those who are most in need are least likely to seek help' (O'Connell-Binns 2009:6). If school-based programs are culturally and socially responsible, they send a message to families that educational settings are places where young children can not only learn, but thrive, and that the family is as valued as the child (Shi et al. 2013). They also place the school squarely at the heart of the community, helping not only children, but their families.

SCHOOL-BASED HEALTH LITERACY

Culturally appropriate, socially just student and family health education that results in physical, intellectual and social wellbeing.

As outlined in Chapter 5, the move towards having local councils more involved in health and wellbeing is a positive step in promoting supportive environments for health, and a sense of belonging, especially at the neighbourhood level. This also helps build trusting, cohesive environments for capacity-building (Lohoar et al. 2013). These environments provide a base of support that can help children overcome the hopelessness of a low socio-economic beginning by helping them strengthen their community identity (Lohoar et al. 2013). A sense of community connectedness is crucial to children's development, and this is entrenched in the International Secretariat for Child Friendly Cities, initiated by the UNICEF Innocenti Research Centre in Florence, Italy, to help shift responsibility for child health, education and protection to municipal councils. This PHC approach sends a message that childhood is integral to community development (UNICEF, Online. Available: www.unicef.org.au, www.childfriendlycities.org [accessed 4 July 2013]). The global statement from UNICEF underlines the importance of the structural supports for child health and wellbeing; the macro forces within a child's environment that predict the extent to which children will do well.

PRACTICE STRATEGY

Community strategies must be inclusive of all members of the community at all stages of development, from implementation to evaluation.

Similar collaborative ventures have seen New Zealand initiatives between health, sport and recreation and local community health, social development and education groups (Jacobs 2009). One example is the iMove Nekeneke Hi! program in the Midcentral region of the lower North Island. The iMove program encourages school students to choose between walking or riding a bicycle to school on a given day for a month. Students receive a trip card which they get signed off and go into a draw to win prizes. The iMove program started as a pilot in two schools in 2006 and by 2013 over 35 schools and ECCE were involved. While initially the project was established by the Roadsafe Central coordinator, the success of the program has been dependent on the collaborative efforts of the police, the Palmerston North City Council, public health services, non-government organisations, local Māori health providers, primary health organisations (PHOs), the media and local sporting organisations (Ferry 2009). iMove now also includes adult cycle safety workshops including workshops exclusively for women. These workshops are designed to promote safe cycling among adults who will then go on to act as role models for children in the community (iMove, Online. Available: http://www.sportmanawatu.org.nz/modules/content/content.php?content.20 [accessed 19 July 2013]).

Comprehensive strategies to provide supportive communities also take into account the increasing levels of migrant, refugee and culturally and linguistically diverse (CALD) families in the neighbourhood. Bringing CALD needs to the intersectoral agenda will help build tolerance in a community across politicians, health and education services, transport, the business community, the community council, consumer organisations, the police, juvenile justice authorities and any service clubs within a community. This type of collaborative approach focuses on ensuring safety and protection for all young people, including refugee children and their families in detention centres. As researchers have shown, the longer young children and their families are detained, the greater the decline in their mental health (Newman 2012). Traumatised children and families often experience confusion about their social marginalisation and then their transition into Australian society, where this occurs. Instead of imprisoning them in dehumanising detention centres, a supportive environment would be community-based, and aimed at assisting the family with trans-generational repair from their traumas (Newman 2012). To change this situation requires strong and sustained community action.

Strengthening community action

Community actions are empowering, particularly if they build partnerships to support children's resilience and capacity (AIHW 2012a; Lohoar 2013). Clear and visible partnerships, with the child at the centre of the community, send a signal to children that their health and wellbeing are central to the way the community sees itself, and it gives them a sense of validation as they move through the various stages of childhood, learning to cope with life's challenges and develop self-confidence and mastery at each stage. Ideally, community action involves a careful blend of voluntary, professional, business, faith-based and family organisations, to nurture children across the spectrum of childhood, irrespective of their abilities or level of disadvantage. To foster this kind of development at the school, neighbourhood, and community level, parents, grandparents, teachers and others need to be made aware of their community's strengths and resources as well as the areas of particular risk to young children.

> ## POINT TO PONDER
> Children learn about society from watching their peers, families and community members act in partnership.

Parent-to-parent programs and ECE programs have in common, a focus on strengthening community action for healthy childhoods, and we have listed a number of these and their websites at the end of the chapter. Programs that use existing networks of volunteers, including grandparents, and health, welfare and education professionals, provide an outlet for new parents to express concerns and to share resources and strategies for parenting, especially in the context of the isolation that new parenting often brings (Horsfall & Dempsey 2011). Grandparents are vital to children's lives, especially those who are in frequent contact with their grandchildren (Horsfall & Dempsey 2011). Where parental separation has occurred those who are available to the children are often able to provide children with a non-judgemental, positive perspective on relationships, and continuity throughout what may be difficult times for them (Deblaquiere et al. 2012).

Researchers have found that the most successful early intervention programs are those aimed at socially disadvantaged families, which use combined strategies for improving both child and parent outcomes (Watson & Tully 2008). One of the most important studies on early intervention has been the work by David Olds and colleagues into home visiting with vulnerable families. The findings from this longitudinal randomised controlled trial found that nurses undertaking intensive home visiting (up to 26 home visits in the first two years of life) resulted in a range of beneficial child health outcomes including children more likely to be enrolled in preschool education, higher intellectual functioning and vocabulary scores, and fewer behavioural problems (Olds et al. 2004a; 2004b). These effects were apparent up to 12 years beyond the end of the nurse visits and were evident in children from a range of social and ethnic backgrounds (although the effects were stronger among children from lower socio-economic backgrounds). The study also found that the home visiting program improved maternal health over the life course and resulted in reduced government spending on the children whose mothers took part in the program at least up until the child's twelfth birthday (Olds et al. 2004a, 2004b, 2010; Kitzman et al. 2010). Interestingly, despite these studies, there is some debate regarding the outcomes of home visiting and this will be examined further in Chapter 15. What is important to recognise is that parenting support should be based on the knowledge that good parenting can compensate for the effects of social disadvantage on the developing child (Marmot et al. 2012). Community programs to help these families are more effective when they begin before the child attends primary school, when the can help develop skills for learning and cognitive development, as well as good health (Brooks-Gunn 2003). The critical moments for childhood risk prevention means that nurses' health guidance for mothers should begin at the earliest part of the continuum, during antenatal care, and extend through childbirth, postnatal and early childhood care (Water 2011).

Early intervention programs are also a vital element in improving the health of first-time Indigenous mothers and their children. The 'asset' or 'strengths-based' approach is acknowledged in programs such as 'Strong Mothers, Strong Babies, Strong Culture', which has been particularly successful in the Northern Territory of Australia (Commonwealth of Australia 2009b). Strategies to overcome disadvantage among these and other disadvantaged children and their families should include adequate health and social protection for women, pregnant women and young families. Women and their partners should have reproductive choices, healthy pregnancies, good parental leave arrangements and affordable and an accessible early years education and child care system. Actions should therefore work towards family empowerment; reducing stress at work, unemployment and any of the causes of social isolation or social exclusion (Marmot et al. 2012).

Developing personal skills

To support child and family health requires ongoing personal development for carers, educators, family members, health professionals and children themselves. Developing children's personal skills extends not only to their intellectual development but to protecting their safety on the internet, which is a cause for concern among some parents. Despite the fact that social network sites try to prohibit young children from participating, many seem to be able to access the sites if their parents do not monitor their online behaviour. This has implications for keeping children safe while helping them participate in digital education.

> ### ASSESSMENT CHALLENGE
> What personal capacities would be a priority in your community?

Mandatory regulatory practices and compulsory in-service sessions for early child care and teaching personnel are designed to protect children, but many programs require only a minimum level of personal development. Community-based programs that help child workers remain connected to one another and maintain currency in their practice are a step further. In an era of evidence-based practice, it is also important that all professionals dealing with children have opportunities to share in the most recent research findings that guide their practices. Universities and colleges can be helpful in this respect, bringing people together as community residents, and providing courses that help them enhance their own capacity by building skills and strengths to cope with the challenges of their work. Personal development courses can also help reduce attrition among child care workers, which is a major problem today, given a rapidly growing need for child care, and a critical shortage of skilled health and welfare workers. The White Paper for Vulnerable Children (Bennett 2012a) called for the development of a tiered set of core competencies and minimum quality standards to be developed for all those working with children by the end of 2015. Health professionals who work with children will be required to demonstrate how they meet the competencies through professional development.

EVIDENCE FOR PRACTICE
Equitable service provision for child health should be planned on the basis of research evidence for the link between services and outcomes.

One of the difficulties of parenting in contemporary society lies in managing child and family roles with formal work patterns. Many parents find themselves returning to work quickly after childbirth with little knowledge of developmental stages or children's needs, and a lack of extended family support. For some of these parents, the opportunity to access group-based positive parenting support programs is a lifeline to the wider community. Parenting programs have been found effective in helping reduce maternal depression and anxiety/stress, and in improving confidence, self-esteem and partner relationships, as well as improving child health outcomes (Fielden & Gallagher 2008). In Australia and New Zealand nurses and other health professionals working in the community have successfully delivered a number of parenting programs, some of which we mentioned in Chapter 5, and others that are listed at the end of this chapter. Most are particularly effective when used in conjunction with individual interventions to support young families in their transition to parenthood. Programs that are embedded in communities, designed with input from the communities where they will be provided, and responsive to community needs have also been found to be most effective (Rumble 2010). Where parenting education is provided in groups within the community, opportunities for interaction, reflection and mutual support enhance the experience for parents (Rumble 2010).

Reorienting health services

In Australia and New Zealand, one of the biggest problems in serving the community is the shortage of health professionals in areas of highest need. Equitable distribution of services is one important way to ensure children and families who are vulnerable to risks and poor health will not be further disadvantaged. Service planning requires evidence of what is feasible, cost-effective, fair, and acceptable to families and communities.

MCFH NURSES

- are there
- are knowledgeable
- are collaborative
- are pivotal to child and family health.

The most definitive evidence of the impact of nursing on children's health comes from a growing body of research into nurse led models of care. Analysis of a 25-year program of research into home visiting for low SES mothers in the US has shown that nurse home-visiting improved parental care, reduced childhood injuries, improved maternal health and workforce participation, and reduced the number of pregnancies and the need for public assistance (Olds 2002). The results of similar studies in the UK have shown improvements in mother-child interactions, better health attitudes and behaviour, improvements to infant health and reduced risk of neglect or abuse (Barlow et al. 2007; Ingram et al. 2011). Studies in Australia and New Zealand have also shown that nurses play a key role in mandated child abuse and neglect cases (Fraser et al. 2009; Rush et al. 2012; Wilson et al. 2008). This type of research should be extended to demonstrate the essential nature of nurse-led care in helping maintain child and family health. Being accessible in the community and home environments provides nurses with the opportunities to observe childhood injuries and provide ongoing monitoring of children's health (Fraser et al. 2009). With new mothers having short hospital stays for childbirth it is usually the maternal child and family health nurses and midwives positioned within the community setting who identify the risk of depressive disorders such as PND (Harvey et al. 2012). In some cases their actions can have a flow-on effect in reducing antisocial and detrimental behaviours such as smoking and substance abuse, simply be helping parents with the stress of early parenting. A new information system developed and trialled by Plunket nurses will see Plunket nurses visiting families equipped with tablet computers that allow them to connect with Plunketline, midwives, the national immunisation database and the national Plunket database. The connectivity of the online system will allow the nurse to make appropriate assessments and referrals instantly and is intended to result in a decrease in the number of children falling through the gaps in health systems (Manchester 2013). Families will also have access to their children's records once it is rolled out nationally. Nurse-led models of care are becoming widely acknowledged by their collaborators in general practice who recognise the importance of early assessment of risk and potential (Harvey et al. 2012; Rush 2012). The guidance and parenting support for new mothers provided by nurses has the potential to affect the health and development of children, enhance the parental life course for mothers, improve father involvement and reduce the risks to children.

With shrinking budgets and fewer personnel to meet family needs, our communities may become increasingly imperilled at the very time as we have determined the most appropriate way to help children. The evidence base indicates that the future of society rests in having all young children equipped emotionally and cognitively for their place in society. This should provoke us to look outside our professional boundaries at the social determinants and conditions that will help children become mentally and socially fit and able to cope with their lives. Health professionals who continue focusing only on illness care and social workers who only focus on crisis events may be doing a disservice to families. Instead, the focus should be on interventions aimed at the whole of the community (Lohoar et al. 2013). This requires comprehensive PHC, with the addition of selective PHC to meet the needs of children with disabilities or special needs by reframing our health care systems toward equity, access, empowerment, cultural sensitivity and intersectoral collaboration. The partnerships between school nurses and teachers attest to the effectiveness of nurses' roles in the early childhood and education systems (see Chapter 5). Collaboratively, the nurse-teacher team can align learning and health resources to make a significant contribution to health in schools. They also work with police and the judicial system that have in the past, focused their efforts on punishing and incarcerating, to develop programs to prevent children's anti-social behaviours.

The LSNZC, which has now reported on the first nine months of the cohort, found that 99% of pregnant women engage with an LMC in their pregnancy, either an independent midwife, obstetrician, hospital midwife or family physician (Morton et al. 2012). At six weeks, three-quarters of the children had been seen by a Plunket nurse and almost 91% of children received all of their well child Tamariki Ora checks. Such high engagement with services suggests they are meeting the needs of most women and children in the early postpartum period in New Zealand. Despite this example, the issue for all involved in child health is to recognise that the organisation of health services continues to value illness care, even though much of the rhetoric proclaims a commitment toward prevention. In the interest of access and equity, all health professionals should work more closely together to ensure that families do not fall through the cracks of service provision. This involves greater teamwork and careful evaluation of services and health outcomes. It also requires examination of the best way to use existing resources. Although there is a significant need to investigate specific health issues related to healthy child development, the need for safe care provision for all is a priority and it is a current and future challenge for researchers because valuing children is valuing the future of society (CSDH 2008).

We now turn to the Smith and Mason families to consider their children's health in the context of their respective situations.

CASE STUDY: Child health for the Smith and Mason families

With Colin absent from the home so much, Rebecca is left to cope with the children's issues, especially Gemma's eczema, which she thinks may be linked to stress as well as an unknown allergy. She is also concerned about Emily's difficulties at school and hesitates to involve Colin too much in her approach to seeking help for her. The school nurse has been to see Rebecca about Emily to try to help her work out some behavioural strategies to help her.

In Pakakura Jake has been admitted to hospital again for an acute asthma attack, which has meant that Huia has had to take time off work and arrange for someone else to care for the other children as Jason is away. Huia's job is under threat because of her frequent absences due to Jake's asthma.

REFLECTING ON THE BIG ISSUES

- The most important investment governments can make is in supporting child and family health.

- The SDH have a profound impact on the health of children and families.

- One of the most significant threats to child health is poverty.

- Healthy pregnancy and antenatal care establish a platform for good health in childhood.

- Breastfeeding is the ideal in nourishing infants.

- The health of children in Australia and New Zealand is at a high standard relative to other countries of the West.
- Family lifestyle and parenting practices have a profound impact on child health.
- Nurse home visiting is one of the most important interventions to provide parenting support and guidance for child health.
- Nursing practice should be evidence-based and connected to child and family outcomes.

REFLECTIVE QUESTIONS: How would I use this knowledge in practice?

1   What are the main priorities you would identify in a first home visit with Rebecca or Huia?

2   How would you assess the Smith and Mason household environments for risks and protective factors for their children?

3   How would your knowledge of Jason and Colin's employment and Huia's role as a teacher change your approach to assessing their needs and that of their children?

4   Which support services in Huia and Rebecca's home communities would be most likely to provide support for their needs and that of their family?

5   What are the most visible effects of the SDH on both families?

6   Explain how you would ensure that both families had sufficient health literacy for their parenting responsibilities.

7   Describe three aspects of their school or recreational setting that would be crucial to providing family support. For each, explain the importance of the setting in promoting child health and its link to primary health care principles.

References

Althabe, F., Belizan, J.U., 2006. Caesarean section: The paradox. Lancet 368, 1472–1473.

Apter, G., Devouche, E., Gratier, M., et al., 2012. What lies behind postnatal depression: Is it only a mood disorder? J. Personal. Disord. 26 (3), 357–367.

Armstrong, M., Birnie-Lefcovitch, S., Ungar, M., 2005. Pathways between social support, family well being, quality of parenting, and child resilience: What we know. J. Child Fam. Stud. 14 (2), 269–281.

Australian Bureau of Statistics, 2010. Population by age and sex, Australian states and territories. Cat No. 3201.0, ABS, Canberra.

Australian Government Department of Education, Employment and Workplace Relations, 2011. Early childhood education. Universal access. AGPS, Canberra.

Australian Government Department of Families, Housing, Community Services and Indigenous Affairs (FAHCSIA), 2013a. The Longitudinal Study of Indigenous Children. AIHW, Canberra.

Australian Government, 2013b. Closing the Gap, Prime Minister's Report. AGPS, Canberra.

Australian Institute of Family Studies (AIFS), 2012a. The longitudinal study of Australian children, annual statistical report 2011. AIFS, Melbourne.

Australian Institute of Family Studies (AIFS), 2012b. Families make all the difference. Helping kids to grow and learn. AIFS, Melbourne.

Australian Institute of Family Studies (AIFS), 2013a. Growing up in Australia, the Longitudinal Study of Australian Families 2012 report. AIFS, Melbourne.

Australian Institute of Family Studies (AIFS), 2013b. Access to early childhood education in Australia, Research Report NO. 24. AIFS, Melbourne.

Australian Institute of Health and Welfare (AIHW), 2009. A Picture of Australia's Children 2009. Cat. No. PHE 112, AIHW, Canberra.

Australian Institute of Health and Welfare (AIHW), 2010. Australia's mothers and babies 2010. AIHW, Canberra.

Australian Institute of Health and Welfare (AIHW), 2012a. A Picture of Australia's Children 2012. Cat. No. PHE 167, AIHW, Canberra.

Australian Institute of Health and Welfare (AIHW), 2012b. Australia's Health 2012. AIHW, Cat. No. AUS 156, AIHW, Canberra.

Australian Research Alliance for Children and Youth (ARACY), 2009. Transforming Australia for our children's future. ARACY National Conference, Sept 4, Melbourne.

Baker, M., Barnard, L., Kvalsvig, A., et al., 2012. Increasing incidence of serious infectious diseases and inequities in New Zealand: a national epidemiological study. Lancet 379, 1112–1119.

Bandura, A., 1977. Self-efficacy: Toward a unifying theory of behavioral change. Psychol. Rev. 84, 191–215.

Barlow, J., Davis, H., McIntosh, E., et al., 2007. Role of home visiting in improving parenting and health in families at risk of abuse and neglect: results of a multicentre randomized controlled trial and economic evaluation. Arch. Dis. Child. 92, 229–233.

Baumrind, D., 1966. Effects of authoritative control on child behavior. Child Dev. 37 (4), 887–907.

Baumrind, D., 1971. Current patterns of parental authority. Dev. Psychol. 4 (10), 1–103.

Bennett, P., 2011. Green paper for vulnerable children. Ministry of Social Development, Wellington, New Zealand.

Bennett, P., 2012a. White paper for vulnerable children. Ministry of Social Development, Wellington, New Zealand.

Bennett, P., 2012b. Children's action plan: Identifying, supporting and protecting vulnerable children. Ministry of Social Development, Wellington, New Zealand.

Bennett, S., Holmes, J., Buckley, S., 2013. Computerized memory training leads to sustained improvement in visiospatial short-term memory skills in children with down syndrome. Am. J. Int. Dev. Disabl. 118 (3), 179–192.

Bloomfield, L., Kendall, S., 2012. Parenting self-efficacy, parenting stress and child behavior before and after a parenting programme. Prim. Health Care Res. Dev. 13, 364–372.

Blythe, S., Halcomb, E., Wilkes, L., et al., 2013. Caring for vulnerable children: Challenges of mothering in the Australian foster care system. Contemp. Nurse 44 (1), 87–98.

Bowlby, J., 1969. Attachment and loss: Vol 1, Attachment. Basic Books, New York.

Brinkman, S., Silburn, S., Lawrence, D., et al., 2007. Construct and concurrent validity of the Australian Early Development Index. Early Educ. Dev. 18 (3), 427–451.

Bronfenbrenner, U., 1979. The ecology of human development: Experiments by nature and design. Harvard University Press, Cambridge.

Brooks-Gunn, J., 2003. Do you believe in magic? What can we expect from early childhood intervention programs? Soc. Policy Rep. 17 (1), 3–14.

Brown, H., Hume, C., Pearson, N., et al., 2013. A systematic review of intervention effects on potential mediators of children's physical activity. BMC Public Health 13, 165–175.

Bryanton, J., Gagnon, A., Hatem, M., et al., 2009. Does perception of the childbirth experience predict women's early parenting behaviors? Res. Nurs. Health 32, 191–203.

Cantor, J., 2001. The media and children's fears, anxieties and perceptions of danger. In: Singer, D., Singer, J. (Eds.), Handbook of children and the media. Sage, Thousand Oaks Ca, pp. 207–221.

Castonguay, G., Jutras, S., 2009. Children's appreciation of outdoor places in a poor neighborhood. J. Environ. Psychol. 29, 101–109.

Chaudhuri, J., Easterbrooks, A., Davis, C., 2009. The relation between emotional availability and parenting style: Cultural and economic factors in a diverse sample of young mothers. Parent. Sci. Pract. 9, 277–299.

Christakis, D., Zimmerman, F., 2007. Violent television during pre-school is associated with anti-social behaviour during school age. Pediatrics 120 (5), 993–999.

Claxton, A., Perry-Jenkins, M., 2008. No fun anymore: Leisure and marital quality across the transition to parenthood. J. Marriage Fam. 70, 28–43.

Clendon, J., 2009. Motherhood and the Plunket book: a social history. PhD thesis, Massey University, Auckland, New Zealand.

Commission on the Social Determinants of Health (CSDH), 2008. Closing the gap in a generation: health equity through action on the social determinants of health, Final Report of the Commission on social determinants of health. World Health Organization, Geneva.

Commonwealth of Australia, 2009a. Report of the maternity services review. Online. Available: <http://www.health.gov.au/maternityservicesreview> 19 October, 2009.

Commonwealth of Australia, 2009b. Australian National Breastfeeding Strategy 2010-2015. AHMAC, Canberra.

Craig, E., Adams, J., Oben, G., et al., 2013. The health status of children and young people in New Zealand. Ministry of Health, Paediatric Society of New Zealand, New Zealand Child and Youth Epidemiology Service, Auckland.

Craig, E., Jackson, C., Han, D.Y., et al., 2007. Monitoring the Health of New Zealand Children and Young People: Indicator Handbook. Paediatric Society of New Zealand, New Zealand Child and Youth Epidemiology Service, Auckland.

Cramp, A., Bray, S., 2011. Understanding exercise self-efficacy and barriers in leisure-time physical activity among postnatal women. Matern. Child Health J 15, 642–651.

Crouch, S., McNair, R., Waters, E., et al., 2013. What makes a same-sex parented family. Med. J. Aust. 198 (9), 1.

Crouch, S., Waters, E., McNair, R., et al., 2012. ACHESS-The Australian study of child health in same-sec families: background research, design and methodology. BMC Public Health 12, 626.

Deblaquiere, J., Moloney, L., Weston, R., 2012. Parental separation and grandchildren. Fam. Matters 90, 68–76.

Dennis, C., Hodnett, E., Reisman, H., et al., 2009. Effect of peer support on prevention of postnatal depression among high risk women: multisite randomized controlled trial. Br. Med. J. 338a, 3064. doi:10.1136/bmj.a3064.

Dockett, S., Perry, B., Kearney, E., 2012. Family transitions as children start school. Fam. Matters 90, 57–66.

Drewnowski, A., 2009. Obesity, diets, and social inequalities. Nutr. Rev. 67 (Suppl. 1), S36–S39.

Dunt, D., Hage, B., Kelaher, M., 2010. The impact of social and cultural capital variables on parental rating of child health in Australia. Health Promot. Int. 26 (1), 290–301.

Edwards, B., Bromfield, I., 2009. Neighbourhood influences on young children's conduct problems and prosocial behavior: Evidence from an Australian national sample. Child. Youth Serv. Rev. 31, 317–324.

Ekeroma, A., Ikenasio-Thorpe, B., Weeks, S., et al., 2012. Validation of the Edinburgh Postnatal Depression Scale (EPDS) as a screening tool for postnatal depression in Samoan and Tongan women living in New Zealand. NZMJ 125 (1355), 41–49.

Emerson, E., 2009. Relative child poverty, income inequality, wealth, and health. Commentary. J. Am. Med. Assoc. 301 (4), 425–426.

Expert Advisory Group on Child Poverty, 2012. Solutions to child poverty in New Zealand: evidence for action. Office of the Children's Commissioner, Wellington, New Zealand.

Families Commission, 2008. Juggling acts: how parents working non-standard hours arrange care for their pre-school children. Families Commission, Wellington New Zealand. Available: <http://www.familiescommission.org.nz/sites/default/files/downloads/juggling-acts.pdf> 28 June 2013.

Ferry, B., 2009. iMove Nekeke Hi! In: Signal, L., Egan, R., Cook, L. (Eds.), Reviews of Health Promotion Practice in Aotearoa New Zealand, 2007–2008. Health Promotion Forum of New Zealand and Health Promotion and Policy Research Unit. University of Otago, Auckland, pp. 69–77.

Fielden, J., Gallagher, L., 2008. Building social capital in first-time parents through a group-parenting program: A questionnaire survey. Int. J. Nurs. Stud. 45, 406–417.

Figueiredo, B., Costa, R., Pacheco, A., et al., 2009. Mother-to-infant emotional involvement at birth. Matern. Child Health J. 13 (4), 539–550.

Fraley, R., 2010. A brief overview of adult attachment theory and research. University of Illinois, Online. Available: <www.internal.psychology.illinois.edu/-rcfraley/attachment htm> 18 June 2013.

Fraser, J., Mathews, B., Walsh, K., et al., 2009. Factors influencing child abuse and neglect recognition and reporting by nurses: A multivariate analysis. Int. J. Nurs. Stud. doi:10.1016666/j.ijnurstu.2009.05.015.

Free, S., Howden-Chapman, P., Pierse, N., et al., 2010. More effective home heating reduces school absences for children with asthma. J. Epidemiol. Community Health 64, 379–386. doi:10.1136/jech.2008.086520.

Gluckman, P., 2011. Improving the transition: reducing social and psychological morbidity during adolescence. Office of the Prime Minister's Science Advisory Committee, Wellington, New Zealand.

Godson, R., Ana, E., Shendell, D., 2011. School environmental health programs and the challenges of achieving the Millennium Development Goals. J. Sch. Health 81 (2), 55–56.

Goldfield, S., Sayers, M., Brinkman, S., et al., 2009. The process and policy challenges of adapting and implementing the Early Development Instrument in Australia. Early Educ. Dev. 20 (6), 978–991.

Goodwin, R., Robinson, M., Sly, P., et al., 2013. Severity and persistence of asthma and mental health: A birth cohort study. Psychol. Med. 43 (6), 1313–1322.

Goodyear, R., Fabian, A., 2012. Household crowding in New Zealand compared with selected countries. Statistics New Zealand, Wellington, New Zealand.

Habib, C., 2012. The transition to fatherhood: A literature review exploring paternal involvement with identity theory. J. Fam. Stud. 18 (2–3), 103–120.

Hackman, D., Farah, M., 2009. Socioeconomic status and the developing brain. Trends Cogn. Sci. 13 (2), 65–73.

Harnack, L., Jeffery, R., Boutelle, K., 2000. Temporal trends in energy intake in the United States: an ecologic perspective. Am. J. Clin. Nutr. 71 (6), 1478–1484.

Harvey, S., Fisher, L., Green, V., 2012. Evaluating the clinical efficacy of a primary care-focused, nurse-led, consultation liaison model for perinatal mental health. Int. J. Ment. Health Nurs. 21, 75–81.

Heckman, J., 2012. The economics of child well-being. IZA Discussion Paper No. 6930, University of Chicago, Chicago, pp. 1–58.

Hector, D., King, L., Webb, K., et al., 2005. Factors affecting breastfeeding practices: applying a conceptual framework. N. S. W. Public Health Bull. 16 (3–4), 52–55.

Hertzman, C., 2001a. Health and human society. Am. Sci. 89 (6), 538–544.

Hertzman, C., 2001b. Determinants of Health. Presentation to the Commission for Children and Young People (CCYP), Queensland Health. 21 November, Royal Children's Hospital, Brisbane.

Hertzman, C., 2012. Putting the concept of biological embedding in historical perspective. Proc. Natl Assoc. Sci. 109 (Suppl. 2), 17160–17167.

Hertzman, C., 2013. Commentary on the symposium: Biological embedding, life course development, and the emergence of a new science. Annu. Rev. Public Health 34, 1–5.

Hertzman, C., Boyce, T., 2010. How experience gets under the skin to create gradients in development health. Annu. Rev. Public Health 31, 329–347.

Hewitt, C., Gilbody, S., 2009. Is it clinically and cost effective to screen for postnatal depression: a systematic review of controlled clinical trials and economic evidence. Br. J. Obstet. Gynaecol. doi:10.1111/j.1471-0528.2009.02148.x.

Heymann, J., Earle, A., McNeil, K., 2013. The impact of labor policies on the health of young children in the context of economic globalization. Annu. Rev. Public Health 34, 355–372.

Hobel, C., Goldstein, A., Barrett, E., 2008. Psychosocial stress and pregnancy outcome. Clin. Obstet. Gynecol. 51 (2), 233–348.

Horsfall, J., Dempsey, D., 2011. Grandfathers and grandmothers looking after grandchildren: Recent Australian research. Fam. Relatsh Q. 18, 10–12.

Hunter, C., 2012. Is resilience still a useful concept when working with children and young people? AIFS, Child

Family Community Information Exchange CFCA Paper No. 2: 1-11.

Ingram, J., Johnson, D., Condon, L., 2011. The effects of Baby Friendly Initiative training on breastfeeding rates and the breastfeeding attitudes, knowledge and self-efficacy of community health-care staff. Prim. Health Care Res. Dev. 12 (3), 266–275.

Jacobs, M., 2009. New Zealand approaches to prevention. Public Health Bull. SA 6 (1), 27–29.

Jacobs, J., Agho, K., Raphael, B., 2012. The prevalence of potential family life difficulties in a national longitudinal general population sample of Australian Children. Fam. Matters 90, 19–32.

Kiernan, K., Huerta, C., 2008. Economic deprivation, maternal depression, parenting and children's cognitive and emotional development in early childhood. Br. J. Sociol. 59 (40), doi:10.1111/j.1468-4446.2008.00219.x.

Kitzman, H., Olds, D., Cole, R., et al., 2010. Enduring effects of prenatal and infancy home visiting by nurses on children: Follow-up of a randomized trial among children at age 12 years. Arch. Pediatr. Adolesc. Med. 164 (5), 412–418.

La Coursiere, D., Hirst, K., Barett-Connor, E., 2012. Depression and pregnancy stressors affect the association between abuse and postpartum depression. Matern. Child Health J 16, 929–935.

Lamont, A., Price-Robertson, R., 2013. Risk and protective factors for child abuse and neglect. Australian Institute for Family Studies, Child, Family Community Australia Online. Available: <www.aifs.gov.au/cfa/pubs/factsheets/a143921/index.html> June 23 2013.

Larkin, H., Shields, J., Anda, R., 2012. The health and social consequences of adverse childhood experiences (ACE) across the lifespan: An introduction to prevention and intervention in the community. J. Prev. Interv. Community 40 (4), 263–270.

Leckman, J., March, J., 2011. Editorial: Developmental neuroscience comes of age. J. Child Psychol. Psychiatr. 52 (4), 333–338.

Li, J., McMurray, A., Stanley, F., 2008. Modernity's paradox and the structural determinants of child health and well-being. Health Sociol. Rev. 17 (1), 64–77.

Li, Z., Zeki, R., Hilder, L., et al., 2012. Australia's mothers and babies 2010. Perinatal statistics series no. 27 Cat. No PER 57. AIHW, Canberra.

Lodge, J., Baxter, J., 2012. Children's experiences of unfriendly behaviour. Longitudinal Study of Australian Children Annual Statistical Report, AIFS, pp. 93–111.

Lohoar, S., Price-Robertson, R., Nair, L., 2013. Applying community capacity-building approaches to child welfare practice and policy. AIFS CFCA Paper No. 13:1-15.

MacKenzie, I., 2006. Induction of labour at the start of the new millennium. J. Reprod. Fertil. 131, 989–998.

Manchester, A., 2013. Plunket plans a plus service. Kai Tiaki Nurs. N. Z. 19 (6), 17.

Manger, W., Manger, L., Minno, A., et al., 2012. Obesity prevention in young schoolchildren: Results of a pilot study. J. Sch. Health 82 (10), 462–468.

Marmot, M., Allen, J., Bell, R., et al., Consortium for the European Review of social determinants of health and the Health Divide, 2012. WHO European review of social determinants of health and the health divide. Lancet 380, 1011–1029.

Martsolf, D., Burke Draucker, C., 2008. The legacy of childhood sexual abuse and adversity. J. Nurs. Scholarsh. 40 (4), 333–340.

Matthey, S., Barnett, B., Ungerer, J., et al., 2000. Paternal and maternal depressed mood during the transition to parenthood. J. Affect. Disord. 60, 75–85.

McCain, M., Mustard, F., 2002. The Early Years Study Three Years Later. Canadian Institute for Advanced Research, Toronto.

McFadden, A., Renfrew, M., Atkin, K., 2012. Does cultural context make a difference to women's experience of maternity care? A qualitative study comparing the perspectives of breastfeeding women of Bangladeshi origin and health practitioners. Health Expect. doi:10.1111/j/1369-7625.2012.00770x.

McMurray, A., 2011. The enabling community for child and family health. Editorial. Contemp. Nurse 40 (1), 2–4.

Mitchell, L., Wylie, C., Carr, M., 2008. Outcomes of early childhood education: literature review. Report to the Ministry of Education. Ministry of Education, Wellington.

Morrell, C., Slade, P., Warner, R., et al., 2009. Clinical effectiveness of health visitor training in psychologically informed approaches for depression in postnatal women: pragmatic cluster randomized trial in primary care. Br. Med. J. 338, a3045. doi:10.1136/bmj.a3045.

Morton, S., Atatoa Carr, P., Grant, C., et al., 2012. Growing up in New Zealand: A longitudinal study of New Zealand children and their families. Report 2: Now we are born. Growing up in New Zealand, Auckland.

Morton, S., Atatoa Carr, P., Grant, C., et al., 2013. Cohort profile: growing up in New Zealand. Int. J. Epidemiol. 42 (1), 65–75.

Mustard, J., 2007. Experience-based brain development: scientific underpinnings of the importance of early child development in a global world. In: Young, M., Richardson, L. (Eds.), Early child development: from measurement to action. World Bank, Washington, pp. 43–71.

Newman, L., 2012. Seeking asylum in Australia: Mental health and human rights of children and families. Fam. Matters 90, 113–114.

New Zealand Ministry of Health (NZMOH), 1998. Child health strategy. MOHNZ, Wellington.

New Zealand Ministry of Health (NZMOH), 2001. The primary health care Strategy. MOHNZ, Wellington.

New Zealand Ministry of Health (NZMOH), 2008. A portrait of health. Key results of the 2006/07 New Zealand health survey. MOHNZ, Wellington.

New Zealand Ministry of Health (NZMOH), 2009. National Breastfeeding Advisory Committee of New Zealand's advice to the Director-General of Health, National Strategic Plan of Action for Breastfeeding 2008-2012. MOH, Wellington.

New Zealand Ministry of Health (NZMOH), 2011. Healthy beginnings: developing perinatal and infant mental health services in New Zealand. Ministry of Health, Wellington.

New Zealand Ministry of Health (NZMOH), 2012a. The Health of New Zealand Children 2011-2012. Key Findings of the New Zealand Health Survey, Ministry of Health, Wellington.

New Zealand Ministry of Health (NZMOH), 2012b. New Zealand Maternity Clinical Indicators 2009. Revised 2012. MOH, Wellington.

O'Brien, M., Buikstra, E., Hegney, D., 2008. The influence of psychological factors on breastfeeding duration. J. Adv. Nurs. 63 (4), 397–408.

O'Connell-Binns, K., 2009. Men's mental health during the first year postpartum. J. Community Nurs. 23 (7), 4–8.

Olds, D., 2002. Prenatal and infancy home visiting by nurses: from randomized trials to community replication. Prev. Sci. 3 (3), 153–172.

Olds, D., Kitzman, H., Cole, R., et al., 2010. Enduring effects of prenatal and infancy home visiting by nurses on maternal life course and government spending: Follow-up of a randomized trial among children at age 12 years. Arch. Pediatr. Adolesc. Med. 164 (5), 419–424.

Olds, D., Kitzman, H., Cole, R., et al., 2004a. Effects of nurse home-visiting on maternal life course and child development: Age 6 follow-up results of a randomized trial. Pediatrics 114 (6), 1550–1559.

Olds, D., Robinson, J., Pettitt, L., et al., 2004b. Effects of home visits by paraprofessionals and by nurses: Age 4 follow-up results of a randomized trial. Pediatrics 114 (6), 1560–1568.

Paterson, J., Taylor, S., Schluter, P., et al., 2013. Pacific Islands Families (PIF) study: Behavioural problems during childhood. J. Child Fam. Stud. 22, 231–243.

Power, C., Kuh, D., Morton, S., 2013. From developmental origins of adult disease to lifecourse research on adult disease and aging: Insights from birth cohort studies. Annu. Rev. Public Health 34, 7–28.

Puterman, E., Epel, E., 2012. An intricate dance: life experience, multisystem resiliency, and rate of telomere decline throughout the lifespan. Soc. Personal. Psychol. Compass 1–19.

Putnam, R., 2005. Civic Renewal and Social Capital Round Table Discussion. Alcoa Research Centre for Stronger Communities, Curtin University, Perth.

Rumble, C., 2010. Moving from the I to we: Effective parenting education in groups. A thesis presented in partial fulfilment of the requirements for the Master of Education. Massey University, New Zealand. Available: <http://www.plunket.org.nz/assets/News–research/ Effective-parenting-education.pdf> 19 July 2013.

Rush, P., 2012. The experience of maternal and child health nurses responding to women with postpartum depression. Matern. Child Health J 16, 322–327.

Salmon, J., Timperio, A., Cleland, V., et al., 2005. Trends in children's physical activity and weight status in high and low socio-economic status areas of Melbourne, Victoria, 1985–2001. Aust. N. Z. J. Public Health 29 (4), 337–342.

Sampson, N., 2012. Environmental justice at school: Understanding research, policy, and practice to improve our children's health. J. Sch. Health 82 (5), 246–252.

Sandlund, M., Waterworth, E., Hager, C., 2011. Using motion interactive games to promote physical activity and enhance motor performance in children with cerebral palsy. Dev. Neurorehabil. 14 (1), 15–21.

Save the Children, 2013. Surviving the first day: State of the world's mothers. Save the Children International, London.

Saxton, M., 2010. Child language. Acquisition and development. Sage, London.

Sayers, M., West, S., Lorains, J., et al., 2012. Starting school. A pivotal life transition for children and their families. Fam. Matters 90, 45–56.

Schmied, V., Olley, H., Burns, E., et al., 2012. Contradictions and conflict: A meta-ethnographic study of migrant women's experiences of breastfeeding in a new country. BMC Pregnancy Childbirth 12, 163–178.

Schumacher, M., Zubaran, C., White, G., 2008. Bringing birth-related paternal depression to the fore. Women Birth 21, 65–70.

Scope, A., Booth, A., Sutcliffe, P., 2012. Women's perceptions and experiences of group cognitive behavior therapy and other group interventions for postnatal depression: a qualitative synthesis. J. Adv. Nurs. 68 (9), 1909–1919.

Seimyr, L., Sjogren, B., Welles-Nystrom, B., et al., 2009. Antenatal maternal depressive mood and parental-fetal attachment at the end of pregnancy. Abstract. Arch. Womens Ment. Health 12 (5), 269.

Shi, X., Tubb, L., Fingers, S., et al., 2013. Associations of physical activity and dietary behaviors with children's health and academic problems. J. Sch. Health 83 (1), 1–7.

Shonkoff, J., Boyce, W., McEwen, B., 2009. Neuroscience, molecular biology, and the childhood roots of health disparities. J. Am. Med. Assoc. 301 (21), 2252–2259.

Shonkoff, J., Phillips, D., 2000. From Neurons to Neighbourhoods: the Science of Early Childhood Development. National Academy Press, Washinton.

Silburn, S., 2003. Pathways to Resilience. Telethon Institute for Child Health Research, Perth.

Stanley, F., Richardson, S., Prior, M., 2005. Children of the Lucky Country. Pan MacMillan, Sydney.

Statistics New Zealand, 2009. New Zealand definition of homelessness Statistics. New Zealand, Wellington.

Steffen, L., Dai, S., Fulton, J., et al., 2009. Overweight in children and adolescents associated with TV viewing and parental weight. Project Heartbeat! Am. J. Prev. Med. 37 (Suppl. 1), S50–S55.

Tanaka, J., Wolf, J., Klaiman, C., et al., 2010. Using computerized games to teach face recognition skills to children with autism spectrum disorder: the Let's Face It! Program. J. Child Psychol. Psychiatr. 51 (8), 944–952.

Thio, I., Oakley Browne, A., Coverdale, H., et al., 2006. Postnatal depressive symptoms go largely untreated. Soc.

Psychiatry Psychiatr. Epidemiol. 41 (10), 814–818. doi: <http://dx.doi.org/10.1007/s00127-006-0095-6>.

Tohotoa, J., Maycock, B., Hauck, Y., et al., 2010. Supporting mothers to breastfeed: the development and process evaluation of a father inclusive perinatal support program in Perth, Western Australia. Health Promot. Int. 26 (3), 351–361.

UNICEF, 2009. Progress for children. A report card on child protection. No. 8 UNICEF Innocenti Research Centre, Florence, Italy.

UNICEF, 2012a. Level and trends in child mortality 2012 Report. UNICEF Innocenti Research Centre, Florence, Italy.

UNICEF, 2012b. Measuring child poverty. New league tables of measuring child poverty in the world's rich countries. UNICEF Innocenti Report Card 10, Innocenti Research Centre, Florency, Italy.

United Nations Family Planning Association (UNFPA), 2000. The State of World Population 2000. United Nations, New York.

Velders, F., Dieleman, G., Henrichs, J., et al., 2011. Prenatal and postnatal psychological symptoms of parents and family functioning: the impact on child emotional and behavioural problems. Eur. J. Adolesc. Psychiatry 20, 341–350.

Waldegrave, C., Waldegrave, K., 2009. Healthy families, young minds and developing brains: enabling all children to reach their potential. Families Commission, Wellington.

Water, T., 2011. Critical moments in preschool obesity: The call for nurses and communities to intervene. Contemp. Nurse 40 (1), 60–70.

Watson, J., Tully, L., 2008. Prevention and early intervention update—trends in recent research. NSW Department of Community Services Centre for Parenting Research, Sydney.

Werner, D., Teufel, J., Holtgrave, P., et al., 2012. Active generations: An intergenerational approach to preventing childhood obesity. J. Sch. Health 82 (8), 380–386.

Whiteside-Mansell, L., Bradley, R., McKelvey, L., et al., 2008. Parenting: Linking impacts of interpartner conflict to preschool children's social behavior. J. Pediatr. Nurs. 2, 1–12.

Wilson, P., Barbour, R., Graham, C., et al., 2008. Health visitors' assessments of parent-child relationships: a focus group study. Int. J. Nurs. Stud. 45, 1137–1147.

World Health Organization (WHO) UNICEF, 2003. Global strategy for infant feeding and young child feeding. WHO, Geneva.

World Health Organization (WHO), 2005. Make Every Mother and Child Count. The World Health Report 2005. WHO, Geneva.

World Health Organization (WHO), 2008a. World Health Report 2008: Primary health care, now more than ever. WHO, Geneva.

Wolrd Health Organization (WHO), 2008b. The World Report on Child Injury Prevention. Online. Available: <http://www.who.int/violence_injury_prevention/child/injury/world_report/en> 4 July 2013.

World Health Organization (WHO), 2009a. Mental health, resilience and inequalitites. WHO regional office for Europe, Copenhagen.

World Health Organization (WHO), 2009b. Breastfeeding guideline. Online. Available: <http://www.who.int/topics/breastfeeding/en/> 21 October 2009.

World Health Organization (WHO), 2010. Background Paper 30, World Health Report 2010. Online. Available: <www.who.int/healthsystems/topics/financing/healthreport/30C-sectioncosts.pdf> (accessed 26 March 2014).

World Health Organization (WHO), Health and Welfare Canada & CPHA, 1986. Ottawa Charter for Health Promotion. Can. J. Public Health 77 (12), 425–430.

Zubrick, S., Smith, G., Nicholson, J., et al., 2008. Parenting and families in Australia, Social Policy Research Paper No. 34. Department of Families, Housing, Community Services and Indigenous Affairs, Australian Government, Canberra.

Useful websites

www.who.int/topics/breastfeeding/en—WHO information on breastfeeding

www.breastfeeding.asn.au—Australian Breastfeeding Association

www.babyfriendly.org.nz—Baby Friendly Initiative

www.lalecheleague.org.nz—La Leche League New Zealand

www.aracy.org.au—Australian Research Alliance for Children and Youth

www.beyondblue.org.au—Clinical depression

www.families.gov.au—Australian Department of Social Services: Families and Children

www.healthinsite.gov.au/topics/Exercise_for_Children—Children's exercise programs

www.refugeecouncil.org.au—Refugee Council of Australia

www.chp.org.au—Australian Council to Homeless Persons

www.plunket.org.nz—Largest provider of well child services in New Zealand

www.paediatrics.org.nz—Paediatric Society of New Zealand

www.kidshealth.org.nz—Information on child health in New Zealand

www.healthinfonet.ecu.edu.au—Government website for health information

www.sidsandkids.org—SIDS information

www.kidshelp.com.au—Kids Helpline

www.moh.govt.nz/moh.nsf/indexmh/breastfeeding—Information on breastfeeding for mothers and health providers in New Zealand

www.cdc.gov/ace—Bibliography of ACE study publications listed by topic area

www.growingup.co.nz—Growing up in New Zealand website

http://aihw.gov.au/closingthegap—Australian Government Closing the Gap Clearinghouse www.adfvc.unsw.edu.au—Australian Domestic and Family Violence Clearinghouse

www.childrenschances.org—Global information on children's health and wellbeing

www.rospa.com/homesafety/adviceandinformation/childsafety/accidents-to-children.aspx—Child safety advice

www.mcafhna.org.au—Maternal, Child & Family Health Nurses Australia

www.ncjrs.gov/internetsafety/children.html—US National Criminal Justice Commission internet safety site for children

www.safekids.com—Information about cybersafety and incivility

www.cybersmart.gov.au—Australian information about cybersafety and incivility

www.parentingrc.org.au—Parenting Research Centre

www.aifs.gov.au—Australian Institute of Family Studies

www.aifs.gov.au/cfca/index.php—Child Family Community Information Exchange

www.bravehearts.org.au—Child abuse advocacy and protection

www.aifs.gov.au/cafca/ppp/profiles/itg_through_looking_glass.html—Through the Looking Glass community partnership in parenting providing intensive psychosocial support, therapeutic assistance and child care for high-risk families

www.tacsi.org.au/families/family-by-family—Family by Family program for families to share their knowledge and skills in modelling 'thriving behaviours' and connecting with the wider community

CHAPTER 9

Healthy adolescents

Introduction

Adolescents—that is, young people in their teenage years—play a vital role in community life, contributing energy and vibrancy to the population through the spirit of youth and a promise for the future. In most cases, their health and wellbeing is focused on school and the developmental tasks and transitions of adolescence. The social sphere within which they interact is predominant. It is the pivot around which their lives and their identity revolves. This chapter begins by addressing social competence, social capital and identity formation, all of which are foundations for healthy adolescence. We then provide an in-depth analysis of the particular risks of adolescence, which often leave parents in a quandary about their competence in guiding their adolescents through the transitions. The chapter outlines the dimensions of adolescent life in the school, home and community context, with an emphasis on the virtual life many young people live through their relational communities on the internet and through instant messaging systems.

Although the adolescent journey is sometimes described as fraught with confusion, conflict and risk, an alternative view sees adolescents 'at promise' instead of 'at risk', and we address the pathway from risk to promise and, ultimately, to resilience. Adolescence is the most dramatic, the most interesting and the most tortuous stage on the journey to adulthood as significant habits of mind and action are formed. We argue for a strengths-based approach to supporting adolescents in all of the contexts in which they stretch towards the future and across all of the social determinants of their lives. Young people on the cusp of adolescence, aged 10–13, and those beyond the teenage years, aged 19–24, also have considerable challenges in negotiating the various stages from childhood to adulthood, but we focus this chapter on the teenage years. From a professional perspective, understanding which risks and assets are modifiable in the world that these adolescents inhabit can be used to plan interventions that will promote and sustain health in this age group. Evaluating nursing's role in the journey toward empowerment and good citizenship is fundamental to community health promotion. We conclude the chapter with specific goals for adolescent health embedded in the ecology of their lives, and health promotion strategies using the guidelines of the Ottawa Charter.

SOCIAL COMPETENCE, SOCIAL CAPITAL AND IDENTITY FORMATION

Adolescence is a period of rapid cognitive, psychological, social, emotional and physical changes in a person's life (Halpern-Felsher 2009). The years from 12–18 are considered a second 'sensitive developmental period' that follows the earlier sensitive developmental period of childhood. During adolescence the transitions of puberty and the maturing brain modify the behaviours and capacities of the childhood trajectory in a way that triggers or

---

OBJECTIVES

By the end of this chapter you will be able to:

1 identify the factors influencing healthy adolescence

2 explain the social ecology of adolescent life

3 analyse the research evidence related to the role of school and family support in influencing adolescent health and wellbeing

4 identify goals for supporting and sustaining adolescents at promise

5 explain how a primary health care framework can be used in planning strategies for adolescent health

6 examine the role of the school nurse in helping students, schools and the community support adolescent health.

enables the requisite transitions to adulthood (Viner et al. 2012). These transitions are influenced by neurocognitive development, which has major effects on decision-making, emotional wellbeing and behaviour (Sawyer et al. 2012). Research into the biology of adolescence has reframed our understanding of how and when young people undergo major changes (Sawyer et al. 2012). In today's society the onset of puberty occurs at a younger age than in the past, while adoption of mature social roles occurs at a later stage. To some extent, these changes are influenced by the fact that many young people spend more years in education and in the family home and are exposed to a wider variety of social factors from peers, school and the media, than in past times (Sawyer et al. 2012). By escalating the speed of communication, new media such as Facebook and Twitter have provided a powerful voice for young people to actively engage with one another. These sites and instant messaging have also changed the speed at which new socio-cultural norms of behaviour become popularised. The frequency and intensity of social influences have also created new risks and problem behaviours such as social contagion (copycat self-harming, suicides, firearms use), sexting (sending sexually explicit messages to one another), cyber bullying and pornography, and these risks have become more of a concern through publicity (Sawyer et al. 2012).

> ## SENSITIVE PERIODS IN BRAIN DEVELOPMENT
>
> 1 Early childhood
> 2 Adolescence

New media have also connected people at a distance, which can enhance communication skills for caring, meaningful relationships. These skills can ultimately help develop young people's capacity for interpersonal intimacy (Whitlock et al. 2006). Virtual and interpersonal social connections contribute to the important tasks of identity formation and the development of autonomy and independent thinking. Sculpting out an adult identity takes precedence over any other issue, as young people 'try on' a range of identities to establish a sense of themselves in relation to the world and various groups of people (Erikson 1963). Identity formation is also a significant step in developing critical thinking ability. Some young people find this difficult, particularly when they are balancing personal changes and aspirations with the influence of family and friends. Peers and other social groups

provide a mirror within which adolescents view themselves, which can have mixed results. Younger adolescents especially develop a heightened sensitivity to socially relevant cues from peers, which can either provide valuable support for adaptive behaviours, or lead to actions that threaten their health and wellbeing (Casey 2013). Although adolescents are just as capable as adults in evaluating risky situations, because of their social bias, the presence of peers 'primes' their motivations to make choices based on friendships (Albert et al. 2013). As a result, those with a tendency to risk-taking may gravitate to other risk takers, whereas those with a tendency towards safer behaviours may align their behaviours accordingly. This type of behaviour has been demonstrated in research showing that adolescents take more risks when they are being observed, in the company of friends, or even when they believe they are being evaluated by peers (Albert et al. 2013; Somerville 2013). Their 'social sensitivity' leaves them 'more emotionally reactive to explicit cues indicative of social inclusion or exclusion' (Somerville 2013:121). Peer rejection is therefore felt deeply, whether it is experience in person, through digital media or simply by suspecting that they are being excluded or rejected (Somerville 2013).

> ## SOCIAL COMPETENCE
>
> • Identity formation
> • Autonomy
> • Independent, critical thinking

> ## SOCIAL SENSITIVITY
>
> • Reactive to cues from peers
> • Influenced by media
> • Reshaped family structures and roles

At the group level, social connections can be seen as dimensions of social capital, which contribute to health literacy and the health, wellbeing and health-related behaviours of adolescents (Morgan & Haglund 2009; Sawyer et al. 2012). Social capital illustrates the importance of a socio-ecological perspective of adolescent life. Everything is connected to everything else in their social world. Family, school, peers and the many contexts in which they interact all have an effect on one another. This includes their virtual social lives on the internet and other electronic media as well as the face-to-face interactions that frame the development of social competence. Positive role models in the home and school environment can help guide adolescents toward behaviours that help them navigate through the changes with a sense of comfort in their identity and relationships (Viner et al. 2012). Without ongoing support from peer groups, families, schools and others within their social and cultural environments, a young person may have conflicting ideas about their identity. They can experiment with different lifestyles and end up feeling isolated, abandoned and without positive role models for successful development (Bronfenbrenner 1986).

Families have a profound influence on adolescent development. Many years ago young people had clear rites of passage from childhood to adult, spouse, parent and worker. In the 21st century, adolescents experience variable transitions in the public eye, which take place over an extended period of time. As we reported in Chapter 7, family structures have changed. Gone are the family norms where a father transferred to his son the means to a livelihood, and a mother passed her skills on to her daughter for a predetermined role as wife or mother. Today, many young people who grow up in families without two biological parents tend to see themselves as adults at a younger stage than those from intact families (Benson & Kirkpatrick Johnson 2009). Assuming a variety of roles in different family structures, households and family groupings can place inordinate pressure on young people to try on different identities. In addition to structural influences, family dynamics and the style of parenting (authoritarian, authoritative or permissive) are also instrumental in identity formation. The major parental influences include the extent to which parents exert social control and monitoring, warmth and closeness, a sense of responsibility and a clear sense of the adolescent's place in the hierarchy of family relations (Benson & Kirkpatrick Johnson 2009).

GROUP EXERCISE: Adolescence

Break into groups of three or four. Try to have at least one member of the group who is aged under 24. As a group, discuss the issues you found (or find) most challenging as an adolescent. Identify the actions that you found provided the most support for you as you faced these challenges and which hindered you. Are these issues and solutions common to the wider group? Are the experiences in your group consistent with what is reported in this chapter?

SOCIAL DETERMINANTS OF ADOLESCENT HEALTH AND RISK

The social ecology of adolescent development can be seen as a matrix of interrelated factors that influence adolescents' health and wellbeing. As with other population groups, the social determinants of their lives present strengths, weaknesses, threats and opportunities. The main strength of adolescents is that most tend to be physically well. The weaknesses or risks inherent in adolescent life generally revolve around the fact that, because they are in the formative stages of development, most adolescents are not yet able to take control of their lives or health-related decisions. But the strongest determinants of adolescent health are not these individual factors, but the structural determinants that provide them with education, employment and the equitable living conditions that will allow them to develop their full potential in adult life (Viner et al. 2012). Education is particularly important, and has been described as the 'engine of opportunity' for the young person, the workforce and the wider society (AIFS 2011:5). To provide a capacity-building transition to adulthood, opportunities to participate in education and the workforce must also be accompanied by safe and supportive families, schools, peers and communities. These are the structural conditions within which young people are exposed to strengths or compromises to health during transitions through school, from education to work, from family dependence to independence, autonomy, partnering and parenthood, and ultimately to responsible citizenship (Viner et al. 2012).

ADOLESCENT TRANSITIONS

- Primary to secondary school to higher education
- Education to workforce
- Family to self-responsibility for health
- Family living to autonomy, partnering, parenthood
- To responsible citizenship

According to the life course theorists (see Chapter 7), there are three ways the SDH affect young people (Viner et al. 2012). First, the 'latent effects' that determine early development occur when a child's biological mechanisms are preset in utero. Second, there are experiences that determine health and wellbeing over the life trajectory, called the 'pathway effects'. Third, there are 'cumulative effects' from the advantages or disadvantages that a person experiences from exposure to unfavourable environments over time (Viner et al. 2012). Years ago the prevailing view was that the young brain was fully developed in childhood, yet research evidence now shows that the brain architecture of both children and adolescents is malleable, and social, emotional and neural development takes place until the early twenties (AIHW 2011). Understanding the second 'sensitive period' in a young person's development has important implications for health promotion, in that some of the negative effects of structural factors in the early years, such as poverty, unemployment, poor housing, cultural or gender-based inequities, or anti-social behaviours at school, can be modified in adolescence, predominantly by strong family and community support (Sawyer et al. 2012; Viner et al. 2012). As health professionals, this leads us to renewed optimism for the success of family and school-based interventions that will help young people navigate their transitions successfully. Contemporary health promotion strategies are also informed by understanding the distinctions between early, middle and late adolescence. Early adolescence involves entering puberty, beginning the process of sexual maturation and shifting focus from family to friends. Middle adolescence sees physical development continue, with increasing reliance on friends and peer groups. This stage is accompanied by the risk of adopting peer-influenced behaviours such as experimenting with drugs and alcohol. In late adolescence, physical changes have levelled off and cognitive development continues, with adult thinking becoming closer to maturity (AIHW 2011).

and one-seventh or 13% of New Zealanders, adolescents in this part of the world experience relatively good health compared to the rest of the population (AIHW 2012; Statistics New Zealand 2012). Most rate their health as good or excellent, and this is reflected in declining rates of hospitalisation for illness or injury (AIHW 2011). Young people today also tend to stay in formal education longer than previous generations, with 72% of Australian adolescents completing school (AIHW 2011, 2012). New Zealand rates, however, remain low with only 43.6% of New Zealand adolescents successfully completing school to university entrance level (Dench 2010). Completion rates in New Zealand also vary by socio-economic status with those from schools in the least deprived areas three times more likely to leave school than those from schools in the most deprived areas (Dench 2010). University access and completion among Australian young people has also increased dramatically, following policy changes encouraging greater participation by students from disadvantaged backgrounds (Foundation for Young Australians [FYA] 2012). In the later stages of adolescence many combine study with part-time work, which helps them develop workplace skills (AIFS 2011). The past decade has also shown some favourable trends in risk and protective factors affecting adolescent health, with decreases in smoking and illicit substance use, greater use of contraception among Year 10 and 12 students and improved survival rates for cancers (AIHW 2011). In New Zealand, weekly smoking rates among adolescents dropped from 16% in 2001 to 5% in 2012, marijuana use dropped from 39% to 23%, and binge drinking dropped from 40% to 23% (Clark et al. 2013a).

STAGES OF ADOLESCENCE

- Early—puberty, sexual maturation, friendships
- Middle—physical development, reliance on friends, peer groups
- Late—cognitive development, adult thinking

Practice challenge

What are the implications of each stage for health promotion?

How young people are faring: good news, bad news

This generation of young people is the largest in history, comprising one-quarter of the world's population (Sawyer et al. 2012). As a group representing one-fifth of the Australian population

THE INDIGENOUS ADOLESCENT DIVIDE

Indigenous adolescents

- Double unemployment rate
- Triple risk of overcrowded homes
- Six times risk of mortality
- 15 times as likely in justice system

Indigenous, non-Indigenous

- One-third are overweight or obese
- Half meet physical activity guidelines
- High road accidents, STIs, diabetes, mental disorders

The transition from school to employment is relatively smooth for the majority of young Australians, although the youth unemployment rate is twice to three times as high as the overall labour force, with young Indigenous Australians twice as likely again to be unemployed or on income support (AIHW 2011; FYA 2012). In New Zealand, the youth unemployment rate is 17.1% (NZ Ministry of Business, Innovation and Employment [MBIE] 2013). The highest rates of young people aged between 15 and 24 years not in education, employment or training (NEET) are among Māori (23.2%) and Pacific young people (19.8%) (NZMBIE 2013). Because of their disproportionate levels of disadvantage Indigenous teens in Australia are also three times as likely to live in overcrowded housing, six times as likely to die from all causes and 15 times as likely to be in juvenile justice supervision or in prison compared with non-Indigenous Australian teens (AIHW 2011). What Indigenous and non-Indigenous adolescents have in common is that over one-third are overweight or obese, less than half meet physical activity guidelines, and most do not eat sufficient fruit and vegetables. There are also rising rates of diabetes and sexually transmissible infections (STIs), as well as high rates of road transport accidents and mental disorders (AIHW 2011; Clark et al. 2013a).

As adolescence is an important period for establishing positive health and social behaviours that will set the stage for a healthy, vibrant society, the issues that concern young people are of interest to all members of society. The most recent Mission Australia survey of young people reflects whole-of-society concerns, as respondents identified their three most important issues as the economy and financial issues, population issues, and alcohol and drugs (Mission Australia 2012). Most felt positive about the future but reported suffering from the stress of trying to cope with study, work and family commitments. A broader set of adolescent concerns have been identified by other researchers and policymakers, which include relationships with family and friends, the integration of mental and physical health, education, employment, income, social participation, the use of technology, civic engagement, risk-taking behaviour and body image (AIHW 2011).

The stress reported by the young people in the Mission Australia study is predictable, as through the evolution from childhood to adolescence, identity formation and other psychosocial challenges place inordinate pressures on adolescents. In some cases these stressors pose threats to mental health. Approximately 9% of Australian adolescents suffer from high or very high levels of psychological distress, with one in four experiencing a mental disorder (AIHW 2011). The most conspicuous mental health issues involve anxiety disorders, substance abuse (primarily alcohol), and affective disorders including depression and bipolar disorder (AIHW 2011). Indigenous youth experience similar problems but at dramatically higher levels, with 31% reporting high or very high levels of psychological distress (AIHW 2011). For young people from disadvantaged families, homelessness is also a problem, especially for the 12–14-year-olds who represent one-third of all homeless people in Australia (AIHW 2011). These young people end up on the streets due to several overlapping causal factors, including family breakdown, conflict, neglect or abuse, mental health issues, unemployment, poverty, alcohol or substance abuse and crime (Australian Government 2012).

New Zealand young people are generally well, have supportive home and school environments and are not involved in serious risk-taking or problem behaviours (Clark et al. 2013a). However, research also shows that young people are increasingly worried their families do not have enough money, they have poorer access to the family doctor and fewer students have part-time jobs (Clark et al. 2013a). It is estimated that 22% of 15-year-olds and 36.6% of 18-year-olds have a mental health problem (Craig et al. 2007), and between 2006 and 2010, 8% of admissions to hospital for young people in New Zealand were for mental health issues (Craig et al. 2013). Unfortunately, although many mental disorders respond to interventions, there are often long-term effects such as isolation, discrimination and stigma which complicate the emotional transitions of adolescence (AIHW 2012). The social determinants of risk explain growing disparities among adolescents, especially the disadvantage experienced by those from Indigenous or refugee backgrounds, and those who are incarcerated or homeless (Sawyer et al. 2012). Certain individual factors such as intelligence, sexual orientation or personality can also attract bullying and discrimination, which, in turn, can lead to substance misuse, unsafe sex, depression, anti-social and illegal activities and dangerous driving (Sawyer et al. 2012). The latter is responsible for many road traffic injuries, which are the leading cause of death among young people worldwide (WHO 2010). Convergence of multiple risk factors show strong behavioural links between motor vehicle accidents, alcohol consumption, substance abuse, attempted suicide, sexually transmissible infections (STIs) and teenage pregnancy. Another pervasive behaviour-linked risk is skin cancer (melanoma). Australia has the highest prevalence of skin cancers in the world, yet 1 in 5 Australian adolescents deliberately lie in the sun to tan (AIHW 2011) and most have a low rate of compliance with sun protection (Williams et al. 2011).

RISKY BEHAVIOURS: SEX, DRUGS AND ALCOHOL, STIS AND PREGNANCY

Analysis of Australian adolescents' sexual behaviours indicates that 78% have experienced sexual activity, with 40% having intercourse and 44% having had oral sex (AIHW 2011). Their lack of knowledge about STIs (chlamydia, gonorrhoea, syphilis, genital warts [HPV] and HIV), and the possibility of lifelong outcomes from risky sexual behaviours are of major concern to health professionals and parents alike (AIHW 2012; East & Jackson 2013). Many young people do not realise that the personal impact on health from STIs can be severe, particularly if the infection is not detected immediately. For example, chlamydia can be asymptomatic for a long period of time, and also increase the risk of HIV, which is a significant risk for older adolescents (Major-Wilson et al. 2008). Some chlamydial infections also progress to pelvic inflammatory disease (PID), which can lead to infertility (AIHW 2009). Although the prevalence of some STIs (HIV/AIDS) has declined in Australia there has been a steady increase in chlamydia and gonorrhoea over the past decade, especially in New Zealand, which has the dubious distinction of being named the 'chlamydia capital of the world' (Braun 2008). Around 32% of Australian and 17% of New Zealand young people have recently reported having unwanted, unprotected sex, sometimes because of pressure from their partner, but primarily because of being intoxicated (AIHW 2011; Clark et al. 2013a). The mix of alcohol and peer pressure to engage in sexual activity can be devastating, with far-reaching consequences. Adolescents as young as 12 and 13 have reported consuming alcohol, and the danger with this group lies in having heightened susceptibility to its effects and in being encouraged to make their sexual debut under the influence of alcohol (Kelly et al. 2012a; Spear 2013). Becoming sexually active at a young age extends the adolescent's vulnerability to STIs over a long period of time, which intensifies the need to address this particular risk factor urgently (Sawyer et al. 2012). Contraceptive use by adolescents is increasing, but condom use has stabilised throughout the past decade, with only half of all adolescents using a condom during all occasions of sexual intercourse in Australia (AIHW 2011). The figures are slightly better in New Zealand with approximately 17% of young people who are currently sexually active not using or only sometimes using condoms or other contraception (Clark et al. 2013a).

Teenage pregnancy is the other main concern from having unprotected sex, posing significant, long-term risks for mothers and their babies. Most teenage mothers have interrupted schooling with a flow-on effect to their career development. Many live their lives as single parents, becoming impoverished from an early age and struggling to provide for their own or their child's health needs, with many experiencing higher rates of mental health problems (AIHW 2011; Craig et al. 2013). Teenage mothers often delay having the pregnancy confirmed or attending antenatal care. Many also engage in risky alcohol or smoking behaviours, which multiplies the risk for miscarriage, preterm birth, low birth weight, SUDI or other complications of pregnancy and birth (AIHW 2011; Graves et al. 2011; Craig et al. 2013). For these babies, there are higher risks of vulnerability to the effects of low socio-economic status, such as housing instability, childhood sexual abuse, absence of a father figure and intergenerational poverty (AIHW 2011).

> ### RISKY BEHAVIOURS
>
> Alcohol + unprotected sex
> = STIs, pregnancy
> intergenerational disadvantage

Although rates of teenage pregnancy are declining in Australia and NZ, there are still 15 births per 1000 teenage females in Australia and 29.5 births per 1000 teenage females in New Zealand (AIHW 2011; Craig et al. 2013). Australia's rate is slightly lower than other OECD countries (AIHW 2011) but New Zealand's is the second highest in the OECD (Zodgekar 2012). In Australia, teenage pregnancy occurs across the socio-economic spectrum and across all cultural groups, with the highest rates among Indigenous and remote-living teenagers (AIHW 2011). In some Indigenous groups, this may be linked to traditional perspectives, where pregnancy and fertility are valued in their culture (Devries et al. 2009). In New Zealand, teenage live birth rates are significantly higher among young Māori and Pacific women and those living in the most economically deprived areas (Craig et al. 2013).

> ### WHAT'S YOUR OPINION?
>
> • Why are teenagers having unprotected sex?
> • What are the social determinants of teenage pregnancy?
> • What are the main influences on reproductive decision-making?

So why are younger teenagers having sex? Besides cultural traditions, peer pressure and the influence of alcohol, some believe it may be linked to poor parent–child relationships, low self-esteem or a lack of personal skills at negotiating sexual behaviour (Devries et al. 2009; Graves et al. 2011). For some time, public speculation has also suggested a link between the highly sexualised images in the media and early sexual activities. Research studies have now confirmed this, demonstrating that sexual content in television programs and digital media is, in fact, a precipitating factor in risky sexual behaviours (Denny 2011). The influence of media images also reflects the importance of peer group norms. An Australian study of adolescents' perceptions of peer sexual attitudes and behaviours revealed that they overestimated the extent to which their peers were sexually active (Lim et al. 2009). This is another aspect of the social sensitivity mentioned above, where young people have not only heightened sensitivity to peers but in many cases, exaggerated assumptions about peers' behaviours.

A number of researchers have focused on the reasons why teenagers shy away from using contraception. Sheeder et al. (2009:302) contend that most adolescents 'are not cognitively and psychosocially mature enough to form intimate, mutually respectful, long-term interpersonal relationships'. Their sexual decisions are made in the moment, intuitively, based on romantic circumstances rather than rational thought. They have no prior experience of what it is like to bear a child, and rarely see the barriers or negative aspects of contraception. Many also have a lack of knowledge or misperceptions about the risk of pregnancy or how it will impinge on their future goals (Haldre et al. 2009; Sheeder et al. 2009). Some scholars argue that developmental imbalance of early adolescence favours behaviours driven by emotion and reward rather than rational decision-making (Sawyer et al. 2012). However, an alternative explanation is that the social context of risk is linked to societal changes such as the visibility and fluidity in sexual identities and relationships, and paradoxically, the attention to sexual issues intended to increase public awareness about prevention (AIHW 2012; Kirby Institute 2011). Research into the experiences of young women in sexual encounters shows that the main barriers to condom use are relationship dynamics, societal norms, personal and cultural beliefs, and the desire for increased intimacy (East et al. 2011). East et al.'s (2011) interviews with young Australian women revealed that even after contracting an STI, they still avoided negotiating the use of condoms with their partners. Some rationalised their behaviour on the basis of gendered relationship dynamics; that is, feeling disempowered in terms of sexual decisions, while others simply trusted their partners to initiate condom use.

Many young people also have a lack of guidance for decision-making, particularly in relation to reproductive choices. Choosing between persevering with or terminating a pregnancy is one of the most difficult issues that confront any woman, especially young adolescents. The teenage mother's developmental stage, her level of self-esteem and her resources have profound effects on her decision-making. Her reproductive choices are also dependent on the social and political context. Social mores and competing views on what is morally right or wrong can conspire against rational reproductive choices, creating highly inflamed debates and polarised opinions. Sometimes this is too difficult an environment for a young person to deal with in such an emotionally charged situation.

THE COMPOUND RISK SYNDROME: ALCOHOL AND SUBSTANCE ABUSE

Alcohol and illicit drugs have a disinhibiting effect on behaviours, many of which create long-term consequences such as those mentioned above. Besides leading to poor decisions, overuse of alcohol can cause or exacerbate diabetes, heart disease, liver disease and a range of other threats to physical health (AIHW 2011). Even though consumption of alcohol has been gradually decreasing over the past 30 years, more than 60% of Australian boys aged 16–17 and 52% of girls of this age ingest alcohol weekly (see Box 9.1). This is higher than the prevalence among New Zealand adolescents, where 45% of high school students drink alcohol regularly and 18% drink weekly (Clark et al. 2013a). However, over 40% of young men and 26% of young women in New Zealand aged 18 to 24 years of age are considered to have hazardous drinking patterns (NZMOH 2013). Adolescents living in the most deprived areas consume the heaviest quantities of alcohol (Vinther-Larsen et al. 2013). Trends suggest that up to 30% of Australian adolescents engage is short-term periods of drinking at high-risk levels, which is even higher than the 20% prevalence among American Year 12 students (AIHW 2011; Spear 2013). The phenomena of binge drinking is also problematic in New Zealand where a survey of high school students found 25% had engaged in binge drinking within the past four weeks, although this has declined since 2001 where 40% reported binge drinking (Clark et al. 2013a). Rates of student and adolescent binge drinking are highest among Māori (31.5%), Pacific (31.6%) and women (28%)

BOX 9.1 **Never drunk enough?**

Rachel Olding from the *Sydney Morning Herald* sat down with a bunch of young male uni students watching the 2013 State of Origin Football match in a pub. After observing their drinking behaviour she asked them about their usual drinking patterns. They described a typical night out as half a case of beer at someone's house to 'pre-load' before they had to buy drinks at the pub, then dropping in to a party for free drinks, hiding a bottle of mixer in the bushes outside the party to prime them for the trip to the city. Once at the pub they could run up a tab for as much as $200 in shots. 'All-nighters, vomiting, unwittingly wetting themselves, and weekend-long benders are not uncommon' they said (Olding 2013:B005). According to experts these young men are the YOLO ('You only live once') generation. They want it all and they want it now. Their brain-behaviour reward system has become so transformed that to have 'fun' they need copious amounts of alcohol.

? What type of evidence could you gather to challenge the notion of drunkenness as fun?

Can you think of a health promotion strategy that would be useful across community-school-family settings to address binge drinking?

(Clark et al. 2013b; Teevale et al. 2012; Collins 2012). Māori students who were heavy binge drinkers (ten or more standard drinks on a single drinking occasion) reported higher rates of unsafe sex, unwanted sex, poor school performance, injuries to themselves and others, and car crashes (Clark et al. 2013b).

A number of social factors are involved in problem levels of alcohol consumption. In rural communities binge drinking is even more prevalent than in the cities, especially for Indigenous young people (AIHW 2011). Rural adolescents are described as consuming alcohol as a way of being socially included, because alternative social activities are often unavailable (Bourke et al. 2009). However, in both rural and urban communities peers are a major factor in problem drinking as it occurs in a social context. For some, social situations where alcohol is consumed can lead to initiating and developing abuse of other substances, especially for young teens who have low family and school connectedness, and those who have sensation-seeking personality traits (Kelly et al. 2012a). In the absence of these family

and social supports young people may progress from one substance to another, with ultimate effects on their mental health. Young people with mental illness are a particular problem, and they report higher rates of drug use, but it is unknown whether the mental illness precedes or follows the drug use (AIHW 2012). The greater availability of alcohol and the marketing of youth-specific beverages (e.g. alcopop drinks) are considered contributing factors to youth drinking in New Zealand (Collins 2012). The lowering of the age at which young people can purchase alcohol from 20 to 18 in 1999 has been attributed with greater rates of hazardous drinking among young people in New Zealand in subsequent years, although the evidence is mixed (Cagney & Palmer 2007). Attempts to change the age back to 20 in 2006 and 2013 were unsuccessful.

In terms of lethal substances, tobacco remains the leading preventable cause of deaths and disease worldwide (AIHW 2012). It is also known to be a 'gateway' drug, which may lead to ingestion of alcohol, cannabis or other harmful substances. Young people who try their first cigarette at the time of adolescence are at the highest risk of becoming daily smokers, and they are the least likely to quit smoking (Sherman & Primack 2009). Although rates of smoking have declined dramatically in Australia and New Zealand, it is still important to be vigilant and communicate the dangers to adolescents who may be on the verge of experimenting with any harmful substances. The risks surrounding substance use continue to be problematic for Australian secondary students, many of whom (19%) have sniffed inhalants, with 17% having used tranquilisers and 14% marijuana/cannabis (AIHW 2012). Approximately 11% of New Zealand secondary students smoke at least occasionally; 23% have tried marijuana and 13% currently use it (Clark et al. 2013a). Other drugs are less commonly used with 4% reporting having used party pills and 3% ecstasy (Clark et al. 2013a). Despite declining rates of drug use, a small proportion of Australian and New Zealand adolescents continue to use 'hard drugs' such as methamphetamine, cocaine, ecstasy, cannabis or other illicit substances (AIHW 2009; Clark et al. 2013a).

PRACTICE STRATEGIES

What health promotion strategies can be undertaken at the population level to prevent the syndrome of risk behaviours?

Adolescent risk-taking in areas such as unsafe sexual behaviour or alcohol and substance misuse has been described as a syndrome of behaviours, wherein engaging in one type of risk makes a person prone to engage in others (Leather 2009). Some risk-taking is thrill-seeking, often aimed at participating in peer group social life. Other risky behaviours are a form of rebellious, reckless or anti-social acts (Leather 2009). Some see adolescent risk-taking as a natural part of development, a type of adolescent play, while others link risky behaviours to the notion of invulnerability, a feeling among adolescents that they are invincible (Leather 2009). Some, especially girls, engage in risky behaviours believing they are not susceptible to negative outcomes, thinking 'it won't happen to me' (Graves et al. 2011:469). Despite these perspectives, it is not always helpful to stereotype reasons for risk-taking, given individual differences (Holland & Klaczynski 2009). What all researchers and scholars of adolescent life agree on is that for some clusters of risky behaviours, there are serious and enduring psychological and social repercussions. These can include threats to mental health, which are manifest in depression, suicide ideation, low self-esteem, poor body image, low social connectedness, a lack of academic performance at school and a poor quality of family life (Holland & Klaczynski 2009).

WEIGHT MANAGEMENT, ACTIVITY AND NUTRITION

The quality of family life has been shown to be the most powerful influence on adolescent health, particularly in relation to nutrition and weight management, which continues to be a problem for adolescents. Around 23% of Australian and 25% of New Zealand adolescents are overweight, with 11% of Australian and 12% of New Zealand adolescents being classified obese (AIHW 2011; University of Otago and Ministry of Health 2011). These rates are twice as high among Indigenous adolescents in Australia (AIHW 2009), but in New Zealand, only 9.4% of Māori males aged 15 to 18 are classified as obese (compared to 10.8% of all males in that age group) (University of Otago and Ministry of Health 2011). For adolescent Māori females, however, 17.2% are obese compared with 13.6% of all adolescent females (University of Otago and Ministry of Health 2011). Comparisons of 15-year-olds in OECD countries show that Australian 15-year-olds are close to the OECD average, but for the same age group of New Zealanders, the risk of being overweight or obese is among the highest in the world, at 37% (AIHW 2011). Being overweight or obese creates risks for cardiovascular disease, diabetes and cancer in adult life, particularly when the risk is compounded by physical inactivity. There is growing evidence that early life environmental signals including stress and nutrition during the perinatal and early childhood period contribute to pathophysiologies including obesity and type 2 diabetes (Sloboda 2011). Interventions that support healthy pregnancy, infancy and early childhood may now be more effective in preventing childhood and adolescent obesity than interventions targeted at children and adolescents themselves (Sloboda 2011). Despite this, there is still evidence that school-based intervention programs are effective in addressing childhood obesity, in particular, those that include family involvement and are of longer duration (Khambalia et al. 2012).

Our young people are not active enough to be considered physically fit. In Australia, only 44% of young people participate in physical activity to the level recommended in Australian national guidelines, a figure that is much lower (14%) among Indigenous or remote-living adolescents (AIHW 2011). In New Zealand, only 10% of secondary school students meet the recommended guideline of 60 minutes of physical exercise per day (Clark et al. 2013a), although 57.5% of New Zealanders aged between 15 and 24 do at least 30 minutes of exercise five times per week with men more likely than women to achieve this (NZMOH 2012). These levels of inactivity run parallel to increasing amounts of 'screen time', as we mentioned in Chapter 8. It is estimated that 71% of Australian adolescents exceed the recommended two hours per day of screen time on weeknights, with 83% exceeding the guidelines on weekends (AIHW 2011). Among New Zealand secondary students, 28% watch more than three hours of television per day (Clark et al. 2013a). Despite considerable media promotion for healthy eating, most young people do not eat fruit and vegetables at the recommended number of serves (AIHW 2011). This combination of poor nutrition, low activity and overweight is an important and complex challenge for health promotion interventions, given the known links between overweight, low self-esteem, stress, a lack of social support and the ultimate risk of depressive illness (Martyn-Nemeth et al. 2009).

There is a strong link between eating behaviours and how young people cope with stress. Adolescents' coping strategies evolve throughout the period of adolescence in response to the stresses of puberty, and the 'in-between' phases of emerging adulthood, which do not always follow a predictable path. For younger adolescents, poor eating habits and overweight can be linked to overscheduling, especially if parents encourage children to become involved in too many after-school activities rather than free play or sports (Brown et al. 2011). These activities can be problematic at a time when the pressures of school may be having a cumulative effect on the young person's stress (Brown et al. 2011). Overscheduling can also interfere with family meal times, which are golden opportunities for sharing ideas, communicating about school issues and conveying family closeness as well as nutritious food. Family mealtime conversations also provide opportunities for parental monitoring of adolescents' views and behaviours. Perhaps more importantly, they are opportunities for young people to disclose information to parents about their lives, which enhances parent–child attachment. Securely attached emerging adults tend to have greater self-worth and personal efficacy (Urry et al. 2011). Sharing a meal can also be an opportunity for parents to share important lessons on how they solve everyday problems and deal with social pressures (Franko et al. 2008). In addition, parents' use of alcohol at mealtimes can also have a major influence on alcohol consumption among adolescents. The combination of role modelling, responsiveness and family connectedness can be a vehicle for ensuring the lines of communication between parents and their adolescent children remain open.

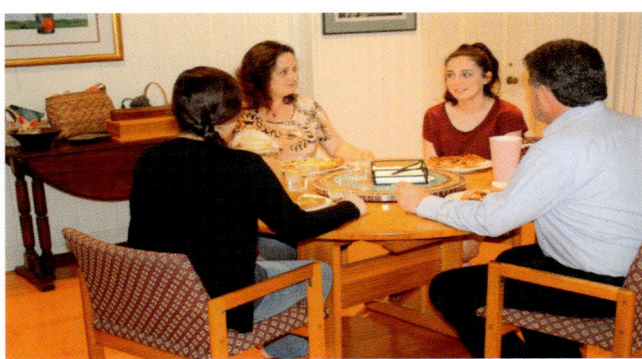

Dinner at the Macdonalds' (photo courtesy of Peter and Nancy Macdonald)

In some cases, parental work schedules reduce adults' control over mealtimes, and this can lead to poor eating habits among their children (Li et al. 2012). Non-standard schedules can prevent parents from spending the quality time with adolescents that help them stay engaged with what is occurring in their child's life and in guiding their lifestyle habits as well as cognitive development (Li et al. 2012). In urban areas, adolescents also tend to gravitate to fast food outlets as a place for socialising, and often substitute high-salt, high-sugar content foods for healthy meals at home with the family. Using food as a coping mechanism or developing fast food habits can lead to overeating as a long-term pattern, especially if there is a lack of family and social support to buffer the effects of stress. This, in turn, can lead to lower self-esteem and depressive mood, which creates a cycle of overeating and weight problems (Martyn-Nemeth et al. 2009). Although rural youth do not have the same access to fast food outlets, many eat because they are bored, feeling emotional or depressed, or because their friends are eating (Bourke et al. 2009). The need to feel connected with peers can also be a potent force in eating behaviours, and a way of feeling included in group activities.

Disordered eating

For some young people, disordered eating patterns may arise from trying to lose weight. Some researchers estimate that around one-half of adolescent girls and one-third of adolescent boys report unhealthy weight loss strategies that include fasting, vomiting or taking laxatives (Choate 2012). These behaviours indicate that too many young people are preoccupied with body image and may be aspiring to unattainable physical ideals, especially if they are subjected to teasing from friends or peers (Lawler & Nixon 2011). To some extent, the media contributes to the prevalence of eating disorders, by reinforcing unrealistic images of what constitutes an ideal body. Images of ultra-thin models and pop stars surround adolescent life, making them difficult to ignore. In the absence of positive role models, young people may adopt a view of their ideal self, based on what they see in magazines and the media instead of what is feasible.

The most common eating disorders are anorexia nervosa (AN), bulimia, and binge eating. These eating disorders are among the most lethal mental health diagnoses, given that 10% of those suffering from AN will eventually die from complications related to the condition (Trepal et al. 2012). The diagnosis of AN is made when someone maintains only 85% of expected body weight, misses three consecutive menstrual cycles and manifests an intense fear of weight gain as well as body image disturbance (Trepal et al. 2012). Some scholars have linked the condition to a variety of life experiences such as childhood traumas, including sexual abuse, while others have focused on the intersection of biological, sociological and psychological factors that maintain disordered eating (Trepal et al. 2012). Feminist interpretations emphasise gender roles, cultural variables, and issues of power, privilege and marginalisation (Trepal et al. 2012).

DISORDERED EATING

Poor body image, unrealistic role models and the desire to 'fit in' with the group can lead to eating disorders, some of which are lethal to adolescents.

Although around one-third of young people with eating disorders recover, many continue to have mental health issues that can manifest in self-injurious behaviours or suicidal thoughts. They are often thought to be obsessed with three forms of control: over their eating, their body weight and food. The individual tends to disconnect from others, including family members, to regain control. In this disconnected state they are not fully aware of their body and their sensations, or the relational pain of conflict or confrontation, because they are consumed with managing their eating disorder (Trepal et al. 2012). Some also exhibit symptoms of depression and anxiety, irritability, mood swings, impaired concentration and a loss of sexual appetite, all of which begins a cycle of social withdrawal and isolation (Fairburn & Harrison 2003). The negative effects include poor physical health, especially oral health and gastrointestinal disorders, which are related to inadequate nutritional status and/or purging after meals.

KATIE'S STORY

Katie was 14 when she was first diagnosed with AN. A short video of her story can be found at:

www.nhs.uk/Conditions/Anorexia-nervosa/Pages/Realstorypg.aspx

---

Early assessment of disordered eating is a critical step in helping young people and their families deal with the problem. In many cases, indicators such as weight loss, listlessness or other behaviour changes are evident in the school setting, which underlines the important role of school nurses and teachers in ensuring appropriate intervention. Although there may be many different factors involved, researchers have linked conditions such as anorexia nervosa and bulimia with family conflicts and parenting styles. The risks of these conditions are heightened when parents are too controlling, where their relationships with their adolescents are lacking in intimacy, and when they communicate inconsistent and irrational messages in relation to weight control (Lock 2011; May et al. 2006). Families are not always to blame for the problems, but they do fall victim to the childlike dependence that occurs in AN, and family members often become medically compromised by coping with the situation (Lock 2011). It is therefore important that solutions to eating disorders are family centred, and work towards empowering the family while focusing on weight restoration (Lock 2011). As mentioned above, family meals have a profound effect on young people's eating patterns through role modelling healthy eating, and promoting family warmth and cohesion (Rodgers & Chabrol 2009). Supporting parents to provide positive role modelling can help establish good nutritional habits for the entire family that tend to endure throughout adult life. Another approach involves cognitive behavioural therapy (CBT) for the person suffering from the eating disorder, which emphasises emotion regulation, combined with relational cultural therapy (RCT) (Trepal et al. 2012). The latter approach encourages the young person to grow through and toward relationships and mutuality through therapeutic collaboration that creates a feeling of safety and mutual empathy (Trepal et al. 2012).

MENTAL HEALTH ISSUES: DEPRESSION, SELF-HARM AND SUICIDE

The psychosocial challenges of adolescents' lives and their behavioural decisions can lead to depression, self-harm and in some cases, suicide. They can also result in some adolescents being subjected to violence, bullying at school and adopting a lifestyle that is detrimental to health. In the 21st century, depression is considered the leading cause of disability throughout the world, affecting 25% of children and adolescents, 10% of whom fulfil criteria for a mental health disorder (Weare & Nind 2011). The prevalence of depression varies with age and gender, with a higher incidence among girls (AIHW

2011). The social determinants of depression include school and peer relationships and family factors, such as having a parent who is mentally ill, a lack of interaction between parent and child, and parental work schedules that prevent family closeness (Hayman 2009; Jui-Han & Miller 2009). Concerns with body image have also been linked to depression in adolescents.

SDH OF ADOLESCENT DEPRESSION

- Structural conditions of disadvantage
- Difficult interactions with others
- Family member with mental illness
- Lack of family, peer, school support
- Hesitancy to seek treatment or lack of access to services

Depression has an impact on every aspect of an adolescent's life, and can have dire consequences, including suicide. Major Depressive Disorder (MDD), or clinical depression, is a state of mental ill health where the emotional lows, often described as sadness, become pervasive (Herman et al. 2009). Besides genetic factors, depression can be the result of an accumulation of stressful life events involving threat, loss, humiliation or personal defeat (Commonwealth of Australia 2008). Clinical depression is often confused with the wide-ranging mood swings and intense emotional highs and lows young people often experience during their teenage years. These mood swings are a normal part of learning to respond to events and other people. However, some events and interactions with others can cause dramatic shifts in emotions that aren't quickly resolved. If these negative responses continue for over two weeks, it may be a sign that the person is slipping into a depressed state. Instead of bouncing back from a reaction or negative mood, the person may continue on a downward slide, often isolating him/herself from others.

MENTAL HEALTH ISSUES

- Anxiety disorders
- Substance abuse (alcohol, marijuana)
- Affective disorders (depression, bipolar)

Depression can be experienced differently by different individuals. It can make a person feel miserable or irritable most of the time. Some feel restless or agitated, while others feel down, and tired all the time. Concentration may be difficult, and they can lose interest in their usual activities, overlook school or work responsibilities, and experience changes in their relationships with family members. They may be overcome by feelings of guilt or worthlessness and ultimately decide life is not worth living. It is alarming that so few cases of clinical depression are detected early, as many young people and their parents or teachers do not recognise that these feelings are not a normal part of growing up. The lack of recognition and personal hesitancy has prevented 80% of young men and 70% of young women in Australia from seeking help (beyondblue, Online. Available: www.beyondblue.org.au/resources/for-me/young-people [accessed 18 July 2013]). For rural adolescents the lack of help seeking is often due to a lack of appropriate services as well as concerns about privacy. In New Zealand, at least one in five young people experience a depressive disorder before the age of 18 and three-quarters of them do not get the treatment they need (Merry & Stasiak 2011; Merry et al. 2012).

WHY DO THEY SELF-HARM?

- Escape from distress, hopelessness
- Anger, frustration
- Relief from tension, conflict
- Punish themselves or others
- Feel alive, in control
- See if someone loves them

One outcome of anxiety or depression can be self-harming behaviours. Self-harm or deliberate self-injury is often a repetitive act of cutting, carving, or burning various parts of the body, pulling out clumps of hair or overdosing on over-the-counter drugs without the intention to commit suicide (Gardner 2008; beyondblue, Online. Available: www.beyondblue.org [accessed 18 July 2013]). The prevalence of self-harm is difficult to estimate as some cases resolve themselves spontaneously, and, except for drug overdoses, many self-harmers are hidden from clinical services (Kolves & De Leo 2013). However, early intervention for those engaged in self-harming behaviours is important, and must be based on expert advice from mental health professionals. A recent survey of secondary school students in New Zealand found that 29% of female students and 18% of male students had deliberately harmed themselves in the previous 12 months (Clark et al. 2013a). Some of these young people report that they self-harm to escape deep distress, hopelessness and misery, to deal with anger and frustration, or to gain relief from inner tension and conflict, to punish others or themselves or to see if someone loves them (Kolves & De Leo 2013). Others report that it is a way of gaining control or feeling alive (Gardner 2008). In some cases self-harm is a way of expressing emotions for a person with a psychiatric or intellectual disability (Australian Government 2012). Researchers have found that the major cause of self-harm today is bullying at school, particularly if there are other risk factors in the young person's life such as a family history of self-harm or suicide, mental health problems or maltreatment by adults (Fisher et al. 2012).

The relationship between self-harm and suicide is complex. Suicide represents the ultimate failure of the transition from childhood to adulthood (Skegg 2011). It is the second most prevalent cause of death among adolescents in Australia after motor vehicle accidents, affecting 10 in every 100 000 young persons (AIHW 2011; Hawton et al. 2012). In Australia the rate of suicide is three times higher for males than females and four times higher for Indigenous young people (AIHW 2011). In New Zealand, suicide is the leading cause of death among young people and New Zealand also has the highest rate of youth suicide in the OECD at 18.2 in every 100 000 young persons (Craig et al. 2013). Although the total rate of youth suicide in New Zealand has halved in the past 10 years, there has been no corresponding decline in rates for Māori (Skegg 2011).

The risks are compounded for those with mental illness, harmful drug use, previous suicide attempts or self-harming behaviours, family history of suicide, socio-economic disadvantage or a low level of education (AIHW 2011). Other adolescent-specific risk factors include parental separation, family discord, child abuse, bullying and peer victimisation (AIHW 2011). The risk of suicide is up to three times greater among those who turn to alcohol, particularly binge drinking, which has been identified as the key differentiating factor in planned and unplanned suicide attempts (Schilling et al. 2009). In some cases a self-harming adolescent will progress to suicide because they have resisted disclosing their feelings for fear of becoming stigmatised (Norman 2009). This makes assessment of the problem difficult for everyone in the young person's web of influence. Self-harm and suicide are familiar concerns for parents, teachers and health professionals, especially with the attention of the mass media. Like substance misuse and other negative aspects of youth culture, media contagion via YouTube or television is a factor in precipitating self-harm or suicide, especially following reports of these behaviours among celebrities (Hawton et al. 2012; Lewis et al. 2012). For

parents, teachers, school nurses and other health professionals, the challenge lies in the fact that each person's experience of distress is highly individual. The causes, extent and intentions of the self-harming individual are variable, and it is extremely difficult to judge which self-harming individuals will progress to the stage where suicide is attempted or completed. Some of the potential causes of self-harm involve individual, family, school and peer-related factors as listed below in Box 9.2.

Recognising the risk of suicide

The treatment for depression typically involves drug therapy, and psychological interventions such as counselling and behavioural therapies. Group programs that provide mutual support and focus on developing life skills can also be effective (Hayman 2009). However, for some, an unknown combination of factors conspires against recovery, and there is a danger of lapsing into hopelessness. An attempt at suicide can be the result of a long history of mental illness or distress, or an impulsive or irrational act (Australian Government 2012). Over the past three

BOX 9.2 Underlying causes of self-harm

- Mental illness such as depression or borderline personality disorder
- Being the victim or perpetrator of bullying at school
- Problems with parents
- Stress surrounding academic performance
- Hypersensitivity, loneliness
- Alcohol or substance abuse
- Family separation and divorce
- Bereavement
- Unwanted pregnancy
- Experiences of abuse
- Problems related to sexuality
- Problems linked to race, culture or religion
- Low self-esteem
- Fears of being rejected
- Exposure to an adverse life event, e.g. a relationship breakdown or trouble with the law
- Exposure to contagion, i.e. knowing friends or family who have committed suicide

(Source: Mental Health Foundation 2006; Rissanen et al. 2009; Skegg 2011)

decades the rates of suicide have declined, with some attributing this to the increased use of antidepressant medications among adolescents (Bursztein & Apter 2008). For those who do attempt suicide there are usually some warning signs that signal their intention. These can include comments about suicide or death, expressions of hopelessness, rage, anger, revenge or comments that they feel there's no way out of the present state. The person may also begin withdrawing from friends or family, or experience abnormal anxiety, agitation or sleep disturbances, either not sleeping or sleeping all the time. They may begin consuming alcohol or other drugs. In some cases, they may begin to give away possessions, say goodbye to people close to them, or make actual threats that they are planning to commit suicide (Commonwealth of Australia 2008).

> ### CAUTION!
> The risk of suicide among young people experiencing depression is high. It is important to recognise the warning signs of an impending suicide attempt.

The 'tipping point' in deciding to commit suicide can be an argument with someone close, a relationship breakdown, a suicide in a family member, friend or associate, hearing a media report of a suicide, recurrence of an illness, an unexpected change in life circumstances or a traumatic event such as bullying, abuse or violence (Australian Government 2012). In preparation for a suicide attempt, some adolescents will begin accessing suicide sites on the internet (Bernsztein & Apter 2008). The most significant preventative measure for parents, teachers, and health professionals is a strong understanding of the adolescent's experiences. To activate protective factors it is important to remain close enough to read the risk factors and warning signs, and to know when it may be time to call for specialised assistance. Precipitating factors or typical triggers are outlined below in Figure 9.1.

ADOLESCENT LIFE IN THE COMMUNITY CONTEXT

To understand adolescent behaviour, Eckersley (2004) suggests it is necessary to disentangle the binary notions that characterise adult perspectives of adolescent life. In his view, we think of young people in terms of differences: between ill and well, marginalised and mainstream, the disadvantaged and the privileged, males and females. Instead, we should be studying young people's ideas, preferences and notions of wellbeing and potential. Researchers tend to over-generalise adolescents' status and behaviours in population approaches that references them to too broad a group (Eckersley 2004). Scientifically measuring adolescents' collective behaviour may not be as helpful as seeing them in the ecological context, which includes the social and environmental determinants of their individual lives. Another flaw in some existing perspectives of adolescence lies in adopting too objective a gaze, trying to understand adolescents and their health risks and potential on the basis of problem behaviours rather than strengths. Assessing their needs from their perspective is a more accurate way of identifying needs and planning any strategies that may be required to support and enhance their health and health literacy. This type of approach is empowering and therefore congruent with a client-centred approach.

Triggers and precipitating events

Risk factors	Warning signs	Tipping point	Imminent risk
• mental health problems • gender – male • family discord, violence or abuse • family history of suicide • alcohol or other substance abuse • social or geographical isolation • financial stress • bereavement • prior suicide attempt	• hopelessness • feeling trapped – like there's no way out • increasing alcohol or drug use • withdrawing from friends, family or society • no reason for living, no sense of purpose in life • uncharacteristic or impaired judgement or behaviour	• relationship ending • loss of status or respect • debilitating physical illness or accident • death or suicide of relative or friend • suicide of someone famous or member of peer group • argument at home • being abused or bullied • media report on suicide or suicide methods	• expressed intent to die • has plan in mind • has access to lethal means • impulsive, aggressive or anti-social behaviour

FIGURE 9.1
Typical triggers or precipitating events to suicide (Commonwealth of Australia 2008)

Identifying strengths and potential includes assessing the contexts of adolescent life. Many activities in the neighbourhood and community play an important role in a young person's sense of self, and therefore in their decision-making. Assessing the extent to which young people participate in community events or volunteer activities can provide a more complete picture of their health and wellbeing than confining assessment to individual issues. Community participation helps foster civic engagement, trust and other aspects of social capital that help young people develop the competence and character to contribute to society (Duke et al. 2009). Strong connections to the broader culture through volunteer work or various forms of community involvement also helps provide a strong grounding for adult life (Duke et al. 2009). The combination of civic engagement, strong family relationships and a caring school environment can help young people believe they are the agents of their own destiny. Developing academic, social and physical competence in the context of supportive family, school and social environments can ultimately lead to empowerment and the self-confidence for successful adulthood.

In maintaining adequate information for helping the adolescent population it is essential to understand the extent to which threats and opportunities are embedded in their social culture. Because the social culture of young people in this century is markedly different to that of their parents, there are often communication dilemmas where parents struggle to encourage disclosure of even the most unremarkable information. Being constantly connected to the external world online or through instant messaging (SMS) can act as a barrier to parental bonding and to interpersonal conversations that open the avenues for help seeking when it is required. The implication for parents, nurses and other health professionals is to seek understanding of the social influences on adolescents by assessing their perspective on these experiences.

WHERE PRACTICE BEGINS

Using assessment tools such as HEEADSSS is the starting point for addressing young people's needs.

A useful assessment tool to help identify young people's needs is the HEEADSSS assessment tool (Eade & Henning 2013; Goldenring & Cohen 1988, see Appendix J). The assessment gathers information on the most common influences on an adolescent's life at home, school and in other social environments. The tool can help nurses gain a multidimensional, yet individual, perspective of adolescent life. The assessment data can be used to foster closer engagement with their world, and ultimately, strategies to help protect and nurture them through uncharted pathways. Assessment can also be collaborative, aimed at helping inform a whole-of-community approach. Teachers, administrators, parents, community members and others can encourage constructive opportunities and validate the adolescent's ability for decision-making. Box 9.3 discusses the importance of being proactive in screening adolescents for health issues.

THE SCHOOL CONTEXT

Schools play a privileged and strategic role in the development of adolescent identity and competence and in helping young people make positive choices for healthy behaviours (Thunfors et al. 2009; Weare & Nind 2011). The school environment also provides a buffer for negative stressors, providing resources

BOX 9.3 Client-centred community practice

Being client-centred in practice does not mean waiting for problems to present themselves, but rather, being proactive in screening for mental and social health issues. Researchers in two community health services in Victoria implemented a screening service for all young people calling their service over a period of five weeks, whether the calls were for appointments, information or primary health care services. By deliberately screening all clients they found a high proportion of young people with problems related to alcohol and drugs, depression and anxiety that would have been otherwise overlooked (Thomas & Staiger 2012). Reflecting on their findings, the researchers concluded that some youth workers are reluctant to ask sensitive questions because of time pressures or their discomfort in managing distress, and this can be a barrier to providing vital guidance and education to young people. They recommended enhanced training for all workers and screening services for all community health centres (Thomas & Staiger 2012).

? What steps would you use to eliminate any gaps in services to adolescents if you uncovered evidence that some health issues are being missed by inadequate screening?

for young people to thrive, even when they come from disadvantaged homes and neighbourhoods (Weare & Nind 2011). A substantial and robust review of the last twenty-five years of research reveals thousands of school-based programs throughout the world that have demonstrated 'clear and repeated evidence of positive impact' on adolescent mental health (Weare & Nind 2011:i63). The success of school-based programs is due to not only teaching students about health issues, but the healthy schools approach that links the school with parents, the community and outside agencies (Weare & Nind 2011). The most effective of these are based on the partnership approach used in Europe and Australia, where school programs emphasise the bottom-up, 'lay voice' rather than the American 'top-down' style of prescribing how programs should be developed (Weare & Nind 2011).

The culture of a school is crucial to a young person's social and psychological development. Schools can provide a training ground for personal assets such as empathy, which is a protective factor for anti-social and aggressive behaviour (Estevez Lopez et al. 2008). Some school health programs are built on the five Cs: 'competence, confidence, character, caring and connections' (Maslow et al. 2012:365). These assets are cultivated through mentoring, parent closeness to school, school connectedness and religiosity. Closeness can help nurture empathy, especially for those who may be suffering a chronic illness or disability. Empathy is shown when a person can understand and imaginatively enter into another's feelings, which is a core skill for developing appropriate friendship networks and partnerships. This helps young people develop mutually respectful relationships and reject those that are aggressive. Teachers play a significant role in helping adolescents develop this level of social competence. Teachers who instil empathy, respect, courtesy, shared responsibility and a sense of community create a culture of reciprocal valuing, which helps prepare adolescents for adult life as workers and citizens (Estevez Lopez et al. 2008). School connectedness is also a predictor of later mental health, acting as a protective factor against mental illness (Herman et al. 2009).

> ## POINT TO PONDER
> School-teacher-parent closeness can help nurture the five Cs: 'competence, confidence, character, caring and connections'.

At school, bonding to others who share the goals of becoming academically competent, respectful and self-motivated reduces the likelihood of young people becoming drawn into substance abuse, smoking or other anti-social behaviours (Haegerich & Tolan 2008; Herman et al. 2009). Peer group norms and values can validate a young person's identity or sanction certain behaviours through criticism or ostracism (Hamilton et al. 2009). For example, ownership of material possessions ('name-brand consumerism') can convey physical attractiveness, athletic prowess and social skills to others in the peer group (Hamilton et al. 2009:1528). Like adults, some students wear or carry name-brand merchandise like a badge of honour. This can define them as part of an in-group culture, or it can be difficult for those whose socio-economic status does not provide the means to access the same consumer goods. Unequal financial status and perceptions of inequality can also widen the gap between the in-groups and out-groups. In most cases, the tensions between these groups are manifest in the school context and linked to their virtual world of social networking.

School, home and social networking

Social media is a universal feature of adolescent life in the 21st century, used by 90% of 12–17-year-olds and 97% of 16 and 17-year-olds (VCOSS 2013). Adolescents rely on technology more than any other population group (Ghaddar et al. 2012). Social websites, texting and instant messaging provide them with instant social communication and access to repositories of knowledge (Thompson & Couples 2008). Being constantly connected can, in some cases, reassure parents that they can contact teenagers wherever they are. However, communication technologies also create *peer contagion*. As social learning theory suggests, a person's emotions, behaviours and moods are strongly influenced by the activities, interactions, thoughts and observations in their social group (Bandura 1977). Where peers are overly critical and unsupportive, young people can develop social anxieties that, unchecked, can ultimately lead to depression. Teachers who try to nurture academic competence and self-determined behaviours and who try to prevent social comparisons can help protect adolescents from such negative outcomes (Herman et al. 2009). But this is increasingly difficult for the digital generation, whose interactions take place in the elusive environment of the internet and instant messaging. In the electronic venue of cyberspace, their language and messages can become transformed. A person's internet identity can be portrayed in photos, affiliations and interests and then socially constructed through feedback from others (Pangrazio 2013). This type of fabrication does not require a person to have a fixed sense of who they really are; instead identity is about a 'series of experimentations' on a digital canvas (Pangrazio 2013:36).

Most adolescents are involved daily in social networking on sites such as MySpace, Facebook and Twitter. For some, these sites provide a virtual community for communicating with their friends about personal behaviours or concerns (Moreno et al. 2009). But these technologies have also changed the rules of mockery, insults and harm, and they can be used as media for deception, cyber bullying and predatory encounters with unsuspecting users (Cassidy et al. 2009; Pangrazio 2013). Abuses include posting defamatory messages on social networking sites, sending a hurtful message to someone by text, instant messaging or email, spreading rumours, stalking, threats, harassment, impersonation, humiliation by editing a picture to distort someone's image or excluding them from an online group (Cassidy et al. 2009). The rise of this type of abuse

has grown over the past two decades since chat rooms first became popular. A further issue concerns the enduring nature of digital messages. Because adolescents do not have the skills for critical engagement with the technologies, they may not consider that the digital fingerprint they place on their social network sites will stay with them forever (Pangrazio 2013). While internet use does pose some risks to adolescent health, there can also be advantages, outlined in Box 9.4.

Bullying and cyber bullying

Bullying has become one of the most pervasive problems for those trying to support children and adolescents in their journey towards adulthood. Although the abuse may technically occur away from school, the presence of bullying can undermine the school climate, interfere with the victim's school performance and cause psychological and emotional harm to the victim, the perpetrator and innocent bystanders (AIHW 2011; Mehta et al. 2013). Bullying occurs in the context of real or perceived power imbalance. The bully victimises another person or

---

BOX 9.4 **The up-side of adolescent internet use**

We are all familiar with the exhaustive amount of information available on the internet and the way it has created a virtual information explosion. A Mission Australia survey revealed that the internet has become the primary source of information for young people (Mission Australia 2012). In addition to information seeking, new ways of using online sites continue to emerge. For example, some adolescents have gone online to share cautionary tales of cyber bullying to protect others, and some have used chat rooms as peer support groups (Yu et al. 2011). Other sites have been designed to promote cultural awareness and inclusive practices in education and health for young people living in rural and remote areas (VCOSS 2013). Some of these sites have proven helpful in adopting a partnership approach to preventing mental illnesses such as depression (Crutzen & Nooijer 2010; Monshat et al. 2011; VCOSS 2013). Young people with highly developed digital skills have been invited to help design an online Mindfulness Awareness Training and Education (MATE) program for their peers (Monshat et al. 2011). Mindfulness training (MT) is a strategy used in counselling to help people regulate emotional control by developing attentiveness or 'mindfulness' of their feelings moment by moment. Internet delivery of this type of program is ideal, because it saves adolescents from the embarrassment of

expressing themselves in person, reduces stigma and loss of privacy, and helps empower them in a way that is tailored to their needs. Although the program continues to be in the development stage, the team researching this development describes this participatory endeavour as an ideal way to use the technology as an asset: 'by adolescents for adolescents' (Monshat et al. 2011). A further example is the development of a computerised cognitive behavioural therapy intervention. Developed in New Zealand expressly for and with adolescents, the interactive online program has been shown to be equally as effective as usual treatment, serves to help reduce the stigma associated with mental illness and could be a successful tool for addressing unmet demand for services (Merry et al. 2012). The internet is also a way of supporting adolescents' health literacy. Although many adolescents do not have the ability to discriminate between accurate and inaccurate information, their technological skills provide a foundation from which health literacy can be developed. Where they have received training in how to access high-level medical evidence, young, internet-savvy adolescents have been able to help family members access information, and make decisions on accessing a health care provider (Ghaddar et al. 2012). This is not only empowering for them, but for their families as well.

group on the basis of ethnicity, age, ability or disability, religion, body size, physical appearance, personality, sexual orientation or socio-economic status (AIHW 2011). The victims are often the unpopular students, those who have poor coping skills and poor relationships, or who are dealing with an emotional episode such as a romantic breakup. Those who are bullied tend to feel less connected to school and attend less often, have lower academic achievement, lower self-esteem, higher levels of alcohol and substance abuse, anxiety, depression, self-harm and the risk of suicide (AIHW 2011). Bullying therefore has a profound effect on the victims, adding another layer of disadvantage to the lives of those who are already vulnerable. It also creates a climate of fear in the school, where students who witness bullying are afraid of being harassed or ostracised, and may do poorly in academic studies, disengage from school activities or simply drop out (Mehta et al. 2013). Both the victim and bully are at risk of dropping out of school, which can lead to reduced opportunities for the future, even a criminal conviction (AIHW 2011). Cyber bullying is particularly toxic, as it is often impossible for victims of this crime to find refuge from the perpetrator(s). When young people are bullied online they often become hyper-vigilant, feeling they cannot relax anywhere, whether they are at school or at home. Their vulnerability to manipulation by those with greater technological skill is exacerbated by their need to remain online, which keeps them from reporting the problem to parents and teachers. Because of their hesitancy to disclose the problem no accurate data are available on either the rates of cyber bullying or effective strategies to deal with the problem (AIHW 2011).

CYBER BULLYING

Cyber bullying is a form of bullying that uses technology as a medium of harassment. Cyber bullying can be pervasive in a young person's life and can be very difficult for a health professional to detect.

Students with a body image or weight problem are a particular target group for cyber bullying. Like other forms of bullying, cyber bullying often attacks the most sensitive students, many of whom are preoccupied with body image and social attractiveness. The teenage years are a time when self-esteem tends to decline, especially in girls who are subjected to diverse and contradictory messages about their role and place in society. Young women are often exposed to gender stereotyping that

suggests they are not good at some things (e.g. science), at the same time as they are challenged to succeed in these areas. These stereotypical pressures set girls up for dissatisfaction with their bodies, which is difficult at a time when their growth defies the idealised body portrayed in the media (May et al. 2006; Rodgers & Chabrol 2009). This has implications for body image and weight management. It also occurs when metabolic changes associated with puberty can cause girls to gain weight and cause boys to shed body mass, both of which can erode self-esteem. In some cases, eating disorders can actually be exacerbated by well-intentioned health educators urging adolescents to exercise and eat healthier foods. The evidence shows that encouraging young people to eat a healthy diet and engage in physical activity requires the support of family, friends, the school, neighbourhood and community (Kelly et al. 2012b). Bullying can act as an impediment to promoting these healthy lifestyle behaviours in all of these settings. A plethora of reviews have shown the effectiveness of school-based health promotion in helping young people develop healthier lifestyles, particularly when a comprehensive, integrated school and community approach is used (Fung et al. 2012). However, these health promotion strategies are open to defeat when the school culture is infiltrated by bullying. Around 6% of New Zealand secondary school students report being bullied at least once per week and this figure has remained approximately the same since 2001 (Clark et al. 2013a), suggesting that current interventions are having little impact. Eliminating bullying is therefore the most urgent priority for schools.

BULLYING AND SELF-ESTEEM

Adolescence is a time where challenges to self-esteem are high. Peers, media images and bullying can all place greater pressure on a young person to attempt to conform to often unattainable standards.

The way body image is handled in the school community can have a marked effect on the outcome. Recognising the importance of the problem has led many schools to develop programs designed to create awareness of the need for an ethic of care surrounding those at risk of all forms of bullying These programs also include websites that have been developed for easy access by students. The Australian Institute of Family Studies has produced a comprehensive list of helplines and telephone counselling services for children and young people as well as a comprehensive set of guidelines for parents and teachers on online safety (AIFS, Online. Available: www.aifs.gov.au/cfca/pubs/factsheets/a143428/index.html, www/aifs.gov.au/cfca/pubs/factsheets/a143367/index.html [accessed 10 December 2012]). In New Zealand, netsafe (www.netsafe.org.nz) has some useful resources on coping with cyber bullying for young people, parents and teachers. A collaborative website between the New Zealand Police and Telecom (www.nobully.org.nz) also provides a range of resources on bullying. These and other online resources are listed at the end of the chapter.

RISK, RESILIENCE AND DECISION-MAKING

Adolescents whose parents remain closely connected with them throughout adolescence have a greater chance of growing into strong, warm, resilient adults. Parenting is a delicate balancing act of providing children with 'roots' and 'wings'; the grounding to know they are safe and loved, but the impetus to individuate, or become their own person and to make good decisions. Parents who negotiate control in a warm and loving environment, and praise their children for the development of competencies, nurture the young person's internalisation of parental standards (Heaven & Ciarrochi 2008). Those who over-monitor their children can constrain an adolescent in trying to develop their personal identity, whereas under-monitoring leaves a young person open to other influences that may not be as safe or as helpful. Adolescents from families that have separated have a particular challenge, in adjusting to changes occurring with their parents, their siblings and their own lives. Separation can be very stressful for young adolescents, especially in the face of family conflict and when they are not quite aware of the reasons for the separation (Lodge 2012). It is therefore important that both parents remain sensitive and responsive to their children's needs, including being flexible with adolescents' schedules of school, friends, work or recreation. Adolescents themselves have expressed the view that in addition to stability and consistency in their lives they need a secure relationship with at least one parent, which is strongly linked to their school achievement, self-confidence and personal happiness (Lodge 2012).

In addition to parental influences, most adolescents make decisions and judgements on the basis of friendships, academic studies, extra-curricular activities, lifestyle and consumer choices. Learning to self-monitor is a deliberate, rational, analytical process that can be critical to developing

as a socially competent, independent person who can cope with stress, which helps build resilience. Even poor decisions can help build resilience if the consequences help an adolescent develop perseverance and strategies for moving on constructively from mistakes. With the support of adults, adolescents' positive risk-taking behaviours (academic pursuits, taking on new challenges) are reinforced, which helps them develop a repertoire of protective factors rather than risky behaviours. Armed with confidence and a sense that they are making their own decisions, young people have a better chance of transforming their lives from risk to promise (see Box 9.5).

Hope and self-esteem

Two important elements along the developmental pathway to maturation are hope and self-esteem (Heaven & Ciarrochi 2008). High self-esteem refers to feelings of wellbeing, positive peer group approval, active coping strategies and the expectation of success in life. Hope is a positive motivational state that comes from setting goals that are seen as

---

BOX 9.5 Adolescents at risk and at promise

Adolescents 'at risk'	Adolescents 'at promise'
Illness/disability	Good physical/mental health
Low self-esteem	Sense of control over life events
Poor coping skills	Good problem-solving skills
Feelings of alienation	Social competence
Family difficulties	Family harmony
Abuse	Love and affection
Poor family communication	Good communication skills
Problems at school	School support
Social or cultural discrimination	Civic engagement
Isolation	Social connectedness
Environmental stressors	Environmental safety, support
Financial difficulties	Academic, job prospects
Neighbourhood violence	Community cohesion
Challenges from peer group	Resilience
Poor nutrition/lifestyle factors	Family mealtimes, role models
Cyber bullying	Vigilance, safe technology

achievable, even when they experience temporary setbacks (Heaven & Ciarrochi 2008). Hope and self-esteem can give a young person a 'future orientation'; that is, aspirations beyond the immediate moment (Haegerich & Tolan 2008). This is linked to impulse control.

> **Hope**—positive goal setting
>
> **Self-esteem**—aspirations beyond the moment

Adolescent decisions to take risks often take place in emotionally-laden and fast-paced situations, where they rely on intuitive rather than rational decision-making, acting on situational cues, emotions, stereotypes, memories and automatic responses (Holland & Klaczynski 2009). Choices may be based on a decision that the perceived benefits (peer approval) are more immediately gratifying than the perceived costs (STIs, pregnancy). This explains why numerous programs focusing on behaviour, such as condom use, have had little effect. The good news is that once adolescents reach adulthood, impulsivity and emotional reactivity decline and most young people develop the cognitive ability for impulse control and better planning (Holland & Klaczynski 2009). The challenge is in supporting adolescents to reach adulthood safely.

Developing social competence for life and resilience in the face of adversity focuses on strengths rather than deficits. The pathway for both implies the presence of both risks and promotive factors that either lead to a positive outcome, or reduce or avoid a negative one. Promotive factors can be either assets or resources. Assets refer to the individual strengths of competence, coping skills and self-efficacy. Resources are supportive elements surrounding the adolescent, such as parental support, adult mentoring, community cohesion and other social environmental influences on adolescent health and development (Fergus & Zimmerman 2005). Resources in the adolescent's home and community environment may be seen as compensatory, such as gaining an education that helps overcome vulnerability or disadvantage, or they may be protective, such as having a highly supportive family.

Countering risk: Healthy adolescence

The major objective for promoting health among today's adolescents should be to create healthy pathways to adulthood that overcome risk and promote resilience. A socio-ecological approach addresses the many dimensions and interrelationships among risk factors and guides best practice in risk reduction, prevention of ill health and promotion of health and wellness. In this respect, any planning strategies to counter risk should be comprehensive, and mindful of how one type of behaviour or environmental situation affects all others. Strategies should also be developed on the basis of a sequential or life course approach, based on an understanding of adjacent stages of development. The settings of adolescent life should also be woven into any strategies, to reflect the environmental influences on behaviours and development and how these vary according to the home, neighbourhood, school, group, physical and broader macro level factors. The objective of programs for improving and maintaining adolescent health and wellbeing is that they should harmonise the needs and aspirations of adolescents within an ecology of youth, one that is empowering and sustainable to develop lifelong habits and habitats of body and mind.

> **RISKS TO ASSETS**
>
> Competence, coping skills, self-efficacy, home, school and environmental factors all contribute to the social ecology of adolescent health.

GOALS FOR ADOLESCENT HEALTH

The major health issues impacting on adolescents include mental and emotional health and maturity, good physical health and safety, academic engagement, minimisation of conditions that create risks to health and wellbeing, sustainable lifestyle habits in healthy environments, adolescent-appropriate nursing and health services, and empowering structures and processes for successive generations. Addressing these goals can help adolescents move from risk to promise. These are all embedded in the ecological framework outlined in Figure 9.2.

Adolescent health begins with the community and society, to create supportive infrastructures for health and wellness. Once again, the strategies of the Ottawa Charter provide a framework for addressing the most salient issues for adolescent health.

Building healthy public policy

Healthy adolescence begins with healthy public policies. These include legislation to control alcohol, tobacco products, cannabis and illicit substances, as well as those that promote healthy nutrition guidelines, mental health and environments

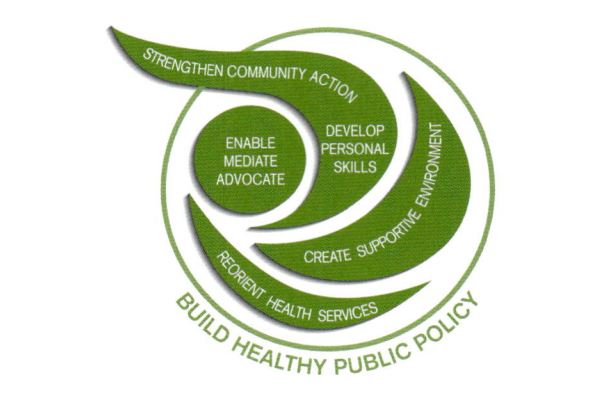

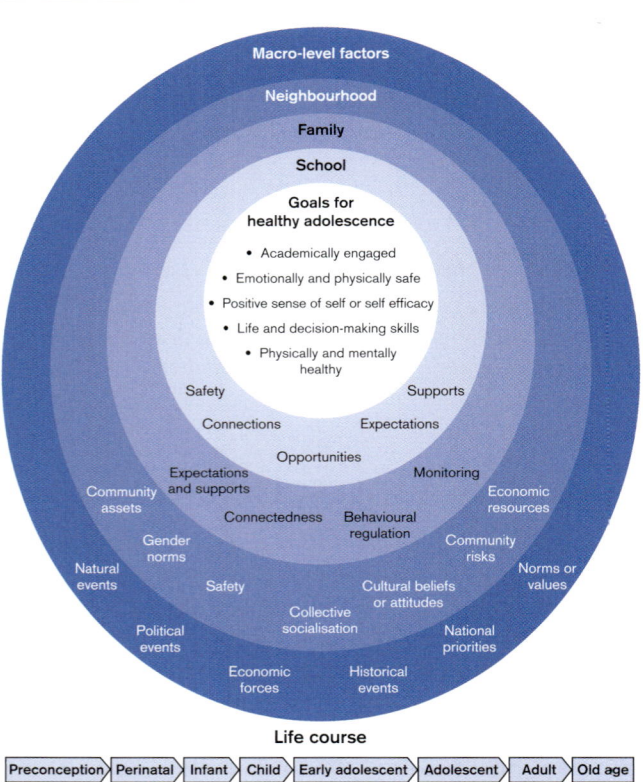

FIGURE 9.2
The ecological framework for adolescent health (Blum et al. 2012)

homeless and those with serious mental health issues.

Among the most important policies are those related to alcohol. Although adolescents consume alcohol for a variety of reasons, especially in response to peer pressure, perceived availability and opportunities to obtain alcohol make it seem more socially acceptable (Kuntsche et al. 2008). Adult role modelling reinforces the acceptability of alcohol consumption. Although it would be unrealistic to create barriers to accessing alcohol there are policies that can help reduce the level of harmful drinking among teenagers. In the US, for example, where the legal drinking age is 21, rather than 18 as it is in Australia and New Zealand, levels of binge drinking are much lower (Olding 2013). The other issue concerns extended availability of alcohol at pubs and clubs, sometimes throughout the entire night. This can be a major risk, given the peer pressure to engage in sustained drinking in the club context. Drinking behaviours are embedded in this culture, while the power of the alcohol industry remains strong. This makes it important to take a wide-ranging response to the problem of adolescent drinking, including advertising policies, restrictions on availability and price, police enforcement and a whole-of-society approach to promoting safe drinking behaviours (ARACY 2009).

Policies governing what is portrayed on television and other media also have an effect on adolescent behaviour. The 'just say no' messages of conservative American governments have driven sexual behaviours below the radar, partly because of the mixed messages adolescents receive from the media. On the one hand, they are bombarded with highly sexualised messages, and on the other, they are cautioned to exercise abstinence. A more reasonable approach is that used in other societies where community awareness campaigns promote a strengths-based, harm-minimisation approach to create positive images of adolescent behaviours.

The harm-minimisation approach is structured around a public health, or morally neutral, approach to policies rather than one that makes moral

conducive to healthy lifestyles. Healthy public policies also include those aimed at reducing health disparities among young people living in disadvantaged or vulnerable circumstances. Policy development is tied to economic conditions, and with shrinking resources, especially in rural and remote regions, certain policies that would support adolescent health have been discarded. These include funding decisions for school health education, child health services, counselling, and community support services that would help the disadvantaged, the judgements about such behaviours as alcohol or drug misuse. This approach precludes thinking about substances within the rhetoric of 'good' or 'bad' substances, refocusing on reducing the harm associated with risky behaviours (Hamilton 2003). Reducing usage is a goal, but the focus remains on protecting individuals and the community from harm. The philosophy underpinning this approach is that permitting access to the substances and teaching safe usage can reduce the likelihood of a young person progressing to more harmful drugs and habits (Beyers et al. 2005). It also protects the community by acknowledging that governments have a responsibility to ensure public safety through such initiatives as injecting rooms or condom dispensaries in places frequented by adolescents.

Tobacco control policies have provided important lessons about the effectiveness of regulation and legislation in creating conditions for better health. The combination of government-mandated smoke-free workplaces, major increases in tobacco taxation, warnings on cigarette packaging and the prohibition of tobacco advertising has dramatically reduced the rate of tobacco smoking in countries like Australia and New Zealand. The returns on government investment in these areas have been extraordinary. Media anti-smoking campaigns have also enjoyed remarkable success, which has made the global anti-smoking movement the most successful of all health promotion interventions, a fitting outcome given that tobacco causes more deaths than any other substance. The lessons from tobacco control could be extended to such issues as obesity control or other population-wide programs. These involve effective clinical intervention and management; individual and population education strategies; regulatory efforts, especially at school level; and economic approaches, through taxation and other incentive schemes (Mercer et al. 2003).

It is essential that any policy changes designed to strengthen adolescent health and wellbeing are effective for the context in which they will be implemented. Evidence-based approaches to policy development, implementation and evaluation along with greater collaboration between the scientific community and policymakers are required to ensure policy regarding adolescent health is robust, effective and safe (Fergusson et al. 2011). We will talk more about prevention science and approaches to policy development in chapters 14 and 15.

Creating supportive environments

Two of the most important environments influencing adolescent health are the school and social environment. The Health Promoting Schools initiatives were begun as part of the World Health Organization (WHO) 'settings' movement, which identified the most influential places to promote health as those places where people work, live, study and play (Kickbusch 1997). Since the early 1990s, networks of Health Promoting Schools have developed worldwide, and these underline the importance of school as an ideal supportive environment. As we reported in Chapter 5, healthy schools combine health and education in components that motivate teachers, parents and students to maintain health and to foster learning in relation to key values, appropriate skills and cultural norms. Young people who do not attend school, or who leave school early to seek employment, are often disadvantaged by a lack of opportunity for this type of support.

SCHOOL-BASED SOCIAL CAPITAL

- Social bonds
- Interpersonal trust
- Norms of reciprocity

At stressful times in a young person's life school connectedness can make the difference between coping and discouragement. School connectedness is the focal point in bringing students, parents, school staff and the community together to develop the social bonds, interpersonal trust and reciprocity that comprise social capital (Rowe & Stewart 2011). It is therefore the most important setting in which young people can be influenced toward positive behaviours and the reduction of risky behaviours (Aspy et al. 2012; Reininger et al. 2012). The whole-of-school approach used in Health Promoting Schools can connect students' lives across all areas of school, including sports, music or art, and academic learning. This integration and coordination conveys an attitude that students are not alone, that someone is always there with support to help maintain their health and safety (Aspy et al. 2012; Marks 2011; Rowe & Stewart 2011). The value of school connectedness has been demonstrated in school-based programs that provide help for students to manage chronic conditions such as asthma (Kintner et al. 2012), healthy eating (Kong et al. 2012), after-school physical fitness and activities (Carter et al. 2007; Kong et al. 2012; Van Acker et al. 2012), sexual health and substance use (Aspy et al. 2012), and positive communication skills (Gleddie 2011).

ACTION POINT

School plays an important role in personal growth and cultural renewal among young people. Facilitate young people's involvement in school activities in order to build resilience.

What all of these programs and initiatives have in common is a commitment to a respectful, tolerant learning environment that celebrates diversity, and empowers students to make appropriate choices for a better, safer life. In the context of promoting health, these schools also promote equity and a greater sense of coherence for young people. Health Promoting Schools therefore play an important role in personal growth and cultural renewal, both of which can be instrumental to building capacity for social competence. Including activities that help shape students' sense of identity and culture, learning, spiritual and moral development (Commonwealth of Australia 2009). One of the most important determinants of whether or not a school environment is able to develop adolescent capacity lies with educational governance. The current worldwide shortage of teachers, partly created by the number of teachers leaving the profession, has drawn attention to the frustration teachers experience when their passion for adolescent development is dampened by restrictive school and government policies. In many cases, teachers would be amenable to extending their role to a stronger focus on mentoring, which would see them using their talents to foster health and wellbeing in adolescents. However, current educational risk management trends have left many good teachers focusing on restraining behaviours around adolescents at the expense of providing the warmth and mentoring that is often needed.

In some cases community groups provide adolescent mentoring schemes such as the Smith Family's Learning for Life Program, the Life is for Living program (Commonwealth of Australia 2009), and the School Volunteer Program in Western Australia. The Achievement in Multicultural High Schools (AIMHI) program is another example of an integrated approach designed to support young people. The AIMHI program targets students at nine high schools throughout New Zealand, and is aimed at improving educational achievement through a range of initiatives such as onsite health and social support services and improving the links between the school and community. Evaluation of the program has found higher retention rates for Pacific students and higher school achievement rates at NCEA Level One and Two (NZMOH 2009).

In Australia and New Zealand, schools with nursing and other health services provide the most timely source of help and guidance for the numerous challenges of adolescent life. However, the distribution and role of the school nurse varies significantly in both countries, depending on whether the school is public or private, independent or faith based, where it is located and who funds the services (Buckley et al. 2012; Bruce et al. 2012; Su et al. 2013). Some nurses conduct school-based groups such as the adolescent girls' group mentioned in Chapter 6 (Garcia et al. 2011). Like other school-based programs this approach capitalises on the peer group, fostering positive group behaviours. Many school-based programs also open the door to intersectoral collaboration with youth-friendly services such as headspace (Muir et al. 2012; Roberts 2012), which can provide opportunities and resources for support for the helper as well as those being helped. In some situations school-based programs can guide a young person to online chat rooms for help with anxiety or depression. As mentioned previously, these online sites have the advantage of anonymity and privacy, but they also afford opportunities to access sites that may not be available at home (Crutzen & De Nooijer 2010). Accessing them at school can promote e-health literacy, which is empowering and can also address and minimise any health disparities that may exist in the school population (Ghaddar et al. 2012). Students choose school nursing services because of their accessibility and confidentiality and nurses providing care are highly qualified and experienced (Buckley et al. 2012). A national strategy for school nursing services in both countries would help address some of the variability in school nursing services and open up services for greater numbers of young people.

Strengthening community action

HELPING PARENTS HELP ADOLESCENTS

Nurses can support parents by providing a bridge between home, school and the community.

Although the primary community for most adolescents is the school, the family environment and family support behaviours are the most powerful influences in helping adolescents through behaviour changes, especially in relation to alcohol and substance use (Ramirez et al. 2012; Riesch et al. 2011). Schools have a vested interest in strengthening family and community support for students because cohesive families that communicate with their young can help maintain a vibrant school environment as well as healthy youth behaviours (Riesch et al. 2011). The myriad of changes to adolescent social life can be difficult for family members, especially in the midst of dramatic changes in family lifestyles. When adolescent children have only one parent available, when both parents work, or where adolescents are in the midst of multiple family transitions, there is an additional layer of intensity and extra challenges for parents, teachers, school nurses and administrators. Because many parents do not have time to be closely engaged with the school or social environment, it is important that teachers, nurses and family support workers take advantage of every encounter, to assess how they are coping with parenting, to keep the channels of communication open and to maintain non-judgemental support and a positive attitude. Helping parents deal with highly emotional issues such as sexuality, eating disorders, substance abuse or self-mutilation requires sensitivity towards their needs as parents and the patience to help them through a period of insecurity and conflicting emotions (Honey et al. 2008; Rissanen et al. 2009). Creating community partnerships that can help support parents as well as their adolescent children helps create social capital by strengthening the bonds that are so necessary to advocate for young people. Encouraging a strengths-based sense of promise, rather than risk, may have a long-term impact on parents and, indirectly, on the health of their children. This can be approached by communicating understanding of the complexity of adolescent issues, and of the importance of building family resilience and a strong sense of place. Resilient children surrounded by resilient families have a greater chance of escaping social and economic disadvantage, lower risks of psychological problems as an adult, and smoother transitions along the life course (WHO 2009).

At the community level, there is also a need to build connections between health and place. The needs of many rural adolescents are unmet by the lack of services, especially mental health services. This situation should be part of any planned attempt to promote mental health literacy and help-seeking behaviour among rural young people (Black et al. 2012). In the cities, many young people are homeless and at risk of becoming caught in a spiral of abuse, risky behaviours, poor nutrition, and physical and mental illness. The community needs to provide sustainable crisis and outreach as well as ongoing support for these young people (Dawson & Jackson

2013). The mark of a civil society is how it cares for the most disadvantaged. In a primary health care, socially just world, community advocates would find solutions to their plight a priority. This requires a concerted effort by all members of society to develop models of intersectoral, coordinated service planning and mentoring programs to help young people receive the basics of shelter, care, personal development, employment and a life worth living. Together all of these outcomes can help build a civil society and stronger communities.

Gay, lesbian, bisexual and transgender/ transsexual/intersex (GLBTI) young people are at particular risk of bullying, verbal and physical abuse, and challenges to their self-esteem due to their sexual orientation (Jones & Hillier 2012). Sexual identity concerns have been identified as major contributors to depression and suicide in adolescence. Being able to engage adolescents in discussion about sexuality is a highly refined skill that needs to be developed in all nurses working with adolescents. Communities, schools and families that are supportive of young people who may identify as GLBTI, or who may be questioning, can make a significant difference in the life of the young person. Groups such as Queer Youth and Rainbow Youth in New Zealand and Minus18 in Australia provide support for young people, their families and their schools to create safe, non-threatening environments in which GLBTI young people can thrive.

Developing personal skills

Adolescents are not a homogeneous group, but they do like to conform to group norms of behaviour. Significant others in their immediate environment can have major influence on their self-esteem and identity formation. As mentioned previously, adolescent life changes throughout the teenage years. Early adolescents (age 13–14) ask 'Am I normal?', middle adolescents (15–16) ask 'Who am I?', and late adolescents (age 17–18) ask 'What is my place in the world?' Understanding the subtle differences between the various stages helps frame adult interactions with adolescents in slightly different ways. For example, early adolescents' fears are generated from wanting to conform to this first step toward adulthood. Sensitivity to their loss of childhood and reassurance in the face of their fear of the future can help build self-esteem by reinforcing the fact that their behaviours, thoughts and feelings are normal. Middle adolescence is the stage of identity formation, and it is here that adolescents need a guide or mentor. This is also the stage of greatest risk-taking, with adolescents testing who they 'really' are. At this stage, adolescents need safe spaces, a secure and trusted significant friend and they need to be listened to, to establish and confirm their uniqueness. During late adolescence, adolescents confront their developing identity, reinventing themselves in terms of the family, back from the isolation of early and middle adolescence (Carr-Gregg & Shale 2002). Relationships with school and teachers are important at all three stages, and nurses can provide helpful support throughout these processes at each step.

PRACTICE STRATEGY

How well do you think motivational interviewing (see Chapter 4) would work with adolescents in helping them change sexual and substance use behaviours?

Some young people seek personal development information online. Many of those who took part in Mission Australia's 2012 survey (31%) reported using the internet as a source of personal advice on health, sexual matters, and financial advice because of the anonymity and accessibility of the internet (Mission Australia 2012). However, the challenge of health literacy looms large for this group, given that many do not have the skills to critically evaluate information on the internet, and may end up with heightened anxiety rather than resolution of their concerns if the websites they are accessing are not providing accurate information (Mission Australia 2012).

Adolescents need to be educated on matters related to their health by those who understand their needs and behaviours, and then supported in changing those they decide to change. This can be nurtured along by helping adolescents integrate functional knowledge (what must be done to improve health or prevent illness), motivational knowledge (how beliefs affect behaviour), outcome expectancy (belief in the effectiveness of preventative action) and self-efficacy (confidence that one can use skills effectively) (Becker 1974). Programs such as the one outlined in Box 9.6 are aimed at enhancing self-esteem. This type of approach has been shown to be effective in helping young girls make healthy decisions, particularly in relation to sexual behaviours (Graves et al. 2011). Suggestions have also been made that motivational interviewing would be effective in helping reinforce young people's positive behaviours in relation to making decisions about substance use; however, there is little research to provide a foundation for recommending this approach (Barnett et al. 2012).

BOX 9.6 SmartGirls

SmartGirls is a program developed by a collaborative group of community, school and academic health professionals aimed at strengthening middle school girls' behavioural choices to maintain positive sexual health and reduce the risk of negative outcomes from sexually risky behaviours. The program is based on Bandura's social learning theory and focuses on enhancing self-esteem, sharpening decision-making skills, setting goals for the future and strengthening family connections. During the eight-week middle school curriculum the girls have the opportunity to develop and practise positive behaviours, observe healthy decision-making by peers, and create positive expectations about sexual activity, the risks of STIs and pregnancy, and consequences of sexual behaviours. They also develop strategies for improving parent-adolescent communication about sexuality. The sessions revolve around self-esteem, values clarification and decision-making, assertiveness, pregnancy, STIs and healthy dating (Graves et al. 2011).

Many school nurses provide individual or group personal development programs such as the one described above. Others focus on 'selective primary health care', where issues of concern to members of the school population are raised. For example, when the issue of self-harm or suicide is raised, schools typically enlist the help of all teachers and the school community to initiate a suicide prevention strategy. These include the universal intervention of media education to counter suicide contagion, restricted access to the means of suicidal behaviours and education about self-esteem and resilience (Kolves & De Leo 2013). Some school programs also include skills training in problem-solving, coping and cognitive skills; awareness training to teach students about mental illness; and steps to reduce bullying, as well as stigma related to mental health problems and sexual orientation. Including teachers and parents in the same programs can help enhance knowledge of risk factors, screening and sources of help (online and individual interventions) (Kolves & De Leo 2013).

Independent, faith-based schools also have initiatives that are focused on spiritual development. Research has shown that 'religiosity'—that is, having beliefs and being involved in religious activities—can support educational attainment by increasing motivation, promoting social networks that provide educational resources and role models, and fostering intergenerational ties (Maslow et al. 2012:365). Religious programs are not typically offered in non-sectarian schools, leaving many adolescents without spiritual nourishment. As Moore (1993) laments, in the busyness of life many of us get so caught up in achievement and the whirlwind of activity that we suffer from a kind of 'heart hunger' that distances us from others and bankrupts the spirit (Moore 1993). At adolescence, it can create a lifelong template for dissatisfaction and longing. Spiritual beliefs and a sense of belonging to a place of worship are considered very important to many young people in New Zealand with over 25% attending a place of worship weekly and 31% reporting feeling that they 'belonged' to a church, mosque or temple (Clark et al. 2013a). When young people are encouraged to feel connected to family, and to something larger than their own lives, they have a better chance of developing into genuine, good-hearted, compassionate people (Fuller 2002). This helps them see relationships in a more positive light than the way the media distorts them, and helps provide nourishment, energy and solace (Fuller 2002). Spirituality has been identified as a protective factor for young people although this can vary in strength and direction and is likely to be strongest for those whose spiritual wellbeing and connection with religion is strong (Smith 2013).

Reorienting health services

One of the most important problems of adolescent life can be alienation from societal institutions, including those that provide health care. In some neighbourhoods, youth-friendly general practices are available to help meet adolescents' health care needs. Practice nurses play an important role in these primary care settings, especially when they are able to link services that are designed for young people (Hart et al. 2012). Attending a general practice for immunisations, general health checks, a Pap smear or family planning can also be an opportunity for health promotion (Hart et al. 2012). Although general practice remains the most common place visited by young people seeking care, barriers such as perceived confidentiality, privacy, accessibility and cost continue to exist (Craig et al. 2013). Improved training and education on adolescent health needs for nurses and doctors in general practice can improve confidence in dealing with adolescents and is recommended for ensuring general practice remains a safe location for young people (Craig et al. 2013). School health centres are also designed to be attractive to teenagers and provide an invaluable teaching and health promotion service. Because of the wide range of needs, adolescent-friendly health services need to be intersectoral, to cut across (or wrap around) institutions for education, employment, human rights and gender equality as well as health (Nicholls et al. 2012; Sawyer et al. 2012). School-based health centres are a common model in the US and are increasingly common in this part of the world. These centres tend to be nurse-led but often include other health practitioners including physicians, counsellors, social workers, mental health workers and occasionally other allied health professionals such as physiotherapists and speech language therapists. Such interdisciplinary approaches are designed to ensure young people have access to the wide range of intersectoral services they need. Intersectoral services are particularly required for young people who, because of disability or illness, need a range of integrated services (Clarke et al. 2011). Some drop-in centres and neighbourhood health clinics provide integrated services, and these are also designed for easy and confidential access.

ACTION POINT

Alienation from societal institutions can be a problem for teenagers. Ensure drop-in centres and local health clinics are adolescent friendly and easy to access.

A review of school-based health services found that those that are provided for all or nearly all school hours increase access for adolescents to health services including primary health care, mental health care and other specialist services, increase school attendance and retention rates, reduce truancy, reduce emergency department visits, and are generally well received by young people, their families and their teachers (Fleming & Elvidge 2010). However, the review also found that such services do not necessarily improve health status among young people (Fleming & Elvidge 2010).

Although schools and general practices can be a good opportunity for nurses to assess and help young people with psychological or emotional problems, designated youth services provide a more youth-friendly atmosphere, where young people can drop in and have a chat about a wide variety of concerns. The most well-known of these is headspace, which has been described as the 'boldest and biggest youth mental health initiative in Australia' (Roberts 2012:320). The headspace model is ideal in that it is a nationwide system of 30 service hubs and networks that offer youth-friendly health care, hot showers, food, art rooms, internet access and referral to a wide variety of services and specialists (www.headspace.org.au). The one-stop shop approach is attractive to young people because they know someone is there to listen to their concerns, irrespective of how diverse these may be. The centres are also free or low cost and have limited waiting times and generous open hours (Muir et al. 2012). The distribution of the centres avoids the practical barriers of transportation or a lack of knowledge of where to seek help for various concerns (Muir et al. 2012). The services are therefore congruent with primary health care in that they are comprehensive, equitable, accessible, intersectoral, affordable and culturally safe.

Places where young people congregate should also be the repository of information on health issues, especially to meet the needs of those who have left school. One of the features of the headspace centres is that young people can receive *esupport* or *etherapy* by accessing the services online (VCOSS 2013). Chat rooms are becoming common throughout the world to promote group interactions in discussions of social behaviour, substance use and other issues where young people explore how they feel about issues concerning their health (Crutzen & Nooijer 2010). Accessing online help or discussions in such a safe environment circumvents the problem of young people having to sift through what is credible or dubious in terms of health information. In some cases, youth-friendly services and sites can be designed in collaboration with teenagers themselves, and some of these programs are now being developed to help homeless youth by including their input on what is needed. As a result there has been greater understanding of the need to progress from meeting immediate needs for shelter to a continuum of care along a series of transitions that include supported accommodation and then independent living (Australian Government 2012). As with other youth-friendly services, these programs operate on the basis of collaborative wraparound services, relationship development that includes families, and a focus on strengths rather than risks (Australian Government 2012).

Another unique example of youth-friendly innovations is the *Boundin* project. *Boundin* is a short film created with and by young people at the Pixar animation studio, which they show at the beginning of the movie *The Incredibles*. It is the story of a young talented lamb who loves to dance, but his peer group makes fun of him and he loses confidence. Another character (a wise jackalope) arrives on the scene and teaches the sheep how to

BOX 9.7 Resilience-building strategies

1   Working on relationships with family
2   Developing a relationship with a mentor
3   Choosing friends who are supportive and responsible
4   Dealing with feelings during times of difficulty
5   Avoiding harmful coping strategies
6   Asking for support during times of need
7   Seeking the support of a group when needed
8   Participation in school and extracurricular activities
9   Engaging in healthful behaviours
10 Serving others

(Source: Cougar Hall & West 2012)

become more resilient and respond to the challenge. Like the programs mentioned above, the film embodies a number of principles that illustrate how young people can respond to and recover from difficult and traumatic events in healthy and adaptive ways (Cougar Hall & West 2012). Ten principles guide these strategies (see Box 9.7).

Electronic media, risk and support

With almost all teenagers communicating online and through instant messaging, and 30% of them seeking health information through the internet, the potential for health education is considerable (Mission Australia 2012). Nurses can support young people as they embrace new communication technologies by growing their own use of technology and online communication skills alongside the young people they work with, using the same technologies to stay in touch with them (Crutzen & Nooijer 2010). All health professionals who work with adolescents also have an obligation to understand the risks involved in online information. For those who post sexual references on their personal site, there is an increased risk of being victimised by sexual predators, especially where there is no parental monitoring of online use (Moreno et al. 2009). The other risk is related to the accuracy of information. Being vigilant and encouraging discussion of what they are learning online is the most useful way to assess the merits of various information resources and helping young people develop health literacy. Since the use of social networking has become so popular, school nurses and others involved in health education have had to shift their assessment style to gather information on the source and types of guidance adolescents are receiving. Many are also establishing networking sites to encourage students to visit them online for appropriate guidance or support. In this respect, social networking can be a valuable tool to provide timely, accurate and individually tailored health advice.

PRACTICE STRATEGY

- How prepared are you for digital communication with young people?
- What research questions might inform ease of this type of communication?

School nurses are also working with young people to help create awareness of the effect sexualised images in the media are having on their decision-making. This issue is also an important topic for child and family health nurses guiding parents on how to deal with early sexualised behaviours. Sexual identity is a topic that adolescents frequently discuss using the internet. A large study in the US investigated online construction of identity and sexuality in a sample of conversations from teen chat rooms. Many who participated communicated information on their gender, physical attractiveness and sexual behaviour. These conversations mirror those that adolescents would be sharing with one another in face-to-face interactions, but the content of their messages was cruder and more explicit, especially in unmonitored chat rooms (Subrahmanyam et al. 2006). The researchers explained this in terms of the disinhibition that occurs in text-based interactions, which are anonymous. Discussing explicit sexual image issues would be like wearing make-up or sexy attire in the real world to declare a sexual identity and demonstrate attractiveness. This can provide an opportunity to compensate for what they lack offline. Clearly, adolescents should be aware of the risks inherent in providing such personal information to strangers.

PRACTICE ALERT!

Sexual identity is an issue of great interest to young people, but it can often be a topic causing embarrassment and shyness, even for health professionals.

What are some strategies to ensure the integrity of your communication with young people about sexuality?

To gain access to screening and comprehensive treatment options, adolescents need to access sexual health clinics, which are usually available in major cities. Rural youth in Australia and New Zealand are often excluded from care because of the difficulties in accessing designated clinics. This creates a double disadvantage because they may delay treatment, and also have no alternative source of information and guidance. In New Zealand, sexual health care is free for all under-22-year-olds at designated providers. The extension of this program to a number of general practices to target under-25-year-olds, along with Māori and Pacific populations, increased screening and testing for STIs, and was particularly successful in detecting chlamydia among young women (Morgan & Haar 2009).

To meet young people's needs health service provision has always been fraught with some degree of fragmentation, especially when services are not integrated with other community health services. A strengths-based approach to services for adolescents should focus on self-esteem and validating an adolescent's ability to make decisions. This approach can be empowering and help them feel confident in dealing with challenges in the future. Strategies will also be more effective if they are linked to peers. Most young people want to feel that their experiences are unique yet have something in

EVIDENCE FOR PRACTICE

The Youth2000 project was set up by the Adolescent Health Research Group (2008) at the University of Auckland to provide accurate and timely information about youth health to policymakers, health and education professionals, schools and parents. The overall goal of the Youth2000 project is to improve the health and wellbeing of all young people in Aotearoa New Zealand. Three national health and wellbeing surveys have been undertaken with young people in 2000, 2007 and 2012. The results from all three surveys have been published widely, providing data on a wide range of health and wellbeing topics affecting young people. Data collected from the study is made available to researchers interested in youth health issues, enabling a wide range of aspects associated with youth health to be examined and published. Research of this type provides a solid foundation for developing evidence-based health promotion projects and nursing and midwifery initiatives that meet the specific needs of young people.

common with others their age. Providing youth-friendly services and accommodating variable schedules to fit with study and social activities sends a message of understanding to those in need of support services. This approach also creates awareness of their need for belongingness. It is also important to connect young people's needs and treatment goals with family expectations. Adopting an approach that is inclusive of parents will help build trust between the health professional and young person. It can also be more effective in ensuring there is family support for whatever intervention has been required. This also conveys the message that the health and wellbeing of the adolescent is everyone's concern. It is important to remember that different types of health services will meet different needs for young people. For injuries and illness, general practice is often the first port of call, for sexual health issues, school-based health centres and one stop shops are more likely to be utilised (Craig et al. 2013). Regardless of which service a young person accesses, it is essential that the service is youth friendly and is aware of the specific needs of young people.

Below we return to the Smith and Mason families to consider the challenges of dealing with current and future adolescent issues to maintain family health and harmony.

CASE STUDY: From pre-adolescence to adolescence in the Mason and Smith families

Jason and Huia's son John is 12 and on the cusp of adolescence. As parents, they were surprised, alarmed, then sad to learn from his teacher that he has just been diagnosed with a learning disability. They are also concerned to know that he has begun hanging out with a group of older boys who are drinking and sniffing glue. John claims that he is not taking part in any of these behaviours but Huia has her doubts. On his return from the Pilbara Jason takes a heavy-handed approach to dealing with John but this only serves to alienate John further. After consulting with Huia John's teacher at the Kurakaupapa has initiated a referral to the child and adolescent mental health service to manage John's behaviour and provide parenting skills for Huia.

Because Jason and Colin have become friends at the mine site, Jason has been confiding in him about his concerns. Colin's attitude is 'just let him be and he'll be right, mate', but Jason is becoming increasingly worried that people around him are too slack and don't understand the needs of teenage boys today.

REFLECTING ON THE BIG ISSUES

- Adolescents are generally healthy but often have psychosocial issues that create risks to their health.
- Adolescents can be seen as 'at promise' as well as 'at risk'.
- Adolescents 'at risk' often engage in a cluster of risky behaviours.
- From a social ecological perspective, home, school and the social environment are closely connected in adolescents' lives.
- The principles of primary health care can be used to ensure that adolescents have access to health and other services, that they develop in equitable life conditions and have culturally sensitive guidance that makes the most appropriate use of technology.
- Although there is considerable research into norms of adolescent behaviour many gaps remain in the nursing research agenda.

REFLECTIVE QUESTIONS: How would I use this knowledge in practice?

1. Explain the main risks of adolescence and how these can be addressed by nurses in a range of settings using a variety of strategies.

2. Describe health promotion resources available to adolescents in your community.

3. Outline a set of strategies for an online program to foster resilience in adolescents based on the social ecology of adolescent life.

4. Design an adolescent suicide prevention program for a local middle school based on the principles of primary health care.

5. Using the HEEADSSS assessment (Appendix J) identify some of the needs that you believe would be revealed by an adolescent. Explain how you would promote a sense of community and school connectedness for this person.

6. Explain the e-health literacy needs of a typical adolescent.

7. Identify one research question to launch an evidence-based agenda for adolescent health.

8. Outline what strategies you would employ to support Jason and Huia in helping John.

References

Adolescent Health Research Group, 2008. Youth'07: The Health and Wellbeing of Secondary School Students in New Zealand. Initial Findings. University of Auckland, Auckland.

Albert, D., Chein, J., Steinberg, L., 2013. The teenage brain: Peer influences on adolescent decision making. Curr. Dir. Psychol. Sci. 22 (2), 114–120.

Aspy, C., Vesely, S., Oman, R., et al., 2012. School-related assets and youth risk behaviors: Alcohol consumption and sexual activity. J. Sch. Health 82 (1), 3–10.

Australian Government Department of Families, Community Services and Indigenous Affairs, 2012. Literature review: Effective interventions for working with young people who are homeless or at risk of homelessness. AGPS, Canberra.

Australian Institute of Health and Welfare (AIHW), 2009. A picture of Australia's children 2009. Cat. NO. PHE 112, AIHW, Canberra.

Australian Institute of Family Studies (AIFS), 2011. Families in Australia: Sticking together in good and tough times. Online Available: <www.aifs.gov.au/institute/pubs/facts/sheets/2011/fw2011a.html> 3 May 2013.

Australian Institute of Health and Welfare (AIHW), 2011. Young Australians, their health and wellbeing 2011. Cat no PHE 140, AIHW, Canberra.

Australian Institute of Health and Welfare (AIHW), 2012. Australia's Health 2012. series no 13. Cat No AUS 156, AIHW, Canberra.

Australian Research Alliance for Children & Youth (ARACY), 2009. Action for young Australians report. Online. Available: <www.aracy.org.au> 12 November, 2009.

Bandura, A., 1977. Self-efficacy: Toward a unifying theory of behavioral change. Psychol. Rev. 84, 191–215.

Barnett, E., Sussman, S., Smith, C., et al., 2012. Motivational interviewing for adolescent substance use: A review of the literature. Addict. Behav. 37, 1325–1334.

Becker, M., 1974. The Health Belief Model and Personal Health Behavior. Charles B. Slack, New Jersey.

Benson, J., Kirkpatrick Johnson, M., 2009. Adolescent family context and adult identity formation. J. Fam. Issues 30 (9), 1265–1286.

Beyers, J., Evans-Whipp, T., Mathers, M., et al., 2005. A cross-national comparison of school drug policies in Washington State, United States, and Victoria, Australia. J. Sch. Health 75 (4), 134–140.

Black, G., Roberts, R., Li-Leng, T., 2012. Depression in rural adolescents: Relationships with gender and availability of mental health services. Rural Remote Health 12, 2092.

Blum, R., Bastos, F., Kabiru, C., et al., 2012. Adolescent health in the 21st century. The Lancet 379, 1567–1568.

Bourke, L., Humphreys, J., Lukaitis, F., 2009. Health behaviours of young, rural residents: A case study. Aust. J. of Rural Health 17, 86–91.

Braun, V., 2008. 'She'll be right'? National identity explanations for poor sexual health statistics in Aotearoa/New Zealand. Soc. Sci. Med. 67, 1817–1825.

Bronfenbrenner, U., 1986. Alienation and the four worlds of childhood. Phi Delta Kappan 67, 430–436.

Brown, S., Nobiling, B., Teufel, J., et al., 2011. Are kids too busy? Early adolescents' perceptions of discretionary activities, overscheduling, and stress. J. Sch. Health 81 (9), 574–580.

Bruce, E., Klein, R., Keleher, H., 2012. Parliamentary inquiry into health promoting schools in Victoria: Analysis of stakeholder views. J. Sch. Health 82 (9), 441–447.

Buckley, S., Gerring, Z., Cumming, J., et al., 2012. School nursing in New Zealand: A study of services. Policy Polit. Nurs. Pract. 13 (1), 45–53.

Bursztein, C., Apter, A., 2008. Adolescent suicide. Curr. Opin. Psychiatry 22, 1–6.

Cagney, P., Palmer, S., 2007. The sale and supply of alcohol to under 18 year olds in New Zealand: a systematic overview of international and New Zealand literature (final report). Research New Zealand, New Zealand.

Carter, M., McGee, R., Taylor, B., et al., 2007. Health outcomes in adolescence: associations with family, friends and school engagement. J. Adolesc. 30 (1), 51–62.

Carr-Gregg, M., Shale, E., 2002. Adolescence: A Guide for Parents. Finch Publishing, Sydney.

Casey, B., 2013. The teenage brain: an overview. Curr. Dir. Psychol. Sci. 22 (2), 80–81.

Cassidy, W., Jackson, M., Brown, K., 2009. Sticks and stones can break my bones, but how can pixels hurt me? Sch. Psychol. Int. 30 (4), 383–402.

Choate, L., 2012. Assessment, prevention, and treatment of eating disorders: The role of professional counselors. Editorial, Special Section. J. Couns. Dev. 90 (3), 259–261.

Clark, T., Fleming, T., Bullen, P., et al., 2013a. Youth'12 Overview: The health and wellbeing of New Zealand secondary school students in 2012. The University of Auckland, Auckland.

Clark, T., Robinson, E., Crengle, S., et al., 2013b. Binge drinking among Maori secondary school students in New Zealand. N. Z. Med. J. 126 (1370), 55–69.

Clarke, S., Sloper, P., Moran, N., et al., 2011. Multi-agency transition services: greater collaboration needed to meet the priorities of young disabled people with complex needs as they move into adulthood. J. Integr. Care 19 (5), 30–40.

Collins, S., 2012. Girls take lead in teen binge-drinking—study. The New Zealand Herald. Online Available: <http://www.nzherald.co.nz/lifestyle/news/article.cfm?c_id=6&objectid=10847267> 16 August 2013.

Commonwealth of Australia, 2008. Living is for Everyone (LIFE): Research and evidence in suicide prevention. Online Available: <http://www.livingisforeveryone.com.au/Research-and-evidence-in-suicide-prevention.h...> 22 July 2013.

Commonwealth of Australia, 2009. Family-school partnerships framework. A guide for schools and families. Australian Government Department of Education, Employment and Workplace Relations, Canberra.

Cougar Hall, P., West, J., 2012. 'Boundin': Responding to life challenges with resilience. J. Sch. Health 82 (4), 196–200.

Craig, E., Jackson, C., Han, D.Y., et al., 2007. Monitoring the Health of New Zealand Children and Young People: Indicator Handbook. Paediatric Society of New Zealand, New Zealand Child and Youth Epidemiology Service, Dunedin.

Craig, E., Adams, J., Oben, G., et al., 2013. The Health Status of Children and Young People in New Zealand. New Zealand Child and Youth Epidemiology Service, Dunedin.

Crutzen, R., Nooijer, J., 2010. Intervening via chat: an opportunity for adolescents' mental health promotion. Health Promot. Int. 26 (2), 238–243.

Dawson, A., Jackson, D., 2013. The primary health care service experience of homeless youth: a narrative synthesis of current evidence. Contemp. Nurse 44 (1), 62–75.

Dench, O., 2010. Education statistics of New Zealand: 2009. Ministry of Education, Wellington.

Denny, S., 2011. Adolescents and the media: consequences and policy implications. In: Gluckman, P. (Ed.), Improving the transition: reducing social and psychological morbidity during adolescence. Office of the Prime Minister' Science Advisory Committee, Auckland, New Zealand, pp. 111–122.

Devries, K., Free, C., Morison, L., et al., 2009. Factors associated with the sexual behavior of Canadian Aboriginal young people and their implications for health promotion. Am. J. Public Health 99 (5), 855–862.

Duke, N., Skay, C., Pettingell, S., et al., 2009. From adolescent connections to social capital: Predictors of civic engagement in young adulthood. J. Adolesc. Health 44, 161–168.

Eade, D., Henning, D., 2013. Chlamydia screening in young people as an outcome of a HEADSS: Home, Education, Activities, Drug and alcohol use, Sexuality and Suicide youth psychosocial assessment tool. J. Clin. Nurs. 22 (23/24), 3280–3288.

East, L., Jackson, D., O'Brien, L., et al., 2011. Condom negotiation: experiences of sexually active young women. J. Adv. Nurs. 67 (1), 77–85.

East, L., Jackson, D., 2013. Sexuality and sexual health: nurses' crucial role. Contemp. Nurse 44 (1), 47–49.

Eckersley, R., 2004. Separate selves, tribal ties, and other stories. Fam. Matters 68, 36–42.

Erikson, E., 1963. Childhood and society, Second ed. Norton, New York.

Estevez Lopez, E., Murgui Perez, S., Musitu Ochoa, G., et al., 2008. Adolescent aggression: Effects of gender and family and school environments. J. Adolesc. 31, 433–450.

Fairburn, C., Harrison, P., 2003. Eating disorders. The Lancet 361 (9355), 407–416.

Fergus, S., Zimmerman, M., 2005. Adolescent resilience: A framework for understanding healthy development in the face of risk. Annu. Rev. Public Health 26, 399–419.

Fergusson, D., McNaughton, S., Hayne, H., et al., 2011. From evidence to policy, programmes and interventions. In: Gluckman, P. (Ed.), Improving the transition: reducing social and psychological morbidity during adolescence. Office of the Prime Minister' Science Advisory Committee, Auckland, New Zealand, pp. 297–309.

Fisher, H., Moffitt, T., Houts, R., et al., 2012. Bullying victimization and risk of self-harm in early adolescence: longitudinal cohort study. Br. Med. J. e2683.

Fleming, T., Elvidge, J., 2010. Youth health services literature review: A rapid review of school based health services, community based youth specific health services, and general practice health care for young people. Waitemata District Health Board, Auckland.

Foundation for Young Australians (FYA), 2012. How young people are faring. FYA, Melbourne.

Franko, D., Thompson, D., Affenito, S., et al., 2008. What mediates the relationship between family meals and adolescent health issues? Health Psychol. 27 (Supp2), S109–S117.

Fuller, A., 2002. Valuing boys, valuing girls: Celebrating difference and enhancing potential. Presentation to the Excellence in Teaching Conference, Fremantle, Western

Australia, Nov. 14, Online. Available: <http://www.andrewfuller.com.au> 20 December 2005.

Fung, C., Kuhle, S., Lu, C., et al., 2012. From 'best practice' to 'next practice': the effectiveness of school-based health promotion in improving healthy eating and physical activity and preventing childhood obesity. Int. J. Behav. Nutr. Phys. Act. 9, 27–36.

Garcia, C., Lindgren, S., Kemmick Pintor, J., 2011. Knowledge, skills, and qualities for effectively facilitating an adolescent girls' group. J. Sch. Nurs. 27 (6), 424–433.

Gardner, F., 2008. Analysis of self-harm. Community Care 1725, 22.

Ghaddar, S., Valerio, M., Garcia, C., et al., 2012. Adolescent health literacy: The importance of credible sources for online health information. J. Sch. Health 82 (1), 28–36.

Gleddie, D., 2011. A journey into school health promotion: district implementation of the health promoting schools approach. Health Promot. Int. 27 (1), 82–89.

Goldenring, J., Cohen, E., 1988. Getting into Adolescents' Heads. Contemp. Paediatr. 75–90.

Graves, K., Sentner, A., Workman, J., et al., 2011. Building positive life skills the smart girls way: Evaluation of a school-based sexual responsibility program for adolescent girls. Health Promot. Pract. 12 (3), 463–471.

Haegerich, T., Tolan, P., 2008. Core competencies and the prevention of adolescent substance use. New Dir. Child Adolesc. Dev. 122, 47–60.

Haldre, K., Rahu, K., Rahu, M., et al., 2009. Individual and family factors associated with teenage pregnancy: an interview study. Eur. J. Public Health 19 (3), 266–270.

Halpern-Felsher, B., 2009. Adolescent decision-making: An overview. The Prevention Researcher 16 (2), 3–7.

Hamilton, M., 2003. Drugs: A contested policy area. In: Liamputtong, P., Gardner, H. (Eds.), Health, social change & communities. Oxford University Press, Melbourne, pp. 306–327.

Hamilton, H., Noh, S., Adlaf, E., 2009. Perceived financial status, health, and maladjustment in adolescence. Soc. Sci. Med. 68, 1527–1534.

Hart, C., Parker, R., Patterson, E., et al., 2012. Potential roles for practice nurses in preventive care for young people. Aust. Fam. Physician 41 (8), 618–621.

Hawton, K., Saunders, K., O'Connor, R., 2012. Self-harm and suicide in adolescence. Lancet 379, 2373–2382.

Hayman, F., 2009. Kids with confidence: A program for adolescents living in families affected by mental illness. Aust. J. of Rural Healh 17, 268–272.

Heaven, P., Ciarrochi, J., 2008. Parental styles, gender and the development of hope and self-esteem. Eur. J. Pers. 22, 707–724.

Herman, K., Reinke, W., Parkin, J., et al., 2009. Childhood depression: rethinking the role of the school. Psychol. Sch. 46 (5), 433–446.

Holland, J., Klaczynski, P., 2009. Intuitive risk taking during adolescence. The Prevention Researcher 16 (2), 8–11.

Honey, A., Boughtwood, D., Clarke, S., et al., 2008. Support for parents of children with anorexia: what parents want. Eat. Disord. 16, 40–51.

Jones, T., Hillier, L., 2012. Sexuality education school policy for Australian GLBTIQ students. Sex Educ. 12 (4), 437–454.

Jui-Han, W., Miller, D., 2009. Parental work schedules and adolescent depression. Health Sociol. Rev. 18 (1), 36–49.

Kelly, A., Chan, G., Toumbourou, J., et al., 2012a. Very young adolescents and alcohol: Evidence of a unique susceptibility to peer alcohol use. Addict. Behav. 37, 414–419.

Kelly, S., Mazurek Melnyk, B., Belyea, M., 2012b. Predicting physical activity and fruit and vegetable intake in adolescents: A test of the information, motivation, behavioral skills model. Res. Nurs. Health 35, 146–163.

Khambalia, A., Dickinson, S., Hardy, L., et al., 2012. A synthesis of existing systematic reviews and meta-analyses of school-based behavioural interventions for controlling and preventing obesity. Obes. Rev. 13 (3), 214–233.

Kickbusch, I., 1997. Health promoting environments: the next step. Aust. N. Z. J. Public Health 21 (4), 431–434.

Kintner, E., Cook, G., Allen, A., et al., 2012. Feasibility and benefits of a school-based academic and counseling program for older school-aged children with asthma. Res. Nurs. Health 35, 507–517.

Kirby Institute, 2011. HIV, viral hepatitis and sexually transmissible infections in Australia Annual Surveillance Report. University of New South Wales, Sydney.

Kolves, K., De Leo, D., 2013. Child and youth suicides: Research and potentials for prevention. Workshop presentations. Australia Institute for Suicide Research and Prevention, Brisbane.

Kong, A., Farnsworth, S., Canaca, J., et al., 2012. An adaptive community-based participatory approach to formative assessment with high schools for obesity intervention. J. Sch. Health 82 (3), 147–154.

Kuntsche, E., Kuendig, H., Gmel, G., 2008. Alcohol outlet density, perceived availability and adolescent alcohol use: a multilevel structural equation model. J. Epidemiol. Community Health 62, 811–816.

Lawler, M., Nixon, E., 2011. Body dissatisfaction among adolescent boys and girls: The effects of body mass, peer appearance culture and internalization of appearance ideals. J. Youth Adolesc. 40, 59–71.

Leather, N., 2009. Risk-taking behaviour in adolescence: a literature review. J. Child. Health Care 13 (3), 295–304.

Lewis, S., Heath, N., Somberger, M., et al., 2012. Helpful or harmful? An examination of viewers' responses to nonsuicidal self-injury videos on YouTube. J. Adolesc. Health 51, 380–385.

Li, J., Johnson, S., Han, W., et al., 2012. Parents' nonstandard work and child wellbeing: A critical review of the existing literature. The Centre for Labour Market Research, Discussion Paper Series 2012/02, Curtin University, Perth.

Lim, M., Aitken, C., Hocking, J., et al., 2009. Discrepancies between young people's self-reported sexual experience and their perceptions of 'normality'. Sex. Health 6, 171–172.

Lock, J., 2011. Family treatment for eating disorders in youth and adolescents. Psychiatr. Ann. 41 (11), 547–551.

Lodge, J., 2012. Parental separation from an adolescent perspective. What do they say? Australian Institute of Family Studies Child Family Community Australia Information Exchange, CFCA Paper No. 5.

Major-Wilson, H., Sanchez, K., Maturo, D., 2008. A collaborative approach to providing care for HIV-infected adolescents. J. Sch. Pediatr. Nurs. 13 (4), 295–296.

Marks, R., 2011. Healthy schools and colleges: what works, what is needed and why? Part 111. Health Educ. 111 (5), 340–426.

Martyn-Nemeth, P., Penckofer, S., Gulanick, M., et al., 2009. The relationships among self-esteem, stress, coping, eating behavior, and depressive mood in adolescents. Res. Nurs. Health 32, 96–109.

Maslow, G., Haydon, A., McRee, A., et al., 2012. Protective connections and educational attainment among young adults with childhood-onset chronic illness. J. Sch. Health 82 (8), 364–370.

May, A., Kim, J., McHale, S., et al., 2006. Parent-adolescent relationships and the development of weight concerns from early to late adolescence. Int. J. Eat. Disord. 39 (8), 729–740.

Mehta, S., Cornell, D., Fan, X., et al., 2013. Bullying climate and school engagement in ninth-grade students. J. Sch. Health 83 (1), 45–52.

Mental Health Foundation, 2006. Truth hurts: Report of the National inquiry into self harm among young people. Mental Health Foundation, London.

Mercer, S., Green, L., Rosenthal, A., et al., 2003. Possible lessons from the tobacco experience for obesity control. Am. J. Clin. Nutr. 77 (Suppl. 4), S1073–S1082.

Merry, S., Stasiak, K., 2011. Depression in young people. In: Gluckman, P. (Ed.), Improving the transition: reducing social and psychological morbidity during adolescence. Office of the Prime Minister' Science Advisory Committee, Auckland, New Zealand. pp. 191–206.

Merry, S., Stasiak, K., Shepherd, M., et al., 2012. The effectiveness of SPARX, a computerized self help intervention for adolescents seeking help for depression: randomized controlled non-inferiority trial. BMJ 344, e2598. doi:10.1136/bmj.e2598.

Mission Australia, 2012. Youth survey 2012. Mission Australia, Sydney.

Monshat, K., Vella-Brodrick, D., Burns, J., et al., 2011. Mental health promotion in the Internet age: A consultation with Australian young people to inform the design of an online mindfulness training programme. Health Promot. Int. 27 (2), 177–186.

Moore, T., 1993. Care of the soul: the benefits and costs of a more spiritual life. Psychol. Today 26 (3), 284–288.

Moreno, M., VanderStoep, A., Parks, M., et al., 2009. Reducing at-risk adolescents' display of risk behavior on a social networking web site. Arch. Pediatr. Adolesc. Med. 163 (1), 35–41.

Morgan, J., Haar, J., 2009. General practice funding to improve provision of adolescent primary sexual health care in New Zealand: results from an observational intervention. Sex. Health 6, 203–207.

Morgan, A., Haglund, B., 2009. Social capital does matter for adolescent health: evidence from the English HBSC study. Health Promot. Int. 24 (4), 363–372.

Muir, K., Powell, A., McDermott, S., 2012. They don't treat you like a virus': youth friendly lessons from the Australian National Youth Mental Health Foundation. Health Soc. Care Community 20 (2), 181–189.

New Zealand Ministry of Business, Innovation and Employment, 2013. Youth labour market fact sheet—March 2013. Ministry of Business, Innovation and Employment, Wellington.

New Zealand Ministry of Health (NZMOH), 2009. Evaluation of Healthy Community Schools Initiative in AIMHI Schools. NZMOH, Wellington.

New Zealand Ministry of Health (NHMOH), 2012. The Health of New Zealand Adults 2011/12: Key findings of the New Zealand Health Survey. NZMOH, Wellington.

New Zealand Ministry of Health (NZMOH), 2013. Hazardous drinking in 2011/12: Findings from the New Zealand health survey. NZMOH, Wellington.

Nicholls, R., Raman, S., Girdwood, A., 2012. Can inter-sectoral collaboration improve adolescent sexual and reproductive health? Discussion paper, Human Resources for Health Knowledge Hub, The University of New South Wales, Sydney.

Norman, A., 2009. First impressions count: Finding ways to support self-harmers. Br. J. Sch. Nurs. 4 (3), 141–142.

Olding, R., 2013. Dead drunk never drunk enough. The Sydney Morning Herald July 20–21, B005.

Pangrazio, L., 2013. Young people and facebook: What are the challenges to adopting a critical engagement? Digit. Cult. Educ. 4 (3), 34–47.

Ramirez, R., Hinman, A., Sterling, S., et al., 2012. Peer influences on adolescent alcohol and other drug use outcomes. J. Nurs. Scholarsh. 44 (1), 36–44.

Reininger, B., Perez, A., Aguirre Flores, M., et al., 2012. Perceptions of social support, empowerment and youth risk behaviors. J. Prim. Prev. 33, 33–46.

Riesch, S., Brown, R., Anderson, L., et al., 2011. Strengthening families program (10–14): Effects on the family environment. West. J. Nurs. Res. 34 (3), 340–376.

Rissanen, M., Kylma, J., Laukkanen, E., 2009. Helping adolescents who self-mutilate: parental descriptions. J. Clin. Nurs. 18, 1711–1721.

Roberts, J., 2012. Improving primary health care services for young people experiencing psychological distress and mental health problems: a personal reflection on lessons learnt from Australia and England. primary health care Research & Development 13 (4), 318–326.

Rodgers, R., Chabrol, H., 2009. Parental attitudes, body image disturbance and disordered eating amongst adolescents and young adults: A review. Eur. Eat. Disord. Rev. 17, 137–151.

Rowe, F., Stewart, D., 2011. Promoting connectedness through whole-school approaches. Health Educ. 111 (1), 49–65.

Sawyer, S., Afifi, R., Bearinger, L., et al., 2012. Adolescent Health 1, Adolescence: a foundation for future health. The Lancet 379, 1630–1638.

Schilling, E., Aseltine, R., Glanovsky, J., et al., 2009. Adolescent alcohol use, suicidal ideation, and suicide attempts. J. Adolesc. Health 44, 335–341.

Sheeder, J., Tocce, K., Stevens-Simon, C., 2009. Reasons for ineffective contraceptive use antedating adolescent pregnancies Part 1: an indicator of gaps in family planning services. Matern. Child Health J. 13, 295–305.

Sherman, E., Primack, B., 2009. What works to prevent adolescent smoking? A systematic review of the National Cancer Institute's research-tested intervention programs. J. Sch. Health 79 (9), 391–399.

Skegg, K., 2011. Youth suicide. In: Gluckman, P. (Ed.), Improving the transition: reducing social and psychological morbidity during adolescence. Office of the Prime Minister' Science Advisory Committee, Auckland, New Zealand, pp. 207–226.

Sloboda, D., 2011. Adolescent obesity: prenatal and early life determinants of metabolic compromise. In: Gluckman, P. (Ed.), Improving the transition: reducing social and psychological morbidity during adolescence. Office of the Prime Minister' Science Advisory Committee, Auckland, New Zealand, pp. 273–286.

Smith, L., 2013. The young person. In: Barnes, M., Rowe, J. (Eds.), Child, youth and family health: strengthening communities. Elsevier, Sydney, pp. 192–209.

Somerville, L., 2013. The teenage brain: Sensitivity to social evaluation. Curr. Dir. Psychol. Sci. 22 (2), 121–127.

Spear, L., 2013. The teenage brain: Adolescents and alcohol. Curr. Dir. Psychol. Sci. 22 (2), 152–157.

Statistics New Zealand, 2012. National population estimates September 2012 quarter—tables. Online. Available: <http://www.stats.govt.nz/browse_for_stats/population/estimates_and_projections/NationalPopulationEstimates_HOTPSep12qtr.aspx> 29 July 2013.

Su, Y., Sendall, M., Fleming, M., et al., 2013. School based youth health nurses and a true health promotion approach: The Ottawa what? Contemp. Nurse 44 (1), 32–44.

Subrahmanyam, K., Smahel, D., Greenfield, P., 2006. Connecting developmental constructions to the internet: identity presentation and sexual exploration in online teen chat rooms. Dev. Psychol. 42 (3), 395–406.

Teevale, T., Robinson, E., Duffy, S., et al., 2012. Binge drinking and alcohol related behaviours amongst Pacific youth: a national survey of secondary school students. N. Z. Med. J. 125 (1352), 60–70.

Thomas, A., Staiger, P., 2012. Introducing mental health and substance use screening into a community-based health service in Australia: usefulness and implications for service change. Health Soc. Care Community 20 (6), 635–644.

Thompson, L., Couples, J., 2008. Seen and not heard? Text messaging and digital sociality. Soc. Cult. Geogr. 9, 95–108.

Thunfors, P., Collins, B., Hanlon, A., 2009. Health behavior interests of adolescents with unhealthy diet and exercise: implications for weight management. Health Educ. Res. 24 (4), 634–645.

Trepal, H., Boie, I., Kress, V., 2012. A relational cultural approach to working with clients with eating disorders. J. Couns. Dev. 90 (3), 346–356.

University of Otago and Ministry of Health, 2011. A focus on nutrition: Key findings of the 2008/09 New Zealand adult nutrition survey. Ministry of Health, Wellington.

Urry, S., Nelson, L., Padilla-Walker, L., 2011. Mother knows best: Psychological control, child disclosure, and maternal knowledge in emerging adulthood. J. Fam. Stud. 17 (2), 157–173.

Van Acker, R., De Bourdeaudhuu, I., De Martelaer, K., et al., 2012. The association between socio-ecological factors and having an after-school physical activity program. J. Sch. Health 82 (9), 395–403.

Victorian Council of Social Services, Youth Affairs Council of Victoria, 2013. Building the Scaffolding, strengthening support for young people in Victoria. VCSS, Melbourne.

Viner, R., Ozer, E., Denny, S., et al., 2012. Adolescence and the social determinants of health. The Lancet 379, 1641–1652.

Vinther-Larsen, M., Huckle, T., You, R., et al., 2013. Area level deprivation and drinking patterns among adolescents. Health Place 19, 53–58.

Weare, K., Nind, M., 2011. Mental health promotion and problem prevention in schools: what does the evidence say? Health Promot. Int. 26 (S1), i29–i69.

Whitlock, J., Powers, J., Eckenrode, J., 2006. The virtual cutting edge: The internet and adolescent self-injury. Dev. Psychol. 42 (3), 407–417.

Williams, M., Jones, S., Caputi, P., et al., 2011. Australian adolescents' compliance with sun protection behaviours during summer: the importance of the school context. Health Promot. Int. 27 (1), 15–22.

World Health Organization (WHO), 2009. Mental health, resilience, and inequalities. WHO Regional Office for Europe, Copenhagen WHO.

World Health Organization (WHO), 2010. Young people: health risks and solutions, fact sheet no 345. WHO, Geneva.

Yu, J., Taverner, N., Madden, K., 2011. Young people's views on sharing health-related stories on the internet. Health Soc. Care Community 19 (3), 326–334.

Zodgekar, N., 2012. Teenage pregnancy and parenting in New Zealand. Families Commission, Wellington, New Zealand.

Useful websites

www.aifs.gov.au—Australian Institute of Family Studies

www.sane.org/information/factsheets-podcasts—SANE Australia, mental health information

www.nzhis.govt.nz—New Zealand Health Information Service

www.spinz.org.nz—New Zealand Youth Suicide Prevention

www.plunket.org.nz—Plunket nurses

www.youthaffairs.govt.nz—Youth affairs

www.mindnet.org.nz—MindNet, New Zealand mental health promotion

www.mhc.govt.nz—Strengthening Families, Family Start programs

www.youthbeyondblue.com—Youth beyondblue, information for Australian youth on depression, emotions and bullying

www.reachout.com—Help for young people in tough times

www.kidshelp.com.au—Kids Helpline

www.lifeline.org.au—Lifeline

www.ncab.org.au/about—Australian National Centre Against Bullying

www.mentalhealth.org.nz—Mental health promotion NZ

www.rainbowyouth.org.nz—Rainbow Youth, an Auckland-based organisation that provides support, information, advocacy and education for queer young people and their families

http://curious.org.nz/nelson-tasman-marlborough/q-youth—Q Youth, support for queer youth in Nelson

http://minus18.org.au—Australia's largest network for gay, bi, lesbian and trans youth.

www.aimhi.ac.nz—Achievement in Multicultural High Schools:collaborative program aimed at educational achievement among multicultural young people

www.youth2000.ac.nz/default.htm—Youth health in New Zealand, a profile of their health and wellbeing

www.vibe.org.nz—Youth Health Service in New Zealand

http://evolveyouth.org.nz—Youth health service in New Zealand

www.nobully.org.nz—New Zealand Police and Telecom website on bullying

www.netsafe.org.nz—Netsafe, internet safety website

www.fya.org.au—Foundation for Young Australians

www.missionaustralia.com.au—Mission Australia

www.reachout.com—Reach Out, Help and advice for adolescent issues

www.aifs.gov.au/cfca/pubs/factsheets/a143367/index.html—Online safety guidelines

www.swytch.org.au—Swytch, online forum for sharing personal stories about accessing mental health support

Helplines and telephone counselling

1800 55 1800 Kids Help Line

13 11 14 Lifeline

1800 737 732—1800 RESPECT

1800 695 463—MYLINE

1800 688 009—Child Abuse Prevention Service

1800 700 357—Children and the media helpline

Healthy adults

CHAPTER 10

Introduction

By the time most people have reached adulthood, they have usually experienced at least one illness or injury serious enough to seek medical help. For the majority of adults these are acute episodes of short duration that are resolved without major intervention or residual effects. For others, however, chronic, disabling conditions cause either premature mortality or compromise the quality of their lives. The difference between these two groups is related to biological, social, cultural and environmental influences and how a person has learned to respond to these influences. Adult health and wellbeing also reflect the culmination of the policy environments that have circumscribed people's lives and constrained or facilitated their choices for health and lifestyles. These include a wide range of policies; for example, those governing taxes on alcohol or tobacco, or workplace policies permitting sick leave when workers are ill or family leave when children need to be cared for. Besides these influences, health in adult life is also a product of family structure, ethnicity, education, employment and place of residence. How an individual has learned to cope with any of these influences, as well as historical illness, injury, disabling conditions or various stressors may be indicative of whether (s)he is able to cope with unexpected events in adult life. Stress and coping are therefore central elements in sustaining health in adult life. Coping strategies also indicate how well an adult is able to continue on the pathway to older age. These issues, which are all linked to the social determinants of health (SDH) will be outlined in relation to various health outcomes throughout the chapter.

The environments surrounding adult life are critical factors in determining their health. This is particularly evident in the effects of the social environment on health and quality of life. A growing body of research linking health to socio-economic disparities, cultural and economic factors sets the stage for greater knowledge of adult health than was available in the past. This chapter will address the effect of these environments on lifestyle choices, especially in relation to the cluster of behaviours that contribute to the burden of ill health from type 2 diabetes, cardiovascular disease and mental illness. The physical environment will also be discussed as part of the ecology of health and wellbeing in adult life. Some aspects of the environment are a cause for urgent concern, with the health effects of climate change and other global changes having a major effect on the way we live our lives in the 21st century. Contemporary lifestyles are also influenced by new developments in research and technology. Unique programs of research are forging ahead in informing health promotion and disease treatments, particularly since the mapping of the human genome and the development of stem cell therapies to respond to errant genes and their expression in the human body. This 'translational' body of research knowledge is an important part of the toolkit for guiding adults toward better health, and it is discussed here in the context of creating and sustaining healthy communities.

THE HEALTHY ADULT

Adulthood is the time of a person's life when the intersecting influences of biology, the environment and lifestyle are most apparent. The years between age 20 to around 50 are concerned with finding one's place in the family, work environment and society, reconciling the needs of various roles and expectations. By the time people have become adults, their innate predispositions combine with their past and current lifestyles and a variety of life circumstances to establish relatively stable patterns for the future. For most, the prospect for a long life free of the burden of illness and disability is good. However, other people achieve less than optimal health because of genetic predisposition, the social determinants of their childhood, or current circumstances. Fortunately for most adults in Australia and New Zealand, the environment provides considerable potential for overcoming vulnerability to ill health and achieving high levels of health and wellbeing.

OBJECTIVES

By the end of this chapter you will be able to:

1   identify the main influences on health and illness in adulthood

2   explain the social determinants of health, illness, injury and disability among adults

3   examine the cumulative effects of interactions between physical, social and cultural environments along the pathway to adult life

4   outline a health promotion intervention for adults focused on reducing multiple health risks through health literacy

5   explain how the health of adults can be improved using the strategies of the Ottawa Charter for Health Promotion

6   identify gaps in our knowledge of adult health that should be addressed through nursing and health research.

Unlike some other parts of the world, most people in this part of the world have access to nutritious food, clean air and water, good housing, education and employment possibilities, scientific and technological expertise, relatively low levels of community violence, and accessible and appropriate health care and social support services. The New Zealand general social survey in 2012 showed that 87% of New Zealanders were satisfied or very satisfied with their lives and 60% rated their health as excellent or very good (Welch 2013). This finding resonates with the findings of the World Happiness Report we mentioned in Chapter 1, which indicates that adult life in our part of the world is more satisfying than in many other countries (Helliwell et al. 2012). However, environmental factors in Australia and New Zealand also create risks emanating from climate change, which is one of the defining challenges of this century, making it a public health priority (Cambell-Lendrum et al. 2009). Climate change risks worsening the health of those already disadvantaged, especially Indigenous people, through natural disasters such as drought, floods and fire, and worsening social inequity (McMichael 2013). As the impact of climate change cascades through daily life, increasing the likelihood of respiratory diseases, housing and food insecurity there is an unprecedented need for intersectoral collaboration. Adding our knowledge base to that of other disciplines will help shed insights into the health implications of policies such as carbon pricing, the increased cost of living from energy, power generation, transport and agriculture, and a need for heightened surveillance of community life (Campbell-Lendrum et al. 2009). The discussion to follow addresses the strengths, weaknesses, threats and opportunities of adult life in this part of the world, and the effect of global influences on health risks and potential.

LIVING THE GOOD LIFE

The health of most Australians and New Zealanders is enhanced by supportive policies, nutritious food, clean air and water, safe housing, education, employment and health services, scientific and technological expertise, and low levels of civil unrest.

RISKS TO ADULT HEALTH

Life expectancy for babies born in this part of the world today is among the best in the world. Non-Indigenous Australian men are expected to live to age 80, women to age 84 (AIHW 2012a), and in New Zealand to age 78 for men and age 82 for women (Statistics New Zealand 2013a). For Indigenous Australians, life expectancy is 12 and 10 years lower respectively for males and females (AIHW 2012a). Māori life expectancy is relatively better compared to Australian Indigenous people, with Māori men expected to live to age 72, and women to age 76 (Statistics New Zealand 2013a).

QUICK FACTS

- The life expectancy of non-Indigenous Australians and New Zealanders born today is among the highest in the world.

- The most common causes of adult *mortality* are cancer, heart disease and cerebrovascular disease (stroke).

- The most common causes of *morbidity* are cancer, cardiovascular disease and mental illness.

Priorities for health interventions are based on data indicating the major causes of morbidity and mortality. In Australia and New Zealand, as in many other countries, the burden of disease is calculated on the basis of the DALY (disability-adjusted life year), representing each year of potential healthy life lost to disease or injury (AIHW 2012a; NZMOH 2013a). Among the 53% of the Australian population who are adults, cancer and cardiovascular disease cause the highest *fatal* burden of disease (mortality), while nervous/sense disorders and mental disorders cause the highest *non-fatal* burden of disease (morbidity). The top three diseases prevalent in the Australian population are ischaemic heart disease, anxiety/depression and type 2 diabetes (AIHW 2012a).

In New Zealand, coronary heart disease followed by anxiety and depressive disorders are the leading causes of health loss (NZMOH 2013a). Health loss is the gap between the population's current state of health and that of an ideal population in which everyone experiences long lives free from ill health or disability (NZMOH 2013a). So while the major causes of death in New Zealand are cancer (28.9%) and ischaemic heart disease (19%) (NZMOH 2012a), it is heart disease and anxiety and depression that cause the most disability.

GROUP EXERCISE: Adult health

In small groups, brainstorm what you think would be the most common influences on adult health. As you work through the chapter identify new or differing items to add to your list. Why do you think some adults maintain health while others struggle?

Cancer

Mortality rates from cancers have declined in recent years throughout the developed world, because of early detection and better treatment. Still, 29% of all deaths in Australia are due to cancers, the most prevalent being prostate, bowel, breast, melanoma and lung cancer (AIHW 2012a, b). Australia and New Zealand are almost identical in the proportion of the population being diagnosed with any type of cancer, which affects 309 people per 100 000 of population (AIHW 2012b). Our cancer rates are among the highest in the world overall, yet deaths from cancer in Australia and New Zealand are slightly below the world average, suggesting that treatment success is relatively high. Regardless of treatment outcomes, Australia has the highest rate of melanoma in the world (more than 12 times the

average world rate), the highest incidence of prostate cancer and the fourth highest rate of breast cancer (AIHW 2012b). The implication of these data is that by the time they reach 75 years of age, 1 in 27 Australians will be diagnosed with melanoma, 1 in 8 men will be diagnosed with prostate cancer, and 1 in 11 women will be diagnosed with breast cancer (AIHW 2012b). In New Zealand, lung cancer is the leading cause of cancer deaths for both men and women, accounting for 18.8% of all deaths from cancer (NZMOH 2012b). This is followed by colorectal (bowel) cancer for men and breast cancer for women. The third most common is prostate cancer for men and bowel cancer for women. These four sites accounted for 48.2% of all deaths from cancer in 2009 (NZMOH 2012b).

GENDER AND LUNG CANCER IN AUSTRALIA AND NEW ZEALAND

Australian women have twice the incidence of lung cancer than males because more women than men have a smoking history. In New Zealand the situation is reversed, as more men than women have been smokers. Smoking rates have declined in both countries, but more women will die from lung cancer because of their longer lifespan.

In the past decade the incidence of new cancer cases in Australia has doubled, due to increases in the population and population ageing and better screening programs. So despite better survival rates, there are more people being diagnosed who also live longer with the disease (AIHW 2012b). Some cancers continue to have low survival rates, including mesothelioma, brain, pancreatic and lung cancer (AIHW 2012b). Lung cancer remains a serious problem for anyone diagnosed with this illness, because it is a preventable cause of death, and because there is a long latency period of around 20 years between the cause (smoking) and the outcome (the disease). Since many men quit smoking in the 1960s the incidence of lung cancer in men has decreased dramatically, however, more women continued to smoke until the 1970s, which has left many of today's older women suffering or dying from lung cancer (AIHW 2012a). Morbidity and mortality from lung cancer are particularly grave issues for Indigenous people, with smoking rates higher among these groups than non-Indigenous people (AIHW 2012a). Others living in remote areas and groups with low socio-economic status also have a higher risk of lung cancer (AIHW 2012b).

Although lung cancer is the leading cause of cancer deaths in New Zealand as a whole, more men than women are diagnosed and die from this form of cancer (NZMOH 2012b). This differs from Australia where more women than men are diagnosed. This is probably reflective of the differing rates of smoking between the two countries. In New Zealand, smoking prevalence among women is lower than among men and has been since at least 1996 (NZMOH 2012c). Rates of smoking have been decreasing for both men and women over the same time period although not as quickly for women (NZMOH 2012c). We may see this slower rate of decrease reflected in increasing lung cancer rates among New Zealand women in the long term. Rates of lung cancer mortality also differ by ethnicity with Māori experiencing 26% greater mortality than non-Māori, with some evidence that this gap may be widening (Soeberg et al. 2012).

After lung cancer, breast cancer is the second leading cause of death among Australian and New Zealand women aged 45–75 (AIHW 2012b; NZMOH 2012b). Breast cancer seems to be increasing among younger women aged 20–40, perhaps because of better surveillance and detection due to national breast screening mammography programs, even though national screening programs do not begin until age 45. However, greater awareness of breast cancer in general, possibly due to advertising of screening programs, may lead younger women to have mammography screening. These younger women have more aggressive forms of disease, lower survival rates than postmenopausal women, and the possibility of infertility and premature menopause (Shaha & Bauer-Wu 2009). For those who survive there are constant reminders of the disease, as they meet requirements for annual health checks and ongoing vigilance by themselves and family members. Because they spend so many years with a history of breast cancer, they often count on nurses in a variety of primary health care settings for guidance and support, especially practice nurses and specialist breast care nurses.

Injuries

Motor vehicle accidents, interpersonal violence and suicide are the major causes of injuries, and represent the leading preventable causes of death and disability (NZMOH and Accident Compensation Corporation [ACC] 2013; AIHW 2012a). Among New Zealanders, males account for nearly three-quarters of injury-related health loss with over half of all injury-related health loss occurring in those under 35 years of age (NZMOH and ACC 2013). Once again, rates of injury-related health loss are greater for Māori than non-Māori with health loss from assault four times higher among Māori (NZMOH and ACC 2013). Alcohol, fatigue, sleepiness and speeding are the main causes of motor vehicle accidents, with young men over-represented among the victims, especially Indigenous men and those from rural and remote areas (AIHW 2012a). Over the past decade, Australia, New Zealand and other Western countries have had significant declines in the rate of motor vehicle injuries due, in part, to improved public education programs, better law enforcement, stricter penalties, better roads and improvement in vehicle safety design. There is also increasing recognition that risky driving behaviours are embedded in a pattern of risky behaviours, as we discussed in Chapter 9. This indicates that the most effective approach for accident prevention is by addressing the cluster of risky behaviours within the context and structures that support them. Ensuring incorporation of all the elements of the Ottawa Charter for Health Promotion will support this approach.

Chronic conditions

Most health concerns revolve around the more insidious conditions of daily life that cause pain, impairments, stress and reduced quality of life. These include asthma, type 2 diabetes, ischaemic heart disease, cerebrovascular disease, arthritis, osteoporosis, chronic obstructive pulmonary disease (COPD), depression and high blood pressure (AIHW 2012a). Respiratory conditions, especially those such as asthma and COPD, create the greatest burden of disease in Australia (AIHW 2012a) whereas in New Zealand it is coronary heart disease (NZMOH 2013a). Respiratory conditions and heart disease often cause lifelong suffering, and are the most commonly managed problems in general practice (AIHW 2012a). These, and any of the other chronic conditions, can cause persistent pain, which affects quality of life in several ways, not only by causing disablement, but in affecting mood, mental wellbeing and disrupted sleep patterns, which, in turn, affects relationships, work and social role participation (Graham & Streitel 2010).

THE BIG PICTURE

Long-term or chronic conditions are the most urgent concern for Australian and New Zealand adults. Many of these are linked to modifiable lifestyle factors.

The global picture of health shows that chronic diseases related to lifestyle factors continue to grow, and are now the most significant cause of mortality worldwide, causing 63% of deaths (WHO 2012). The tragedy is that people everywhere are dying from preventable causes such as unhealthy diets, physical inactivity and tobacco use. Cardiovascular disease is the number one cause of death globally, obesity has doubled in the past 30 years, more than 347 million people worldwide have diabetes and mental ill health is often comorbid with each of these conditions (WHO 2012). It is estimated that 35% of the Australian population and 49.5% of the New Zealand population has at least one chronic condition, increasing to 78% among those over age 65 (AIHW 2012a; Holt 2010). Asthma and depression are the most common comorbid conditions among younger adults, with arthritis and high blood pressure the most common for those over age 45 (AIHW 2012a; Holt 2010).

THE TOP 2 RISKS: CARDIOVASCULAR DISEASE (CVD) AND TYPE 2 DIABETES

THE DEADLY RISK CLUSTER

- Tobacco smoking
- Inactivity
- Overweight, obese
- High-fat, high-salt diet
- High alcohol consumption
- High blood pressure
- High cholesterol (LDL)

Cardiovascular disease (CVD) includes all diseases and conditions of the heart and blood vessels, such as coronary artery disease (CAD) and stroke, which are responsible for the largest proportion of deaths throughout the world, including Australia and New Zealand (AIHW 2012a; Hamerton et al. 2012). Most of the SDH affect a person's risks or assets in relation to these diseases. Important structural determinants of CVD and type 2 diabetes include economic resources, education, living and working conditions, social support and access to health care (AIHW 2012a). Some members of the population also have inherent risks of developing either or both of these diseases because of age, sex, family history or ethnicity; however, the cluster of factors that create the highest risks are those that are modifiable through healthy lifestyles. The cluster is composed of tobacco smoking, physical inactivity, being overweight or obese, having a diet high in saturated fats, high alcohol consumption, high blood pressure and hyperlipidemia (high LDL cholesterol) (AIHW 2012a). These lifestyle factors create co-morbid risks, as those with type 2 diabetes are also at risk of coronary heart disease (CHD) and stroke (AIHW 2012a). These conditions are of serious concern to health planners, particularly with increasing rates of chronic conditions among Indigenous and Māori populations in Australia and New Zealand (AIHW 2012a; Hamerton et al. 2012). The prevalence of diabetes has doubled in the Australian population over the past 15 years, to 4.1% of non-Indigenous adults, with rates among Indigenous people three times greater. More than half of Indigenous diabetics also have CVD, and, like other Australians, many also experience mental illness (AIHW 2012a). In New Zealand, the overall prevalence of diabetes is 7% with the rate for Māori at 9.8% and for Pacific people at 15.4% (Coppell et al. 2013). While the rates for Pacific people are particularly high, of greatest concern is the ratio of undiagnosed to diagnosed diabetes among Pacific people at 5:4. This compares to 10:3 among Māori and 10:1 among New Zealand European and other groups (Coppell et al. 2013), suggesting that significant work remains to be done in terms of diagnosing and supporting Pacific people with diabetes in New Zealand.

LIFESTYLE AND THE CLUSTER OF RISKS

Although there have been some improvements in lifestyle behaviours since the new century, around 99% of adults have at least one risk factor; most have three, and 17% of men and 11% of women have five or more, with the largest proportion being those who live in disadvantaged areas (AIHW 2012a). Many adults in Australia and New Zealand continue to smoke and drink alcohol at excessive levels, especially young Indigenous people living in rural and remote areas (AIHW 2012a). Although levels of smoking have decreased to less than 20% of the adult population, alcohol consumption continues to be problematic. Harmful consumption of alcohol is a risk factor for 1 in 5 members of the adult population, which is a severe risk, given that alcohol is a causal factor in 60 types of diseases and injuries (AIHW 2012a). Alcohol is also a factor in a considerable number of assaults, including intimate partner violence (IPV), which makes alcohol consumption not only risky for the drinker but dangerous for other victims.

In our obesogenic environments, the level of physical activity continues to decline, especially among women, with 60% of all Australian adults and 46% of New Zealanders failing to meet the national guidelines of 30 minutes a day of exercise (AIHW 2012a; NZMOH 2012c). Interestingly, in New Zealand there are only negligible differences between Māori and non-Māori adults in their level of physical activity, with 53.5% of Māori adults meeting physical activity guidelines compared with 52.6% of Pacific peoples and 48.9% of European New Zealanders (Hamerton et al. 2012). In Australia, participation in sport and physical recreation is declining each year, which is concurrent with an increase in leisure time spent watching TV or other screen activities. Many people do not adhere to a nutritious diet, with insufficient daily fruit and vegetables, and a propensity to drink whole (rather than skim) milk products (an indicator of saturated fat) (AIHW 2012a). In New Zealand, seven in ten adults eat the recommended number of vegetable servings per day and six in ten meet the recommended fruit intake (NZMOH 2012c). People living in more deprived areas are less likely to eat the recommended fruit and vegetable intake (NZMOH 2012c), suggesting that the high cost of fruit when compared with other, less nutritious foods may have an impact on this. With busy lives, many urban dwellers especially, access fast food outlets, consuming too many high-salt, high-fat, energy-dense foods. These factors, combined with the implications of poverty in New Zealand, have led to overweight and obesity in epidemic proportions (WHO 2012). Australian and New Zealand men have the second highest rate of obesity among OECD countries. Australian women have the fifth highest rate, with New Zealand women slightly higher still (AIHW 2012a). This includes 25% of Australian adults, most of whom live in disadvantaged conditions, including 34% who are Indigenous (AIHW 2012a). Although individual behaviours play a major role in lifestyles, social conditions in the community and social environment determine the extent to which different groups are able to make lifestyle changes.

PRACTICE STRATEGY

Nurses who are overweight are often criticised by their peers on the basis that they should be better role models.

How do you think the profession should deal with both sides of this issue?

THE COMPLEX PROBLEM OF OBESITY

The 'obesity epidemic' is placing large numbers of adults at risk for metabolic syndrome, type 2 diabetes and cardiovascular disease (CVD) as well as some cancers (WHO 2012). As we mentioned above, overweight and obesity are at epidemic proportions among the Australian and New Zealand populations. In most Western countries the indicators of overweight and obesity are calculated as a simple index of weight-for-height—as weight in kilograms divided by the square of height (kg/m^2). The benchmark for overweight is a Body Mass Index (BMI) between $25 \ kg/m^2$ and $30 \ kg/m^2$ and for obesity, a BMI greater than $30 \ kg/m^2$ (WHO 2012). The prevalence of overweight and obesity is alarming because of the relationship between high BMI and CVD, type 2 diabetes, musculoskeletal disorders and some cancers (WHO 2012). Obesity creates a multiplier effect to these diseases by creating disability that lasts for many years.

Obesity is not only a constraint on the health, wellbeing and quality of life of the population, but also presents a significant drain on health care resources (WHO 2012). This is expected to worsen with higher rates of obesity among children and younger adults creating a longer term, and therefore more costly, burden for the health system (WHO 2012). The need for behavioural interventions to help stem the epidemic of overweight and obesity is clear, particularly in balancing exercise and a healthy diet. However, as with smoking, obesogenic environments influence lifestyle choices. Globalisation and technological innovations have transformed work processes into passive, monitoring-type activities. Together with shrinking spaces in our communities for parks and bicycle pathways, we are confronted with a protracted, serious population health issue. Disparities in access to culturally appropriate supports in the physical environment also play a part in whether or not people can take advantage of resources (Hamerton et al. 2012).

The obesogenic factors in our environments are compounded and reinforced when calorie-dense foods are marketed and accessible throughout the community (WHO 2012). These conditions need to be recognised by all members of the general public, to counter the stigma attached to obese people in the community. Stigmatising people for being overweight is based on a common view that weight is easily controlled by disciplined individual decisions to exercise more and eat less. This type of discrimination is personal and it can evoke strong emotions (Walsh & Fahy 2012). The diet industry has some responsibility for marketing appropriate foods, and food labelling is sometimes misleading. It is important to recognise that there is variable quality among fats and carbohydrates, which can play a role in the development of type 2 diabetes (Hu 2011). For example, 'low fat' may not mean 'low salt' or 'low sugar', which can create a false sense that there are no harmful ingredients in the product. Some breads and cereals contain inordinate amounts of salt, trans fats or high glycemic loads, yet these are advertised as health foods. A large meta-analysis of studies showed how important it is to use discretion when selecting foods, finding that a two-serving-per-day increment in whole grain intake was associated with a 21% lower risk of diabetes (de Munter et al. 2007). In addition to checking individual food items, some diets are better than others. For example, the typical Mediterranean diet is known to have a higher protective effect against CVD risk factors compared with a low-fat diet, because of what it contains, as well as the cultural context of healthy eating patterns. The Mediterranean diet consists of high consumption of olive oil, legumes, unrefined cereals, fruits, vegetables, moderate consumption of dairy products (cheese and yogurts), moderate to high consumption of fish, low consumption of meat and moderate wine consumption (Martinez-Gonzalez et al. 2009). Equally as important is the fact that Mediterranean families tend to have regular family mealtimes, which also illustrates the cultural context of healthy eating (Martinez-Gonzalez et al. 2009).

For people who are already obese or who have been diagnosed with chronic illnesses, nutrition counselling is often a first step in making lifestyle improvements. Advice needs to be tailored to individual needs, as a one-size-fits-all prescription for healthy eating may present barriers for certain individuals. Many people live in circumstances that prevent them from adopting healthy lifestyle practices that may be appropriate for someone else. Some of these circumstances that act as barriers to change include pregnancy, living in a situation where they have little personal support or are subjected to ridicule from family members or close friends, or having co-morbidities. Any of the chronic conditions may change a person's appetite and attitude to food as well as their access to preferred products. Some diabetics, for example, have difficulty with the constant food vigilance that can be involved in managing their condition. They may feel uncomfortable eating with others, or have variable treatment regimes. Statin treatments for lowering cholesterol also come with contraindications for certain foods because they effect changes to metabolism. Motivation can also be a barrier to behaviour change. Many people live alone these days and those with chronic disease, limited finances, functional difficulties or who suffer from loneliness, anxiety or depression may simply fail to take the time to prepare appropriate meals.

STRATEGY FOR ACTION

Nutrition counselling needs to be tailored to meet individual needs. Cultural imperatives, the social context of eating and motivation influence the ability of individuals to make the dietary changes they need to maintain good health.

Social, cultural and environmental factors are important in promoting lifestyle changes, especially those intended to increase exercise and other activities. Organised physical activities at the neighbourhood level can provide opportunities to develop supportive social networks as well as helping manage chronic conditions, or preventing further deterioration once a person has experienced an acute episode such as a cardiac event. The environmental determinants for healthy lifestyles include safe walkways, cycleways and well-lit streets to allow working people to exercise and socialise after working hours. Intersectoral planning by engineering, transportation, recreation, health and education professionals can help make neighbourhoods conducive to activities. Studies have shown that group exercise programs for cardiac rehabilitation are effective in improving physical and mental wellbeing, reducing anxiety and isolation and enhancing quality of life (Shepherd & While 2012). These programs are crucial for those having suffered a heart attack, who are often either tentative about exercising because of fear, or who over-exercise to show that they have recovered. In some cases, cardiac survivors become anxious, depressed and socially isolated, which can affect their family and other relationships (Shepherd & While 2012). Structured group exercise programs tend to create a feeling of wellbeing that can enhance value, belongingness and attachment to others, which builds social capital. At a personal level, exercise boosts immune functions, enhances anti-tumour activity and has shown positive effects on depression, anxiety, stress, self-esteem, Alzheimer's disease, pain and premenstrual syndrome (Street et al. 2007). For this reason, 'sweat' has been called the natural antidepressant. It is visible in the group photographed below, who meet twice weekly for free Tai Chi sessions on Burleigh Beach, courtesy of Gold Coast Council's commitment to an 'Active and Healthy Gold Coast'. Box 10.1 discusses research into the various factors that contribute to the positive impact of exercise.

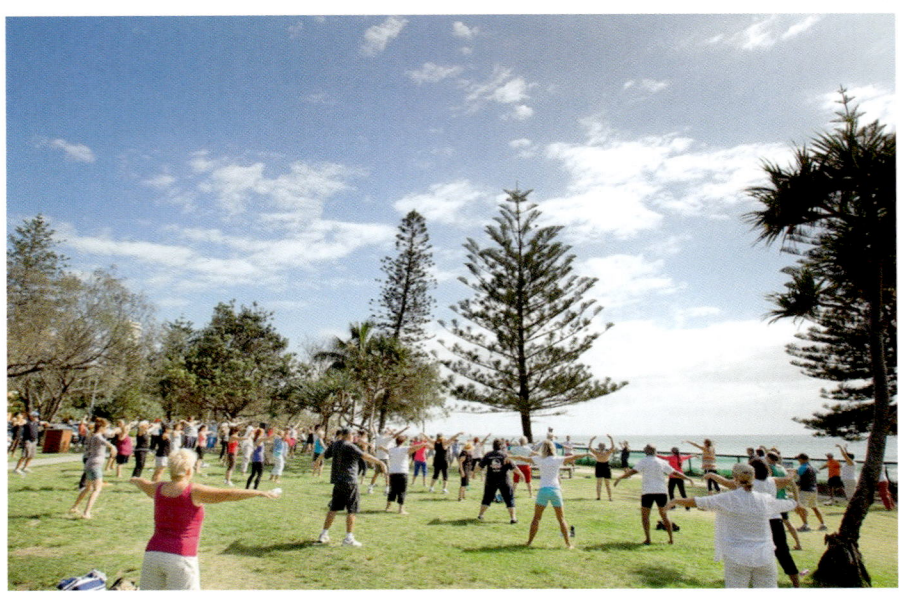

Tai Chi on Burleigh Heads (photo courtesy of Gold Coast City Council)

BOX 10.1 **Exercise: is it physical?**

Despite years of research, much remains to be learned about exercise: what works, for whom, in what context. In comparing the impact of exercise in different groups of people, a meta-analysis of quality-of-life improvements from exercise interventions showed that exercise had less effect on those with chronic disease than rehabilitation patients or well adults (Gillison et al. 2009). Researchers have also compared individually based programs with group programs aimed at weight control and activity (Critchley et al. 2012). Despite a burgeoning personal trainer industry, group programs seem to have better outcomes, as they have also been associated with changes in mood, cognition, motivation and self-efficacy about participants' ability to make changes (Critchley et al. 2012). However, it is yet to be shown whether mood is the only mediating factor or whether there are combinations of psychological factors that lead to changes in diet and exercise (Critchley et al. 2012). Critchley and colleagues conducted a randomised control trial (RCT) to compare group versus individual interventions in a sample of pre-diabetic Australian adults, and found that group

programs had better outcomes in terms of healthy lifestyle improvements. They then used Prochaska et al.'s (1992) Stages of Change theory (see Chapter 6) to examine the pathways to change. They found that education was a significant aspect of the program as it increased knowledge of diabetes as well as improving mood. Together these factors enhanced weight control. The research team concluded that education can help people feel more positive (improved mood), which motivates them to act on their knowledge. It is possible that the two factors (education and mood) go hand in hand. Their findings concur with a previous study of Australian men who reported that just exercising was not as enjoyable as sports, explaining that sporting activities had the added advantage of the team spirit and obligation to team-mates (Burton et al. 2008). The implication for health promotion suggests a 'common sense' approach; that is, exercise programs need to be socially contextualised and fun.

? What do you think would help advance this body of evidence?

RURAL LIFESTYLES: HEALTH, PLACE AND RISKS

The relationship between health and place is an important element of the social context that creates lifestyle risks. Urban living has risks from crime, neighbourhood violence, various air, water and food pollutants, motor vehicles and a proliferation of fast food outlets. However, compared to urban dwellers, people living in regional or rural areas, many of whom are Indigenous, are at significantly higher risk of chronic illness through being overweight or obese (AIHW 2012a). Some of the factors related to high rates of obesity in rural areas include low education and health literacy, inherited behaviours, consumption of processed rather than fresh foods, a shortage of dieticians and other health professionals, insufficient resources to support maternal and child health, and a lack of funding and personnel available to run exercise and other health promotion activities (Berends et al. 2011).

Responses to these issues require political commitment to ensure that adequate nutritious foods are not only available but affordable for rural people. Health promotion strategies that revolve around health literacy and empowering people to take control over their lifestyles are important, but these are often hampered by a lack of access to resources. Unlike urban dwellers many rural people do not have opportunities for group sports or other activities, and many regional towns and rural areas do not have access to green parks, exercise playgrounds for children or safe walking trails close to schools. When they need assistance, there are few specialists available to treat chronic illnesses or to offer them preventative programs. In addition to supportive services and programs, the 'digital divide' between those with and without access to internet information can worsen inequities by preventing the level of education enjoyed by people in the city.

LIFESTYLE, HEALTH AND PLACE

High rates of obesity in rural areas can be linked to low education and health literacy, a shortage of dieticians and other health professionals, inherited behaviours and few opportunities to participate in healthy lifestyle groups.

As we mentioned in Chapter 2, where patients need to travel for treatments such as dialysis, cancer care or treatment for mental health problems, there is also social, emotional and cultural isolation as well as economic pressures. Rural people also have considerable lifestyle stress due to their occupations, which can be dependent on the vagaries of the weather as well as the economic uncertainty of their lifestyles. For young adults, the loneliness of life in rural and regional areas can lead to relationship breakdown and depression, which can set individuals on a path to over-consumption of alcohol or other substances (Berends et al. 2011). Rural residents with same-sex preferences can also be alienated from others in the community, especially given the cultural dominance of values such as masculinity and rugged individualism. Mental health issues emanating from their feeling of social exclusion are often ignored by rural residents who tend to be stoical, believing they can take care of things themselves, or can be hesitant to seek help in a small community, where others would take note of their actions. In some cases, unacknowledged depression and other mental health issues can lead to suicide, especially where firearms and poisons such as pesticides are readily available. These reasons are often cited as explanations for the relatively high rate of suicide among rural males (Farmer et al. 2012). Box 10.2 discusses the work of Federated Farmers New Zealand in increasing awareness of mental health issues in rural communities.

THE GLOBALISATION OF LIFESTYLE RISKS: EAST MEETS WEST

Another link to health and place lies in the globalisation of diabetes (Hu 2011). The global economy has dramatically accelerated the growth in obesity to such a degree that Asia is now the global epicentre of diabetes, containing 60% of the world's diabetics (Hu 2011). Trade liberalisation has inadvertently contributed to this epidemic through making edible oils and sugar more accessible and cheaper than in the past, which has encouraged greater consumption of sugar and fats among Asian populations (Hu 2011). Rapid economic development and urbanisation in countries like China have led to lower physical demands, as the workforce moves from agricultural to manufacturing and technological jobs that require less energy expenditure. The dietary transitions and decline in physical activity have led to insulin resistance, which is accompanied by a shift in metabolism to an adverse resistance to carbohydrates, including white rice, which is a staple of the Asian diet (Hu 2011). A further metabolic risk

BOX 10.2 Federated Farmers New Zealand

Federated Farmers is a New Zealand organisation that lobbies on farming issues both nationally and within each province. Membership of the organisation is voluntary and there are over 26 000 members. One of Federated Farmers most recent campaigns is the 'Life's a bitch' campaign aimed at increasing awareness of mental health issues among farmers. Federated Farmers not only want better resources for mental health in rural communities, but they are also providing farmers with wallet cards on the signs and symptoms of mental health issues and where to go for help. A number of farmers have come forward to share their stories as part of the campaign. Paul Bourke, a farmer from rural Taranaki who suffered from depression, is highly supportive of the campaign and says mental health is about caring for your mates (O'Dowd 2013). Often, farmers find it easier to discuss weather or grass growth rather than issues such as the loss of loved ones to cancer, accidental road death or the death of a child, making campaigns such as this one important for raising community awareness. Further information on the campaign can be found at: www.fedfarm.org.nz/advocacy/National-Policy/Rural-Mental-Health.asp.

? So what does this tell us?

Depression is an insidious problem throughout society, and it is affecting many farmers and their families. Caring for rural communities first requires understanding of the many aspects of society that affect their lives.

Is there an appropriate program or initiative that would help draw attention to the health promotion needs of a rural community in your region?

is related to biological embedding and the pathway to adult development. The dramatic transition from severe undernutrition in utero to a nutritionally rich environment in later life as people adopt Western diets creates metabolic and structural changes that increase the risk of insulin resistance (Hu 2011).

Genetics and ethnicity also play an important role in the cycle of risk. The Asian body phenotype does not resemble other ethnic groups who tend to accumulate larger masses of abdominal fat from Western diets. Instead, many Asian people have a higher ratio of abdominal fat and a lower muscle mass, which elevates the threshold for developing insulin resistance, increasing the risk of diabetes at a lower BMI than Europeans (Hu 2011). The effect of this increased threshold is that many Asian people develop diabetes at a younger age and with lower weight gain than other ethnic groups. Asian women also have a higher risk for gestational diabetes, which puts their children at risk of type 2 diabetes in later life (Hu 2011). Adding to this dilemma is the fact that many Asian people continue to smoke, especially in China, which is the greatest producer of cigarettes in the world. Smoking can promote abdominal fat accumulation and further insulin resistance, which compounds the level of risk for these people (Hu 2011).

These changes, and Western dietary practices being adopted on migration to Western countries, have created a high level of risk for many Asian cultures migrating to Australia and New Zealand. Asian people constitute 33% of the overseas born migrants in the Australian community, and approximately 9.2% in the New Zealand community (ABS 2013; Statistics New Zealand 2013b). With the length of time these people live in our countries, the 'healthy migrant effect'—that is, the health advantage seen in immigrants who have been selected for migration on the basis of good health— disappears, and their health becomes more closely aligned with other Australians and New Zealanders (AIHW 2012a; Davidson et al. 2011; Hajat et al. 2010). As a result, our Asian migrants tend to experience declining health over time. Another layer of risk is created by the tendency to avoid seeking help. Although various cultural groups are not homogeneous, Western dietary patterns, low levels of physical activity in the workplace and community can be exacerbated by cultural predispositions to avoid seeking care from Western health care providers (Davidson et al. 2011). Many older Asian migrants are passive in expressing their needs; they may hesitate to seek or adhere to advice or care, preferring instead to retain traditional

A VICIOUS CIRCLE OF MIGRANT RISK

- Global trade reducing the cost of sugars and fats
- Genetic, biological factors
- Western dietary practices
- Low physical workplace demands
- Inadequate public transportation
- Few cycleways, walkways
- Cultural preferences for traditional health practices

family-oriented solutions to health issues (Davidson et al. 2011). To provide help at the individual, community and societal levels it is important to conduct careful, culturally sensitive assessment of intergenerational lifestyle patterns as a basis for developing solutions that are tailored to their individual and collective needs.

Stress, Mental Health and the SDH

Psychosocial stress, especially chronic stress, is a significant risk factor for many illnesses (Frisvold et al. 2012). Stress emanates from many areas of daily life and can be both a cause and consequence of mental illness (WHO 2009). From a socio-ecological perspective, stress needs to be seen less in terms of individual pathology and more as a response to relative deprivation and social injustice (Viner et al. 2012; Wilkinson 1996; WHO 2009). As we have discussed previously, inequalities along a social gradient are created when the SDH are distributed unevenly, leaving some people living in disadvantaged conditions. The stress of social injustice affects many people across the settings of their lives, creating the risk of depression, anxiety and a range of other responses. Stress is even greater for those with chronic conditions, disabilities or those without transportation, as they rely more heavily than others on local services and facilities. For these groups, the effects of incivilities such as neighbourhood crime, vandalism and conflict, are also experienced more intensely than others (Raphael 2009; Warr et al. 2009).

At the individual level, chronic stress 'gets under the skin' through neuro-endocrine, cardiovascular and immune systems (WHO 2009). This occurs through disruptions to neuro-endocrine and metabolic systems from the constant stress of living disempowered lives (Raphael 2009). These responses can elevate cortisol, cholesterol, blood pressure and inflammation. Psychosocial reactions such as anger and despair related to occupational insecurity, poverty, debt, poor housing, exclusion or other indicators of low status can lead to health-damaging behaviours such as smoking, alcohol consumption or poor dietary habits as well as having a negative impact on intimate relationships, self-care and the care of children (WHO 2009). In addition, many health services struggle to put equity principles into practice meaning those experiencing these difficulties are further disadvantaged by poor access to care (Sheridan et al. 2011). This insight into the psychobiological pathways to ill health highlights the integral nature of mental and physical health.

Mental health is a feeling of wellbeing, perceived self-efficacy, autonomy, competence, intergenerational dependence and recognition of the ability to realize one's intellectual and emotional potential. It has also been defined as a state of wellbeing whereby individuals recognize their abilities, are able to cope with the normal stresses of life, work productively and fruitfully, and make a contribution to their communities.

(WHO 2003:7)

Health, wellbeing, stress and the family

> **TRUE OR FALSE?**
> Is it marriage that creates better health?

Among the most pronounced sources of stress in adult life are those related to family events such as separation, divorce, death or illness of a family member, abuse or economic hardship. Early family life can have a cumulative effect across the adult lifespan, particularly if the marital relationship is not satisfying for both partners. Poor relationships can have a negative influence on cardiovascular, endocrine, immune and neurosensory function, while positive relationships can provide a supportive context for dealing with stress or illness (Windsor et al. 2009). Social scientists have gathered considerable research demonstrating that married people enjoy better mental health than people who are separated, divorced or have never been married (Uecker 2012). Adults in marriage and de facto relationships tend to have fewer mental health issues and a lower rate of suicidal thoughts and behaviours than those who live their adult lives alone (Johnston et al. 2009). The marriage advantage is a result of social attachment and support, which seems to create psychological wellbeing; that is, positive affect and the absence of distress (Uecker 2012). The effect of mutual support is related to the *interdependency*, rather than *dependency* of the relationship, wherein people are able to develop a sense of control or mastery over their environments (Windsor et al. 2009). However, some people suffering from anxiety or depression find family relationships difficult, and they tend to disengage, rather than draw on family resources, which can exacerbate rather than ameliorate stress (Wadsworth et al. 2011). This is particularly problematic for parenting, where children need the warmth and attentiveness of their parents.

MENTAL HEALTH, ILLNESS AND THE SDH

Health, wellbeing and how people think, feel and relate to one another are socially determined. These outcomes are linked to social position and people's sense of coherence or meaning in life, as well as their cognitive, emotional and social relations with others (Henderson 2012). Unequal life conditions can have a major impact on a person's mental health, if how they think, feel and relate causes low self-esteem, shame and disrespect (Raphael 2009; WHO 2009). Feeling disempowered or unsupported can lead to discouragement about seeking an education, low perseverance in overcoming workplace or social relationship difficulties, general hesitance to participate in community life and low use of health services. The effects can be profound, as psycho-social factors such as mood disorders, lack of social support and isolation create the same level of risk to health as smoking, high blood pressure and elevated cholesterol (WHO 2009).

PSYCHOLOGICAL WELLBEING

- Positive affect
- Absence of distress

Worldwide, there is a rising prevalence of persistent mental illness, particularly depression, which is a major contributor to the global burden of mental illness (Holm & Severinsson 2012; Thorpe 2012). As many as 45% of Australian adults to age 85 have experienced a mental illness at some time in their lives, with 1 in 9 having a comorbid mental and physical disorder, the most common being CHD, type 2 diabetes and depression or anxiety (AIHW 2012a). In New Zealand 1 in 7 adults report they have been diagnosed with a common mental health disorder (NZMOH 2012c). Women and those living in more deprived areas are more likely to have been diagnosed with a mental health disorder and, as is

---

MENTALLY ILL AT WORK

- High demands
- Job insecurity
- Low reward or opportunity to use skills
- Low authority
- Interpersonal relationships
- Inadequate support
- Discrimination

---

evidenced elsewhere, these figures are increasing (NZMOH 2012c).

The cycle of disadvantage for the mentally ill is particularly evident in the world of work (OECD 2008, 2011). Those with a mental disorder are twice as likely as others to be unemployed, which is a greater risk to health than 'killer' diseases such as CHD (Thorpe 2012:S15). For those who do have a job, their mental health problems can be exacerbated in the workplace by high psychological demands, job insecurity, lack of reward or opportunity to use skills, low decision-making authority, difficult relationships and inadequate support (OECD 2008; Pasca & Wagner 2011). Workers with mental illness also suffer disproportionately from casual employment, discrimination or attitudinal barriers to inclusion, particularly immigrant workers, leaving them at risk of chronic disability or suicide (OECD 2008; Pasca & Wagner 2011). In the face of discrimination, those with mental illness tend to underperform in their jobs rather than take sick leave when they need it (OECD 2008, 2011). Mental health issues have thus become the second most frequent occupational health issue worldwide, after musculoskeletal conditions, affecting 1 in 5 workers (OECD 2008, 2011). This is because workers spend so much of their lives in the workplace, with little respite from stressful situations.

STIGMA, SOCIAL EXCLUSION AND MENTAL ILLNESS

STIGMA

- Ignorance
- Prejudice
- Discrimination

Some social conditions surrounding adult life can cause stress and stress-related disease for disadvantaged individuals, not only through economic deprivation, but through disproportionate exposure to prejudice and discrimination (Meyer et al. 2008). These attitudes usually arise from ignorance, failing to understand the notion of 'difference' (SANE 2013). Obvious examples of discrimination are perpetrated on the basis of race, gender, mental illness or other personal characteristics. Stigma against those with mental illness is common. It stops people from seeking help, finding accommodation, a job, mortgage, insurance, friends and self-belief (SANE 2013). People with a mental illness are discriminated against by media images of stereotyped, dangerous, violent mentally ill people perpetrating all kinds of bad behaviour on the rest of society. The effect of stigma can be destructive and life changing, as surveys of the mentally ill in Australia by the Wesley Mission and in New Zealand by the 'Like Minds, Like Mine' anti-discrimination campaign (discussed below) have found. Both studies revealed that the social exclusion experienced by those with mental illness had severe impacts on their personal, family and community life (SANE 2013).

CONSIDER THIS

A job applicant who explains a two-year gap in their resume by mentioning chemotherapy is treated differently than one who explains it on the basis of a psychiatric hospitalisation (SANE 2013).

In the absence of social support, some people are socially excluded on a number of fronts. They may be marginalised through exclusion from certain social activities in their local community because of non-conformity or personal behaviours. At a societal level, they may be excluded from secure, permanent employment, sufficient earnings, access to credit or land; housing and adequate consumption of necessities; education, skills and cultural capital; welfare, citizenship and legal equality; democratic participation, public goods, family and sociability, humanity, respect, fulfilment and understanding (Meyer et al. 2008; SANE 2013). Further, the nature of the neighbourhood in which people live may compound the impact of mental illness: increased social fragmentation in communities is associated with poorer mental health—particularly for women (Ivory et al. 2011). Mental health patients also encounter stigma in the health care system, with many being either 'shunned' or told to lower their expectations (Mental Health Council of Australia 2011). All of these aspects of social exclusion constitute institutionalised stressors. Yet few disclose their condition or complain, some because of self-stigmatising (see Box 10.3), and others hesitating because it is too difficult to work through agencies such as the Australian Human Rights Commission or other bureaucracies that are mired in complexities (SANE 2013).

WHAT'S YOUR OPINION?

Culture and cultural beliefs can have a profound impact on mental health. Is this a positive or negative impact, or both?

In some cases, cultural norms may exacerbate states of mental ill health. Certain cultures recognise anxiety, depression, grief, stress or worry as merely problems in living, and therefore they do not warrant help seeking (Davidson et al. 2011). Other cultures have a broader perspective on mental health and ill health. An Australian study of people's perceptions of mental health found that the three most common factors contributing to positive mental health were having good friends to talk problems over with, keeping an active mind and having control over one's life (Donovan et al. 2007). The same cohort described being mentally *unhealthy* in terms of excessive use of alcohol or drugs, having no friends or support network, and life crises or traumas (Donovan et al. 2007). At the extreme end of the continuum is homelessness, where those disadvantaged by a lack of employment and housing live in a vicious circle of vulnerability to ill health, injury, violence and a lack of social support.

In 1997, New Zealand began a publically funded campaign called 'Like Minds, Like Mine'. The campaign was one of the first in the world aimed at reducing discrimination and stigma associated with mental illness. Using a combination of community action at a local level with nationwide strategies and media advertising, the campaign has led to increased acceptance and openness in the community about mental illness (NZMOH 2007). A cost-benefit analysis of the campaign looking specifically at the effect on employment and use of primary care services has found a 13.8 : 1 benefit; that is, the $52 million dollars spent on the campaign has generated an economic benefit of approximately $720 million (Vaithianathan & Pram 2010). Although change has occurred in people's attitudes toward those with mental health issues, the campaign continues today to ensure changes in behaviour, policies and practice follow the changes already achieved in attitudes (NZMOH 2007; SANE 2013). This is important as a survey of mental health service users in New Zealand in 2010 found that 70% had experienced moderate levels of unfair treatment from family and friends (Wyllie & Brown 2011). New initiatives to help those with mental illness have followed in Australia, with the Better Access and Personal Helpers and Mentors programs, beyondblue and headspace, which we mentioned in Chapter 9, and early intervention centres such as Mindful Employer, a program to improve understanding and reduce stigma in the workplace. However, at the highest level, the mental illness share of the Australian budget continues to shrink, which in itself is discriminating (SANE 2013).

The recommendations outlined in Box 10.3 apply to all settings in our communities but are

BOX 10.3 Solutions to the revolving door of self-stigma

The New Zealand report on self-stigma *Fighting Shadows* has drawn attention to the fact that many people with mental illness self-stigmatise and become isolated, alienated and withdrawn (SANE 2013). The report identified eight recommendations to disrupt the cycle of stigma and discrimination as follows:

- Recognise the contribution of the mentally ill and foster leadership.
- Celebrate and accept difference.
- Affirm human rights.
- Encourage disclosure.
- Encourage recovery-oriented practices.
- Encourage empowerment.
- Support peer support services.
- Challenge attitudes and behaviour

(Source: Peterson et al. in SANE 2013)

particularly relevant for those in the workplace who experience discrimination. Many of these recommendations are also applicable to non-mentally ill workers who may be experiencing stress and dysfunctional workplace relationships.

WORKPLACE STRESS

Workplace stress is a serious problem in today's society, incurring a cost to industry and the health system, as well as the personal costs of distress. Because it affects adults at all stages of their working life, it is also becoming an increasing issue for nurses working in home, family and community settings. Sources of job stress can include overwork, shift work or irregular schedules as well as workplace relationships. Shift work has the additional disadvantage of compromising workers' lifestyle behaviours by reducing access to good nutrition and opportunities for physical activity. A study that looked specifically at nurses aged over 50 and their experiences of shift work found that while shift work suited many, for others it had deleterious effects on family and social relationships, and physical and mental health (in particular sleep patterns and fatigue). In addition, participants indicated they experienced decreasing tolerance for shift work as they aged (Clendon & Walker 2013). Irregular schedules and shift work can also cause chronic fatigue, sleep disturbances and other stress-

related illnesses (Huntington et al. 2011). Bambra et al. (2008) explain the problem as psychological and social desynchronisation, where the worker experiences disharmony, or is 'out of sync' within their body.

WHAT'S YOUR OPINION?

One of the most stressful workplaces is the health care environment. Why do you think health care professionals who are educated to promote health are at risk of experiencing the greatest levels of stress?

The nursing profession has a level of risk that is among the highest of all occupations (Frisvold et al. 2012), due to 'compassion fatigue', work intensification practices, and high workloads as well as variable schedules (Preston 2009). In 2007 New Zealand introduced flexible working arrangements with the passing of the *Employment Relations (Flexible Working Arrangements) Amendment Act* (NZ Govt, Online. Available: www.dol.govt.nz/er/bestpractice/worklife/flexiblework/ [accessed 26 August 2013]). The Act gives people the right to negotiate flexible working arrangements under certain circumstances. In 2010 Australia followed suit by introducing National Employment Standards that do the same thing (ABS 2010). This initiative is intended to help workers meet their family needs, but sometimes flexible schedules can create difficulties by preventing the type of respite that can be gained from a whole day or weekend off work. The need to negotiate can also be difficult for those who are not used to dealing with managers and who prefer to just take whatever work they can do to prevent any future difficulties. Some stressors in the health care environment also come from violent patients, or exposure to allergens and harmful chemicals as well as infectious agents.

Stress is also generated from organisational climate, especially where work objectives are unclear, unattainable, not shared or visionary, and where workers are not involved in decision-making (Ylipaavainiemi et al. 2005). Studies of nursing in a positive work climate where the leadership cultivates feelings of common beliefs and values have found that nurses engage in 'discretionary performance'; that is, they go the extra mile because they feel good about being in the organisation (Snow 2002). Positive work environments are also related to better patient outcomes—patients are significantly less likely to die in hospitals with higher nurse work environment quality than in hospitals with lower ratings (Schubert et al. 2012). Nurses' decisions and professional behaviours are also not as careful when the organisational climate is stressful (King 2010). A stressful or careless organisational climate can have serious outcomes, including medication errors (Symons & McMurray 2013), failing to establish a supportive environment for new graduates (Laschinger et al. 2013), or a general inattentiveness to patient safety (King 2010). A healthy workplace climate is characterised by mutual support. Helping others cope with existing stress or preventing stress from causing unhealthy behaviours is also personal. For both formal and informal caregivers, a stressful environment can lead coping reserves to be tapped to the limits (Frisvold et al. 2012). Stress is particularly hard on caregiving women, including nurses, who often find themselves part of the 'sandwich generation' caring for both their children and their ageing parents. The high levels of caregiving stress experienced during this time often coincide with the perimenopause decade of their lives, when they are most at risk of cardiovascular disease and other stress-linked conditions (Frisvold et al. 2012). Some also have the multiple risks of poor diets, inactivity, alcohol and tobacco consumption, all of which add to their stress rather than relieving it.

Workplace stressors affect members of cultural and socio-economic groups differently, but in general, workplace stress is becoming more prevalent across all categories of workers. This is linked to changing social conditions. Life in the 21st century has become fast-paced for many adults, with resounding effects on the family, the workplace and society. The 'busyness' of lifestyles and changes in workplace demands, such as intermittent schedules, and workplaces that demand total absorption on the job, are major sources of stress (Bianchi & Milkie 2010). Workplace policies also affect home life. Some, but not all, countries have flexible workplace policies, where employers are obliged to continue a person's employment if they have experienced illness. Without workplace policies that provide income security, workers hesitate to take sick leave, even in the face of severe illness or injury. This creates additional stress, especially with the threat that the worker may be dismissed without explanation or financial compensation, which affects the entire family (Lander et al. 2009). On the other hand, positive work experiences can have an additive effect on physical and psychological wellbeing, and help buffer the effects of personal stress. This can occur through role enrichment that flows from being satisfied with both the work role and family relationships (Bourne et al. 2009).

> ## REMINDER
>
> Spillover occurs when there is an imbalance between work and home life.

As we mentioned in Chapter 7, in some cases the logistical difficulties of managing 'spillover' between work and home creates harmful psychological health effects, especially for women (Glavin et al. 2011). Despite changing role responsibilities many young mothers continue to feel guilty at not being able to meet family needs, which emanates from feeling their employment is 'symbolically in competition with their ability to feel like good mothers' (Glavin et al. 2011:54). Research from many fields has shown that the stress of balancing work and home is increasing and causing lost productivity as well as emotional stress (Bianchi & Milkie 2010; Glavin et al. 2011). High workloads and work stressors can place pressure on family relationships, especially where the worker comes home stressed or where (s)he receives little social support from a spouse or partner (Michel et al. 2009). Likewise, family conflicts can cause problems in the workplace by influencing organisational performance (Beauregard & Henry 2009). In addition to the role-strain and role-spillover effects, many people experience work-family *role blurring*, which arises from having nonstandard work hours and communications technologies (email, mobile phones) that allow work to be performed anytime, anywhere (Glavin et al. 2011). The interdependence and integration of work and family demands are a 'boundary-crossing' issue that arises when people bring paid work into the home, which forces people to transition quickly from a family to a work mindset, virtually being in two places at the same time (Glavin et al. 2011: 45).

Workplace incivility and bullying

Some stressors in the workplace arise from interpersonal behaviours, such as bullying and intimidation. These are antisocial behaviours that reflect a power imbalance in the working relationships, where an employee may be victimised by co-workers or a supervisor. A broader construct for this type of effect is commonly referred to as *incivility*, which refers to unfairness or insensitivity of supervisors to employees (Cortina & Magley 2009; Laschinger et al. 2013). It constitutes behaviours that violate norms of interpersonal respect, workplace morality and a sense of community (Cortina & Magley 2009). Employees subjected to uncivil treatment in the workplace experience high levels of stress, cognitive distraction, lower job satisfaction, higher levels of sickness absence and reduced creativity (Cortina & Magley 2009; O'Donnell et al. 2010). Incivility is increasing in many workplaces, partly because of casualisation and job insecurity, and as a reaction to the work intensification caused by staff shortages and/or employer competitiveness.

Uncivil behaviours such as bullying are often the result of multi-layered work systems where each layer of management tends to micro-manage the next level down, keeping tighter and tighter control over each person's work. Micro-managing leaves little room for creativity or lateral thinking. Instead, the objective of the day's work becomes appeasement of the person above. This occurs in hospitals and health organisations, as well as in other workplaces as we outline in Box 10.4.

WORKPLACE BULLYING

Incivility and bullying are pervasive in Australian and New Zealand workplaces.

As a new graduate how would you respond to incivility?

PRACTICE STRATEGY

Occupational health nurses have a key role to play in reframing a toxic workplace culture into one that embraces equity, diversity and tolerance.

Research into incivility among nurses revealed that new graduates are particularly vulnerable, given their novice status and the challenges they face in adapting to the workplace (Laschinger et al. 2013). Bullying seems to occur more frequently in organisations with rigid hierarchical lines of responsibility, such as in the public service. In Australia, the public service has proliferated at all levels to where State and Commonwealth Government departments constitute many layers of bureaucrats working towards endless circles of reporting. Bullying is rife, and, in some cases, it has become transformed into an insidious epidemic of 'mobbing' behaviour (Shallcross et al. 2008). Workplace mobbing is where several people in the workplace 'gang up' on someone, usually to try to bring about their expulsion or resignation. It can begin with gossip, innuendo and malicious accusations about a person, intended to discredit

BOX 10.4 Workplace incivility in the UK

Between 2005 and 2008, exceptionally poor standards of care occurred at the two major hospitals that make up the Mid Staffordshire NHS Foundation Trust in Birmingham, UK. These poor standards of care were characterised by high mortality rates, reported breaches in standards of care and serious patient complaints. There were numerous warning signs indicating that a problem existed during the 2005–09 period including highly critical peer reviews and audits, whistleblowing by staff and highly critical reviews by the Health Care Commission (HCC), but no action was taken. Two further reviews were commissioned by the Department of Health which gave rise to widespread public concern and loss of confidence in the Trust. Following these reviews, a first inquiry into individual cases of care was undertaken by Robert Francis QC, to allow those most affected by poor care an opportunity to tell their stories, followed by a second inquiry into the role of commissioning, supervisory and regulatory bodies. The second inquiry found a culture of negativity was pervasive throughout both hospitals, staff were required to focus on achieving narrow financial targets, and there was a disconnect between the Department of Health, management and staff to the extent that even well-intentioned directives were construed as bullying. Community trusts also failed to make their concerns known. It was estimated that up to 1500 patients lost their lives as a result of the situation at Mid Staffordshire (Francis 2013; Clendon 2013).

? Could such a situation occur in Australian or New Zealand hospitals? What would prevent this type of situation from arising?

them or their work. Because this type of behaviour has created toxic work environments that threaten employees' mental health, mobbing is an important topic for workplace research (Shallcross et al. 2008). The behaviour tends to move through five phases. First there is a conflict or critical incident, followed by a campaign of psychological abuse. The next phase involves reporting negative comments to the person's manager with the objective of further isolating her/him from the work group. As the target person, usually a relatively weak female employee, reacts, they are accused of being difficult or even mentally ill. The fifth phase culminates in the employee's resignation, as (s)he finds the workplace unbearable.

One of the relevant issues uncovered in the research on mobbing is related to diversity and gender roles in the workplace. In workplaces with high levels of diversity and gender balance, mobbing is less likely (Shallcross et al. 2008). However, where there is high occupational segregation with gender and ethnic power imbalances, conformity rules. This has been identified as part of the problem in Australian public sector workplaces. Australia ranks highest among all OECD countries for occupational segregation, where males and females tend to work in different sectors (Shallcross et al. 2008). Women are frequently in the lower paid ranks of education, health and social welfare, and are, more often than males, casual staff, especially in those sectors experiencing downsizing. Women are therefore easier targets for bullying and mobbing, scapegoating and manipulating, especially if they are seen to be different from the norm, or if they try to assume masculine management behaviours. The issue is not always gender based, as women managers can also be perpetrators as well as victims. But it is an important part of workplace culture, and therefore workplace health.

Reframing a toxic workplace culture into one where equity, diversity and tolerance are pre-eminent is a challenge for occupational health nurses. At the primary level, the objective is to identify, reduce or eliminate the causes of stress in the working environment. Secondary interventions involve teaching employees coping strategies, and, where necessary, tertiary interventions include psychological therapy and guidance (Bamber & McMahon 2008). Another aspect of the role is networking with other community-based nurses to provide continuity of care for the family, and referral to community resources and support. All of these roles merge into a common need for nursing advocacy, for workers, their families, and a socially cohesive community.

OTHER WORKPLACE HEALTH AND SAFETY ISSUES

Because 80% of the adult population is employed, health and safety in the workplace is a major risk to adult health (AIHW 2008). Illness and injury at work has the potential for long-term disability, which can affect not only the worker, but his/her family and community. Workplace events also cause losses in worker productivity which, in cases where a worker does not have job security, can exacerbate socio-economic disadvantage. Accidents and injuries also incur costs to businesses and the health care system.

Workplace accidents are highly variable, depending on the type of work and the workplace culture, particularly in terms of safety and support. Most are sprains and strains of joints and muscles, primarily back and hand injuries. Musculoskeletal injuries are the most common work-related injuries, with around 20% affecting long-term health (AIHW 2008). Despite the implementation of extensive health and safety laws in the early 1990s, New Zealand's workplace injury and death rate remains one of the highest among developed countries. In a comparison of nine countries including New Zealand, Australia, Canada, the UK, Finland, France, Norway and Spain, New Zealand ranked last for overall occupational safety performance with an average of 4.2 occupational fatal injuries per 100 000 person years (Lilley et al. 2013). Deaths are most common in the forestry and mining industries exemplified by the deaths of 29 men in the Pike River mining disaster in 2010. New legislation was introduced in 2013 designed to address the high rates of occupational injury and death.

Another prevalent work-related injury is hearing loss, caused by excessive noise in the workplace. In some cases, workplace injuries are linked to individual worker characteristics as well as the work environment, including the worker's commitment to health and safety. For example, the consumption of alcohol or substances, either during or before work, can interfere with jobs that require the operation of machinery or intense concentration.

Other factors affecting health and safety in the workplace include the type of work undertaken, the pressures placed on the workers to meet productivity targets, and exposure to hazardous substances or safety risks. Productivity pressures can cause biologic, physical or psychosocial risks or a combination of these. For this reason, primary prevention activities include a hazard or risk assessment in the workplace. This begins with an ergonomic assessment of the workplace, and the working conditions. Ergonomic assessment involves examining the engineering aspects of the relationship between the worker and her/his work environment. Ergonomic hazards are those that induce fatigue, boredom, or glare, or tasks that must be conducted in an abnormal position. Examples include work that causes vibration, repetitive motion, poor workstation–worker fit and lifting heavy loads. Biologic hazards can include exposure to bacteria, moulds, insects, viruses or infectious co-workers. Chemical hazards can include exposure to dangerous liquids, gases, dust, vapour or fumes. Examples of physical hazards are extremes of temperature, noise, radiation, poor lighting or exposure to unprotected machinery. A survey of New Zealand nurses undertaken in 2013 found that 11% had required time off work in the previous two years with a workplace acquired infection or injury. The most common causes were influenza, norovirus and back, knee, wrist and shoulder injuries. Only 41.5% of survey respondents felt their employer was fully compliant with occupational health and safety standards (Walker & Clendon 2013).

WHAT'S YOUR OPINION?

To what extent do you think technology has reduced versus increased work stress?

In addition to physical and chemical hazards, psychosocial hazards are those that produce an inordinate amount of stress. As a response to the competitiveness of global markets, downsizing, rightsizing and streamlining work processes have become the norm. Performance-based human resource policies and management structures have increased job demands, task reorganisation, restructuring of work teams and work intensification, all of which create pressures on the family as well as the worker (Beauregard & Henry 2009). These demands are not always accompanied by supportive co-workers or managers, as we mentioned above, which can erode workers' respect and dignity as well as other indicators of psychosocial health (Lawson et al. 2009). The problems become worse for casual employees or those without long-term contracts, as well as for those with the added stress of family responsibilities. For these employees, non-standard working hours create additional pressures. Unlike other countries, there is no cap on working hours in Australia, and workers now work an average of 70 minutes unpaid overtime per day, which is among the longest working hours in the Western world (The Australia Institute 2009). In New Zealand, three out of ten full-time workers work 50 or more hours per week—again, very high by international standards (Families Commission 2009).

The World Health Organization has done significant work on supporting the development of healthy workplaces, developing a set of criteria for a healthy workplace. The imperative to address the health needs of workers was reinforced at the World Health Assembly in 2007. The Assembly endorsed the WHO Global Plan of Action on Workers' Health 2008–17 (WHO 2007), which emphasises the need to address all aspects of workers' health, including

ACCIDENT PROTECTION AT WORK

New Zealand's Accident Compensation Corporation (ACC) provides comprehensive no-fault personal injury cover for all New Zealanders including for accidents that occur at work. In Australia, each state has an agency that provides a similar workplace service. In 2009, a new statutory body called Safe Work Australia was created to compare performance and worker's compensation outcomes across states. The ACC and various state programs also provide comprehensive injury prevention programs to support employers in preventing workplace injuries, and help return injured employees back to work as soon as possible.

health promotion at work, protection of workers' health and primary prevention of occupational hazards (see Box 10.5).

POSITIVE MENTAL HEALTH AND WELLBEING

One of the approaches to helping people cope with work stress or personal issues is to concentrate on a combination of psychological strategies called primary and secondary control coping. *Primary control coping* involves direct efforts to manage stress through emotional expression, emotional regulation and problem-solving. *Secondary coping* involves adapting to stressful situations by acceptance, cognitive restructuring, distraction and positive thinking (Wadsworth et al. 2011). These personal strategies become habits, or assets that can

BOX 10.5 **The healthy workplace**

Healthy workplaces:

- create a healthy, supportive and safe environment
- ensure that health promotion and health protection are integral to management practices
- foster work styles and lifestyles conducive to health
- ensure total organisational participation
- extend positive effects to the local and surrounding community and environment.

(Source: WHO 1999)

mobilise positive health behaviours through bolstering resiliency and resourcefulness (Rotegard et al. 2010). Teaching people these psychological techniques helps position mental health interventions within a positive paradigm (Wand 2012). Thinking positively includes contemplating a 'best-possible self', cultivating gratitude and kindness, recalling happy rather than difficult experiences and using a strengths-based approach. Together these can help individuals work towards small gains that lead to a sense of wellbeing, resilience and hope (Wand 2012). Another approach uses 'Mindfulness-Based Stress Reduction' (MBSR), wherein people are taught to respond to stress rather than react to it (Frisvold et al. 2012). Mindfulness, which has been used to help nurses cope with stress, helps the individual achieve balance by reflecting on how stress is affecting them, and then developing ways to acknowledge the stress and react in a way that is not self-destructive (Frisvold et al. 2012). It is also a good way to live a harmonious life, being mindful of who to be and how to be in one's own skin.

REMINDER: Resilience

The ability to engage in competent, adaptive functioning despite exposure to risk or adversity.

Positive mental health has a powerful effect on individuals and the community. People with positive mental health tend to be more socially connected, to volunteer, to have better social networks and high health assets, or quality of life. Mental wellbeing has a powerful effect on job performance, worker productivity, creativity and absenteeism (WHO 2009). Workers who feel in control over their work life, and who feel they are treated fairly at work, have been found to have lower stress levels (Bianchi & Milkie 2010; WHO 2009). This has a reciprocal effect on the workplace, as individual employees engage in the 'discretionary participation' we mentioned previously. When employees feel empowered to participate in decision-making, they tend to provide mutual support, engage in employee health promotion programs and work toward achieving team goals. Together with others in the workplace, they have a better chance of developing skills such as resilience, optimism, self-esteem and self-efficacy, which can help buffer stress. As a result, individuals are seen to have high emotional and cognitive capital. When these positive personal assets are spread among neighbourhoods and

communities, they create high social and environmental capital, which can also buffer the cumulative effects of deprivation with feelings of hope, trust and social support (WHO 2009).

SOURCES OF STRESS

- Caregiving
- Family responsibilities
- Workplace
- Lifestyle risks

To redress the disadvantage of inequity or social exclusion, redistributing wealth to provide food, housing and material resources seems like an appropriate solution. However, simply providing resources would not be effective without opportunities for disadvantaged people to achieve equity in social status, friendship, social capital and sense of control (Pickett & Wilkinson 2009; Raphael 2009). Opportunities to fully participate in society by accessing education and employment help generate social cohesion (norms of trust, reciprocity at work and in the community), social integration (networks, activities), and social support (care and loving relationships) (Song 2010). When conditions can be rearranged to reduce the gap between the rich and poor so that everyone has a chance at succeeding, there is a greater likelihood that social pathways will have a protective effect on the whole population. This pathway to social capital can help reduce the prevalence of violence, bullying, teenage births, rates of imprisonment, low educational attainment, social mobility and trust, and workplace stress (Pickett & Wilkinson 2009). Box 10.6 lists the 10 ways social capital protects health (Song 2010).

ENVIRONMENTAL FACTORS AFFECTING ADULT HEALTH

Our environment includes all external elements surrounding and affecting life (AIHW 2012a). These include natural and built features such as temperature, ultraviolet radiation, homes, transport and climate change, all of which affect clean air, water, food, vector populations and planning for extreme weather events and pandemics (AIHW 2012a). Modifiable aspects of the environment are primarily aspects of the built environment; our homes, schools, workplaces, recreation areas, and infrastructure for transport, energy and waste disposal. Australia has some remarkable hazards to health because of our built environment. For example, we have one of the highest rates of

BOX 10.6 **How social capital protects health**

1   Influencing macro level policymaking decisions, micro-level sense of control and access to health resources

2   Providing health-related informational support

3   Acting as social credentials in accessing health resources

4   Reinforcing psychological resources such as self-esteem

5   Supplying emotional support

6   Delivering health-related material support

7   Encouraging engagement in healthy norms and behaviours

8   Decreasing exposure to stressors like involuntary job disruptions

9   Increasing the use of quality health services by strengthening access to insurance and care

10 Reinforcing subjective social status

(Source: Song 2010)

asbestos-related deaths in the workplace (AIHW 2012a). We have families who live in overcrowded conditions, many of whom are Indigenous, rural or remote-area residents. Our cities also have high exposure to aircraft noise, which can cause high blood pressure and stress, and like New Zealand, we have communities with damp and mouldy homes, which place people at risk for asthma and other respiratory conditions (AIHW 2012a).

WHAT'S YOUR OPINION?

Biotechnology will have an increasing role to play in future health outcomes. How will you guide community members to stay abreast of this knowledge?

The extended changes in weather patterns that we call climate change have become an issue of major concern in the 21st century. Climate change science has revealed that human activities have led to increases in global average air and ocean temperature, along with rising sea levels and widespread melting of snow and ice (AIHW 2012a). The direct effects of climate change include ill

health, injury and mortality associated with extreme temperatures such as heat waves, bushfires, floods and cyclones. Air pollution has also increased from larger motor vehicle usage, mining, energy production and agriculture. Indirect effects of climate change are thought to be responsible for increased rates of diseases such as Ross River virus and dengue fever, changes in food quality and availability because of poorer crop yields, increased rates of foodborne diseases caused by rising temperatures, such as salmonellosis and campylobacteriosis, and increased rates of post-traumatic stress disorder among those exposed to natural disasters (AIHW 2012a).

Global warming has displaced many people, causing poverty through loss of their livelihood, malnutrition or diseases. It places pressure on global migration, especially among people from countries that are ravaged by weather events or where their own environment has already been damaged beyond sustainable levels. This is a problem for international migrants, who all live in unhealthy environments for varying periods of time. Climate change is therefore a cause for concern for all health professionals advocating for communities. The health impacts of climate change are not pre-destined; in fact, there are many outcomes that are as yet speculative. What is known, however, is that there is an urgent and unconditional need to work towards preservation of current environments to safeguard the future. Together with reduction in unhealthy and unsafe behaviours, sustainable environments will ensure the next generations have at least the potential to achieve the state of health to which they aspire.

WISE CHOICES

- Excellent science
- Compassionate values
- Effective communication
- Cultural inclusiveness
- Openness to new knowledge
- Commitment to prevention
- Health promotion

The ecology of adult health also includes attention to new biotechnologies that are changing patterns of risk and potential. Since the Human Genome Project (HGP), there has been a clearer understanding of the influence of genetic factors on health, which is helping to inform some people's treatment decisions. Stem cell research has reached the stage where, in future, an individual's genes will be transformed for therapeutic advantage in treating certain long-term disease states, such as Parkinson's Disease. As knowledge provides greater clarity on how nature and nurture interact at the cellular level, families and communities will have many decisions to make about their ecosystems and exposures, the risk/reward ratios of different activities and even whether and when to alter their genetic make-up (Fielding et al. 2000). Some of these developments have been rapid, challenging people's level of health literacy. A major role for nurses will therefore involve staying well informed to keep abreast of the new developments so that they can make informed choices. As Omenn (2000:10) suggests, wise choices for future generations will depend on 'excellent science, compassionate values, effective communication, appreciation of diverse cultures and preferences, openness to new knowledge and alternative views, commitment to disease prevention and health promotion'. The first challenge lies in reframing goals for health within both visionary perspectives and creative approaches to identifying and defending scientific evidence as a basis for community health research.

HEALTHY ADULTHOOD

The best approach for adult health is community participation in all matters concerning health and wellbeing, irrespective of whether the objective is to overcome risks or enhance the quality of people's lives. The most pertinent issues in planning for healthy adulthood are social: to overcome inequity and inequality. The focus of today's health promotion agenda for adults should be to address the social determinants of health, to reduce risk, to improve the quality of work and family life, to prevent and better manage chronic diseases, including mental health, and to respond capably to current and future threats including both infectious diseases and threats to the environment. To address these issues requires public awareness of the seriousness of each, and dissemination of accurate information that will be both instructive and supportive. The focus should remain on communities in creating and maintaining health to decrease the incidence of chronic diseases, develop safer workplaces, living spaces and societies, and provide greater opportunities for people to achieve better physical, mental, spiritual, environmental and culturally sensitive health.

At the individual level, expert opinion has a set of specific recommendations (Box 10.7)

> ### BOX 10.7 **What the experts say about healthy living**
>
> - Eat two serves of fruit and three serves of vegetables a day.
> - Drink no more than two standard alcoholic drinks on any day.
> - Do 30 minutes of moderate to vigorous activity per day.
> - Maintain a healthy weight (BMI 18.5–25kg/m^2).
> - If sexually active, practise safe sex.
> - Get regular health checks.
> - Get screened for breast, cervical and bowel cancer.
> - Reduce and manage your stress.
> - Include yourself in your community as a volunteer or get involved in sport or community groups.
> - Practise road safety—helmets, seatbelts, child restraints, speed limits.
> - Don't smoke.

GOALS FOR ADULT HEALTH

The major goals for adult health include:
- ensuring an appropriate balance between comprehensive and selective primary health care (PHC), particularly in addressing chronic conditions for disadvantaged populations
- providing political support for health in all policies
- integrating primary, secondary and tertiary intervention for adult health in the workplace and community
- adopting a life course approach for the prevention of chronic conditions
- promoting an ecological risk-reduction approach by focusing on the environments for good health
- using intersectoral collaboration to address physical and mental health issues comprehensively
- ensuring cultural sensitivity in all interactions
- designing health promotion strategies that are empowering, with people and families as partners at the centre of care
- using health resources efficiently and effectively, eliminating boundaries between professionals
- using the Ottawa Charter as a guideline for health promotion.

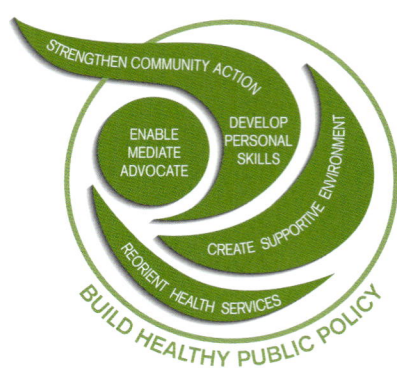

Building healthy public policy

Public policies to support adult health should be aimed at providing enabling environments and structures that support personal and community capacity for good health. These personal capacities are embedded in health literacy, opportunities for community engagement and capacity development. Multidimensional policies are seen as more effective than those supporting single agencies working from single government departments on single issues. At the highest level of government there should be a shift from disease-focused funding to health promotion and prevention of lifestyle diseases that leave many people chronically ill over long periods of time (WHO 2012). The policy focus should begin with the environment. First, the physical environment should be preserved for a sustainable future. Initiatives such as the National Climate Change Adaptation Framework have begun to outline the agenda for long-term adaptation to climate change (AIHW 2012a). Some of the recommendations for adapting our environments are also targeting better health through reducing obesogenic factors: encouraging bicycle paths (see Box 10.8) as well as reducing greenhouse gas emissions (AIHW 2012a). These multidimensional policies have a greater likelihood of sustainability. The other obesogenic conditions that create risky behaviours also require our ongoing advocacy; the fast food outlets and television advertising that promote consumption of high-energy dense foods, the regulatory conditions that prevent people from accessing affordable, healthy foods and the streets that are unsafe because of high speed limits or other factors (Allender et al. 2011).

In 2009, the Australian National Preventative Health Taskforce made a series of policy recommendations to promote healthier lifestyles (Kirby 2009). These include increasing taxes on cigarettes and alcohol, and eliminating advertising for both, as well as reducing media promotion of

BOX 10.8 Melbourne: Australia's best cycling city

In a search for Australia's best cycling city Melbourne wins hands down. City Councillors in Melbourne have recognised the impact of the obesogenic environment on health outcomes and are taking steps to make cycling the transport option of choice for commuters, sightseers and those with business in the city. Using a combination of on and off road cycle paths, access to cheap rental bicycles and helmets at purpose-built stations across the city, making cycling safer, and providing showers and bike racks at key locations, the city aims to increase bicycle use over the next four years by 50% on weekdays. The most astonishing development has been removal of a vehicle lane as part of a trial to make more room for cyclists on Princes Bridge. Although other cities like Brisbane have added public rental bicycles to the downtown area it is impossible to connect up the cycleways to replace coming into the city in a car. As a result, Brisbane is one of the most car-dependent places on earth. Canberra, Perth, Darwin, Sydney and Hobart have all made progress in creating cycleways but the long-term goal of Melbourne city council to create a 'cycling city' is exemplary. Melbourne, give yourself a pat on the back! (City of Melbourne 2012).

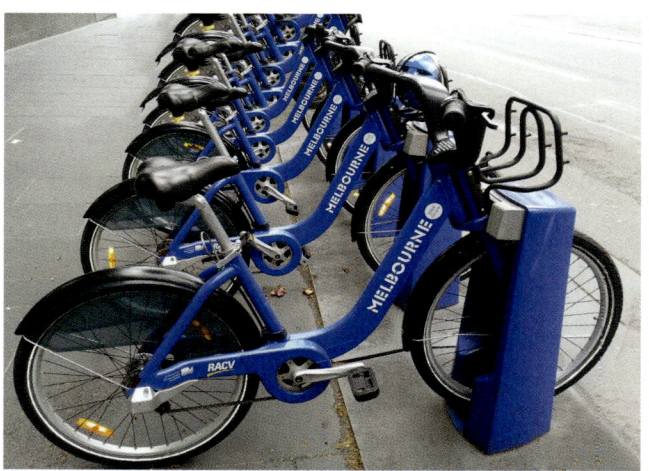

Photo: City of Melbourne

unhealthy food. In New Zealand similar initiatives have focused on addressing obesity issues in the same way that smoking has been addressed—with a multi-pronged approach to prevention, including public policy changes, taxation and creating environments that support people to make healthy food choices (Pearson 2009). These initiatives respond to the WHO's mandate for pressure to be brought to bear on food producers to ensure reductions in the fat, sugar and salt content of processed foods, that healthy and nutritious choices are available and affordable, and that responsible marketing practices are upheld (WHO 2012).

WHAT'S YOUR OPINION?

- How effective is taxing carbon emissions?
- What if every citizen paid an annual transportation levy of $25 per year to enable everyone to ride on public transport, anytime, anywhere, at no cost?
- Which would improve the carbon footprint more?

Besides comprehensive, population-level policies, some public policies target health and wellbeing in specific settings. For example, occupational health and safety policies in Australia and New Zealand are aimed at the working population. These policies are governed by national agencies such as Safe Work Australia (SWA, Online. Available: www.safeworkaustralia.gov.au/sites/SWA/ [accessed 5 August 2013]), and the New Zealand Workplace Health and Safety Council (NZWHSC, Online. Available: www.dol.govt.nz/whss/whsc/index.asp [accessed 22 August 2013]). These agencies provide national guidelines to improve health and safety at work, and provide information for workers and their representatives, including the trade unions. One of the historical problems with occupational health and safety policies is that they have tended to have a singular biomedical focus rather than linking workplace health and safety to the social determinants of worker health and lifestyle balance. However some changes have been made in the last few years, including the SafeWork Australia Mentally Healthy Workplace Alliance, an intersectoral collaboration between government, business and numerous mental health agencies, to drive sustainable changes in business culture and practices.

As part of the mental health agencies as well as in the occupational setting, nurses have a role to play in ensuring that the SDH are included in all programs. Nurses are also advocates for the 'Health in all Policies' initiatives, in the workplace and in the community. Policies that reflect understanding of the SDH are those that provide income security and appropriate wages, housing for those with disabilities, employment, adequate provision for

carers, and cross-cultural and gender considerations in helping people cope with their life situations (Raphael 2009). A further challenge in today's work environment is to ensure the sustainability of the workforce, by long-term planning for workers once the baby boomer generation retires. This is a major issue for the health workforce, with existing shortages of health professionals (Forbes & While 2009) that are likely to rise. A study of nurses over 50 in New Zealand found 53% of nurses working in primary health care settings intended to retire in the next 10 years (Walker & Clendon 2012). This has major implications for the sustainability of the nursing workforce in primary health care long term unless action is taken now to encourage more nurses into primary health care work. The development of policies designed to recruit and retain nurses and doctors in rural and remote settings, including voluntary bonding schemes and postgraduate study opportunities (Health Workforce New Zealand, Online. Available: http://healthworkforce.govt.nz/our-work [accessed 23 August 2013]) will hopefully assist in alleviating long-term health workforce shortages in these areas.

Mental health policy development is a critical area requiring attention in Australia, which has one of the highest rates of suicide in the world. The national framework presented in Chapter 9 'Life: A framework for preventing suicide and other self-harm in Australia' (Commonwealth of Australia 2009), and the National Mental Health Strategy, provide examples of bipartisan collaboration in addressing a problem of national significance (SANE 2013). Beyondblue, the national depression and anxiety organisation, provides a biannual Depression Monitor survey to measure changes in community awareness, knowledge and understanding of these conditions (SANE 2013). In addition, the Mindframe National Media Initiative is an intersectoral collaboration developed by the Australian Government National Suicide Prevention Program, aimed at influencing the media to encourage responsible reporting and education about mental health and suicide prevention (SANE 2013). Queensland's 'Change our Minds' and South Australia's 'Let's Think Positive' are also media campaigns with the same intention. Australia's report card on mental health—'A Contributing Life'—identified stigma reduction in the community as a key priority for action (National Mental Health Commission 2012). In response, the SANE Media Centre has a one-stop-shop to provide information, expert comment, advice and referral on mental health, stigma and suicide prevention. SANE has a specific program called StigmaWatch, which voices community feedback on media reports that inadvertently promote self-harm and suicide (SANE 2013).

New Zealand has a long history of strong national commitment to mental health, including funding to address social exclusion and addiction. The Ministry of Health's policy *Te Tahuhu-Improving Mental Health 2005–2013* declares that these problems erode an individual's sense of belonging and participation in society, calling for cultural awareness, sensitivity and promoting access to the resources of mainstream society to encourage full participation by all New Zealanders (SANE 2013). Since 2001 the New Zealand Government has extended the 'Like Minds, Like Mine' project by providing national funding to entrench this as a core public health activity (SANE 2013). The most recent policies focus on youth mental health through the provision of school-based, nurse-led services, vulnerable children, a drivers of crime work program targeted at conduct disorder and addictions, suicide prevention, Whānau Ora initiatives, and welfare reforms that encourage people into work (NZMOH 2012d, 2013b).

ACTION POINT

Some nurses lead from behind, supporting community advocates with information and guidance on lobbying for policy change.

Nurses working in the community play an important role in informing policy development, particularly practice nurses (PNs), public health nurses and those working in home care settings. Because they have knowledge from the operational level, their voices should be heard at the policy table. Many nurses support community members in their networking and advocacy to lobby policymakers for comprehensive approaches to public health. As nurses know, comprehensive policies have the best chance of success for community health. Although some situations require selective attention and resources, it is important to integrate mental health policies with those intended to promote physical health and prevent chronic illnesses.

WHAT'S YOUR OPINION?

Given Allender et al.'s findings, what other reasons might exist for local councils supporting one type of policy but not another when they are both aimed at improving health?

One of the issues with healthy public policy concerns the evidence base, which is less than optimal. Although there is a growing body of research into policymaking it is important to consider the political and social influences (Allender et al. 2011). For example, Melbourne researchers found that there was considerable political support for healthy walking, cycling and active recreation, but not for healthy eating initiatives. They hypothesised that this situation may be due to a number of things: the contextual or regulatory difficulties of mandating healthy food environments, reticence by the policymakers to seem like they were being intrusive or coercive, or their hesitancy to set legislative parameters around a broader SDH agenda (Allender et al. 2011).

Creating supportive environments

Supportive environments are those that promote equitable access to resources at the local level, where people live, work and play. They are also sustainable across the life course and across generations. To sustain community life, as well as personal health and wellbeing, children and their families need access to safe spaces for family life, adequate education and opportunities for community engagement. Safe, vibrant, inclusive spaces for living, working and playing require multisectoral, interagency partnerships and collaboration with the focus on community residents (WHO 2009). Given that the risks of chronic illness are greater among those from disadvantaged backgrounds all measures to create supportive environments should be designed to help the most vulnerable in the community (Allender et al. 2011). A major focus for environmental planning concerns the obesogenic environments that are problematic in most cities. Supportive environments should shape people's choices, making healthy food choices and physical activity accessible, available and affordable (WHO 2012). They should also consider mental wellbeing as integral to good physical health. This is acknowledged in the intersectoral collaboration being undertaken by the Mentally Healthy Workplace Alliance, but it is also important that workers' community health and social services are integrated with occupational health services. By acting as a conduit between work and the community, nurses can help ensure that supervisors and work team members are educated and empowered to be of assistance to the worker when help is needed (OECD 2011).

CARERS AND VOLUNTEERS

The voluntary sector of the community provides an invaluable contribution to social capital.

What aspects of community nursing do you think could be outsourced to volunteer carers?

Working towards sustaining the community also brings a set of personal values to the community. These enrich the community-health professional partnership with respect, support and mutual caring (Hill 2009). At the centre of all issues is a commitment to enabling, preserving and celebrating community strengths. The social-ecological approach also includes recognition of the individuals who are at the vanguard of community life; the volunteers and the large number of informal caregivers (12% of the population) who are at risk themselves from weariness, anger and resentment, sleep deprivation and stress-related illness (AIHW 2012a). These are the individuals who make a difference to the quality of life of those most in need. As carers, they need ongoing encouragement and support from others, and a healthy environment within which they can undertake their important roles.

PRACTICE STRATEGY

Try the SDH community assessment process we outlined in Chapter 3 to identify and build on community strengths.

Many carers are also living in economically disadvantaged situations, with no chance of improving their circumstances because of their caring responsibilities (AIHW 2012a). Like those they care for, they often have reduced earnings, no opportunity for self-improvement through education, and no income security. As with many other groups in the community, carers can become socially isolated, which is a particular problem for those without access to transportation (WHO 2009). Legislation in New Zealand has seen the inclusion of family carers as recipients of welfare benefits improving their standard of living and access to the determinants of health. Inclusive approaches to planning bring members of different ethnic groups or migrant groups together with long-term community residents, which enhances opportunities to develop social capital as well as culturally competent care (Peckover & Chidlaw 2007).

Strengthening community action

Community action is necessary to support people in sustaining their community. This can be guided by the assessment model we introduced in Chapter 3 to assess community strengths and weaknesses. Once you have analysed the impact of the SDH on the community it is a simple step to conduct a SWOT analysis of the community's health and wellbeing. This type of foundation for planning can be invaluable to strengthening community action. To tailor interventions to the community, nurses need to acquire local knowledge as well as awareness of current research. This information can then be translated into plans that will suit the local context. Plans for community action should also be based on current awareness of what is being disseminated in the media, to clarify any public misperceptions or expectations. This helps strengthen health literacy, particularly critical health literacy.

SWOT

Strengths
Weaknesses
Opportunities
Threats

Some members of the community may need help to understand the politics of health. Because urbanisation and technology have created an overwhelming amount of information for the average family to sift through, translating research findings to the community can help promote discretion and fully informed choice. At the community level, for example, it makes no sense to teach people about the need for good dietary practices, and then have them confronted with blatant commercial messages urging them to eat calorie-dense, low-nutrient foodstuffs. To be empowered to take action, it is important that they understand both the products being advertised, and the powerful vested interests that shape their lives (Choi et al. 2005). They also need to know the practicalities of nutrition, where to access healthy foods that are affordable, and what lifestyle supports may be available through the local council, or what income support may be available through welfare agencies. Providing accurate and appropriate information will help ensure a level of authenticity of information that extends beyond the 'bytes' offered to them in the popular media.

Many people are also unaware of the policies that govern the health care system and how to access appropriate services. This may be particularly important for the large number of people who live alone at all stages of adult life. They may not have opportunities to engage with others or be hesitant to seek advice, yet they need to know the potential impact of current government debates on various health initiatives, treatments and pharmaceuticals, and how these affect their health. Members of the public also need to understand the impact of political lobby groups who may be more inclined to encourage spending health funds on new hospitals and monopoly services, rather than on health promotion, or continuing care for those with illnesses or disabilities. Partnerships with local community members can promote the type of citizen engagement that leads to community action and achievement of goals, such as those listed in Box 10.9 for supporting those with mental illnesses.

Developing personal skills

Providing support for people to improve their health literacy is one of the most important ways nurses can help them develop personal capacity. Some community residents may have moderate levels of health literacy, but generally, low levels of health literacy are found among those who have migrated from non-English speaking countries, and those with advanced age, lower educational attainment, poorer health, and less social participation (Barber et al. 2009). Homeless people also have a need to develop sufficient health literacy to survive, and to navigate informal, as well as formal systems, that can help

them cope with chronic illness, injuries and mental illness. The role of nurses in supporting them includes being sensitive to the shame, embarrassment and discrimination they experience when they attempt to secure care and support. These are also issues for other hard-to-reach groups, including the prison population (AIHW 2012a). Despite the barriers to bringing disenfranchised people such as the homeless into care, neighbourhood-based nursing activities have been found to be effective by providing primary care and social support (Montemurro et al. 2013). For those who have been subject to social exclusion for any reason, the sensitivity of health professionals can make the difference in whether or not they are able to engage in capacity building. A deliberate, incremental approach is to help people by first networking, then engaging in information exchange, partnering, priority setting, planning/implementing changes, then supporting and sustaining those changes (Montemurro et al. 2013).

PRACTICE STRATEGY

Use a partnership approach to support people to develop personal capacity.

Helping people develop personal capacity is a central goal of PNs and others working with adults who attend general practice or community clinics. A partnership approach works well with people seeking lifestyle changes, and this begins with an exploration of their personal health goals. Assessing their preferences allows a program to be customised to their needs. It also acknowledges their need for autonomy in working towards health improvements, or maintenance of ongoing conditions. In effect the nurse is then the 'guide on the side', available with resources and referrals as well as engaged in their networks to gain community insights into what works, for whom, and in what circumstances. Once programs have been deemed acceptable and effective, they can be embedded within community agencies or organisations to broaden supports and ensure sustainability (Montemurro et al. 2013).

Reorienting health services

The worldwide shift in health services from episodic care to chronic disease management has continued, and this is entrenched in national initiatives such as the primary health care strategies of New Zealand and, more recently, Australian governments. The PHC approach is responsive to the community, particularly in the role encompassed by practice

BOX 10.9 Community support for the mentally ill

- Encourage direct personal contact with those suffering from mental illness.
- Use creative arts and multi-media to help change attitudes.
- Mental health problems are best framed as part of our shared humanity.
- Create a simple and enduring national vision.
- Support grassroots, local programming.
- Plan strategically at the national level.
- Support those living with mental illness in active leadership.
- Target programs at influential groups.
- Assist media to play a significant role.
- Use evidence for programs and practice.

(Source: SANE 2013)

nurses (PNs) and those working in child, family and home care (Parker et al. 2012). These nurses practise from the knowledge that many people can be prevented from progressing from one chronic condition to another by ensuring that their encounters in primary care are carefully planned and focus on developing the interpersonal skills will assist early identification of problems (Walsh & Fahy 2012; WHO 2012). Yet studies in Australia and overseas show that around 50% of people with chronic illnesses do not receive best practice in managing their condition (Holden et al. 2012; Parker et al. 2012). The Chronic Disease Management (CDM) plans instituted by Medicare to address the needs of Australian patients with chronic illness were intended to improve chronic care management, particularly with extra funding provided to general practices to employ a PN to assist with the process (Holden et al. 2012). However, a study of GP practices indicates that few have taken up the opportunity to implement CDMs (Holden et al. 2012). Explanations given for the lack of uptake of the program have included being too busy, the complexity of the process, a lack of information on patient eligibility, fear of being audited and not having a PN (Holden et al. 2012).

This situation is untenable in terms of prevention and management of chronic conditions, which represent the most significant burden of illness (80%) in Australia. International studies have found that, in many cases, GPs fail to initiate discussions of weight and exercise with people having multiple risk factors, especially people who are obese or those who have had chronic conditions over time (Walsh & Fahy 2012). Their failure to discuss these issues places the onus on nurses in PHC, especially PNs, to undertake surveillance and monitoring of their condition as well as providing guidance and weight loss counselling (Parker et al. 2012). Although some PHC nurses are hesitant to confront lifestyle issues because of inexperience or inadequate knowledge, it is critical to do so, especially in the case of survivors of a heart attack or stroke, where 1 in 4 are at risk of recurrences, especially having a second heart attack, which is often fatal (Redfern 2013; WHO 2012).

The Care Plus program in New Zealand is a primary health care initiative aimed at improving the management of long-term conditions, reducing inequalities in health, improving primary health care teamwork and reducing the cost of services to high-need primary health care users (NZMOH 2004). People who meet specific eligibility criteria have low or reduced cost access to a nurse and/or doctor, receive a comprehensive assessment and care plan, receive advice on improving health outcomes through better self-management and receive support to meet their health goals (NZMOH 2004). These are people most in need: those experiencing two or more long-term conditions, a person with a terminal illness, a person who has had two acute medical or mental health admissions to hospital in the past year, a person who has had six or more visits to primary health care in the past year, and/or someone who is on active review for elective surgery. Evaluation of Care Plus demonstrated that people in the program believed their care had improved and that it was more structured. People also appreciated dedicated time to talk about their condition with a health professional (CBG Health Research Limited 2006). However, evaluation also showed that admissions to hospital for those on a Care Plus program had increased 40% in the following year although this may have been due to improved care and early intervention as a result of the program (CBG Health Research Limited 2006). More recent evaluation of the program is required, as is the need to address the variability in the way it is provided. In some areas nurses take on the bulk of Care Plus work using tools such as the Flinders Program™ to support self-management (Roy et al. 2011), whereas in other areas it is doctors who provide care under the program. More collaborative approaches that draw on the respective skills of both nurses and doctors in an interdisciplinary way may prove more successful than the existing variability. Recent funding increases for Care Plus provision demonstrate the government's commitment to the program (Care Plus, Online. Available: www.nzdoctor.co.nz/in-print/2013/may -2013/22-may-2013/budget-tops-up-vote-health-and -gives-boost-to-care-plus.aspx [accessed 23 August 2013]), but evaluation has not been built into this funding stream.

Nurse-led models of chronic illness care have become increasingly evident throughout the global community, particularly those focusing on Self-Management Support (SMS) interventions aimed at empowering people with skills and confidence to manage their condition in the community (Johnston et al. 2012; Kawi 2012; Wallace et al. 2010). Self-management can be approached by helping people set goals, following up on their progress, linking them to community resources and ensuring the delivery system helps develop health literacy (Wallace et al. 2010). These programs involve collaboration with the multidisciplinary team to encourage people to participate in interactive learning, timely follow-ups and long-term supportive care (Kawi 2012; Wallace et al. 2010). Although some research has shown that people who are more engaged in self-care have better outcomes (Wallace et al. 2010), the lack of a consistent evaluation strategy has failed to produce evidence for the viability of the nurse-led SMS approach (Johnston et al. 2012). As in the New Zealand example of Care Plus outlined above, this gap in our research agenda warrants a long-term program of study in this important area, including studies of the process of multidisciplinary and intersectoral collaboration.

To date, there has been little translation of research findings into practice, yet knowledge of the cycle of risk for chronic conditions is growing exponentially. Evaluation of supportive interventions has proven problematic in many programs, given that the evidence tends to be cross-sectional and of limited applicability across settings. Community-based participatory research (CBPR) is an ideal approach to research that integrates research with capacity building and incorporates meaningful input from those with chronic conditions and their family members (Raine et al. 2010; Schulz et al. 2011). CBPR partnerships for research respond to the need for an ecological perspective, promoting co-learning, equalising power and integrating knowledge acquisition and interventions as well as preventative practices (Hu 2011; OECD 2011; Schulz et al. 2011).

The determinants of chronic diseases underline the need for an integrated approach to health services rather than focusing on heart health, or diabetes care or mental health (Raine et al. 2010). Good and best practice in community nursing means assessing and providing care for those with chronic conditions on two levels: horizontally and vertically. Horizontal care accommodates people's needs between systems and settings, to ensure continuity of care. Vertical care management involves preventative care, self-care support and education. This includes identification of problems (such as obesity), managing care across the continuum of different therapies, and establishing ongoing support and rehabilitation, which can involve case management in complex cases for people with multiple needs (Forbes & While 2009).

BEST PRACTICE

Horizontal care—between systems and settings.

Vertical care—preventative, self-care support and education at primary, secondary and tertiary levels.

The multidisciplinary approach is particularly important in helping people with mental illness achieve appropriate, ongoing accessible care. Many nurses in general community practice do not tend to screen for mental illnesses (Allen et al. 2012). Clinical interventions in primary care are typically aimed at successful maintenance of blood pressure,

cholesterol management and early signs of diabetes side effects such as foot care or kidney disease (WHO 2012). To take these a step further and encourage client self-management, nurses need to be knowledgeable about the risks and dimensions of chronic conditions, and the motivational strategies that will help people make healthy choices for self-management. These require a personal attitude of respect, cultural sensitivity, attention to disparities, and a genuine interest in the impact of chronic illness and the challenges faced by those who live with these conditions (Kawi 2012). Because many chronic physical illnesses are comorbid with mental health problems such as depression, services need to embrace a collaborative approach that values relationships, teamwork and coordination of services for both primary and specialist care (Holm & Severinsson 2012). Allen et al. (2012) developed and evaluated a clinical pathway for generalist community nurses to screen for mental health difficulties with a focus on war veterans and war widows. Their analysis showed how research can be used as a basis for changing practice, using an evidence-based clinical pathway to appropriate referrals to maintain continuity of care for this important group of people (Allen et al. 2012). The approach they advocate also helps family caregivers, who find service discontinuities challenging.

Many community nursing roles have adopted a comprehensive, primary, secondary and tertiary approach to health promotion. For example, occupational health nurses balance individual and population-based strategies for healthier workplaces. This begins with assessment and surveillance of the work environment, often in collaboration with the safety officer. At the primary level, occupational issues and problems are assessed and triaged, identifying strengths, weaknesses, opportunities and threats. This is called a hazard audit. Primary prevention for reducing stress includes attention to ergonomics, work and environmental design, and organisational and management development. At the secondary level, the nurse can help identify appropriate interventions for modifying the environment to support worker health and safety. Extensive liaison with others is the key to tertiary-level activities. These can be aimed at reducing the impact of stress through more sensitive and responsive management and occupational health and safety programs (WHO 2007). Tertiary interventions can also include collaboration with general practitioners, PNs, nurses working in family and community roles, and other rehabilitation personnel involved in planning. A major part of tertiary interventions is liaison with management to ensure successful implementation of programs, and ongoing evaluation of effectiveness.

Health professionals have always been challenged by the need to help individuals develop strategies to foster better personal health and wellbeing. In our market-driven economies, weight loss, for example, has become a major growth industry and it has become the norm for people to outlay large sums of money to be urged to lose weight and take up physical activity. This has created a decline in health education services offered by governments and community agencies. It would seem fairer to society if members of the public were offered supports for living healthy lives. This could include public health assistance for trying to achieve health and fitness, rather than punitive initiatives to cast blame. This type of approach represents a de-commodification of health, which places community needs at the heart of the community, instead of at the centre of the health services bureaucracy (Raphael 2009).

Below we return to the case study to consider issues related to the health of the adults in the Smith and Mason families.

CASE STUDY: Healthy adults in the Mason and Smith families

The occupational health nurse has been developing health promotion materials for the miners on a variety of health issues, including heart disease, depression, stress and diabetes. She is finding that the materials provoke some discussion but continues to offer personal assistance to those who don't seem to find the materials helpful.

Rebecca has been developing her health knowledge about her pre-metabolic syndrome and has become quite health literate in the process. Working with the practice nurse to manage her diet and lifestyle she has brought her blood sugar and weight into a healthy range.

Jason has been finding the health promotion material provided by the occupational health nurse helpful in managing his blood pressure, but the diet provided in the mining camp makes his health management difficult. Huia is worried about losing her job because of Jake's asthma and although the family doesn't need the extra income she finds the work rewarding and stimulating. She has not shared her concerns with Jason.

REFLECTING ON THE BIG ISSUES

- Adult health is socially determined and needs to be seen in the context of a person's life course development.
- Adult health can be compromised by unhealthy behaviours.
- The physical environment has a major influence on health behaviours, suggesting an important relationship between health and place.
- The major burden of disease in the 21st century comes from lifestyle factors such as poor nutrition, inactivity and stress.
- Chronic physical conditions are often co-morbid with chronic mental health problems.

- Equity is a major factor in adult health, with chronic illnesses experienced more intensely by those who are disadvantaged.
- As most adults spend the majority of their time in the workplace, the health of both worker and workplace is a major focus for intervention.
- The work-home life nexus can create major stress, especially for women trying to lead a balanced life.
- Workplace relationships can be a source of psychological ill health.

REFLECTIVE QUESTIONS: How would I use this knowledge in practice?

1   What would be the most important priorities for Colin and Jason's health and wellbeing at work? What would you include in an occupational health care plan for each of them?

2   What information would you need to know to conduct a comprehensive workplace health assessment of their manager in the mine, aged 50, who suffers from clinical depression?

3 Identify five important issues that must be addressed in a program to encourage positive mental health among 40–50-year-olds with a family history of cardiovascular disease.

4 Design a set of strategies for guiding someone who has been victimised by workplace bullying.

5 What components would you include in a health literacy project designed to help empower residents of a migrant community?

6 In the research on balancing family and home responsibilities, no mention is made of the triple responsibility of work-study-home balance. What research does this suggest to you? How would you go about such a study? What variables do you think should be included?

7 How do you think nursing education programs can help prevent incivility in the health workplace?

References

Allen, J., Annells, M., Clark, E., et al., 2012. Mixed methods evaluation research for a mental health screening and referral clinical pathway. Worldviews Evid. Based Nurs. doi:10.1111/j.1741-6787.2011.0026x.

Allender, S., Gleeson, E., Crammond, B., et al., 2011. Policy change to create supportive environments for physical activity and healthy eating: which options are the most realistic for local government? Health Promot. Int. 27 (2), 261–274.

Australian Bureau of Statistics (ABS), 2010. Labour force, Australia. Cat. No. 6291.0.55.001. ABS, Canberra.

Australian Bureau of Statistics (ABS), 2013. Reflecting a nation: Stories from the 2011 Census. Online. Available: <www/abs.gov.au/ausstats/abs/Lookup2071.0main+features902012-2013> 29 July 2013.

Australian Institute of Health and Welfare (AIHW), 2008. Australia's Health 2008 Cat No AUS 99. AIHW, Canberra.

Australian Institute of Health and Welfare (AIHW), 2012a. Australia's Health 2012 Series no 13,Cat No AUS 156. AIHW, Canberra.

Australian Institute of Health and Welfare (AIHW), 2012b. Cancer in Australia: an overview 2012, Cancer Series No. 74, Cat no. CAN 70. AIHW, Canberra.

Bamber, M., McMahon, R., 2008. Danger-early maladaptive schemas at work!: the role of early maladaptive schemas in career choice and the development of occupational stress in health workers. Clin. Psychol. Psychother. 15, 96–112.

Bambra, C., Whitehead, M., Sowden, A., et al., 2008. 'A hard day's night?' The effects of compressed working week interventions on the health and work-life balance of shift workers: a systematic review. J. Epidemiol. Community Health 62, 764–777.

Barber, M., Staples, M., Osborne, R., et al., 2009. Up to a quarter of the Australian population may have suboptimal health literacy depending upon the measurement tool: results from a population-based survey. Health Promot. Int. 24 (3), 252–261.

Beauregard, T., Henry, L., 2009. Making the link between work-life balance practices and organizational performance. Hum. Resour. Manage. Rev. 19, 9–22.

Berends, L., MacLean, S., Hunter, B., et al., 2011. Implementing alcohol and other drug interventions effectively: How does location matter? Aust. J. Rural Health 19, 211–217.

Bianchi, S., Milkie, M., 2010. Work and family research in the first decade of the 21st century. J. Marriage Fam. 72, 705–725.

Bourne, K., Wilson, F., Lester, S., et al., 2009. Embracing the whole individual: Advantages of a dual-centric perspective of work and life. Bus. Horiz. 52, 387–398.

Burton, N., Walsh, A., Brown, W., 2008. It just doesn't speak to me: mid-aged men's reactions to '10 000 steps a day'. Health Promot. J. Austr. 19 (1), 52–59.

Campbell-Lendrum, D., Bertollini, R., Neira, M., et al., 2009. Heath and climate change: a roadmap for applied research. Lancet 373, 1663–1665.

CBG Health Research Limited, 2006. Review of the implementation of care plus. Ministry of Health, Wellington.

Choi, B., Hunter, D., Tsou, W., et al., 2005. Diseases of comfort: primary cause of death in the 22nd century. J. Epidemiol. Community Health 59, 1030–1034.

City of Melbourne, 2012. Bicycle plan 2012-2016. City of Melbourne, Melbourne.

Clendon, J., 2013. NZNO analysis of the Mid Staffordshire NHS Foundation Trust public inquiry. New Zealand Nurses Organisation, Wellington.

Clendon, J., Walker, L., 2013. Nurses aged over 50 and their experiences of shiftwork. J. Nurs. Manag. doi:10.1111/jonm.12157.

Commonwealth of Australia, 2009. A healthier future for all Australians—final report of the National Health and Hospitals Reform Commission, Publications No. P3-5499. AGPS, Canberra.

Coppell, K., Mann, J., Williams, S., et al., 2013. Prevalence of diagnosed and undiagnosed diabetes and prediabetes in New Zealand: findings from the 2008/09 Adult Nutrition Survey. N. Z. Med. J. 126 (1370), 23–42.

Cortina, L., Magley, V., 2009. Patterns and profiles of response to incivility in the workplace. J. Occup. Health Psychol. 14 (3), 272–288.

Critchley, C., Hardie, E., Moore, S., 2012. Examining the psychological pathways to behavior change in a group-based lifestyle program to prevent Type 2 diabetes. Diabetes Care 35, 699–705.

Davidson, P., Daly, J., Leung, D., et al., 2011. Health-seeking beliefs of cardiovascular patients: A qualitative study. Int. J. Nurs. Stud. 48, 1367–1375.

DeMunter, J., Hu, F., Spiegelman, D., et al., 2007. Whole grain, bran, and germ intake and risk of type 2 diabetes:

a prospective cohort study and systematic review. PLoS Med. e, 261.

Donovan, R., Henley, N., Jalleh, G., et al., 2007. People's beliefs about factors contributing to mental health: implications for mental health promotion. Health Promot. J. Austr. 18 (1), 50–56.

Families Commission, 2009. Finding time: parents' long working hours and time impact on family life. Families Commission, Wellington New Zealand. Online. Available: <http://www.familiescommission.govt.nz/research/work-life-balance/finding-time> 26 February 2010.

Farmer, J., Bourke, L., Taylor, J., et al., 2012. Culture and rural health. Aust. J. Rural Health 20, 243–247.

Fielding, J., Lave, L., Starfield, B., 2000. Preface. Annu. Rev. Public Health 21, v–vi.

Forbes, A., While, A., 2009. The nursing contribution to chronic disease management: a discussion paper. Int. J. Nurs. Stud. 46, 120–131.

Francis, R., 2013. Report of the Mid Staffordshire NHS Foundation Trust public inquiry: executive summary. The Stationary Office, United Kingdom.

Frisvold, M., Lindquist, R., Peden McAlpine, C., 2012. Living life in the balance at midlife: Lessons learned from mindfulness. West. J. Nurs. Res. 34 (2), 265–278.

Gillison, F., Skevington, S., Sato, A., et al., 2009. The effects of exercise interventions on quality of life in clinical and healthy populations; a meta-analysis. Soc. Sci. Med. 68, 1700–1710.

Glavin, P., Schieman, S., Reid, S., 2011. Boundary-spanning work demands and their consequences for guilt and psychological distress. J. Health Soc. Behav. 52 (1), 43–57.

Graham, J., Streitel, K., 2010. Sleep quality and acute pain severity among young adults with and without chronic pain: the role of biobehavioral factors. J. Behav. Med. 33, 335–345.

Hajat, A., Blakely, T., Dayal, S., et al., 2010. Do New Zealand's immigrants have a mortality advantage? Evidence from the New Zealand Census-Mortality Study. Ethn. Health 15 (5), 531–547.

Hamerton, H., Mercer, C., Riini, D., et al., 2012. Evaluating Maori community initiatives to promote Healthy Eating, Healthy Action. Health Promot. Int. doi:10.1093/heapro/daso48: 1-10.

Helliwell, J., Layard, R., Sachs, J. (Eds.), 2012. World happiness report. New York. Online. Available: <www.earth.columbia.edu/worldhappinessreport> 13 January 2013.

Henderson, G., 2012. Why the way we are living may be bad for our mental well-being, and what we might choose to do about it: Responding to a 21st Century public health challenge. Public Health 126, S11–S14.

Hill, S., 2009. Social ecology as future stories: An Australian perspective. University of Western Sydney, Sydney.

Holden, L., Williams, I., Patterson, E., et al., 2012. Uptake of Medicare chronic disease management incentives. A study into service providers' perspectives. Aust. Fam. Physician 41 (12), 973–977.

Holm, A., Severinsson, E., 2012. Chronic care model for the management of depression: Synthesis of barriers to, and facilitators of, success. Int. J. Ment. Health Nurs. 21, 513–523.

Holt, H., 2010. Health and labour force participation. New Zealand Treasury working paper 10/03. New Zealand Treasury, Wellington.

Hu, F., 2011. Globalization of diabetes. Diabetes Care 34, 1249–1257.

Huntington, A., Gilmour, J., Tuckett, A., et al., 2011. Is anybody listening? A qualitative study of nurses' reflections on practice. J. Clin. Nurs. 20, 1413–1422.

Ivory, V., Collings, S., Blakely, T., et al., 2011. When does neighbourhood matter? Multilevel relationships between neighbourhood social fragmentation and mental health. Soc. Sci. Med. 72 (12), 1993–2002.

Johnston, A., Pirkis, J., Burgess, P., 2009. Suicidal thoughts and behaviours among Australian adults: findings from the 2007 National Survey of Mental Health and Wellbeing. Aust. N. Z. J. Psychiatry 43, 635–643.

Johnston, S., Liddy, C., Mill, K., et al., 2012. Building the evidence base for chronic disease self-management support interventions across Canada. Can. J. Public Health 103 (6), 462–467.

Kawi, J., 2012. Self-management support in chronic illness care: A concept analysis. Res. Theory Nurs. Pract. 26 (2), 108–125.

King, C., 2010. To err is human, to drift is normalization of deviance. AORN J. 91 (2), 284–286.

Kirby, T., 2009. Australia considers string of preventive health measures. Lancet 374, 963.

Lander, F., Friche, C., Tornemand, H., et al., 2009. Can we enhance the ability to return to work among workers with stress-related disorders? BMC Public Health 9, 372–378. doi:10.1186/1471-2458-9-372.

Laschinger, H., Wong, C., Regan, S., et al., 2013. Workplace incivility and new graduate nurses mental health. The protective role of resiliency. J. Nurs. Adm. 43 (7/8), 415–421.

Lawson, K., Noblet, A., Rodwell, J., 2009. Promoting employee wellbeing: the relevance of work characteristics and organizational justice. Health Promot. Int. 24 (3), 223–233.

Lilley, R., Samaranayaka, A., Weiss, H., 2013. International comparison of International Labour Organisation published occupational fatal injury rates: How does New Zealand compare internationally? Injury Prevention Research Institute, University of Otago, Dunedin.

Martinez-Gonzalez, M., Bes-Rastrollo, M., Serra-Majem, L., et al., 2009. Mediterranean food pattern and the primary prevention of chronic disease: recent developments. Nutr. Rev. 67 (Suppl. 1), S111–S116.

McMichael, A., 2013. Why climate change should be a key health issue this election. Online. Available: <www.theconversation.com/why-climate-change-should-be-a-key-health-issue-this-election-15761> 29 July 2013.

Mental Health Council of Australia, 2011. Consumer and carer experiences of stigma from mental health and other health professionals. Mental Health Council of Australia, Melbourne.

Meyer, I., Schwartz, S., Frist, D., 2008. Social patterning of stress and coping: Does disadvantaged social status confer more stress and fewer coping resources? Soc. Sci. Med. 67, 368–379.

Michel, J., Mitchelson, J., Pichler, S., et al., 2009. Clarifying relationships among work and family social support, stressors, and work-family conflict. J. Vocat. Behav. 76 (1), 91–104.

Montemurro, G., Raine, K., Nykiforuk, C., et al., 2013. Exploring the process of capacity-building among community-based health promotion workers in Alberta, Canada. Health Promot. Int. doi:10.1093/heapro/dat008.

National Mental Health Commission, 2012. A Contributing Life: the 2012 National Report Card on Mental Health and Suicide Prevention. National Mental Health Commission, Canberra.

New Zealand Ministry of Health (NZHOH), 2004. Care plus: An overview. Ministry of Health, Wellington.

New Zealand Ministry of Health (NZHOH), 2007. Like minds, like mine national plan 2007-2013: Programme to counter stigma and discrimination associated with mental illness. Ministry of Health, Wellington.

New Zealand Ministry of Health (NZHOH), 2012a. Mortality and demographic data 2009. Ministry of Health, Wellington.

New Zealand Ministry of Health (NZHOH), 2012b. Cancer: New registrations and deaths 2009. Ministry of Health, Wellington.

New Zealand Ministry of Health (NZHOH), 2012c. The Health of New Zealand Adults 2011/12: Key findings of the New Zealand Health Survey. Ministry of Health, Wellington.

New Zealand Ministry of Health (NZHOH), 2012d. Rising to the challenge: The mental health and addiction service development plan 2012–2017. Ministry of Health, Wellington.

New Zealand Ministry of Health (NZHOH), 2013a. Health loss in New Zealand: A report from the New Zealand burden of diseases, injuries and risk factors study, 2006–2016. Ministry of Health, Wellington.

New Zealand Ministry of Health (NZHOH), 2013b. New Zealand suicide prevention action plan 2013–2016. Ministry of Health, Wellington.

New Zealand Ministry of Health (NZHOH) and Accident Compensation Corporation (ACC), 2013. Injury-related health loss: A report from the New Zealand burden of diseases, injuries and risk factors study 2006–2016. Ministry of Health, Wellington.

O'Donnell, S., McIntosh, J., Wuest, J., 2010. A theoretical understanding of sickness absence among women who have experienced workplace bullying. Qual. Health Res. 20 (40), 439–452.

O'Dowd, S., 2013. Farmers 'need help to talk about their pain'. stuff.co.nz. Online. Available: <http://www.stuff.co.nz/taranaki-daily-news/news/8271236/Farmers-need-help-to-talk-about-their-pain> (accessed 5 April 14).

Omenn, G., 2000. Public health genetics: an emerging interdisciplinary field for the post-genomic era. Annu. Rev. Public Health 21, 1–13.

Organisation for Economic Co-operation and Development (OECD), 2008. Policy Brief, Mental Health in OECD Countries. OECD, Washington.

Organisation for Economic Co-operation and Development (OECD), 2011. Sick on the job? Myths and realities about mental health and work. Factsheet. OECD, Washington.

Parker, D., Clifton, K., Shams, R., et al., 2012. The effectiveness of nurse-led care in general practice on clinical outcomes in adults with type 2 diabetes. Joanna Briggs Library of Systematic Reviews 10 (38), 2514–2558.

Pasca, R., Wagner, S., 2011. Occupational stress in the multicultural workplace. J. Immigr. Minor. Health 13, 697–705.

Pearson, J., 2009. Fags and fat: nutrition sector looks to learn from smokefree successes. Press release. Online. Available: <http://www.obesityaction.org.nz/media/091206FagsandFat.pdf> 8 December 2009.

Peckover, S., Chidlaw, R., 2007. The (un)-certainties of district nurses in the context of cultural diversity. J. Adv. Nurs. 58 (4), 377–385.

Pickett, K., Wilkinson, R., 2009. Greater equality and better health, Editorial. Br. Med. J. 339, b4320. doi:10.1136/bmj.b4320.

Preston, B., 2009. The Australian nurse and midwifery workforce: Issues, developments and the future. Collegian 16, 3–9.

Prochaska, J., DiClemente, C., Norcross, J., 1992. In search of how people change. Applications to addictive behaviors. Am. Psychol. 47, 1102–1114.

Raine, K., Plotnikoff, R., Nykiforuk, C., et al., 2010. Reflections on community-based population health intervention and evaluation for obesity and chronic disease prevention: The Healthy Alberta Communities project. Int. J. Public Health 55, 679–686.

Raphael, D., 2009. Restructuring society in the service of mental health promotion: Are we willing to address the social determinants of mental health? Int. J. Ment. Health Promot. 11 (3), 18–31.

Redfern, J., 2013. A five-point plan to reduce heart attack deaths in Australia. Online. Available: <www.theconversation.edu.au/a-five-point-plan-to-reduce-heart-attack-deaths-in-australia-11908> 21 February 2013.

Rotegard, A., Moore, S., Fagermoen, M., et al., 2010. Health assets: A concept analysis. Int. J. Nurs. Stud. 47, 513–525.

Roy, D., Mahony, F., Horsburgh, M., et al., 2011. Partnering in primary care in New Zealand: clients' and nurses' experience of the Flinders Program™ in the management of long-term conditions. J. Nurs. Healthc. Chronic Illn. 3 (2), 140–149.

SANE, 2013. A life without stigma. A SANE Report. SANE Australia, Melbourne.

Schubert, M., Clarke, S., Aiken, L., et al., 2012. Associations between rationing of nursing care and inpatient mortality in Swiss hospitals. Int. J. Qual. Health Care 24 (3), 230–238.

Schulz, A., Israel, B., Coombe, C., et al., 2011. A community-based participatory planning process and multilevel intervention design: Toward eliminating cardiovascular health inequities. Health Promot. Pract. 12 (6), 900–911.

Shaha, M., Bauer-Wu, S., 2009. Early adulthood uprooted. Transitoriness in young women with breast cancer. Cancer Nurs. 32 (3), 246–255.

Shallcross, L., Sheehan, M., Ramsay, S., 2008. Workplace mobbing: experiences in the public sector. J. Organ. Behav. 13 (2), 56–70.

Shepherd, C., While, A., 2012. Cardiac rehabilitation and quality of life: A systematic review. Int. J. Nurs. Stud. 49, 755–771.

Sheridan, N., Kenealy, T., Connolly, M., et al., 2011. Health equity in the New Zealand health care system: a national survey. Int. J. Equity Health 10, Online.

Snow, J., 2002. Enhancing work climate to improve performance and retain valued employees. J. Nurs. Adm. 32 (7/8), 393–397.

Soeberg, M., Blakely, T., Sarfati, D., et al., 2012. Cancer Trends: Trends in cancer survival by ethnic and socioeconomic group, New Zealand 1991–2004. University of Otago and Ministry of Health, Wellington.

Song, L., 2010. Social capital and psychological distress. J. Health Soc. Behav. 52 (4), 478–492.

Statistics New Zealand, 2013a. New Zealand period life tables: 2010-2012. Online. Available: <http://www.stats.govt.nz/browse_for_stats/health/life_expectancy/NZLifeTables_HOTP10-12.aspx> 28 October 2013.

Statistics New Zealand, 2013b. Births and deaths: Year ended 2011. Online. Available: <m.stats.govt.nz/browse_for_stats/population/births/BirthsandDeaths_HOTPYeMar11/Commentary.aspx> 24 June 2013.

Street, G., James, R., Cutt, H., 2007. The relationship between organised physical recreation and mental health. Health Promot. J. Austr. 18 (3), 236–239.

Symons, V., McMurray, A., 2013. The factors influencing nurses to withhold surgical patients' oral medications pre- and postoperatively. Collegian 20 (3).

The Australia Institute, 2009. Something for Nothing. Unpaid overtime in Australia. Policy Brief No. 7. Online. Available: <http://www.actu.asn.au> 23 November, 2009.

Thorpe, A., 2012. Health and work: Progress and priorities in 2011. Public Health 126, S15–S18.

Uecker, J., 2012. Marriage and mental health among young adults. J. Health Soc. Behav. 53 (1), 6–83.

Vaithianathan, R., Pram, K., 2010. Cost benefit analysis of the New Zealand national mental health destigmatisation programme ("Like-Minds programme"). Phoenix Research and Ministry of Health, Auckland.

Viner, R., Ozer, E., Denny, S., et al., 2012. Adolescence and the social determinants of health. Lancet 379, 1641–1652.

Wadsworth, M., DeCarlo Santiago, C., Einhorn, L., et al., 2011. Preliminary efficacy of an intervention to reduce psychosocial stress and improve coping in low-income families. Am. J. Community Psychol. 48, 257–271.

Walker, L., Clendon, J., 2012. Ageing in place: retirement intentions of New Zealand nurses aged 50+. Proceedings of the New Zealand Labour and Employment Conference. Wellington, New Zealand.

Walker, L., Clendon, J., 2013. Our nursing workforce: 'for close observation'. The third NZNO biennial employment survey. New Zealand Nurses Organisation, Wellington.

Wallace, A., Carlson, J., Malone, R., et al., 2010. The influence of literacy on patient-reported experiences of diabetes self-management support. Nurs. Res. 59 (5), 356–363.

Walsh, M., Fahy, K., 2012. Interaction between primary health care professionals and people who are overweight or obese: A critical review. Aust. J. Adv. Nurs. 29 (2), 23–29.

Wand, T., 2012. Positioning mental health nursing practice within a positive health paradigm. Int. J. Ment. Health Nurs. 22, 116–124.

Warr, D., Feldman, P., Tacticos, T., et al., 2009. Sources of stress in impoverished neighbourhoods: insights into links between neighbourhood environments and health. Aust. N. Z. J. Public Health 33 (1), 25–33.

Welch, D., 2013. New Zealand general social survey: 2012. Statistics New Zealand, Wellington.

Wilkinson, R., 1996. Unhealthy societies: the afflictions of inequality. Routledge, London.

Windsor, T., Ryan, L., Smith, J., 2009. Individual well-being in middle and older adulthood: do spousal beliefs matter? Journal of Gerontology. Psychol. Sci. 64B (5), 586–596.

World Health Organization (WHO), 1999. Regional Guidelines for the Development of Healthy Workplaces. WHO, Manila.

World Health Organization (WHO), 2003. Investing in mental health. World Health Organization, Geneva. Online. Available: <http://www.who.int/mental_health/en/investing_in_mnh_final.pdf> 18 November, 2009.

World Health Organisation (WHO), 2007. Workers health: global plan of action. Online. Available: <www.who/int/occupational_health/publications/global_plan/en/> 6 August 2013.

World Health Organization (WHO), 2009. Mental health, resilience and inequalities. WHO Regional Office for Europe, Copenhagen.

World Health Organization (WHO), 2012. Chronic diseases. Online. Available: <www.who.int/mediacentre/factssheets/fs317/en/index.html> 26 July 2013.

Wyllie, A., Brown, R., 2011. Discrimination reported by users of mental health services: 2010 survey. New Zealand Ministry of Health, Wellington.

Ylipaavalniemi, J., Kivimaki, M., Elovainio, M., et al., 2005. Psychosocial work characteristics and incidence of newly diagnosed depression: a prospective cohort study of three different models. Soc. Sci. Med. 61, 111–122.

Useful websites

www.aci.health.nsw.gov.au/chronic-pain—Website for self-help in managing chronic pain

www.asthma.org.au—Asthma Foundation Victoria

www.diabetescontrol.com—Diabetes

www.beyondblue.org.au/—beyondblue (Australia)

http://depressionet.com.au/resources/services/nat/lifeline.html—Lifeline's rural mental health information service (also their helpline 1300131114)

www.SANE.org.au—SANE Australia

www.healthdirect.gov.au—Variety of topics on Australia's health

www.heartfoundation.com.au/sepa/index_fr.html—Supportive Environments for Physical Activity—SEPA

www.inclusivecities.org/—Inclusive cities

www.moh.govt.nz—Ministry of Health, New Zealand

www.sparc.org.nz—Obesity Action Coalition, NZ

www.worklifebalance.com.au—Managing Work Life Balance

www.business.gov.au—Business topics, occupational health

www.likeminds.org.nz—Like Minds, Like Mine: reducing the stigma and discrimination associated with mental illness

www.acc.co.nz—Accident Compensation Corporation: New Zealand accident insurance scheme

http://nhc.health.govt.nz/archived-publications/phac-publications-pre-2011/re-thinking-urban-environments-and-health—Useful readings on urban planning and health

Healthy ageing

CHAPTER 11

Introduction

This chapter addresses the health of older persons in the context of community. The central challenge for healthy ageing lies in creating the conditions for people to age with optimal health and wellbeing and a good quality of life. But what is ageing? In the 21st century, social commentators quip that 40 is the new 20, and 60 the new 40. Does this make 80 the new 60, and if so, what does that mean for the way we nurture health and wellbeing along the latter stages of life's pathway? We know that the quality of ageing depends on the cumulative effects of social determinants in the earlier years. But there are also developmental changes that occur in the years from 65 to 90 and beyond, and these have not often attracted the attention of health care planners. Instead, planning has tended to revolve around population trends towards disease states, and how to prevent, treat and palliate these. This 'illness' rather than 'wellness' focus, is disempowering for older people, especially for those trying to cope with the cumulative effects of lifelong disadvantage. Community-based actions to support and enhance healthy ageing should revolve around health promotion; improving the social, physical, economic and policy environments within which older people can enjoy good health into the years of the 'oldest old', and engage in healthy lifestyles.

COMMUNITY ACTION

The most important challenge for healthy ageing is creating the conditions for people to age well.

Communities for healthy ageing need to acknowledge the extent to which older persons contribute to the social, cultural and geographical life of the community. People over the age of 65 are vital to child care and other aspects of family life, particularly for their grown children who may be living in busy, dual-earner families. Many older persons are also carers for family members with disabling conditions. Importantly, older citizens are also a viable economic force. Some continue in the workplace longer than their forebears, bringing wisdom to a wide range of industries, including health care. Older adults also have the potential to dominate shifts in the economy through their spending, investments and service requirements. They are a political force through the sheer weight of numbers, capable of swaying the policy climate for health, the environment and their grandchildren's educational future. In some communities, older people help calm the social climate through their understanding, and by having a more emotionally balanced perspective that comes with the patience of ageing. Others' lives may be destitute and lonely. The combination is unique for every person and experienced differently, depending on social and environmental supports. This chapter examines the continuum of ageing across different experiences and contexts, with a view toward establishing community and societal goals for health and wellbeing in the latter stages of life. First and foremost among these goals is empowerment, to nurture older citizens' participation in community life and in their health care decisions.

AGEING AND SOCIETY

The terms 'ageing' and 'elderly' were once used to indicate that a person had begun the journey to the end of life. Yet today, as the world experiences a proliferation in medical and health-sustaining knowledge and technology, and as older people embrace vibrant lifestyles, ageing has taken on a new connotation: that of unexplored possibilities. Many people over the age of 65 in Australia and New Zealand lead healthy and productive lives, some thriving in ways they could not during their middle years, when their life circumstances prevented them from achieving a balance between work, recreation and family responsibilities. A large number of older people are also unwell, suffering from chronic diseases or conditions that limit their mobility or sense of wellbeing. But these two groups are not polar opposites. There are numerous older people whose health lies between the extremes of high-level wellness and immobility. The challenge for nurses and other professionals working with older persons is to see each person in terms of individual strengths and needs, and in the context of the environments that support or constrain their health and wellbeing. This includes understanding their individual journey, and what it has meant for the way they experience health. From this understanding, plans can then be implemented to provide community supports that enable the highest level of health and capacity possible.

This generation of older people born in Australia and New Zealand live in relative peace and harmony. The lives of most of those approaching their 70s in the 21st century have not been without conflicts, including the Vietnam war of the 1960s and 70s. Some have also been beleaguered by the global financial crisis of 2008–09 that eroded their retirement income, causing uncertainty about the future. Conflicts and disrupted living circumstances have also affected the earlier years of many immigrants and refugees who are ageing in both countries. Ageing is also proving difficult for lesbian, bisexual, gay and transgender/transsexual/intersex (LBGTI) elders, some of whom have suffered the cumulative strains of lifelong discrimination. The older years are also challenging for Indigenous people who live in remote areas with few services or supports. But most people aged 65–75 are ageing well, perhaps because they have not lived in the deprivation of the first and second World Wars, like the 'oldest old' in society, and because society has responded to their needs with age-friendly living spaces, technologies, and supports tailored to their needs and lifestyles. For this, and other reasons, they tend to have a more optimistic outlook on life than their parents.

AGEIST ATTITUDES

Despite today's older adults having grown up in an era of experimentation, dramatic social change and relative prosperity, they are still subject to ageist attitudes, behaviours and stereotypes from those younger than themselves.

As a group, today's over-65s have lived their lives around values of hard work and industriousness. Many have a strong spiritual connection to place, either to the land or to the community and its ability to provide employment. In their younger years, they entered married life to raise a family, then went through some of the most dramatic social changes of any generation before them. They were the first generation to experience the women's movement and the subsequent changes to marriage and family life. Their relative prosperity meant that they were well nourished, but often with too many high-fat, high-salt foods, and perhaps too much meat. Most smoked and many drank alcohol. Some also experimented with marijuana and other drugs that created altered states of consciousness. But somewhere along their adult lives, they likely discovered the error of their ways, and stopped smoking. With their grandchildren in mind, they took up the green agenda, becoming advocates for preserving the environment. Many began to eat yogurt, a habit that would have been unheard of among their parents. Some also adopted new ways of thinking and got in touch with their feelings, engaging in meditation, Tai Chi and a plethora of techniques to create harmony in their lives. These too, are aspects of social life that were not part of their parents' generation. Yet, despite being unique, interesting, socially engaged, balanced, yet rebellious at times, they are often the subject of discrimination and ageist attitudes.

Ageism is a type of discrimination against older adults on the basis of misconceptions about their characteristics, attitudes, abilities and capacity. Describing older persons as a 'demographic time bomb' or as universally and exclusively needy, dependent and ill negates their diversity and varied outcomes (Garner 2009). The global state of alarm at population ageing may therefore be the most 'pernicious' example of ageism (Garner 2009:5). With so much attention drawn to population ageing, it is common to hear younger people make disparaging comments about older people being non-productive, resistant to change or a liability to society. This type of comment causes older people to worry about health-related decisions that might affect their future, including the possibility that a younger generation might ration their health and social services (Fairhurst 2005). Insensitive comments often draw undue attention to an older person's memory slip, labelling it as dementia or Alzheimer's disease, when it may be due to other factors such as motivation, the saliency of remembering or personal interest (Wilkinson 1996). In many cases, where ageist remarks are made, there is little consideration of personality characteristics, or personal responses to provocation, pain, disability or recent life events. Instead, the older adult's concerns are often stereotyped as if they were typical of the entire demographic group.

Stereotypes of older persons include negative impressions of their cognitive function (senile versus wise), physical functions (decrepit versus spry), and social lives (boring, perhaps) (Levy & Leifheit-Limson 2009; Sanchez Palacios et al. 2009). Stereotypes include assumptions that being older causes illness and irritability; that older people are lonely and devoid of affective links, or that they are disinterested in sexual activity (Sanchez Palacios et al. 2009). These negative stereotypes can be insulting to older people, and they can also be barriers to adequate care and support (Reyna et al. 2007). Garner (2009:6) notes that there is 'greater individual variability between 70 year olds than among 17 year olds'. Older people also continue to develop and evolve into their oldest years. Some do not cope well with ageing because of negative beliefs about self-efficacy, but others thrive, especially those who remain connected to family, social activities in the community (such as those of the Ulysses Club, described in Box 11.1), or volunteer activities, which are the lifeblood of community services.

DON'T WORRY, BE HAPPY

Despite dramatic increases in the oldest old and the imminent retirement of 'baby boomers', fears of decreased tax intake and increasing health care costs may be exaggerated.

TRENDING NOW: OVER 65s

- Social networking in cafes, sharing grandchildren photos
- Planning adventure holidays several years in advance
- Retiring
- Volunteering
- Caring for children, others
- Staying socially connected
- Exercising

GROUP EXERCISE: Ageism

In small groups, discuss your thoughts on older people's contribution in the workplace. Have you ever seen ageism toward older people in the workplace? How has this been manifest? What would you do about it if you saw it in your place of work or as a nurse?

Although widely recognised by demographers, the dramatic effects of population ageing have yet to be adequately acknowledged by health and social planners. The 'baby boomers' born between 1946 and 1964 seem to be wealthier than their parents, but with increased longevity, they will live longer in a state of poor physical health, with fewer family members to support them in their old age (Robotham 2011). Among this generation are the 'leading edge' group born between 1946 and 1954, who have protested against inequities in society, challenging 'the system' throughout their lives. They have campaigned against discrimination, and for the rights of the disempowered in society. The most notable of these campaigns include the civil rights movement, the gay rights movement, the sexual revolution, the feminist movement and the environmental movement. They have been the architects of many innovations, including television, oral contraceptives, the internet and personal computers. The 'trailing edge' group born between 1955 and 1964 also contains many social activists, and some hold politically influential positions in contemporary society (Robotham 2011). Together

BOX 11.1 Growing old disgracefully (with apologies to those who choose to grow old gracefully!)

The Ulysses Club is a motorcycling club for people aged over 40 that goes by the motto of 'Growing Old Disgracefully'. The club was formed in Australia in 1983 with the intention of providing ways in which older motorcyclists can get together for companionship and mutual support; to show by example that motorcycling can be an enjoyable and practical activity for riders of all ages; and to draw the attention of public and private institutions to the needs and views of older riders. With branches throughout Australia, New Zealand and South Africa, with more to follow in Canada, Germany, the UK and the US, the club demonstrates that growing older does not have to mean giving up activities that might have traditionally been associated with youth. Many members are returnees to motorcycling, having ridden in their younger days but given it away as family and work commitments got in the way. With the freedom of retirement, many can now return to motorcycling with the support of a club that meets their specific needs.

(Source: UMC, Online. Available: www.ulysses.org.nz/about.html [accessed 11 September 2013])

(Photo: Ulysses Club. www.ulysses.org.nz)

they are having a profound effect on social norms as well as health care. First, the leading edge of the boomers are relatively wealthy with low debts, but the trailing edge have experienced the recession of the 1980s and may not have the same resources as those born earlier throughout their later years (Marmot 2010). Second, the baby boomers have taken a strong stance against ageism, which will influence the way services are organised to support their needs as they age. Third, they have had smaller families and are more mobile than other generations, and may find difficulties in maintaining face-to-face relationships with close family and friends at the time they need them the most. Fourth, as they survive to be the 'oldest old', they may suffer from more years of disability. Fifth, they have stayed in the workforce longer than previous generations, and will continue to engage in part-time work, often simultaneously with volunteer activities, which have important implications for productivity (Robotham 2011).

BABY BOOMERS

- Some are relatively wealthy
- Vocal about ageism
- Smaller families, less contact
- Longevity means some disability
- Longer in workforce
- Retirement: risk or potential?
- Risk of frailty or illness
- Less workplace stress
- Time for exercise, fitness
- More social connectedness
- Sufficient financial resources
- Skills shortages, fewer role models

Despite the uniqueness of the baby boomers, concerns persist about their imminent retirement from full-time employment. Some policy experts have argued that retirement is a risk factor for illness or frailty, while others have mounted a counter-argument—that leaving the stress of the workplace and assuming a healthier lifestyle during retirement has major health benefits. Some older workers prefer to remain in the workforce, as a way of remaining connected with their colleagues and their self-identity. Others stay for financial reasons, primarily to maintain a preferred standard of living. Brockmann et al.'s (2009) research conducted on a large cohort of retirees indicates that early retirement lowers mortality risks. Those with poorer health self-select themselves out of the workplace, leaving a healthier workforce behind, thereby reducing their risk for mortality or further morbidity. Retired life also provides more opportunities for healthy lifestyles, which improves health and quality of life. This is often more likely for those of higher socio-economic status (SES). Those wealthy enough to retire early enjoy healthier ageing because of their opportunities for healthy lifestyles as well as the protective effect of financial security (Brockmann et al. 2009).

The main public concerns about the exit of the older generation from the workplace are centred on skills shortages, a lack of mentors for young people, and erosion of the tax base, as retired people pay much less in tax than those employed in paid work. However, these concerns may be exaggerated by younger people. Because the current generation of older people have greater wealth than their parents, many will be self-funded retirees, rather than relying on government support in their older years. In addition, many also enjoy better health than their age group has in previous eras, so the strain on health care systems may not be as great as some imagine. Financial security also permits greater opportunities for social engagement, which is a critical element for both retirees, and those who choose part-time employment in their older years. Social engagement in the workplace is a lifeline for many older people who, like a large proportion of others in the population, may be living alone. For some older people the family remains the centre of their social life, but for others, the freedom that comes from retiring and having fewer family responsibilities can open up new social networks, which are fundamental to health and wellbeing.

As we mentioned above, the generation of people who are approaching their 70s in the second decade of the 21st century are unique in their social and marital history, and this affects their patterns of social activity. They were the first generation of married couples to be offered and, in some cases, encouraged by no-fault divorce. As young adults, their lives were bombarded by the 1970s public media that promoted self-involvement and constant questioning of the status quo. Some resisted, and lived their mid-adult lives as married couples, but others have experienced multiple divorces and family combinations. As older citizens, members of this group tend to be more self-aware, more adaptable to new situations, and capable of living independently. Others, who have lived a more conservative lifestyle, may experience social life in their older years entirely differently. But for both groups, maintaining connectedness to family and community is a priority.

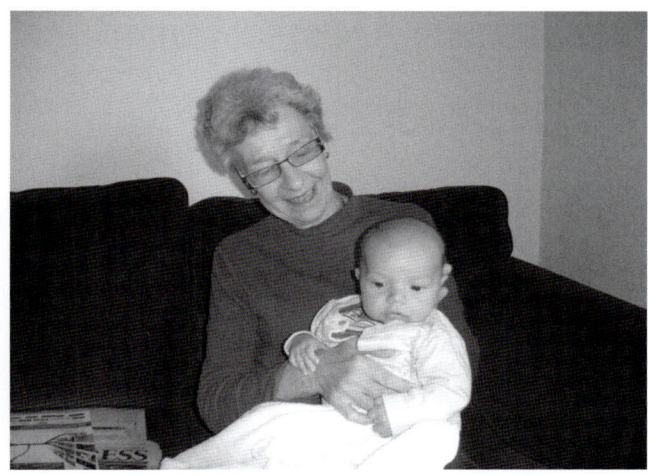

Grandparenting provides many rewards (photo: Jill Clendon)

QUALITY OF LIFE IN OLDER PERSONS

Despite individual differences in lifestyles, many older people rate their quality of life as satisfactory, and this has been linked to their current rather than past circumstances (Brett et al. 2012). In New Zealand, 91% of adults over 65 are satisfied or very satisfied with their lives compared to only 84% of adults aged between 45 and 64 (Statistics New Zealand 2013a). Although people age and mature in different ways, many begin to develop a more balanced perspective of life as a function of getting older. Psychological changes include a greater capacity for delayed gratification, and a greater valuing of relationships (Garner 2009). These traits evolve through acquired knowledge, and the recognition that internal resourcefulness and a sense of humour are critical to ageing well; that is, maintaining a high quality of life. Placing a high value on relationships also fosters greater tolerance of difference, which is important in an era where there is such diversity in community life. In the cities, especially, older people can be an anchor for newcomers such as migrants, with the time and tolerance to help ease their transitions and changes in the social fabric of their community. In the context of volunteering to help newcomers or simply in sharing stories of resilience, older citizens exert a powerful effect on the community.

> ## WHAT'S YOUR OPINION?
>
> Activity theory describes formal, informal or solitary activities as having differential effects on successful ageing.
>
> Do you think these act individually or in combination?
>
> To what extent are these linked to personality?

During the retirement or semi-retirement phase of life, increased leisure time provides opportunities for closer social engagement than during a person's working life. Many older people experience high levels of participation in social activities that are a type of role replacement for previous occupational roles. The activity theory of ageing describes these as informal, formal or solitary activities (Betts Adams et al. 2011). Research conducted in the 1970s and 80s has shown that informal social activity tends to influence wellbeing more than formal or solitary activity, but more recent studies indicate that a combination of both formal and informal activities, including physical activities, have a strong association with wellbeing, health and survival (Betts Adams et al. 2011). Social engagement helps maintain emotional closeness, or social intimacy, as well as instrumental assistance, which is usually seen in having greater social support for times when it is needed. Role replacement or, in some cases, role continuity through the familiarity of collegial relationships, can help an older person maintain a sense of meaning, purpose and identity. Participating in social activities tends to help people feel they have maintained mastery over their life; that they continue to accomplish things despite any constraints associated with ageing such as functional impairments, widowhood or lack of family support. This embodies the positive psychology concept of increasing self-efficacy or self-esteem through physical and mental stimulation, a sense of purpose and having choices and control (see Chapter 9). In

older people, the emphasis is on happiness, contentment and satisfaction with the past, current and future (Betts Adams et al. 2011).

EVIDENCE FOR PRACTICE:
Happiness-enhancing activities

Understanding the factors that enhance happiness in the latter part of life could be the key to promoting and sustaining quality of life in older people. Based on activity theory, New Zealand researchers conducted interviews with 23 seniors (aged 56–76) to explore their happiness-enhancing activities. They categorised the findings into four main themes: other-focused (time with significant others, meeting others, helping others); personal recreation and interests (hobbies, entertainment, relaxation, external engagement); thoughts and attitudes (giving thanks, constructive thinking); and achievement related (small achievements, longer term goal progress). Other themes, such as 'spiritual activities' and 'self-concordant work', cut across these four basic themes. They found differences between their participants in how they valued solitary versus social activities, and the types of things they saw as a 'happiness-enhancing' activity. This led the researchers to consider their findings in terms of 'person-activity fit'; a theoretical perspective that some people find a better fit with various activities than others (Henricksen & Stephens 2010).

So what does this tell us?

Research into something as subjective as happiness can be difficult to interpret. Henricksen and Stephens (2010) cited previous research that had identified a set of fundamental happiness 'techniques', which include spending more time socialising, stopping worrying and developing positive, optimistic thinking. They also identified factors such as 'counting one's blessings' or 'performing random acts of kindness' as having an association with happiness. These positive psychology concepts may be the key to happiness in the older generations, or they may operate selectively in certain types of people. Individual variability is also a factor in research undertaken from a quantitative approach, which can be fraught when measuring concepts such as quality of life, spirituality or happiness, because the measurements do not always tell us how these are experienced.

 What would you consider in developing a happiness-enhancing project in your community as a health promotion initiative for seniors?

GLOBAL POPULATION AGEING

With longevity at an all-time high, the world is ageing rapidly, especially with lower fertility rates in many countries. Population ageing is therefore the culmination of fewer babies being born and older people living longer. The WHO (2013) reports that for the first time in history there will soon be more older than younger people in the world, half of whom will be living in urban areas. Throughout the world, thousands of older people live in poverty and conditions of disadvantage, particularly in countries where infectious diseases like HIV/AIDS and malaria have caused deaths in family members. In these families ravaged by disease, there are fewer middle-aged adults to guide and support younger generations through their transitions into adult life. Older people in these families may be the only ones available to care for young children. As a result, in the case of many developing countries, their lives may be difficult not only from caregiving, but also overwork, a lack of food security, environmental degradation, civil conflicts or family displacement (WHO 2011). As we have mentioned previously, even in wealthy countries such as our own, levels of disadvantage among certain groups of people have seen older grandparents with responsibility for child care. Their input to family life is crucial, in the case of Indigenous people, often providing 'cultural sanctuary' for younger family members (Milroy 2013:43). Global concerns are the same as those we are considering in Australia and New Zealand; namely prevention of chronic disease, access to age-friendly primary health care, and creation of age-friendly environments (WHO 2013).

GLOBAL AGEING CONCERNS

- Prevention of chronic disease
- Access to age-friendly PHC
- Creation of age-friendly environments
- Culturally appropriate care

Cross-cultural perspectives on ageing are also at the forefront of health and social planning. Migration and other environmental concerns are relevant to the global dialogue on ageing, especially with so many families being displaced and relocating with their elders. Comparing health and social life between countries and between ethnic groups within a country can illuminate the strengths, weaknesses, threats and opportunities of ageing in different environments, especially in planning for social policies that will govern people's lives and the health care systems that will sustain them. Sometimes these comparisons can reveal unexpected differences and similarities among people. For example, researchers studied the experience of pain among older Italian immigrants and a cohort of Australian-born older men, expecting to find differences on the basis of ethnicity. However, the differences they found were minor, and only remarkable in relation to socio-economic factors such as years of education and occupational history (Stanaway et al. 2011). This is interesting in relation to the social determinants of health (SDH), in that older people's needs should be considered in relation to their environments, their cumulative histories and their support systems as well as their culture. Clearly, the SDH can vary widely between different stages of the older years, between different settings and life conditions such as employment history. It is also important to know how successful communities help their elders financially and socially, and where intervention may be required to rearrange circumstances for those living more challenging lives and promote citizenship. Supporting the ageing population requires knowledge of the individual, intergenerational sensitivity and consideration of the relationship between health and place, as older people's needs are accommodated differently in various communities and workplaces.

HEALTH AND PLACE

People develop ways of adjusting to the challenges of their lives in a variety of ways. Some of these differ by gender or other factors, but some differ according to the environmental or circumstantial aspects of their lives. 'Place' holds a pre-eminent position in the lives of many older adults, beyond the space where they live. The place or setting where people grow old usually has meaning for them, in that it shapes the intimate relations between people, and the broader processes of social relations that comprise social capital (Cagney & Cornwell 2010). As they go through the many transitions of ageing, their places, whether these are homes or institutional environments, are constantly being negotiated as a kind of personal geography. This includes where they live, how they move about and how they experience and understand their surroundings (Wiles 2005). Many older people are 'ageing in place', remaining in the community, neighbourhoods and households where they have spent most of their life (Cagney & Cornwell 2010; Ryan et al. 2012). In some cases the neighbourhood can intensify other stressors if they are unsafe or do not have supports that encourage healthy lifestyles. Older people often spend more time in their homes than during their earlier adult lives. Some have declining immune function, chronic illnesses or poor nutrition. These factors can leave them physiologically vulnerable to hazardous exposures, toxic emissions, infections or stressful environments (Cagney & Cornwell 2010). Mobility limitations can leave them fearful about neighbourhood crime or other safety concerns.

PLACE AND AGEING

The 'place' where people grow old has significance to an individual beyond its physical boundaries, providing meaning to the older person, through the creation and maintenance of broader interpersonal and inter-generational relationships.

Rural and urban environments for ageing

The most visible influence of place on health is in rural-urban comparisons. Ageing in each of these contexts has unique challenges. Independent-living older people with the financial means to be selective often gravitate to inner city living, where services such as the medical practitioner, pharmacist, physiotherapist, grocer or newsagent are readily available. Safety and accessibility are the most important issues for these urban older people, so the features they look for if they are choosing a neighbourhood are well-maintained, interconnected footpaths, lighting, safe traffic conditions, safe, warm shelter and green spaces (Burton 2012). Other independent-living people may wish to remain in their more suburban homes. Their environmental concerns may be focused on transportation, and ensuring there is someone to monitor their safety, health and wellbeing, especially if they live alone. A lack of transportation can be a barrier to accessing health care, insurance, dental care, rehabilitation programs or follow-up by health professionals (Corcoran et al. 2012).

Certain aspects of the built environment have an effect on all older urban dwellers. For example, to promote social engagement in the neighbourhood, low fences can help keep neighbours connected (Burton 2012). It is also important that houses are warm and dry in winter, cool in summer and well ventilated, especially if outside air may be polluted from traffic. Older houses tend to have narrow stairs or uneven rises, which may need to be revamped to prevent falls. Falls prevention is a high priority in promoting the health of community-dwelling seniors. A Cochrane review of falls-prevention strategies revealed that falls tend to occur because of problems with balance, poor vision and dementia, with some medications (such as psychotropic medications) also increasing the risk of falling (Gillespie et al. 2012). Poor lighting, clutter, torn carpets or noise can also increase the likelihood of falls (Cagney & Cornwell 2010). Natural lighting is important for those without clear vision, as is having a clear line of sight or 'surveillance zone' outside windows (Burton 2012; Ryan et al. 2012). Most injuries from falls are minor, and include bruising, abrasions, strains or sprains, but they can have a profound impact on a person's confidence in living alone. Major injuries from falls can have a major effect on people's lifestyles, often precipitating admission to hospital or residential care (AIHW 2012). Those in residential care have a greater risk of falling for the same reasons as those who fall in the community, but with the additional risks of wearing slippers or crowded environmental conditions in the residential care facilities.

Rural people also need supports from the built environment. Rural older people have been reported as having strong community and personal support and connectedness, low psychological distress, and good overall mental health, relationships and life satisfaction (Inder et al. 2012). In some cases, they have even greater needs for safe environments and timely access to services than urban-dwelling older people, because of distance and the sparse distribution of services (Ryan et al. 2012). Few people are able to live alone throughout their entire older years in their home because of the isolation, but many rural older residents have strongly perceived ideas of independence. Like people in urban areas, safety and access to services are paramount. Rural living also carries a higher risk for families caring for older people. This is related to a lack of transportation and assistance to move elder family members when they need care, a lack of emergency or specialist services, or the type of supports for various disabilities that may be available in the cities or regional areas. In addition, carers usually have no access to respite services in rural or remote areas. This becomes most stressful when their older family members return home after an acute episode of illness that may see them requiring rehabilitation over a long period of time. As there are few rehabilitation specialists in rural areas, this situation can hasten their admission to residential care. Once they are at a stage of dependency when they need residential care, an additional burden may be placed on family members if the facility is not available locally (Ryan et al. 2012).

Many older adults experience 'displacements' through multiple relocations; from their own home to the residence of a family member and sometimes back and forth between the homes of family members. They may also experience relocations between residential facilities, health care institutions and their usual residence. Each of these moves adds stress to older adults' lives, especially if they have been forced by illness or family circumstances to leave a home in which they have spent a substantial portion of their lives. For some, the stress is exacerbated by the unpredictability of the move, either because of its location or duration, or because it signals that the family has become scattered, and there may be no one to take care of them. Relocation stress is influenced by several factors: the person's characteristics prior to the move, their attitudes toward moving, their preparation for the move, their physical and cognitive status and the extent to which they feel they have control over the move. The stress is magnified for those who have had to dislocate because of the death of a spouse or partner.

Being from a culturally or linguistically diverse (CALD) background can add another dimension to the stress of dislocation, especially if the individual has difficulties in communicating with family or staff members in their new location or if they are unaware of the services provided (Yeboah et al. 2013). For rural people, successful transition into an aged care facility is dependent on whether or not they are able to maintain local social and family ties. Because of the outmigration of young rural people into the cities, there is a larger proportion of older people left in rural communities, many of whom are ageing without family support (Inder et al. 2012; Parmenter et al. 2012). The emphasis on ageing in place has also increased the age at which people are admitted to residential care, so there are more frail elderly in care who may not have many visits from family living at a distance (Parmenter et al. 2012). Those suffering from dementia are often neglected, with family members believing they have a decreased responsibility for connecting to someone with whom they can't always communicate (Parmenter et al. 2012).

At some point, most people experience a loss of place in both the material and emotional sense. Some have an extended period of grieving, which can be a very intense personal experience. Besides losing the material comforts of their home, they may also be grieving for the symbolic meaning of their sanctuary, the place where they have established and sustained the family. Home is often a source of satisfaction in having provided a protective environment for loved ones. It is where possessions and personal touches mark significant family moments and memories. Dislocation from the family home because of financial peril causes extraordinary stress for some people, and brings with it concerns about becoming homeless, or dependent on institutionalised care. Some people also worry about losing their home if it will leave their children financially liable, or in difficult circumstances following their death.

PRACTICE STRATEGY

Assess personal geographies, family supports, coping, self-care abilities, preferences.

DISPLACEMENT STRESS

- Situation/health prior to move
- Attitude towards move
- Unfamiliarity with services
- Shortages of caregivers
- Culturally inappropriate care
- Disconnection from family, friends
- Loss of material supports
- Financial strain

The relationship of personal geographies to health and wellbeing has implications for both home and community care. Unlike rural people who tend to live with family until they need residential care, many urban elderly live alone, and with greatest access to home care services, their proximity to family members is not as critical as for rural dwellers (Borowiak & Kostka 2012). However, home care may violate a person's sense of personal space by the intrusion of caregiving devices and external caregivers, or it may be readily accommodated and help define a person's sense of place. These reactions are variable. Models of shared care involving one or more outsiders and someone in the family setting may be received differentially, depending on the older person's connection with others, and how they choose to negotiate the relationships involved in both care and domestic living (Sebern 2005). The nurse–client relationship is often pre-eminent. Older people attending general practice or other PHC settings typically rely on nurses for advice and support for their self-management of chronic conditions. Nurses also provide the first line of support for caregivers,

The experience of ageing is typically characterised by some or all of the following:

- normative declines in health, physical and cognitive abilities and the likelihood of developing ill health or chronic diseases
- greater salience of health concerns in life
- diminishing time left to live
- the experience(s) of bereavement
- having more restricted but intense social relationships and networks
- being perceived or treated in ageist ways
- increasing interiority (looking inward), desire for integrity and search for meaning in life
- greater acceptance of what cannot be controlled and greater fear of losing control over one's life.

(Source: Settersten 2005:S175)

particularly in the context of home visiting. In this context, the privacy of the home becomes public, and home visiting nurses must bridge the gap between formal and informal caregiving (Bourgeault et al. 2010). In doing so, they may be the most trusted health professional in an older person's network of support. The most important resources they bring to these visits are a respectful attitude, diplomacy, and a commitment to working in partnership with the older person and/or family to identify strengths and potential, risks and needs (see Box 11.2). Their assessments, advocacy and plans for care are then tailored to the older person and their caregiver's needs and preferences.

AGEING IN AUSTRALIA AND NEW ZEALAND

Despite the inherent declines of ageing, older people in the 21st century have the potential for a long life, and better health status than the generations before them. Australians over age 65 comprise 14% of the population, and this is expected to double over the next four decades (AIHW 2012). Their life expectancy is second only to Japan, at 81.4 years. In New Zealand, 14% of the population are over age 65, and this is expected to double by 2040 (Statistics New Zealand 2013b). Life expectancy in New Zealand, at 81 years, has improved since 2010 though still does not quite match Australia's. There

is a 3.7 year difference between male and female life expectancy, with males lagging behind females (StatisticsNZ, Online. Available: http://www.stats.govt.nz/browse_for_stats/health/life_expectancy/period-life-tables.aspx [accessed 27 August 2013]).

Most people over age 65 consider themselves to be in good health, and in Australia over half (53%) remain in part-time employment (AIHW 2012). Most older Australians (94%) live in the community in private homes or self-care accommodation (AIHW 2012). Around 44% of those aged 65–74 and 81% of those over age 85 have a disability, the most common being vision or hearing loss, arthritis or other musculoskeletal problems, and elevated blood pressure or cholesterol levels (AIHW 2012). The figures are not dissimilar in New Zealand. Over 80% of older New Zealanders consider themselves in good health (NZMOH 2012), with one in five remaining in the workforce (Bascand 2012). While the majority of older New Zealanders are reliant in some way on the New Zealand superannuation scheme (NZS) for their livelihood, mortgage-free home ownership is high among the current cohort (Perry 2010). This means that the impact of lower income is mitigated to some extent by lower housing costs. Around 45% of those aged over 65 have some type of disability (Office for Disability Issues and Statistics New Zealand 2013). Musculoskeletal conditions, vascular disorders and cancers are the leading contributors to health loss among New Zealanders aged over 65 (NZMOH 2013).

QUICK STATS

Life expectancy in Australia is currently at 81.4 years—up from 77.1 years in 1990. In New Zealand, life expectancy has increased from 75.3 years in 1990 to 81 years in 2012.

Despite better prospects for healthy ageing, some changes are predictable in the latter part of a person's life. Physical changes reduce the body's physiological reserve, presenting a range of obstacles to healthy ageing, more serious for some than others. All older people experience some loss of skin resilience and moisture. Most develop more pronounced facial features from the loss of subcutaneous fat and skin elasticity. Changes in vision and hearing are typical. Respiratory muscle strength tends to decrease, and there may be decreased cardiac output due to decreased cardiac muscle strength. There may also be changes in mass, tone and elasticity of breasts, the abdomen, and the reproductive system. The urinary and musculoskeletal systems function less efficiently, and there may be some loss of balance, due to neurological changes. Some problems affect quality of life more profoundly than others. Incontinence, for example, can be a major problem for older people, as it is surrounded by stigma and can rapidly lead to social isolation, with those who are incontinent becoming less inclined to venture out of their homes. These conditions are not always life-threatening, but in combination they can work against a person's attempts to remain energised and vital, so they are often important areas for community nursing assessment.

MORBIDITY

The most important causes of morbidity in older adults in Australia and New Zealand are depression, diabetes, cardiovascular disease, cancer and injuries.

As we mentioned above, the SDH also play a part in the risk, potential and quality of a person's older years. Worldwide, urbanisation, ageing and globalised lifestyle changes have combined to make chronic and non-communicable diseases—including depression, diabetes, cardiovascular disease and cancers and injuries—the most important causes of morbidity (WHO 2011). Many older people live with the dual burden of social disadvantage and chronic diseases. Among older Australians, 49% of those aged 65–74 suffer from five or more long-term conditions, rising to 70% of those aged 85 and over (AIHW 2012). Those who live in disadvantaged circumstances also tend to have poor oral health, especially the loss of teeth, which can have a long-term effect on their nutritional status, self-confidence and quality of life (AIHW 2012). People over age 65 also have the highest proportion of hospitalisations. Although many of these are short-stay hospital visits, the longer hospital episodes are usually for joint replacement surgery for hip and knee replacements or revisions of previous surgery. Falls-related injuries account for around 72% of all hospitalisations for this age group, more commonly for women (AIHW 2012). The chronic disease burden in ageing is caused by the same group of diseases as are manifest in adulthood (see Chapter 10), as identified in Box 11.3. These are the leading causes of death, mainly coronary heart disease, stroke and lung cancer (AIHW 2012; NZMOH 2013).

BOX 11.3 Common chronic diseases of ageing

- Cardiovascular diseases
- Hypertension
- Stroke
- Diabetes
- Cancer
- Chronic obstructive pulmonary disease
- Musculoskeletal conditions (arthritis, osteoporosis)
- Mental health conditions (dementia, depression)
- Blindness and visual impairment

(Source: AIHW 2012)

SAFE ENVIRONMENTS FOR AGEING

Safety is a priority in home, community and residential care. Protecting older people from harm throughout ageing begins with attention to the community environment, and the structural features of their lives. Maintaining a safe environment at home includes falls-prevention strategies, ensuring the home is safe and secure from intruders, and assessing the need for physical supports. Home visits can be an opportunity for surveillance of the immediate home environment and the neighbourhood, with a view toward determining whether they need mobility supports to prevent falls, or any modifications that would help with any hearing or vision problems. Safety surveillance outside the home includes ensuring safe walkways, transportation systems and measures to ensure road safety. Well-maintained parks and footpaths with good lighting are crucial to keeping older people mobile and independent as well as providing an incentive for exercise.

HEALTH LITERACY

Involving older people in health promotion and community planning can help build health literacy.

Evaluating health literacy is also a component of safety surveillance. Identifying information needs can help promote self-awareness of any strengths or constraints that may influence a person's capacity for independent living. This includes helping them understand any physical or mental condition that might influence their ability to continue driving, or engaging in other activities of community life. Older people also need information and support to take precautions against violence, or other community crimes that may place them at risk. This information can be shared with others in community planning forums, gathering input from those with a wide variety of needs for services and support. Sharing information is invaluable for older people who may be unaware of how to access services or manage liaison across services, from primary care to acute and home care. Their involvement in planning can help promote awareness of the type and location of services available, and how they can be accessed.

An important objective of assessing the home and community environments is to help people stay in their own homes as long as possible. This is also the focus of various government support programs for healthy ageing. These include the Australian National Injury Prevention and Safety Promotion Plan (NPHP 2004–2014) and the New Zealand Injury Prevention Plan (NPHP, NZIPS, Online. Available: www.health.gov.au/internet/main/publishing.nsf/Content/health-pubhlth-strateg-injury-index.htm, www.nzips.govt.nz [accessed 12 August 2013]), both of which outline measures for falls prevention, and support national and state-run programs. Specific to older people, the National Falls Prevention plans in Australia and New Zealand ('National Falls Prevention for Older People' in Australia, and New Zealand's 'Preventing Injury from Falls') have been effective in reaching more people about the importance of preventing falls, and reducing the number of falls in our communities that require hospital treatment (ACC 2013; AIHW 2012).

These preventative programs are intended to keep older people on their feet at home and in the community, to prevent hospital admissions for falls injuries. All provide information for older people and their carers. Some programs, such as the 'Stay on Your Feet Canterbury' in New Zealand and Australian 'Healthy@Home' programs, provide a range of services that include volunteer exercise trainers, falls assessment and physiotherapy services. Multiple agencies in both countries are working on falls prevention as part of their national injury prevention strategies, and these are listed at the end of the chapter. Positive Ageing Strategies developed by the national governments of Australia and New Zealand are also aimed at extending health protection and risk management by promoting positive and active ageing (Australian Government, NZ Government, Online. Available:

www.health.gov.au/internet/ministers/publishing.nsf/Content/mr-yr08-je-je099.htm, www.msd/govt.nz/what-we-can-do/seniorcitizens/positive-ageing/strategy/ 12 August 2013). The goals and initiatives of the Australian Government program include supports for older people maintaining their health, physical activity, recreational and community engagement, as well as their contribution to the paid and unpaid workforce. The New Zealand Positive Ageing Strategy (NZ Ministry of Social Policy 2001) extends this type of commitment to monitoring older people's living standards, health, housing, transport, cultural diversity, access to services (especially in rural areas), and employment circumstances. The New Zealand strategy is also expansive in promoting community attitudes toward positive ageing, valuing older people's wisdom and providing opportunities for personal growth and community participation.

MENTAL HEALTH: ANXIETY, DEPRESSION, DEMENTIA AND COGNITIVE DECLINE

In general, mental health seems to improve with age, and this is the case for most Australians and New Zealanders (AIHW 2012; Dulin et al. 2011). The relatively quiet life of the older years leads many people to feel more content, focusing on emotionally meaningful and satisfying goals and activities as they confront the notion of a limited time horizon (Dulin et al. 2011). However, this type of peacefulness is not necessarily the case for those who suffer from various forms of stress, which can result from multiple losses that may be financial, psychosocial, personal, or a decline in health or mobility (Lavretsky 2012). Some older adults are better able to cope with stressors because of previous experiences with stress, whereas others succumb to anxiety and/or depression, particularly where they have serious or chronic illnesses requiring major adjustments in lifestyle (Lavretsky 2012; Rybarczyk et al. 2012). Depressive disorders and anxieties can occur on a continuum where some people develop minor depression triggered by stress, which can then develop into major depressive illness and functional impairment over time (Rybarczyk et al. 2012). Some progress to suicidal ideation, and the increasing rates of suicide among those over age 75 are a concern for families as well as health professionals (Schuler et al. 2012). Caregiver stress is particularly difficult for most people who are responsible for another's wellbeing, often causing anxiety and depression, particularly for women who are themselves ageing. However the way people react to stress and their ability to be resilient depends on individual predisposition or temperament, the severity and nature of the stressors, and the duration of exposure (Lavretsky 2012; Rybarczyk et al. 2012).

Besides caregiver stress, other stressors include being homeless, or in permanent residential care (AIHW 2012). It is estimated that as many as 60–80% of all aged care residents having some cognitive impairment related to dementia (Ervin et al. 2012, Forsman et al. 2011). In terms of the overall population of older Australians, 4.4% of those aged 75–84 and 11.2% of those over age 85 suffer from dementia or Alzheimer's disease (AIHW 2012). Alzheimer's New Zealand estimates that 48 000 New Zealanders currently suffer from Alzheimer's; with 300 000 affected by dementia (Alzheimers New Zealand 2013). Diagnosed dementia increased by 18% from 2008 to 2011 in New Zealand, and although improved diagnosis is thought to have contributed to these figures, it is estimated that 2.6% of the population will have some form of dementia by 2050. Up to 41 000 new cases of dementia will be diagnosed each year (Deloitte Access Economics 2012). As the prevalence of dementia increases, nurses will see more and more patients with dementia across all settings. Recognising dementia and ensuring appropriate care and treatment is in place will be essential to ensure patients receive the best possible care.

Research has shown that dementia is the result of more than 100 illnesses and conditions. These include Alzheimer's disease, which involves abnormal plaques and tangles in the brain; vascular dementia, which is brain damage from cerebrovascular disease or a stroke; dementia with Lewy bodies, or abnormal proteins, which affect brain cells and therefore a person's ability to function; and frontotemporal lobe dementia, in which the front part of the brain is affected, causing personality and behavioural symptoms. Other types of dementia are associated with Parkinson's disease, Huntington's disease, alcohol or drug-induced dementia, or dementia from head injury (AIHW 2012). Dementias such as Alzheimer's disease can affect language, memory, visual-spatial skills, personality or emotional state, and cognitive functions such as planning, abstraction or judgement (Gavan 2011).

Dementia is the most significant cause of disability at older ages, but it can also affect people under age 65 (Alzheimer's Australia 2013; Alzheimer's New Zealand 2013). It is a progressive, incurable condition that is highly disabling and, because it is more prevalent among the oldest old, it affects more women than men. Even moderate dementia can cause severe impairments in judgement and the ability to function independently, which renders the condition a major cause of stress for both the person suffering from the condition and their carers. Carers are often older people themselves, and the strain of caregiving can be detrimental to their health, especially those without access to respite services, or who hesitate to avail themselves of respite because of embarrassment, fear of abandoning their loved one or other reasons (Robinson et al. 2012). Some report sleep disturbances, depression, poor overall health and higher mortality than non-carers (Rose & Lopez 2012). The source of these pressures is intense as caregivers try to support the person with dementia through the initial diagnosis, the transition to advanced planning for financial and health care matters, driving cessation, and preparing for end-of-life (Romero-Moreno et al. 2010; Rose & Lopez 2012). Memory loss tends to be the first sign of dementia, and this is disconcerting for all involved. Caregivers also have to deal with the major challenges of mobility and communication, and these become more intense in cases where their loved one develops psychotic symptoms and aggressive behaviours. Often this is a response to being placed in an alienating environment, or because of the frustration of not being able to communicate their needs. Nurses in the community play an important role in helping these families assist their older members, either in adult day care settings, home visits or practice nursing (PN), where they may be responsible for coordinating care (Loge & Sorrell 2010; Moyle et al. 2010).

Although the majority of people with dementia are living at home, most people with dementia eventually display behavioural and psychological symptoms severe enough to warrant admission to residential care (Gavan 2011; Robinson et al. 2012). Nurses are pivotal to successful transition to residential care, especially in allaying caregivers' fears as well as those of the person being admitted (Bramble let al. 2009). A partnership approach can be instrumental to empowering carers as they work through the trajectory of the illness and decisions that have to be made, including those surrounding psychological as well as pharmacological treatments (Rose & Lopez 2012). Care in the residential context often revolves around anti-psychotic drugs, but research suggests that a more person-centred, recovery approach has had promising results (Ervin et al. 2012; Gavan 2011). This approach is aimed at examining assets and constraints in a person's environment that could be arranged to promote behavioural, cognitive, stimulation and emotional support rather than over-reliance on pharmacological management (Ervin et al. 2012). Maintaining independence in home and care settings can be assisted through the use of monitored dispensing systems for medicines. Monitored dispensing systems use blister packs (also known by brand names such as Webster Paks or Medico Paks) for supplying and dispensing medicines and are prepared by a community pharmacist. These systems involve dispensing a client's medicine into a special container with sections for days of the week and times within those days. The person does not need to remember which medicine to take, but simply what time medicines must be taken.

PERSON-CENTRED CARE

- Relational
- Empowering
- Refocuses care on interpersonal relationships rather than interventions

Person-centred care emphasises relational processes, and seeing the person with dementia as a unique, valued, empowered member of the community (Gavan 2011). Recovery-based approaches do not have the connotation of physical illnesses, where 'recovery' is seen as 'curative'; instead recovery implies identifying aspects of a person's life that they can actually 'recover'. In the case of someone with dementia this may involve recovering identity or some control over their life by being included in planning to manage the condition. It is a more optimistic outook than considering dementia as steady deterioration (Gavan 2011). In some residential facilities, nurse practitioners (NPs) act as expert resources to other nursing staff, helping them deal with the behavioural and psychological symptoms of dementia while building evidence-based staff capacity; that is, promoting person-centred, recovery-based care (Borbasi et al. 2011; Moyle et al. 2010). Support for staff includes attention to broader mental health terms, including the environment, which should be empowering to help families and the person in care through the different stages and experiences (Moyle et al. 2010).

DEMENTIA CARE

- Anti-psychotic drugs
- Person-centred care—empowering patient, carers
- Recovery-based care—recovering aspects of life that can be retained
- End-of-life care

Besides dementias, cognitive decline can also be related to having a smaller working memory, reduced processing speed and inattentiveness to fewer extraneous environmental stimuli. These cognitive effects result from the pathway effect of genetic factors combined with cumulative life experiences, including social determinants (Williams & Kemper 2010). People with cognitively stimulating occupations or who actively engage in stimulating activities may be able to overcome the effects of cognitive inability in early life and retain a high level of functioning (Williams & Kemper 2010). Recognising cognitive decline can be frustrating for older people. Like chronic pain or loss of mobility, compromised cognitive ability can lead to poor mental health as well as difficulties with health literacy, especially in maintaining their ability to manage medications or navigate the health care system (McDougall et al. 2012). Anxiety and depression can also be a cause or a consequence of loneliness or social isolation, especially in environments with low social capital and restricted social networks and support (Forsman et al. 2011). Depression is an interesting phenomenon in older people, thought to arise from the cumulative effect of chronic stressors and negative life events, including both health and non-health-related events. However, depression may also arise as a response to behaviour patterns established in earlier life stages that trigger stressors. This works like a feedback loop, in that stressors trigger depressive symptoms, which continue to elicit behaviours such as antagonistic interpersonal interactions that generate more stressors. Once this self-perpetuating loop is set in motion, it may endure for years, because of relatively stable personality and interaction patterns among older adults. One of the risks of suffering from depression or other chronic conditions is elder abuse.

ELDER ABUSE AND NEGLECT

Alarmingly, some older people are abused or subjected to bullying in their homes, in relatives' home or in care facilities, especially the frail elderly. With increased frailty comes the threat of harm by a caregiver who may have become overwhelmed with the pressures of caregiving, unable to cope, or simply malicious. An older person who does not see, hear or think as clearly as when they were younger may leave openings for unscrupulous people to take advantage of them either financially, emotionally or physically (Helpguide 2013). The most common types of elder abuse are financial and psychological, and these are most likely to be perpetrated by a family member (Families Commission 2009).

Financial exploitation can involve misusing personal funds, stealing, forging a signature, identity theft, investment fraud or seeking funds for a phony charity. Physical abuse includes non-accidental use of force, assault or inappropriate use of drugs, restraints or confinement.

ELDER ABUSE

- Financial
- Physical
- Emotional
- Sexual
- Neglect

Emotional abuse often includes intimidation, humiliation and ridicule, blaming and scapegoating, but it can also involve ignoring the person, isolating them from friends or activities, menacing or terrorising them. Sexual abuse may be overt or involve forcing the person to watch pornographic material or sex acts. Neglect or abandonment can be intentional or non-intentional, with some caregivers failing to understand the extent of assistance required (Helpguide 2013). Nurses may be the first to recognise signs or symptoms of abuse and are in a key position to provide support, guidance and resources to the older person. Important first steps in supporting an older person experiencing abuse include establishing a trusting relationship, and conveying respect and a non-judgemental attitude. Nurses also have a role in developing evidence-based policies and procedures within their organisations, to ensure older adults experiencing abuse are identified and supported. Box 11.4 lists resources to help detect and report elder abuse (Helpguide, Online. Available: www.helpguide.org/mental/elder_abuse_physical_emotional_sexual_neglect.htm [accessed 28 March 2014]).

STAYING WELL, STAYING PHYSICAL, STAYING CONNECTED

Because so many older people suffer from chronic illnesses such as heart disease, diabetes and depression, helping them achieve a healthy lifestyle is the great challenge of health promotion. Joint pain, decreased mobility and activity intolerance can also contribute to an inactive lifestyle, and lead to overweight or obesity (Newman 2009). Obesity in particular creates a cycle of disadvantage for those who are trying to maintain a healthy lifestyle. Obesity in older age is often related to a decrease in

---

BOX 11.4 Indicators for elder abuse

- Changes in personality or behaviour in the elder
- Discrepancy between observations made by the health professional and information from the older person
- Discrepancy in perceptions of the older person and the suspected abuser
- Incongruity between an injury and the history, there are unexplained injuries, restraint marks, conflicting stories, vague or bizarre explanations, or denial
- Frequent requests for care or treatment for relatively minor conditions
- Delay in seeking care or reporting an injury
- The older person is described as 'accident prone' or has a history of injury, untreated injuries and multiple injuries, broken eyeglasses, sexual injuries
- Repeated accident or emergency attendances of the older person from the same care setting
- Manifestations of inadequate care, including poor hygiene or nutritional status, poorly controlled medical conditions, frequent falls or confusion
- A relative or carer appears overly protective or controlling, or the older person displays unexplained anger or fear toward the carer or relative
- Desertion of an elder in a public place
- Suspicious changes in financial activity, wills, titles, power of attorney
- An apparent inability to afford food, clothing housing or social activities or questionable use of the older person's possessions/property/funds

(Source: Adapted from Glasgow & Fanslow 2006; Helpguide 2013)

---

energy expenditure, with hormonal changes causing an accumulation of fat, and metabolic changes that decrease a person's ability to regulate appetite (Newman 2009). In addition, environmental and social factors include concerns about safe places to walk, a lack of recreational spaces, safety fears because of neighbourhood hazards, and the tendency to eat out or from vending machines, for those without someone to share mealtimes (Newman

2009). Being overweight or obese can exacerbate arthritis and osteoarthritis by increasing the load on knee and hip joints, causing deterioration of the cartilage. Although mobility in joints should be maintained by stretching and strengthening exercises, these may cause pain that often prevents older persons with even mild levels of joint deterioration from continuing to be active (Newman 2009). People in pain often have poor sleep patterns, which can also cause people to eat more than usual. For those who become mired in a cycle of sleeplessness and depression, antidepressants can do as much harm as good, stimulating the appetite, causing water retention or slowing metabolism.

Based on the research evidence, most countries have introduced national guidelines for 30 minutes of exercise per day for all adults, including older people. However, only 38% of men and 28% of women over 75 meet these guidelines in New Zealand (NZMOH 2012). One of the interventions introduced to address physical inactivity in New Zealand is the 'Green Prescription', which is an activity prescription provided by primary care providers, including nurses (Elley et al. 2003; Kolt et al. 2009; NZ Ministry of Social Policy 2001; Sinclair & Hamlin 2007). Prescribing the exercise regime helps motivate a person to achieve the requisite level of activity by drawing attention to the benefits of exercise at the primary care visit, then intermittent telephone support by exercise professionals from the Regional Sports Trust. The program has already been deemed effective in terms of maintaining physical fitness, and it has proven cost effective (Dalziel et al. 2006; Elley et al. 2003, 2004; Kerse et al. 2005). More recent research has started to explore the various ways in which the program is offered and has had useful findings.

A study examining the use of pedometer-based versus time-based green prescriptions among low-active community-based adults over the age of 65 has found that while the costs of both are similar, the pedometer group showed significantly increased leisure walking time (Leung et al. 2012). Over the course of one year, the pedometer-based Green Prescription program reduced the percentage of those physically inactive by a further 6.7% compared with the standard Green Prescription (Leung et al. 2012). Leung et al. (2012) suggest this new approach is an effective approach to increasing physical activity and health-related quality of life among older adults. With nurses prescribing Green Prescriptions, this type of research demonstrates the importance of remaining up to date with the most effective approaches to exercise-based prescriptions. Nurses must also remain cognisant of the

JOINT AND MOBILITY PROBLEMS

Ageing, genetics, obesity, hormonal changes, intergenerational effects and the cumulative effects of lifelong exposure to environmental factors increase the risk of joint and mobility problems.

Physical activity and ageing

Maintaining physical activity is one of the greatest challenges of ageing. Although joint pain and a lack of muscle strength can be a deterrent to regular exercise, it is important to help maintain joint mobility. Combined with pain management techniques, regular exercise can help sustain quality of life throughout the older years. However, the exercises must be carefully planned to improve strength and balance, which, together with safe home and environmental modifications, can help prevent falls (Gillespie et al. 2012). Gillespie et al.'s (2012) review revealed that footwear assessment for aged care residents and exercise programs containing balance and strength training or Tai Chi are most appropriate in helping with balance and developing muscle integrity. This knowledge underpins evidence-based planning for preventing falls, which are one of the most frequent reasons for hospitalisation among older people. Age-appropriate physical activity also provides social opportunities, whether through interactions at a gym or other facility, walking or cycling groups. Maintaining 30 minutes of exercise a day helps prevent physical deterioration and prevent lifestyle-related diseases in all adults. International studies have shown that this level of exercise has been responsible for reducing coronary artery disease, some cancers, type 2 diabetes, obesity, osteoporosis and injury from falls (Kolt et al. 2009). Regular activity also improves quality of life and cognitive function by increasing cerebral blood flow and oxygen to the brain, which has been shown to reduce the risk of dementia (Williams & Kemper 2010). When exercise is undertaken in a social context the impact on cognitive decline is even greater, especially for women who tend to start at lower baseline exercise levels (Williams & Kemper 2010).

PHYSICAL ACTIVITY

- Maintains balance
- Prevents falls
- Enhances social life
- Provides feeling of wellbeing
- Reduces cognitive decline

importance of assessing the differing needs of the individual. Although pedometer-based approaches may suit many, it is important to offer a variety of options to individuals based on their personal preferences (see Box 11.5). For example, research into the outcomes of Green Prescription programs that offered phone-based support versus support provided through a community-based face-to-face support group found that although the proportion of people who completed the phone-based support program was greater, the face-to-face program had greater uptake by Māori and Pacific people (Foley et al. 2011). These groups are at particular risk of physical inactivity and the group-based approach used in combination with a pedometer may be particularly useful.

CRITICAL PATHWAYS TO AGEING

By the time a person reaches age 65, the cumulative risks from all earlier stages of life are usually evident. These risks accumulate from hereditary predispositions and conditions in the womb; childhood illnesses and injuries; immunisation status; access to education; growth and developmental issues; coping styles; diet and activity patterns; obesity, smoking, other risky behaviours; exposure to harmful substances or traumatic events; socio-economic status in childhood, adolescence and adult life; and a host of circumstances in the home, family, community and occupational environments. Just as these can be mapped across the pathway of childhood development, they also provide a pathway to healthy ageing, as depicted in Figure 11.1.

The 'critical pathways across the life course' model illustrates the parallel influences on achieving health and wellbeing at either end of the developmental continuum. From this perspective, ageing can be seen as a process incorporating events and predispositions from a person's earlier life, rather than a specified stage of life. This 'long view' of ageing seeks to understand accumulated risk and potential from childhood throughout the life course. Tracking the effects of the many and varied influences on a person's life provides insight into the social meanings they hold in their later years and how these have been shaped by their biological, psychosocial and environmental experiences. An individual's journey along the pathway is also indicative of how their personal history affects the world around them as they continue to make transitions to the end of life.

BOX 11.5 Evidence-based fitness: the Health Ventures program

A unique program of physical activity was established on the Gold Coast by Sue Vaughan, a nurse, psychologist, fitness specialist and manager of a fitness organisation. The program was advertised in the local papers as exercise for people over age 40, as part of the 'Active and Healthy'program of the Gold Coast City Council, which subsidised attendance to keep the cost down and encourage participation by older residents. Sue's program was immediately successful, and she attributes this to several things: it is fun; she is highly trained in exercise techniques, and has classes with participants at various levels of strength and balance; their activity level is individually assessed before they move to another activity; the classes are conducted to music, which changes weekly but is a combination of familiar 60s and 70s songs (by The Beatles, Tina Turner, etc.), and the popular music of today. With this formula, Sue's program quickly expanded from one venue to five, holding early morning classes with a range of people from aged 55–91. After two very successful years, she decided to conduct a research study based on the hypothesis that regular exercise over a period of 16 weeks would improve cognitive as well as physical ability. She enrolled 49 women aged between 65 and 75 in a 60-minute multi-modal class twice each week, which included cardiovascular, strength and motor fitness (balance, coordination, flexibility and agility) training. Another group (the control group), who were waitlisted to enter the program once the research study was completed, were asked to maintain usual lifestyle and activity levels. She conducted a number of neuro-cognitive tests on participants and gathered a biochemical measure of their cognitive functioning. In addition, she interviewed participants about their lifestyle and self-perceptions. The women were overwhelmingly satisfied with their renewed fitness and improved mental sharpness. One diabetic woman had come into the program unable to feel her feet and was doing foot exercises by the end of the program. Another diabetic had ceased insulin injections since completing the program. Many others related their feelings of vitality, self-esteem, fun and social enjoyment. The study measures showed significant improvements in psychological and cognitive test results and biochemical markers relative to the measurements taken at the beginning of the study (Vaughan et al. 2012, 2014). In particular, there were improvements in memory, concentration and thinking speed.

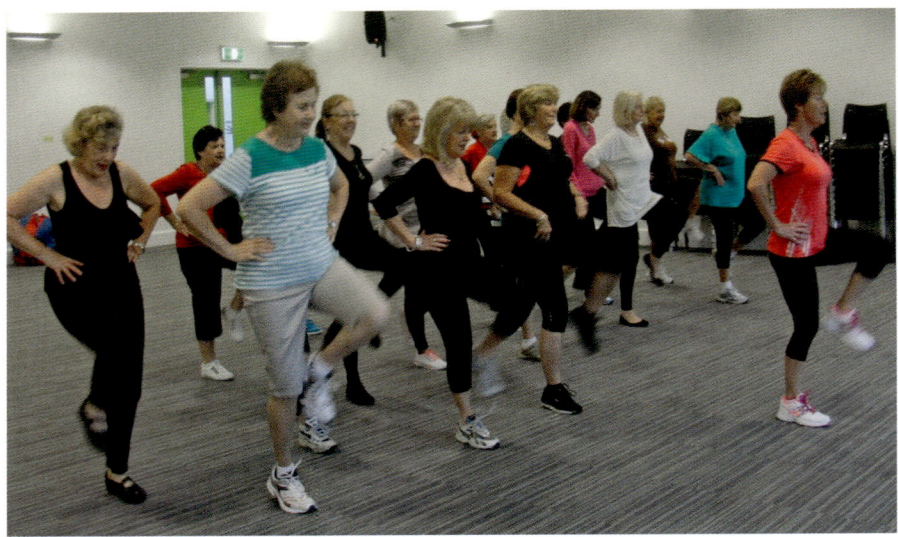

Health Ventures (photo courtesy Sue Vaughan)

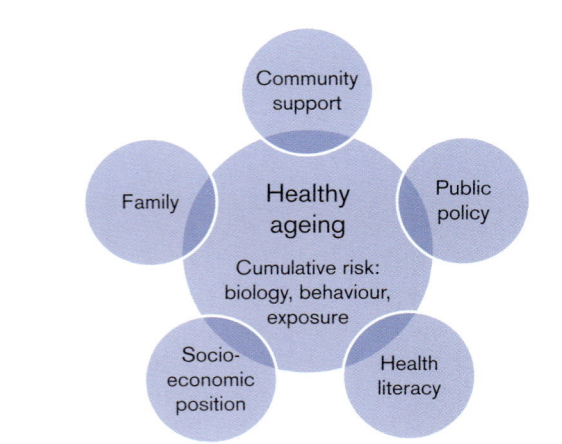

FIGURE 11.1
Critical pathways to healthy ageing

TRANSITIONS: CHALLENGES AND OPPORTUNITIES

The critical pathway approach to ageing incorporates various views of ageing. Erickson's (1963) model of human life cycle stages contends that we all have certain characteristic 'crises' to resolve at various stages of development. In the context of this theoretical framework, the major life crisis of old age is the struggle between integrity and despair, the resolution of which is expected to produce wisdom. But this may be a generalisation of what actually occurs, because of wide variability among people's individual responses to the circumstances of their lives (Wilkinson 1996). Some older individuals

experience entirely different life crises. Attitudes vary widely, and while some people do not consider themselves old at 80, others believe they are old at age 50. Others do not experience transitions as 'crises', but as opportunities to refresh their lifestyle.

Workplace and retirement transitions

A large, but not exclusive component of adults' self-esteem is developed in the context of work roles. Occupational roles give people a sense of presence and place. For this reason, the sting of ageism in the workplace cuts deep, and some feel it for a period of years leading up to their actual retirement and beyond. It is also surprising to ponder ageist attitudes in the workplace, given widespread recognition of our need for the skills and wisdom of older adults in many fields of work. Despite the need for older adults' mentorship, and a general recognition that older workers are honest, dependable and stable, many workplaces continue to discriminate against older workers (Berger 2009). The six major stereotypes held by employers are that older workers are less motivated, less willing to participate in career development, resistant to change, less trusting, less healthy and more vulnerable to work-family imbalances (Ng & Feldman 2012). These attitudes become a self-fulfilling prophecy where older workers are overlooked for employer training programs and promotion. With population ageing many workplaces have a large proportion of older workers. To counter stereotypes researchers suggest that human resources managers work proactively to raise consciousness in the workplace of the particular assets and needs of older workers, and work towards balanced work groups of young and old working together (Ng & Feldman 2012). For the older worker, being relegated to a passive rather than active role in the workplace diminishes their opportunities to remain socially engaged, especially for those whose lives have revolved around their work role. For those over age 65 the risk of being displaced from the workplace can be traumatic because of the lack of mobility, education and training (Berger 2009). One of the most important strategies for preventing ageism is managing a multi-generational workforce effectively.

WHAT'S YOUR OPINION?

- Less motivated
- Less participation in career development
- Resistant to change
- Less trusting
- Less healthy
- More vulnerable to work-family imbalances

Are these stereotypes of older workers typical of older nursing colleagues?

Nursing is a good example of where four generations of worker are frequently working in a single team; and when each generation brings their own communication styles, work preferences and attitudes to the workplace, a lack of understanding of the differing perspectives of each generation can see the sparks fly. For older nurses, this can mean experiencing ageism and bullying in the workplace. This type of antagonistic work culture does not help with retention of nursing staff, as researchers have found that older workers who feel they have been subject to discrimination are more likely to retire early (Graham & Duffield 2010). A study of nurses aged over 50 in the workplace in New Zealand found that many had experienced ageism with participants giving examples of where they had poorer access to educational opportunities because of their age (Clendon & Walker 2012). Study participants also noted difficulties in the workplace that had increased with age including managing shift work, being able to read medication labels, struggling with new technology and finding the physical nature of nursing more and more difficult (Clendon & Walker 2012). With 3.5% of the New Zealand nursing workforce already over 65

years of age (Clendon & Walker 2012), the health care sector, along with many other sectors, faces some important challenges in managing an older workforce. Recommendations for managing a multigenerational workforce include ensuring older workers are valued and given opportunities to mentor younger colleagues, educating workforces on the differing approaches to work that different generations may have, and ensuring a workplace culture that values all workers (Dols et al. 2010; Clendon & Walker 2012).

One of the major challenges for employers of older workers is to rearrange health and safety aspects of the workplace to accommodate employees' needs. Older workers may need to work at slower speeds, with fewer extremes of posture and less cardiovascular stress. They can also have lower tolerance to extremes of temperatures and may need intermittent breaks throughout their shift. However, studies have shown that even though work tasks may take more time, workers in their 60s tend to have equivalent or superior decision-making and other cognitive skills. They are also exposed to the same stressors as younger workers, which, as we mentioned in Chapter 10, are considerable. Some older workers are content to stay in the workplace and plan a slow, graduated transition into retirement. They tend to anticipate retirement as a reward for growing older, embracing retirement without looking back wistfully, as if they were losing a major part of their lives. Many seek this transition as an opportunity to engage in desirable and valued non-work activities, which can balance a number of different dimensions of a person's life and promote personal self-esteem, a sense of social engagement or belongingness, and greater satisfaction with life. (see Box 11.6). Many retirees gravitate to volunteer activities and those with some economic or social benefit that are closely aligned with their previous roles. These often reflect the need to respond to expectations of success and competency, just as they have done in the workplace (Hall et al. 2007).

Transitions to single ageing or widowhood

The most significant transition for many older people is the change from a long-term partnership to being alone. In some cases, this occurs because of a partner's death, while in other cases, it may arise from divorce or a partner's placement in long-term care. Although couples have varied life histories, many older people in this generation have been partnered for most of their adult life, and find the transition from being part of a couple to being alone devastating. It is unknown whether this is more

BOX 11.6 Maz who lives life

As a woman in her 60s, Maz recounts her life plan. 'It is interesting,' she says, 'to muse upon how one identifies oneself or how society identifies us as women. Throughout life we evolve from being known as "so-and-so's daughter" to "someone's wife/partner" to developing a significant professional identity—something you do in your own right, earned, and not assigned to you. My experience has led me to be known as "Maz from Curtin", "Maz the midwife". Socially, I was "Maz the yachtie". As I travelled and sailed for many years aboard a yacht I was "Maz from Ironbark" (name of the yacht). During this phase of my life I was meeting many people for the first time and became aware of folks trying to categorise me or work out which box to put me in. My appearance, price of shoes, clothes etc. provided them with a framework. Asking "What do you do?" and expecting a work-related identity created confusion when I said "I enjoy life". Some people would just avoid eye contact, casting about for somewhere safe or someone else to talk to. Others would pursue it, "tell me more", and then we'd go on to have stimulating conversations.

'Returning to "home in the burbs" I faced another major transition, as I was no longer engaged in the workforce. I felt comfortable in who I was, someone who works hard in community and family life, and began to envision who I would become in my 80s—like the eccentric little old lady down the road with an extensive herb garden, speaking her mind, dispensing advice on all sorts of issues, whether solicited or not. Hopefully I would be a wise old woman who would be approachable to share her wisdom, adventures and life experience to the benefit of others. At 50 I thought maybe some doors were closed to me. Maybe I should modify my behaviour/dress codes/activities or aspirations. Then I examined the longevity on both sides of my family and reckoned I hadn't lived half my life yet. It was an exhilarating, liberating feeling. "The world is my oyster". Now I can do anything I choose. I am comfortable in my skin, and continue a nurturing, permission-giving and sometimes challenging role in different ways.

'I have taken up belly dancing, enjoying the interaction and friendship of a special group of women of all ages and backgrounds. When I dance in public performances with joy and confidence, it doesn't matter that I am older and don't have the body of most of the other dancers. I am at ease with my body. I hope it inspires other women to "have a go" at something outside their comfort zone they may have been hesitant about. I am also the Queen of the Red Hat Society chapter, a community service where women get together for fun and friendship—simply coming together to share frivolity as well as develop caring, supportive relationships and networks. I am Maz who lives life. It is good, full, challenging and rewarding.'

(Source: Maz Osborne, citizen of Western Australia, sailor of the world, queen of the Rockingham Red Hat Rockettes, Arabian Nights Dancers performer)

---

difficult the longer a couple has been together, because couples go through variable adaptations in their lives. Some older people grow comfortably content with one another, while others find their relationship more difficult with the passing of time. The latter situation can occur if a couple has enjoyed an active life together, then experience a dramatically changed lifestyle because of ill health in one partner. The healthy partner may actually anticipate the loss of their partner because of the demands of caregiving, seeing the closure that comes with the definitive moment of loss as a step towards a better quality of life. Another dramatic transition occurs in older singles who, after many years alone, have partnered only to find the new relationship short-lived, because of the death or disablement of their new spouse or partner. Included in the anguish of these two situations is the loss of intimacy and sexuality.

GENDER AND WIDOWHOOD

Men tend to rely on long-standing friendships for support, while women rely on existing friendship networks. Women nurture themselves, while men tend to neglect themselves and their home. Responses depend on structural, process and contextual factors, including the relationship.

Transitions in intimacy and sexuality

Intimacy is an important aspect of self-esteem. For some people intimacy may simply mean feeling close to another and gaining the mutual benefits of closeness. Similarly, social intimacy can be immensely rewarding in bringing together members of a friendship group (Betts Adams et al. 2011).

These groups can be seen in the 'third places' where people congregate; those places that are neither home nor workplace, but cafes, clubs, the beach or settings where the opportunity for social engagement is always available. But for most people, intimacy includes romance, companionship, communication, touching, affection, and a sense that they are attractive and sexually desirable (Rheaume & Mitty 2008). Widowhood is often an intense loss of this type of intimacy.

Both widows and widowers suffer loneliness from losing their partner, but the cause and consequences differ for each. The 'widowhood effect', where a widowed spouse is thought to be more likely to die soon after losing their partner, has been disputed in recent research suggesting that only a minority of 15–30% of bereaved spouses progress to significant depressive symptoms, or that they go through predictable stages of grief (Carr & Springer 2010). Variations in responses are often due to structural, process and contextual aspects of the relationship. These include the nature of the transition; whether death was anticipated or not; whether it was preceded by stressful spousal caregiving or any other condition that may have impinged on the surviving spouse's health and wellbeing; and factors such as age and the length and type of the relationship (Carr & Springer 2010). Some widows and widowers become so distressed over time that they suffer from *complicated grief*, which is intense distress that interferes with functioning. Symptoms can progress from sadness to intense yearning to despair and suicide (Sorrell 2012; Schuler et al. 2012). Suicide rates among older New Zealanders are concerning, with men over 85 having the highest rate of suicide of all age groups in 2013 (McCracken 2013). Suicide among older people can be difficult to distinguish from euthanasia or simply self-neglect. Choosing not to take prescribed medications, poor nutrition or simply giving up the will to live can have significant implications for the health of the older person and can ultimately result in death.

Loneliness plays a key role in a person's response to the lack of intimacy. Psychologists define loneliness as 'a discrepancy between one's desired and actual relationships' (Carr & Springer 2010:754). It is a subjective state, experienced differently by those who consider their relationship highly desirable and those who do not (Carr & Springer 2010). For those who are lonely, bereavement may have a profound effect, creating social isolation or lifelong loneliness after a long-term marriage or partnership. Loneliness is also linked to risk factors for ill health such as sleep problems, poor cardiovascular health and elevated blood pressure (Carr & Springer 2010). The presence of friends or a confidant, children, good health and a social network are protective factors against loneliness (Grenade & Boldy 2008). Conversely, having no family or surviving children, living alone or having poor health can all be risk factors for loneliness.

People cope with loneliness in different ways, depending upon factors such as their personality, self-esteem, capacity for resilience and style of relating to others. Access to friends, self-help support groups, home visiting services or community social activities can be helpful, especially if a person is bereaved (Grenade & Boldy 2008; Sorrell 2012). Men and women experience sources of help differently, and tend to cope with loss and loneliness in the way they have coped with other stressors in their lives. The marital relationship tends to provide the closeness and support men need throughout their married life, and they are often more devastated by their partner's death than women. Men often find their home unbearable, and spend most of their time away from it, sometimes neglecting even the basic housework. For many women, once they overcome their fear of being alone, they tend to nurture themselves, after spending their life caring for others. What both have in common is a dislike for the terms 'widow' and 'widower', believing that the label isolates them at a time when they most need nurturing (Sorrell 2012). Reminiscence with friends or carers can be helpful (Forsman et al. 2011), as can becoming engaged in meaningful activities. This type of activity can also provide an incentive to adjust to the lack of intimacy. An important element of the loss of intimacy is the loss of sexuality and its contribution to a sense of personhood. Not all older people are as interested in sexual expression in the same way as they may have in their younger years, but their desire for closeness and intimacy is usually unchanged (Rheaume & Mitty 2008).

POINT TO PONDER

Intimacy and sexuality are as important at older ages as they are at younger ages.

As acknowledged by the WHO, everyone has a right to intimacy and sexuality throughout their lifespan. What nurses can do to support healthy sexual expression in older people is to support their right to a pleasurable sexual relationship without fear, shame, violence or coercion (Rheaume & Mitty 2008). In residential care, this can be challenging, especially for those with cognitive impairment, but in the community, nursing interventions may be more focused on permission-giving and health literacy. People who may have grown up in a culture where sexuality was suppressed often find ageing confusing, in terms of understanding their bodily changes, and what they believe is appropriate behaviour. Nurses working in primary care or community settings are the first person with whom they can discuss these issues, usually in the context of a home visit. A holistic health assessment may reveal a need for information about sexual behaviour or changing sexual function. This can often include information on the effects of chronic conditions, normal hormonal changes, and/or medications on sexual desire or performance. Any of these factors may affect the health of one or both partners, and their goals for a continuing sexual relationship (Rheaume & Mitty 2008).

SEXUALITY (WHO)

'Sexuality is a core dimension of life that incorporates notions, beliefs, facts, fantasies, rituals, attitudes, values, and rights with regard to gender identity and role, sexual acts and orientation, and aspects of pleasure, intimacy, and reproduction.'

(in Rheaume & Mitty 2008:342)

For many older people, having a partner become dependent on them for caregiving represents a loss of intimacy, sexuality, self-identity and a sense of the future. In New Zealand, 11.8% of people aged over 65 years provide unpaid care for a family member in their own household who is ill or disabled (Statistics New Zealand 2007). In Australia, more than 2.6 million Australians care for others because of disability or old age, most (78%) in their own homes (AIHW 2012). More than half of these carers are women, many of whom have care needs themselves. Caring often takes up to 20 hours a week, which severely compromises carers' financial status as well as the opportunity to engage in paid work outside the home. It is a demanding role, often causing difficulties with physical, mental and emotional health and wellbeing because of caring responsibilities (AIHW 2012).

As mentioned previously, caregiving can be a frequent source of chronic stress among women, who often go through transitions from child-carer to parent-carer without respite as they are ageing

themselves. Many of these 'sandwich carers' combine caring for both children and parents at the same time. Widowhood compounds caregiver stress by causing depression or anxiety, or a sense of worthlessness. At the time of widowhood and beyond, self-esteem tends to suffer. Some people neglect their health or discontinue healthy behaviours they may have shared as part of a couple. Their needs at this time revolve around social support, and regaining a sense that there is a future to look forward to, and opportunities to continue developing physically, emotionally and spiritually. Interestingly, a New Zealand study of family caregivers found those over 65 years of age, despite experiencing high levels of stress and depression, experienced less stress and depression than those under 65 (Jorgensen et al. 2010), suggesting that older caregivers cope better with this role than their younger counterparts. This could be due to the lack of other commitments such as a job or other family members to care for, or could simply demonstrate the resilience (or possibly resignation) of this age group to taking on a caregiving role with their partner or spouse. In the same study, less than 4% of all caregivers of older people were happy with the support they received for their caregiving role (Jorgensen et al. 2010).

SANDWICH CARERS

Many older women become 'sandwich carers', caring for both children and parents simultaneously.

Transitions to the end of life

Nurses play an important role in helping people as they near the end of their lives, most often, older people. Community nurses typically have an in-depth understanding of end-of-life experiences, but equally as important, they often act as the point of access to the private spaces where people and their family members prepare for this stage (O'Connor & Alde 2011). A person who knows death is near can become overwhelmed with making end-of-life decisions about symptom management for pain, physical, psychosocial, spiritual or socio-legal issues, and those related to palliative care. Palliative care is generally considered specialist care aimed at maintaining the highest quality of life possible in the circumstances rather than continue efforts to have the person survive at any cost. Palliative care therefore begins when a person's condition is no longer amenable to cure. The way we think about palliative care is important. Dying is a normal process, so a dying person should have relief from pain and other distressing symptoms and each person's care should be assessed and managed in a holistic way that includes support for the family as well as the individual (O'Connor & Alde 2011).

The palliative care movement has seen the development of palliative care homes or hospices in many communities. These offer an attractive alternative to hospital care at the end of life, but they are not widely available in all areas (O'Connor & Alde 2011; Payne 2009). To redress this gap in services an innovative web based program called the virtual hospice has been developed by Dr Susan Neuman and her team at the Maitland Palliative Care Service in NSW. The site provides contacts and advice for patients, carers, health professionals and community members to promote health behaviours around death, dying, bereavement and end-of-life care (www.virtualhospice.com.au). Australia's National Palliative Care Strategy conveys a commitment to the principles of palliative care for all, but because of shortages of specialist practitioners, care is usually provided by primary care providers or an interdisciplinary palliative care team. Despite the sparsity of palliative care centres, research comparing the 'quality of death' among 30 OECD countries revealed that Australia and New Zealand are ranked second and third after the UK as places where quality care at the time of death is entrenched in government policy and provided as widely as possible (OECD, Online. Available: www.eiu.com/site_info.asp?info_name+qualityofdeath_lienfoundation&page+noads [accessed 15 August 2013]).

The objective of palliative care is to work towards close engagement with the patient and family for healing and harmony at the end of life, especially in accommodating family members' burden of care and cultural needs (Chater & Tsai 2008). Palliative care nurses are highly trained in psychosocial skills, to respond to anger and a range of emotions that might occur from family members who are hesitant to let go of their loved one (Pavlish & Ceronsky 2009). Their main objectives are to care for the person in a way that provides comfort, dignity, involvement in decision-making, symptom support and bereavement support (O'Connor & Alde 2011). Nurses can help enhance personal growth for the surviving family members if they are treated as partners in care, rather than as merely visitors, throughout this stage of their elder's illness (Whitaker 2009). Because palliative care nurses are

specialists in family relationships they can act as a resource for others, to ensure that a partnership model is implemented. This type of approach to care includes teaching, caring, coordinating, advocating and mobilising resources (Pavlish & Ceronsky 2009). These outcomes are accomplished with personal attributes that include maintaining clinical expertise, honesty, having a family orientation, perceptive attentiveness, being present, calm and connected, collaborating with others in a way that would provide a cohesive plan for care, and being purposeful and deliberate in their preparation (Pavlish & Ceronsky 2009).

PALLIATIVE CARE PRINCIPLES

- Dying is a normal process.
- Care is provided for comfort, dignity, symptom relief, bereavement support.
- Care is holistic, based on assessing and managing individuals and their family as partners in decision-making and care.

Palliative care is also guided by a set of ethical and cultural principles as identified in Box 11.7.

Advance care planning (ACP) is another process that supports people on the pathway toward the end of life. ACP is a process of discussion and shared planning that enables the individual to identify and incorporate their personal beliefs and values into their future health care (NZMOH 2011). ACP allows individuals to express their preferences for care and usually includes writing an advance care plan and/or an advance directive. Some may also take the opportunity to appoint an enduring power of attorney. Expressing their end-of-life care preferences gives older people and their families the opportunity to discuss and plan care to ensure that the wishes of the individual are met by care providers when they may no longer be able to express those preferences themselves. It is estimated that being given the opportunity to undertake advance care planning may be offered to as few as 2% of people who may benefit from this approach in Australia (Jeong et al. 2011). While advance care planning can be seen as a difficult process for some, Jeong et al. found both older people and their families participating in the process came to accept it as the right thing to do despite their initial misgivings. A number of barriers to ACP exist including a lack of knowledge and

BOX 11.7 Ethical and cultural issues in palliative care

- Respect for the patient's and family's choices
- Advanced care planning
- Integrity and selflessness in caring
- Open communication, relevant, appropriate message at the right pace
- Agreed goals of care, negotiated between patient, family, primary care provider and multidisciplinary team
- Attentiveness to bereavement concerns, cultural differences in the requirement for religious and spiritual support
- Regular assessment and review of goals and preferences
- Inclusion of those who are resource poor
- Consideration of rural populations and those without access to care
- Providing care for the caregivers, such as those who are caring for orphans or children caring for children
- Tailoring care to the needs of children where appropriate
- Meeting special requirements of those with special needs such as those with learning difficulties, mental health problems, refugees, prisoners, internally displaced people
- Addressing the needs of minority and ethnic groups
- Advocating for policy and funding support for palliative care

(Source: Adapted from O'Connor & Alde 2011; Payne 2009)

RESILIENCE AND EMPOWERMENT IN OLDER PEOPLE

Resilience in ageing can be part of the developmental continuum, if adequate and appropriate supports are provided and if an individual has developed the inner resources to transcend some of the difficult situations they have encountered in their life. Contrary to ageist stereotypes, many adults cope well with normative declines as they grow older, particularly when they occur gradually (Ramsey 2012). But the experience of pain, of not being able to drive or otherwise navigate the environment, or interact with others, are the adversaries of healthy ageing, because these are seen as signs that the body is deteriorating. Pain, in particular, has a profound impact on quality of life. Pain changes a person's lifestyle, as it can cause or exacerbate immobility and dampen chances of remaining physically active. Being immobile is a barrier to social relationships that could be energising in an otherwise difficult lifestyle (Ziegler & Schwanen 2011).

POSITIVE AGEING

- A sense of humour
- Philosophical stoicism
- Selective optimisation
- Intellectual curiosity
- Mobilising latent resources by positive reframing and psychological flexibility
- Mindfulness, spirituality
- Affirmative decision-making, bouncing back from adversity
- Hope
- Social support

uncertainty of ACP processes among practitioners, legislative barriers and procedural issues, uncertainty among patients and their families, and questions about roles and responsibilities (Boddy et al. 2013). Nurses can help to alleviate these barriers by facilitating ACP, both by brokering the process for patients who may not have considered undertaking ACP (Jeong et al. 2007) and also by educating colleagues about ACP and its benefits. Nurses working in primary health care settings interviewed about their experiences with ACP believed the most important aspect of successfully working with patients and their families around ACP was building trust and rapport, and being aware of their own beliefs in relation to end-of-life care (Davidson et al. 2013).

Positive ageing includes the ability to mobilise one's latent resources, be psychologically flexible, use an affirmative decision-making style, and generate an optimistic response even in the context of age-related decline (Hill 2010). The wisdom and emotional regulation that comes with advanced age can lead a person to transcend earlier experiences and to be more selective about the things that hold meaning (Rybarczyk et al. 2012). Spirituality and 'selective optimisation' are protective factors that help people become resilient, bouncing back in the face of longstanding pain, chronic illness, grief or any other adversity (Rybarczyk et al. 2012; Windle

2012). Older people who have cumulative stressors from traumas such as abuse, bereavement, social disadvantage or the onset of ill-health may have the capacity to be resilient, but not all are able to do so (Windle 2012). Cultural considerations play a part in coping with ageing (Dulin et al. 2011). Some families may not encourage help-seeking because of a cultural value of self-sufficiency, while others may be more inclined to seek assistance early for any difficulties (Romero-Moreno et al. 2010). However, there are ways to reinforce the importance of self-efficacy and developing a philosophical stoicism about what can, and what can't, be changed. Nurses and other health professionals can help older people with whom they interact to see that their sense of humour, intellectual curiosity and maturity are all assets. Guiding people to develop mindfulness, positive reframing and hope can all reinforce self-efficacy, especially if social support is also available (Rybarczyk et al. 2012). Psychological techniques such as positive reframing involve rational explanations of life such as focusing on how well they have survived. For those who hesitate to be reliant on others for support, the emphasis can be shifted to seeing how they can remain independent for much longer if they are willing to accept support from others (Rybarczyk et al. 2012). These are person-centred techniques that can help counter a person's fear of progressive decline.

> ### HELPING PEOPLE COPE
> * Encourage reminiscence.
> * Use motivational interviewing.
> * Encourage participation.
> * Identify personal assets.
> * Guide people toward mindfulness.
> * Reinforce self-efficacy.

Coping can be a pervasive challenge for older people, who often live with a subterranean stream of grief for their earlier life, whether this is grieving for a partner, children, a career or a mark of relevance in the world. For some people reminiscence can be helpful in helping them develop a coherent personal narrative about why certain things eventuated in their life, and helping them reconcile some of the tensions between joy and sorrow (Ramsey 2012). Nurses can use motivational interviewing (see Chapter 4) to help people shift from negative to positive coping strategies, encouraging reflection on the past and consideration of the future. Reflections late in life can be affirming if they bring happy memories of an accomplishment, an insight or a shared moment (Stovall & Baker 2010). Alternatively, feeling their life has not been validated by others or themselves, or experiencing a sense of loss of all that is familiar can lead to a loss of control over a person's life, and their sense of the future. Some of the things older people worry about during their various transitions are whether or not they can retain personal space, whether they will be cared for according to the traditions of their faith, whether they will be honoured as a unique individual and the extent to which they will have choices, such as having a drink when they want one (Bano & Benbow 2010). The difference between those who become resilient and those who sink into depressed states may be due to empowerment, the extent to which they feel in control of their lives and able to participate in creating positive outcomes (Shearer et al. 2012).

Shearer and her team of nurse researchers explored a number of theoretical positions that could underpin empowerment in older people. One is the 'lifespan developmental perspective', where people have an inherent potential to participate in the changes that affect their lives in the context of dynamic, supportive environments. Another is 'critical social theory', which contends that people become aware of the social constraints under which they live, and this frees their thinking, establishes unconstrained communication, and encourages them to participate in creating change. A third approach, 'feminist theory', argues that empowerment is choice and freedom, while a fourth approach, 'Bandura's self-efficacy theory' (see Chapter 6), revolves around a person's belief from previous experiences that they can succeed or adapt to life, and develop a sense of mastery, control and choice (Shearer et al. 2012). These understandings of empowerment suggest that nurses can play an important role in helping people cope with chronic illnesses of ageing by using multilevel interventions that address a combination of personal, cultural, contextual and sustainability issues (Shearer et al. 2012).

Social and spiritual support

Spirituality is an important factor that helps many older people find a larger frame of reference and imagine a positive future when they must cope with the stresses of ageing (Ramsey 2012). Private expressions of spirituality, or the communal sharing of religious rituals such as attending church services, can be a source of comfort and hope for those with

EVIDENCE FOR PRACTICE:
The health empowerment intervention

Shearer et al. (2010) used their knowledge of empowerment to develop a nurse-led program called the Health Empowerment Intervention (HEI) to nurture wellbeing among a group of older chronically ill, homebound people. Their program was based on the relationship between personal and social resources and involved weekly visits for six weeks. The objective of each visit was to engage participants in activities that would help them recognise personal and social contextual resources, and to identify desired health goals, as well as the means to attain these goals. A comparison group received a weekly newsletter with information on home safety, medication safety, ageing and skin care, vision, dental care and bone health. The intervention group who received the HEI program were visited by the nurses and helped through specific goals for each week as follows:

1   personal resources and building self-capacity

2   recognising one's strengths, self-talk, purpose in life, personal growth and self-acceptance

3   building social networks to enhance awareness of and access to social supports

4   identifying and building social service use

5   communicating to build social networks and access service providers

6   reviewing progress toward goal attainment and goals for the future.

Participants in the program found it acceptable, and reported to the researchers that it increased their self-capacity. They saw themselves as growing and expanding, being open to new experiences, realising their potential, improving and changing in ways that reflected self-knowledge. Older, frailer participants with more chronic conditions and less money, and men, seemed to benefit the most from the program.

So what does this tell us about working with older people?

The findings led the nurses to conclude that this type of intervention that focuses on a strengths-based, empowerment approach could lead to a more effective way of working with older people.

? How would you go about lobbying for resources to conduct such a program? Who in your community would benefit most from the HEI intervention?

disabling or life-threatening physical conditions or the emotional despair that comes from loneliness (Mazzotti et al. 2011; Ramsey 2012). Faith-based communities promote common bonds of hope and faith, a kind of spiritual solidarity, which can be integral to preventing or recovering from illness, or mediating end-of-life anxiety (Ramsey 2012). Church groups can also act as a buffer for the adverse effects of stress, anger, disappointment, loss and bereavement (Chatters 2000). Collective worship promotes a sense of community in helping people feel they are not alone, even when life circumstances seem to leave them feeling abandoned. This type of communal activity, warmed by positive interpersonal behaviours, can be a source of solace to older adults. Many therefore turn to religion in their older years, to work through life's transitions within a community of people who are spiritually similar, comfortable and caring. In some cases, use of the word 'reconciliation' in the religious context is used to introduce spiritual compatibility, or consistency in thoughts and deeds. This helps shape interpersonal behaviours that promote warmth, friendliness, love, compassion, harmony, tolerance and forgiveness (Chatters 2000).

> **Religion**—adherence to beliefs and practices of an organised religious institution
>
> **Spirituality**—how people understand their lives in view of their ultimate meaning and value

Faith-based communities can also be instrumental in shaping behaviours that determine risk-taking or health maintenance, which may include dietary restrictions, prohibition against alcohol or tobacco, or promoting healthy patterns of activity and the values of moderation and conformity (Chatters 2000). However, some aspects of the relationship between religion and health remain ambiguous, especially if they become engulfed in a group and its traditions instead of flourishing in support of their spiritual development (Ramsey 2012). Religious groups that are inclusive of the personal spiritual journey are those that service the dual purpose of a bonding community and support for older people in a way that maintains their dignity.

Maintaining dignity in coping

Dignity is also an issue for those ageing in conditions of social disadvantage. Being poor increases a person's vulnerability to the effects of ageing, and constrains their coping ability. Clearly, it is easier for those with sufficient resources to access the social activities they need. For people living in disadvantaged circumstances, being able to connect with others in the community can be a greater challenge. With adequate financial resources, there are more opportunities to access social support, which helps people develop a sense of mastery over their lives (Gadalla 2009). Social disadvantage creates even more difficulties in coping with ageing for women, and those with low educational levels (Rueda et al. 2008). Many women continue to have responsibility for the household into old age, and this can place a burden on their health. Those without transportation are also at a disadvantage in not being able to get out and interact with others. Another layer of disadvantage for women occurs among those living in rural areas. As high users of health services, older, rural women have poorer health and lower survival rates from disease, because of their lack of access to services (NRHA 2013; Vagenas et al. 2009).

> ### POINT TO PONDER
>
> Being poor increases an older person's vulnerability to the effects of ageing, and may result in ineffective coping strategies.

Personal coping behaviours can also be problematic. Some older adults regularly use alcohol in combination with other drugs to manage pain, the frustrations of disabling conditions and loneliness. In many cases, the alcohol consumption remains hidden unless it is detected in diagnostic tests, which may not occur until later in life. For some, consuming alcohol may be a lifelong coping mechanism. Over-consumption of alcohol is responsible for a large proportion of the burden of cirrhosis of the liver, primarily in men (AIHW 2012). Alcohol also has a compound effect if it is mixed with other medications, and this is often the case with older people. Many older people suffering from even mild depression are treated with antidepressants. Others may be on analgesics for pain relief, and also on medications for metabolic disorders or cardiovascular conditions. This 'polypharmacy' creates the risk of overdosing, when alcohol is added to the daily intake of substances. Being in an altered state from alcohol can also create a risk of falling, losing awareness of the immediate environment, or having an accident such as a burn

injury, because of a lack of attentiveness. Many people who consume alcohol also ignore their diet, which compounds their level of risk for illness.

The attraction of alcohol is that it works so well. For those with sleep problems, as often occurs in older people, alcohol has a relaxing effect, helping a person get to sleep, even though it is usually a restless sleep. When mixed with antidepressants or other medications, alcohol becomes antagonistic to sleep, and can start a cycle of sleeplessness that is difficult to resolve. However, alcohol can help numb the pain of aching joints, and alleviate loneliness where this is an issue. So although it is a perverse solution, it remains a constant in many older people's lives, especially if it has played a major role in a person's social life in their younger years. One of the dangers of continuing to drink large amounts of alcohol during the older years is that a person's tolerance may change. Smaller amounts of alcohol can cause headaches, frequent memory lapses and reduction of mental abilities (Flood & Buckwalter 2009). Those particularly at risk are those who are trying to cope with a transition such as retirement, relocation, or the loss of a spouse, friend, or family member.

Polypharmacy is a significant issue among older people in Australia and New Zealand. As previously noted, older people have high rates of chronic disease and are frequently taking multiple medications in order to manage their condition/s. However, older people on multiple medications are also more prone to drug-related complications due to the complex medicine regimes they may be required to adhere to and the physiological changes associated with ageing. Adverse events and interactions associated with this polypharmacy can lead to a greater risk of falls, fractures, confusion, incontinence, constipation and other issues that can cause distress. These events can also lead to admission to hospital or residential care facilities (Central Region District Health Boards 2012). Nurses have an important role in ensuring older people are managing their medicines well, providing education and support in the home or clinic. Identifying where polypharmacy may put an older person at risk and putting in place appropriate strategies to manage this including regular medicine reviews, referral and reconciliation is important. Often older people may also be taking over-the-counter medicines or complementary and alternative medicines and may be reluctant to share this with their doctor. Careful assessment can help identify where this may be occurring and allow preventative strategies to be put in place early.

The most significant societal level challenge for the next decades will be how to best care for the over-85 age group, which is the fastest growing group globally (WHO 2013). Population ageing will require adjustments in pension and income security schemes, to support the ageing population. Health care systems will also have to accommodate changing needs. Acute care hospitals will be populated by a large proportion of the oldest old, many of whom will experience multiple health problems. With shortened hospital stays, nurses practising in the community have already begun to provide the bulk of care across extended periods of time for a wide range of acuity. In the near future, evolving technologies and therapeutic techniques will transform home care. Nurses will be part of the rapidly developing models of care that will see treatments customised to individual needs. Their roles will be central to caring for the communities where ageing takes place, supporting health-promoting behaviours, and advocating for environmental supports for lifestyle modifications.

Goals for healthy ageing

Healthy and successful ageing provides:

- access, equity, empowerment and cultural safety
- physical, emotional and spiritual health
- intersectoral collaboration for services and resources based on individual needs and strengths
- a balance between independent living and adequate service provision based on appropriate technologies
- acknowledgement of the relationship between health and place
- a place to feel safe and comfortable in living a dignified life
- adequate financial and health care resources to sustain the latter stages of life irrespective of geographic location
- policies to promote social inclusion, social engagement.

Once again, the strategies of the Ottawa Charter for Health Promotion provide a guide to implementing these health goals.

Building healthy public policy

Involving older persons as partners in health is crucial to developing age-appropriate health care systems and healthy ageing. Older persons consume more health care than any other demographic group. They carry the major burden of chronic diseases and primary care services. But they also contribute to the overall care of the population, especially for those with disabilities. This unpaid work should warrant a greater voice in health care planning, and some older

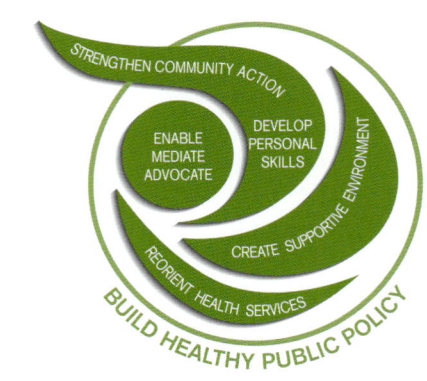

persons do participate in this type of planning. But, far too often, older people are excluded from participating in meaningful ways for service improvements. As a numerically dominant group they should be given greater opportunities to influence models of health care, based on their experiences and needs. This will become even more important in future, with the development of personalised therapies from genomics and molecular biology on the horizon. Today's older people may be the first trial recipients of stem cell transplants and other new therapies.

ACTION POINT

Providing links for older people to connect with organisations that advocate for older people's rights can empower them to become involved in policymaking.

It is important to recognise the strengths older people bring to community life, to balance the perspective purveyed in policy debates and the media that population ageing is a threat to Western society. Like children, older adults are often dependent on others and this does not always offer them a voice at the policy table. One of the most important outcomes of this dependency is that their health, wellbeing, security and wishes are often subjected to the decisions of others. Policies governing the way older adults will spend the last years of their lives should be inclusive, equitable and participatory. Some progress has been made in this direction over the past two decades, particularly with the development of global organisations such as the Associations of Retired Persons, Age Concern, Grey Power and others, to advocate for their rights. Some of these organisations are listed at the end of the chapter, particularly those that draw attention to the most pressing problem for community-living older people; falls prevention.

New Zealand's Positive Ageing Strategy (New Zealand Ministry of Social Policy 2001) and subsequent action plans (NZMOSP, Online. Available: ww.msd.govt.nz/about-msd-and-our-work/publications-resources/planning-strategy/positive-ageing/action-plan-and-annual-report/index.html [accessed 4 September 2013]), along with the Family Violence Intervention Guidelines Elder Abuse and Neglect (Glasgow & Fanslow 2006) also support the promotion of positive experiences for older people as vital to healthy communities. New Zealand also has a Minister for Senior Citizens and an Office for Senior Citizens who work together to ensure the voice of senior citizens is heard at all levels. In 2006 the New Zealand Government also developed a Health, Work and Retirement Study (HWR) with data collection every two years, focusing on the health and wellbeing of New Zealanders aged 55–70 (Dulin et al. 2011). First wave results showed optimal ageing among the population except for Māori, who scored lower on physical and mental health, related to economic living standards and a propensity towards less physical activity. The researchers concluded that culture and ethnicity are important in age-related decline because of socio-economic position. The Positive Ageing Strategy is therefore aimed at optimising the wellbeing of New Zealanders within their socio-cultural context and with culturally embedded supports (Dulin et al. 2011).

Policies affecting the older population should also be intergenerational. As Settersten (2005) suggests, policies must move away from the 'zero-sum logic' of political decisions which see expenditures for one age group construed as competing with, or draining support from, another. Having a voice at the policy table may help ensure this perspective is maintained. Health policies for older people also include those governing safe food and water, clean air and safe accommodation. One of the most important policy decisions impacting on the health of the ageing population relates to housing, and other types of accommodation for the elderly. Many older adults move from home to hospital, hostel or palliative care environment and back to home. These multiple transitions and relocations have distressing effects, particularly if financial support for accommodation is inadequate. Some government schemes have persuaded older adults to sign away their homes to secure residential care. Imbalances in services and funding arrangements have placed many older adults at risk of chronic illness and impoverished large numbers

of families. The lack of personal financial security will place an indeterminate burden on society in the future, as larger numbers of people require care that is effective, age-appropriate and allows maximum levels of health with minimal risk to both health and finances.

The level of care provided to older people in residential care in New Zealand is an area of particular concern. A 2010 report found that low numbers of registered nurses and trained caregivers was the likely cause of increased reports of neglect, injury and falls in residential care facilities (New Zealand Labour Party, Greens and Grey Power 2010). A subsequent inquiry in 2012 by the Human Rights Commission also found that the low levels of pay received by caregivers in the industry reflected a lack of respect and valuing of older New Zealanders and that urgent action was needed (Human Rights Commission 2012). Ironically, the New Zealand Government funds the aged-care sector to the tune of millions of dollars each year to provide care for those who need it; however, much of this funding goes to privately owned for-profit companies that make millions of dollars per year from the ownership of such facilities, with much of the profit going offshore. A failure by government to implement compulsory safety standards and require such organisations to improve the level of care they provide does a disservice to the many older people affected and who are frequently powerless to do anything about it.

Creating supportive environments

The emphasis in health care has shifted from stemming the tide of disability to examining what will help older people develop their potential for health and wellbeing. Today, society is gradually becoming aware of the need to value older people as instrumental to sustaining community capacity. Older people themselves are also more inclined to consider the potential of modifying their environments and engaging in robust personal behaviours for healthier lives. These include healthy nutrition, physical exercise, low-risk personal habits and coping styles and a general refocusing on what can enrich, rather than compromise, their health and happiness in the later years.

PRACTICE STRATEGY

Nurses can advocate for environmental policies and supports for healthy environments that support healthy ageing.

Healthy lifestyles among older people are visible in communities that provide environmental supports, such as the beach communities on Queensland's Gold Coast, which attract a large number of retirees. The local Gold Coast Council has established walking trails alongside the beaches, with exercise stations approximately every 10 metres. The stations are equipped with weather-resistant gym equipment that is shared by young and old people on a daily basis. The equipment represents a small investment in the health and fitness of citizens that might otherwise be precluded from exercising because of a lack of transportation or finances. The Council's commitment to fitness among the older generations provided the inspiration for the Health Ventures program described earlier in the chapter. At a global level, the Global Network of Age Friendly Cities was instituted by WHO to help older city dwellers share information and experiences and to provide city planners with technical support and training for safe, healthy urban environments for ageing (Parry 2010). Their recommendations for things such as safe housing, walkways and good lighting can be used as a model for PHC in other urban, ageing environments. Similarly, those in rural areas need special attention. The shrinking of the rural sector is an issue that has caused many older rural people considerable stress. Away from their familiar space and sense of independence, many experience the crowding and financial stress of the cities for the first time, during and after retirement. Many of these people have led self-reliant and independent lives, yet find their preferences subsumed within lifestyles unfamiliar to them, and they often have the added misfortune of suffering from dementia, depression or other chronic diseases. Often it is these chronic and long-term conditions that contribute to older people making the move from their rural homes to cities, to be closer to health services. Age-friendly community networks, especially for the large proportion of women caring for family members and their caregivers, can help rural people remain connected and feeling valued until the end of life. Health professionals have an important role to play in the more immediate environment of the home by monitoring the health and wellbeing of caregivers for early detection and intervention for stress.

As people remain in the workforce longer, employers will need to accommodate any declines in older workers' capacity, including work content or physical loading, stressful work environments, and the psychosocial elements of good work practices. They will also need to ensure there is a culture that supports worker interaction and social engagement. Vulnerable groups among older generations in need of supportive environments include the migrant population, the rural population, the economically disadvantaged and those attempting to fulfil casual employment positions. Strategies for mentoring young workers can have maximum value for both the mentors and the mentees, as older people are encouraged to pass on their experience to those who need to develop knowledge and skills.

Strengthening community action

One of the greatest community assets in many cities and communities today is the vast array of volunteer networks that often provide a critical link to social life and social services. These networks often comprise numerous people having reached older age themselves. Their guidance is often invaluable in helping others make the transitions from rural to urban, home to community or residential care, or to services and facilities they need. Volunteering is one of the most rewarding activities for older adults, as it helps build a strong sense of control. Often volunteers have a deep understanding of older adults' problems from first-hand experience, and they often recognise the type of information or assistance that is needed. They may also have the time and patience to listen when it is most needed, especially for people who may be suffering from depression or other mental illness. Volunteers also develop a sense of self-esteem through their actions, especially knowing the extent to which their input is valued.

ACTION POINT

Encourage volunteering or educational opportunities as a means of increasing self-esteem and maintaining cognitive ability.

One of the most vital movements of current times is the response to widespread recognition of the need for lifelong learning, through courses such as those in the University of the Third Age (U3A). Older students are often willing to share life experiences, integrating their insights into course material. Older people also approach learning in unique ways, using new knowledge to forestall deterioration of their cognitive abilities, eager to build linkages between old and new knowledge. Studying and learning helps build cultural bridges, linking personal and public perspectives, blending emotional insights with enhanced awareness of the world. The advent of the internet has also provided some older persons with a thirst for even more knowledge, and different ways of exploring the world. Organisations such as SeniorNet (www.seniornet.org.nz) provide opportunities for older people to learn internet skills at a pace that is appropriate to their needs. Evaluation data show that SeniorNet has not only enhanced older people's use of the internet to find information and to engage with organisations and agencies online, but has also decreased the sense of isolation older people can feel as they age, increased mental stimulation and improved contact with family and friends (Federation of New Zealand SeniorNet Societies 2009).

One way to promote connectedness within the ageing community is to reinforce the value of religious institutions, where this is appropriate to community members. Relocation to a different environment may cause older adults enormous stress if they are unable to retrieve the familiarity of the church, temple or synagogue, or those who provide religious support. Our role as health advocates should include assessing older community members' needs for communication and spiritual worship. This may involve arranging transportation, social networks of lay people with similar religious affiliations or visits by members of the church, especially for older adults who are incapacitated and cannot meet the obligations of their faith.

Developing personal skills

Building personal health capacity in the later years should be multidimensional, addressing psychosocial health issues and health literacy, as well as any risks related to disability or poor general health. Effective pain management strategies can support older people to overcome the impact of pain on their lives and develop the resiliency needed to age well. One of the most useful resources is a website developed in Western Australia to help people understand and manage pain, Pain Health: http://painhealth. csse.uwa.edu.au. The website explains different types of pain, provides various personal stories of pain and outlines ways of coping with pain through techniques such as mindfulness and goal setting as well as medication management.

Promoting healthy behaviours at this stage of life can be more effective if a positive ageing approach is used to entrench the notion that the person is valued as an individual, that their life history is relevant, meaningful and included in the social fabric of the community. There are many ways older people continue to develop personal skills. When confronted with a serious illness, some will change their lifestyle habits, not always for the better. For some individuals, their decision to become inactive, or to drink alcohol or engage in other risky behaviours, may be a result of loneliness. Some older adults, especially men, shy away from close connections and withdraw from social activities after losing a partner or family member. They often have fewer activities to distract them when they are trying to make major lifestyle changes, and also have a longer history of the behaviour(s) than young people.

It is difficult to understand the challenges and obstacles involved in trying to unlearn, then relearn ways of behaving. Patience is crucial, and this helps older adults feel that they are being taken seriously. For some, massage, therapeutic touch and alternative therapies provide a remedy to counter unhealthy lifestyles or loneliness. Others respond to a more cognitive, rational approach and can be convinced to reframe the negative lifestyle practice as a threat to their longevity or to the quality of their life. The most successful techniques to help build personal strengths capitalise on both the unique and shared characteristics of people attempting to change. They also place at least equal emphasis on community infrastructure that would support the change. The most important determinant of change is a sense of control: believing you can change, and that the community is there to support you. Supportive communities are empowering, and aimed at nurturing health literacy. Understanding an older person's need for knowledge to maintain personal capacity begins with a comprehensive assessment of personal strengths and barriers to change. This information can then be used to validate their existing knowledge and direct them to access any further information that will help support choices for health and wellbeing.

Many older people are embracing technologies, and these can be used to optimise care. Computer training, memory tapes and video games are also strategies for helping older people retain cognitive function (Williams & Kemper 2010). Many older people are internet savvy, some using social networking to stay in touch with family members, and others using it to search for services or supports. Developing internet literacy can help people remain

PRACTICE STRATEGY

Motivational interviewing may be one way of helping people develop or extend healthy lifestyles during ageing.

in their homes safely, access groceries and other services, and prevent deterioration in their health. For example, there are electronic devices now with motion and vibration sensors that can detect falls. Other mobile devices connect health professionals with older people living alone to collect information about their medical condition or alert authorities when they have a problem. Technological devices can also monitor sleep, toileting, and urinary tract infections (Tsang 2012).

Reorienting health services

Older people are often inappropriately admitted to acute hospitals due to delays in diagnostic tests, specialist consultations and discharge, and the lack of appropriate post-acute and community care services. The widespread attention to acute health care for older adults has also deflected attention from their health promotion needs. For years, community health professionals have been relentlessly urging governments to deploy resources into community and home supports for healthy ageing, but still, most resources continue to go to the hospital sector. The Australian National PHC Strategic Framework is aimed at addressing the ageing population in recommending greater emphasis on primary prevention (Commonwealth of Australia 2013), but there remains uncertainty as to how the recommendations will be implemented in future. Declaring a policy commitment to ageing in place but allocating the lion's share of funding to hospital and specialist care is inherently contradictory, and may not best serve the needs of older people, especially those suffering from chronic illness. One area where community-based care is well serviced is falls prevention. In New Zealand and Australia, Commonwealth, state and territory governments have deployed significant resources to keep older people mobile, especially the frail elderly. Many caregivers may be unaware of these resources, so it is important to maintain a working knowledge of new developments and supports for falls prevention. Dissemination of this information is expedited by numerous online sites, as we have listed at the end of the chapter.

For those ageing in rural and remote areas, community services are often absent in rural areas, leaving them at a disadvantage. Nurses and other health professionals working with older people in the community need to be vigilant to ensure that rural voices are heard, and that policies include strategies for implementation with a focus on the specific needs of elders (NRHA 2013). The National Rural Health Alliance argues that the introduction of the new Australian National Disability Scheme in 2014 should be accompanied by a new health professional to service rural areas; the 'Community Rehabilitation Worker'. This could be a paraprofessional who lives locally and would be educated to provide rehabilitation and case management under the guidance of specialist allied health and medical professionals. Developing this role would be a major new initiative in caring for older rural residents who currently must either access rehabilitation services at a great distance from their homes, or forego the opportunity for rehabilitation (NRHA 2013).

TRENDING NOW—AGED CARE

- Evidence-based practice
- Systematic assessments
- Health risk appraisal
- Health promotion
- Care based on PHC principles
- Multi-professional team care
- Person-centred care
- Recovery-based care

Mental health services for older people continue to be sporadic, especially in regional and rural areas, and community mental health nurses remain the best source of assistance for families trying to manage dementia-related behaviours. These nurses are also an ideal support for family members trying to manage their own anxieties related to caregiving. Working as specialist practitioners, community mental health nurses are committed to evidence-based approaches to care, particularly in systematically screening older people for mental conditions such as depression and anxiety (Thompson et al. 2008). Using tools to gather accurate data can provide the best foundation for a personalised, solution-focused approach to care. Evidence-based, solution-focused care includes the perspectives of the individual and family members to ensure that their preferences and needs are acknowledged (Adams & Moyle 2007). This

PRIMARY HEALTH CARE

Using the principles of PHC and focusing health care on the socio-ecological environments for healthy ageing can have a major effect on community-dwelling seniors.

information can then provide a foundation for creative and imaginative solutions. Another important role for nurses working in home and community care is to help older people manage chronic conditions and prevent deteriorating health (Mason 2009). Ideally, this is achieved in collaboration with practice nurses who adopt a PHC approach to encouraging client self-management.

Some general practices are now adopting a Health Risk Appraisal (HRA) system for older people that can help identify risk factors for disability, ill health and social isolation (Iliffe et al. 2010). This systematic approach has been trialled on the basis that older people themselves could complete interactive computer-based HRAs, yet, because of some difficulties in using the technology, support from health professionals remains the key to successful implementation (Iliffe et al. 2010). A multi-professional, collaborative team approach with personal involvement from nurses, pharmacists and dietitians may be better able to focus comprehensively on risk reduction, educating people about diet and exercise, monitoring and adjusting drug therapy, and helping motivate them to adhere with prescribed medications (Horgan et al. 2009; Mason 2009). The multi-professional approach should also extend across the continuum of care, to include acute care episodes and palliative care, involving the older person and family members as partners in care with specialist support as required from palliative care professionals (O'Connor & Alde 2011).

Nurses and/or nurse practitioners are also among the most frequent visitors to long-term care homes, and in this capacity they can help promote continuity between services and caregivers and decrease hospital admissions (Dening & Milne 2009; Peri et al. 2013). These nurses play an important dual role in helping create awareness of the range of issues that may be challenging in care, as well as encouraging evidence-based practice and the translation of new information into practice changes such as person-centred care (Moyle et al. 2010). Research into the types of skills required of nurses working with older people in residential care settings shows that they need advanced assessment skills, the ability to manage complex care, and a focus on PHC and keeping people well (Clendon 2009). Nursing plans should also be mindful of people's sense of place. Older adults living in residential care settings are, in essence, at 'home'. Nurses can help others in the aged-care setting work within a PHC approach that includes social inclusion, connectedness, cultural safety, person-centred care, health literacy, and appropriate use of technology to tailor plans to people's multidimensional needs. Recent directions for care include the 'recovery-based' approach to helping those suffering from dementia as well as other mental illnesses to eliminate stigma and marginalisation (Gavan 2011). Encouraging a reflective partnership approach to caregiving can help those with dementia maintain hope and a sense of optimism, even as they recognise changes in their condition (Gavan 2011)

Another aspect of service provision demanding attention is the need to tailor services to the needs of different community groups of older citizens. Older adults are not a homogeneous group, nor do they represent a common culture, or common experiences of illness or disability. It is therefore important to assess people's individual needs before assigning them to one type of care. Care facilities are already being redesigned to accommodate various subgroups within residential and semi-residential care, and this is a step in the right direction. Home to residential care will probably be the most problematic transition for the oldest old, and current initiatives for 'ageing in place' need to be customised to individual preferences and needs, particularly for older people from a CALD background (Yeboah et al. 2013). Understandings of ageing and generational considerations for people of various cultures can help ensure that language and cultural barriers do not prevent appropriate care (Bourgeault et al. 2010). Ageing in place in the community will work for some, but not all people, and services should accommodate a range of preferences and choices where possible.

In an era of protracted economic restraint, increasing emphasis on community and home care inadvertently increases the burden on family caregivers. These people need ongoing support, and education that provides a base of information on rehabilitation strategies, as well as the intervention technologies planned for their family member. There is also a significant need for respite care to prevent situations where they are overcome by the stress of caregiving. Caring for our ageing population requires careful deliberation of the mix that constitutes optimal conditions for health enhancement. Included is access and equity in service provision, empowerment for older adults and their families and a physical and social environment within which health can be achieved until the end of life within a milieu of encouragement and caring. Australia has made improving older people's health a national priority, and developed the Living Longer Living Better site (www.livinglongerlivingbetter.gov.au) to provide easy access to information and guidance for older people, their caregivers and those who organise aged care. We now turn to our case study to identify any issues related to ageing in the Smith and Mason families.

CASE STUDY: Older workers, older Mason and Smith family members

Some of the occupational health nurses are working with older mining managers, many of whom had not expected to continue working after age 65. They are addressing the special needs of the older worker in the context of not only chronic illness management but preventative care and the effect of shiftwork on older workers.

Rebecca's mum has developed breast cancer and is having to travel to the city for chemotherapy. During those weeks of treatment she is staying in Rebecca's home, and this is causing some problems with the young children disturbing her mother's rehabilitation and adding to the pressure on Rebecca of maintaining family harmony.

Huia's mother has recently had a heart attack and moved into the family home for Huia to look after, which is normal practice for Māori families. This has created additional pressures on her and now she has become one of the sandwich carers who are dealing with both children and parents. Although her mum has tried hard to help around the house, her recent illness hampers her ability to contribute much. Huia has spoken with the Māori nurse practitioner who works in Papakura and she has promised to make a home visit.

REFLECTING ON THE BIG ISSUES

- Although there are some common influences on ageing, it is an individual experience, dependent on a person's social, physical and psychological history.
- Older people are often the subject of stereotypical age discrimination in the workplace, in social life and in health care.
- Older people need to be valued for their wisdom, calmness and ability to see life in perspective.
- An older person's health and wellbeing is the product of cumulative experiences, indicating the need for a life course approach in evaluating health and wellness.
- Older people undertake a disproportionate amount of family caregiving and community volunteer work.
- Nursing research has primarily focused on illness and disability in ageing, leaving gaps in our knowledge of the evidence base for healthy ageing and health promotion for older people who are ageing in place in the community.

REFLECTIVE QUESTIONS: How would I use this knowledge in practice?

1. What social, physical and psychological influences have the most important effects on healthy ageing?

2. How does the environment affect older people's risk and potential in relation to falls prevention?

3. What are the unique health literacy needs of older people living alone?

4. How would you promote healthy ageing in the Maddington and Papakura communities using the Ottawa Charter for Health Promotion as a guide?

5. Discuss how the relationship between health and place might affect Huia and Rebecca's mothers as they relocate for assistance.

6. How can primary health care principles be used to guide a holistic assessment of their needs?

7. What strategies could you use to promote resilience in older residents of the community?

8. What gaps exist in our nursing research on community-based chronic illness management?

References

ACC, 2013. Vitamin D supplements linked to big drop in falls in aged care facilities. Online. Available: <www.acc.co.nz/news/WPC119005> 12 August 2013.

Adams, T., Moyle, W., 2007. Transitions in aging: a focus on dementia care nursing. In: McAllister, M. (Ed.), Solution-focused nursing: rethinking practice. Palgrave Macmillan, Basingstoke, pp. 154–162.

Alzheimer's Australia, 2013. Your Brain Matters. Online. Available: <www.alzheimer's.org.au> 13 August 2013.

Alzheimers New Zealand, 2013. Who we are. Online. Available: <www.alzheimers.org.nz> 13 August 2013.

Australian Institute of Health and Welfare (AIHW), 2012. Australia's Health 2012, Cat. No. AUS 156. AIHW, Canberra.

Bano, B., Benbow, S., 2010. Positive approaches to the fourth age. Qual. Ageing Older Adults 11 (2), 29–34.

Bascand, G., 2012. National labour force projections: 2006 (base)—2061 (August 2012 update). Statistics New Zealand, Wellington.

Berger, E., 2009. Managing age discrimination: An examination of the techniques used when seeking employment. Gerontologist 49 (3), 317–332.

Betts Adams, K., Leibbrandt, S., Moon, H., 2011. A critical review of the literature on social and leisure activity and wellbeing in later life. Ageing Soc. 31, 683–712.

Boddy, J., Chenoweth, L., McLennan, V., et al., 2013. It's just too hard! Australian health care practitioner perspectives on barriers to advance care planning. Aust. J. Prim. Health 19 (1), 38–45.

Borbasi, S., Emmanuel, E., Farrelly, B., et al., 2011. Report of an evaluation of a nurse-led dementia outreach service for people with the behavioural and psychological symptoms of dementia living in residential aged care facilities. Perspect. Public Health 131 (3), 124–130.

Borowiak, E., Kostka, T., 2012. Comparative characteristics of the home care nursing services used by community-dwelling older people from urban and rural environments. J. Adv. Nurs. 69 (6), 1259–1268.

Bourgeault, I., Atanackovic, J., Rashid, A., et al., 2010. Relations between immigrant care workers and older persons in home and long-term care. Can. J. Aging 29 (1), 109–118.

Bramble, M., Moyle, W., McAllister, M., 2009. Seeking connectioon: Family care experiences following long term dementia care placement. J. Clin. Nurs. 18 (22), 3118–3125.

Brett, C., Gow, A., Corley, J., et al., 2012. Psychosocial factors and health as determinants of quality of life in community-dwelling older adults. Qual. Life Res. 21, 505–516.

Brockmann, H., Muller, R., Helmert, U., 2009. Time to retire—Time to die? A prospective cohort study of the effects of early retirement on long-term survival. Soc. Sci. Med. 69, 160–164.

Burton, E., 2012. Streets ahead? The role of the built environment in healthy ageing. Perspect. Public Health 132 (4), 161–162.

Cagney, K., Cornwell, E., 2010. Neighbourhoods and health in later life: The intersection of biology and community. Annu. Rev. Gerontol. Geriatr. 30, 323–348.

Carr, D., Springer, K., 2010. Advances in families and health research in the 21st century. J. Marriage Fam. 72, 743–761.

Central Region District Health Boards, 2012. Multi interventional approach to reducing polypharmacy in the central region. Central Region District Health Boards, Wellington.

Chater, K., Tsai, C., 2008. Palliative care in a multicultural society: a challenge for Western ethics. Aust. J. Adv. Nurs. 26 (2), 95–100.

Chatters, L., 2000. Religion and health: Public health research and practice. Annu. Rev. Public Health 21, 335–367.

Clendon, J., 2009. Enhancing preparation of undergraduate students for practice in older adult settings. Nelson Marlborough Institute of Technology, Nelson.

Clendon, J., Walker, L., 2012. Research advisory paper: late career nurses in New Zealand. New Zealand Nurses Organisation, Wellington. Online. Available: <http://www.nzno.org.nz/services/publications> 30 August 2013.

Commonwealth of Australia, 2013. National primary health care Strategic Framework. AGPS, Canberra.

Corcoran, K., McNab, J., Girgis, S., et al., 2012. Is transport a barrier to healthcare for older people with chronic diseases? Asia Pac. J. Health Manage. 7 (1), 49–56.

Dalziel, K., Segal, L., Elley, C., 2006. Cost utility analysis of physical activity counseling in general practice. Aust. N. Z. J. Public Health 30, 57–63.

Davidson, R., Banister, E., de Vries, K., 2013. Primary healthcare NZ nurses' experiences of advance directives: understanding their potential role. Nurs. Prax. N. Z. 29 (2), 26–33.

Deloitte Access Economics, 2012. Updated dementia economic impact report, 2011, New Zealand. Alzheimers New Zealand. Deloitte Economic Access Pty Ltd, Auckland.

Dening, T., Milne, A., 2009. Depression and mental health in care homes for older people. Qual. Ageing 10 (1), 40–46.

Dols, J., Landrum, P., Wieck, K., 2010. Leading and managing an intergenerational workplace. Creat. Nurs. 16 (2), 68–74.

Dulin, P., Stephens, C., Alpass, F., et al., 2011. The impact of socio-contextual, physical and lifestyle variables on measures of physical and psychological wellbeing among Maori and non-Maori: the New Zealand health, Work, and Retirement Study. Ageing Soc. 31, 1406–1424.

Elley, C., Kerse, N., Arroll, B., et al., 2003. Effectiveness of counseling patients on physical activity in general practice: Cluster randomized controlled trial. Br. Med. J. 326, 793–796.

Elley, R., Kerse, N., Arroll, B., et al., 2004. Cost effectiveness of physical activity counseling in general practice. N. Z. Med. J. 117 (1207), 1–15.

Erickson, E., 1963. Childhood and Society, second ed. Norton, New York.

Ervin, K., Finlayson, S., Cross, M., 2012. The management of behavioural problems associated with dementia in rural aged care. Collegian 19, 85–95.

Fairhurst, E., 2005. Theorizing growing and being older: Connecting physical, well-being and public health. Crit. Public Health 15 (1), 27–38.

Families Commission, 2009. Family violence statistics report: a Families Commission report. Families Commission, Wellington.

Federation of New Zealand SeniorNet Societies, 2009. Improving our understanding of older person's needs in learning new technologies. Online. Available: <http://www.seniornet.org.nz/researchreport.asp> 22 December 2009.

Flood, M., Buckwalter, K., 2009. Recommendations for mental health care of older adults Part 2-An overview of dementia, delirium, and substance abuse. J. Gerontol. Nurs. 35 (2), 35–47.

Foley, L., Maddison, R., Jones, Z., et al., 2011. Comparison of two modes of delivery of an exercise prescription scheme. J. N. Z. Med. Assoc. 124 (1338), Online. Available: <http://journal.nzma.org.nz/journal/124-1338/4757/> 30 August 2013.

Forsman, A., Nordmyr, J., Wahlbeck, K., 2011. Psychosocial interventions for the promotion of mental health and the prevention of depression among older adults. Health Promot. Int. 26 (S1), doi:10.1093/heapro/dar074:i85-i107.

Gadalla, T., 2009. Sense of mastery, social support, and health in elderly Canadians. J. Aging Health 21 (4), 581–595.

Garner, J., 2009. Considerably better than the alternative. Qual. Ageing 10 (1), 5–8.

Gavan, J., 2011. Exploring the usefulness of a recovery-based approach to dementia care nursing. Contemp. Nurse 39 (2), 140–146.

Gillespie, L., Robertson, M., Gillespie, W., et al., 2012. Interventions for preventing falls in older people living in the community. Review, The Cochrane Collaboration, Issue 11. Wiley.

Glasgow, K., Fanslow, J., 2006. Family violence intervention guidelines: elder abuse and neglect. Ministry of Health, Wellington.

Graham, E., Duffield, C., 2010. An ageing nursing workforce. Aust. Health Rev. 34, 44–48.

Grenade, L., Boldy, D., 2008. Social isolation and loneliness among older people: issues and future challenges in community and residential settings. Aust. Health Rev. 329 (3), 468–478.

Hall, C., Brown, A., Gleeson, S., et al., 2007. Keeping the thread: Older men's social networks in Sydney, Australia. Qual. Ageing 8 (4), 10–17.

Helpguide, 2013. Online. Available: <www.helpguide.org> <www.helpguide.org/mental/elder_abuse_physical_emotional_sexual_neglect.htm> 14 August 2013.

Henricksen, A., Stephens, C., 2010. An exploration of the happiness-enhancing activities engaged in by older adults. Ageing Int. 35, 311–326.

Hill, R., 2010. A positive aging framework for guiding geropsychology interventions. Behav. Ther. 42 (1), 66–77.

Horgan, S., LeClair, K., Donnelly, M., et al., 2009. Developing a national consensus on the accessibility needs of older adults with concurrent and chronic, mental and physical health issues: A preliminary framework informing collaborative mental health care planning. Can. J. Aging 28 (2), 97–105.

Human Rights Commission, 2012. Caring counts: Report of the inquiry into the aged care workforce. Human Rights Commission, Auckland.

Iliffe, S., Swift, C., Harari, D., et al., 2010. Health promotion in later life: public and professional perspectives on an expert system for health risk appraisal. Prim. Health Care Res. Dev. 11 (2), 187–196.

Inder, K., Lewin, T., Kelly, B., 2012. Factors impacting on the well-being of older residents in rural communities. Perspect. Public Health 132 (4), 182–191.

Jeong, S., Higgins, I., McMillan, M., 2007. Advance care planning (ACP): the nurse as 'broker' in residential aged care facilities. Contemp. Nurse 26 (2), 184–195.

Jeong, S., Higgins, I., McMillan, M., 2011. Experiences with advance care planning: older people and family members' perspective. Int. J. Older People Nurs. 6 (3), 176–186.

Jorgensen, D., Parsons, M., Jacobs, S., et al., 2010. The New Zealand informal caregivers and their unmet needs. J. N. Z. Med. Assoc. 123 (1317), 9–16.

Kerse, N., Elley, C., Robinson, E., et al., 2005. Is physical activity counseling effective for older people? A cluster randomized, controlled trial in primary care. J. Am. Geriatr. Soc. 153, 1951–1956.

Kolt, G., Schofield, G., Kearse, N., et al., 2009. The Healthy Steps study: A randomized controlled trial of a pedometer-based Green Prescription for older adults: trial protocol. BMC Public Health 9, 204. doi:10.1186/1471-2458-9-404.

Lavretsky, H., 2012. Resilience, stress, and mood disorders in old age. Annu. Rev. Gerontol. Geriatr. 32, 49–72.

Leung, W., Ashton, T., Kolt, G., et al., 2012. Cost-effectiveness of pedometer-based versus time-based Green Prescriptions: the Healthy Steps Study. Aust. J. Prim. Health 18 (3), 204–211.

Levy, B., Leifheit-Limson, E., 2009. The stereotype-matching effect: greater influence on functioning when age stereotypes correspond to outcomes. Psychol. Aging 24 (1), 230–233.

Loge, J., Sorrell, J., 2010. Implications of an aging population for mental health nurses. J. Psychol. Nurs. 48 (9), 15–18.

Marmot, M., 2010. Fair Society, Healthy Lives, Strategic Review of Health Inequities in England Post 2010. Department of Health, London.

Mason, C., 2009. Preventing coronary heart disease and stroke with aggressive statin therapy in older adults using a team management model. J. Am. Acad. Nurse Pract. 21 (1), 47–53.

Mazzotti, E., Mazzuca, F., Sebastiani, C., et al., 2011. Predictors of existential and religious well-being among cancer patients. Support. Care Cancer 19, 1931–1937.

McCracken, H., 2013. Suicide rates rise for women, drop for men. The New Zealand Herald. Online. Available: <http://www.nzherald.co.nz/nz/news/article.cfm?c_id=1&objectid=11114600> 30 August 2013.

McDougall, G., Mackert, M., Becker, H., 2012. Memory, performance, health literacy, and instrumental activities of daily living of community residing older adults. Nurs. Res. 61 (1), 70–75.

Milroy, H., 2013. Beyond cultural security: towards sanctuary. Ed. Med. J. Aust. 199 (1), 42.

Moyle, W., Hsu, M., Lieff, S., et al., 2010. Recommendations for staff education and training for older people with mental illness in long-term aged care. Int. Psychogeriatr. 22 (7), 1097–1106.

National Rural Health Alliance (NRHA), 2013. Health and disability service models in rural and remote areas. Online. Available: <www.ruralhealth.org.au/news/health-and-disability-service-models-rural-and-remote-areas> 8 June 2013.

Newman, A., 2009. Obesity in older adults. Online Journal Issues Nurs. 14 (1), 1–8.

New Zealand Labour Party, Greens and Grey Power, 2010. A report into aged care: What does the future hold for older New Zealanders. New Zealand Labour Party, Greens and Grey Power, Wellington. Online. Available: <https://www.greens.org.nz/agedcare> 4 September 2013.

New Zealand Ministry of Health (NZMOH), 2011. Advance care planning: A guide for the New Zealand healthcare workforce. Ministry of Health, Wellington.

New Zealand Ministry of Health (NZMOH), 2012. The Health of New Zealand Adults 2011/12: Key findings of the New Zealand Health Survey. Ministry of Health, Wellington.

New Zealand Ministry of Health (NZMOH), 2013. Health Loss in New Zealand: A report from the New Zealand burden of diseases, injuries and risk factors study, 2006–2016. Ministry of Health, Wellington.

New Zealand Ministry of Social Policy, 2001. The New Zealand Positive Ageing Strategy. New Zealand, Wellington.

Ng, T., Feldman, D., 2012. Evaluating six common stereotypes about older workers with meta-analytical data. Pers. Psychol. 65, 821–858.

O'Connor, M., Alde, P., 2011. Older persons' health and end-of-life care. In: Kralik, D., Van Loon, A. (Eds.), Community Nursing in Australia, second ed. John Wiley & Sons, Milton, Queensland, pp. 354–386.

Office for Disability Issues and Statistics New Zealand, 2013. Disability and formal supports in New Zealand in 2006: Results from the New Zealand disability survey. Statistics New Zealand, Wellington.

Parmenter, G., Cruickshank, M., Hussain, R., 2012. The social lives of rural Australian nursing home residents. Ageing Soc. 32, 329–353.

Parry, J., 2010. Network of cities tackles age-old problems. Bull. World Health Organ. 88, 406–407.

Pavlish, C., Ceronsky, L., 2009. Oncology nurses' perceptions of nursing roles and professional attributes in palliative care. Clin. J. Oncol. Nurs. 13 (4), 404–412.

Payne, S., 2009. The role of the nurse in palliative care settings in a global context. Cancer Nurs. Pract. 8 (5), 21–26.

Peri, K., Boyd, M., Foster, S., et al., 2013. Evaluation of the nurse practitioner in aged care. Central PHO and Mid Central District Health Board, Palmerston North.

Perry, B., 2010. The material well-being of older New Zealanders: Background paper for the Retirement Commissioners 2010 review. Ministry of Social Development, Wellington.

Ramsey, J., 2012. Spirituality and aging. Annu. Rev. Gerontol. Geriatr. 32, 131–150.

Reyna, C., Goodwin, E., Ferrari, J., 2007. Older adult stereotypes among care providers. J. Gerontol. Nurs. 33 (2), 50–55.

Rheaume, C., Mitty, E., 2008. Sexuality and intimacy in older adults. Geriatr. Nurs. (Minneap) 29 (5), 342–349.

Robinson, A., Lea, E., Hemmings, L., et al., 2012. Seeking respite: issues around the use of day respite care for the carers of people with dementia. Ageing Soc. 32, 196–218.

Robotham, D., 2011. Ageing well in the 21st century. Qual. Ageing Older Adults 12 (3), 133–140.

Romero-Moreno, R., Marquez-Ganzalez, M., Losada, A., et al., 2010. Motives for caring: relationship to stress and coping dimensions. Int. Psychogeriatr. 23 (4), 573–582.

Rose, K., Lopez, R., 2012. Transitions in dementia care: Theoretical support for nursing roles. Online Journal Issues Nurs. doi:10.3912/OJIN.Vol17No02Man04.

Rueda, S., Artazcoz, L., Navarro, V., 2008. Health inequalities among the elderly in Western Europe. J. Epidemiol. Community Health 62, 492–498.

Ryan, A., McKenna, H., Slevin, O., 2012. Family care-giving and decisions about entry to care: a rural perspective. Ageing Soc. 32, 1–18.

Rybarczyk, B., Emery, E., Guequierre, L., et al., 2012. The role of resilience in chronic illness and disability in older adults. Annu. Rev. Gerontol. Geriatr. 32, 173–187.

Sanchez Palacios, C., Trianes Torres, M., Blanca Mena, M., 2009. Negative aging stereotypes and their relation with psychosocial variables in the elderly population. Arch. Gerontol. Geriatr. 48, 385–390.

Schuler, T., Zaider, T., Kissane, D., 2012. Family grief therapy. Fam. Matters 90, 77–86.

Sebern, M., 2005. Shared care, elder and family member skills used to manage burden. J. Adv. Nurs. 52 (2), 10–179.

Settersten, R., 2005. Linking the two ends of life: What gerontology can learn from childhood studies. J. Gerontol. 60B (4), S173–S180.

Shearer, N., Fleury, J., Belyea, M., 2010. Randomized control trial of the health empowerment intervention. Nurs. Res. 59 (3), 203–211.

Shearer, N., Fleury, J., Ward, K., et al., 2012. Empowerment interventions for older adults. West. J. Nurs. Res. 34 (1), 24–51.

Sinclair, K, Hamlin, M., 2007. Self-reported health benefits in patients recruited into New Zealand's 'Green Prescription' primary health care program. Southeast Asian J. Trop. Med. Public Health 38 (6), 1158–1167.

Sorrell, J., 2012. Widows and widowers in today's society. J. Psychosoc. Nurs. 50 (9), 14–18.

Stanaway, F., Blyth, F., Cumming, R., et al., 2011. Back pain in older male Italian-born immigrants in Australia: The importance of socioeconomic factors. Eur. J. Pain 15, 70–76.

Statistics New Zealand, 2007. New Zealand's 65+ population: a statistical volume. Statistics New Zealand, Wellington.

Statistics New Zealand, 2013a. New Zealand general social survey: 2012. Statistics New Zealand, Wellington.

Statistics New Zealand, 2013b. National population estimates: At 30 June 2013. Statistics New Zealand, Wellington.

Stovall, S., Baker, J., 2010. A concept analysis of connection relative to aging adults. The Journal of Theory Construction & Testing 14 (2), 52–56.

Thompson, P., Lang, L., Annells, M., 2008. A systematic review of the effectiveness of in-home community nurse led interventions for the mental health of older persons. J. Clin. Nurs. 17, 1419–1427.

Tsang, M., 2012. Connecting and caring: Innovations for healthy ageing. Bull. World Health Organ. 90, 162–163.

Vagenas, D., McLaughlin, D., Dobson, A., 2009. Regional variation in the survival and health of older Australian women: a prospective cohort study. Aust. N. Z. J. Public Health 33 (2), 119–125.

Vaughan, S., Morris, N., Shum, D., et al., 2012. Study protocol: a randomised controlled trial of the effects of a multimodal exercise program on cognition and physical functioning in older women. BMC Geriatr. 12 (60), 1–11.

Vaughan, S., Wallis, M., Polit, D., et al., 2014. The effects of multi-modal exercise on cognitive and physical functioning and BDNF in older women: a randomised controlled trial. Age Ageing. 0, 1, 1-6 doi: 10.1093/ageing/afu10.

Whitaker, A., 2009. Family involvement in the institutional and eldercare context. Towards a new understanding. J. Aging Stud. 23, 158–167.

Wiles, J., 2005. Conceptualizing place in the care of older people: the contributions of geographical gerontology. Int. J. Older People Nurs., 14(8b) in conjunction with J. Clin. Nurs. 14 (8b), 100–108.

Wilkinson, J., 1996. Psychology 5: implications of the ageing process for nursing practice. Br. J. Nurs. 5 (18), 1109–1113.

Williams, K., Kemper, S., 2010. Interventions to reduce cognitive decline in aging. J. Psychosoc. Nurs. 48 (5), 42–51.

Windle, G., 2012. The contribution of resilience to healthy ageing. Perspect. Public Health 132 (4), 159–160.

World Health Organization (WHO), 2011. Hidden Cities: Unmasking and overcoming health inequities in urban settings. Online. Available: <http://hiddencities.org/downloads/WHO_UN-HABITAT_Hidden_Cities_Web.pdf> 21 January 2013.

World Health Organization (WHO), 2013. Population ageing. Online. Available: <www.who.int/features/qu/72en> 12 August 2013.

Yeboah, C., Bowers, B., Rolls, C., 2013. Culturally and linguistically diverse older adults relocating to residential aged Care. Contemp. Nurse 44 (1), 50–61.

Ziegler, F., Schwanen, T., 2011. 'I like to go out to be energized by different people': an exploratory analysis of mobility and wellbeing in later life. Ageing Soc. 31, 758–781.

Useful websites

www.advancecareplanning.org.nz/—Advance care planning in New Zealand

http://www.respectingpatientchoices.org.au/—Advance care planning in Australia

www.fightdemential.org,au—Alzheimer's Australia (Hotline—1800 100 500)

www.alzheimers.org.nz—Alzheimer's New Zealand

www.carers.net.nz—Carers New Zealand

www.dementiacareaustralia.com—Dementia Care Australia

www.vuw.ac.nz/ageing-institute/nzag/nzag.htm—New Zealand Association of Gerontology

www.nphp.gov.au/publications/a_z.htm—Australian National Injury Prevention Strategy

www.osc.govt.nz/positive-ageing-strategy/index.html—New Zealand positive ageing

www.greypower.co.nz—Political lobby group those 50+

www.ageconcern.org.nz—Organisation supporting older people in New Zealand

www.ruralhealth.org.au—Australian Rural Health Alliance

www.livinglongerlivingbetter.gov.au—Living Longer Living Better, aged-care reform

http://.painhealth.csse.uwa.edu.au—information on chronic pain

www.virtualhospice.com.au—Information on palliative care, end of life issues

Falls-prevention agencies

www.anzfallsprevention.org/resources.html

www.nzips.govt.nz/priorities/falls.php

New Zealand

Accident Compensation Corporation

Age Concern New Zealand (with regional offices)

Alcohol Advisory Council of New Zealand (ALAC)

Building Industry Authority

Cultural Strategies Management, ACC

Pacific Representative from the Disabled Persons Assembly

District Health Boards

Department of General Practice and PHC, University of Auckland

Injury Prevention Research Centre, University of Auckland

Falls Prevention Research Group, University of Otago Medical School

Grey Power

Māori Health Providers

Pacific Health Providers

Minisdtry of Consumer Affiars

Ministry of Health

NZ Institute of Sport and Recreation Research, AUT

NZ Orthopaedic Association

Office for Senior Citizens, Ministry of Social Development

Royal NZ College of General Practitioners

Royal NZ Plunket Society

Safe Waitakere (Waitekere City Council)

Safekids

Sport and Recreation NZ (SPARC

Stay on Your Feet Canterbury

Australia

Aged Care Victoria Falls Prevention

Australian Commission on Safety and Health

Australian and New Zealand Falls Prevention Society (ANZFPS)

Australian Centre for Evidence Based Aged care (ACEBAC)

Australian Resource Centre for Health Innovations (ARCHI) Falls Prevention

Centre for Physical Activity in Ageing (SA)

Clinical Excellence Commission (NSW Falls Prevention)

Council on the Aging (COTA)

Falls Prevention Research Unit, MOnash University

Home Modification Information Clearing Warehouse

Independent Living Centre NSW

Injury Control Council of WA

Injury Prevention in Australia Department of Health and Ageing

The Joanna Briggs Institute

National Aging Research Institute

National Injury Surveillance Unir

NSW Injury Risk Management Research Centre

Osteoporosis Australia

PEDro: Physiotherapy Evidence Database

Neuroscience Research Australia, Falls and Balance Research Group

Queensland Injury Surveillance Unit

Queensland Stay on Your Feet Falls Prevention

Quickscreen Information, Falls and Balance Research Group

Research Review Australia

SA Falls Prevention and Management

Stay on Your Feet WA

Vision Australia

SECTION 3
Inclusive Communities and Societies

Introduction to the Section

This section begins with an explanation of what is meant by an inclusive community and society, and how these concepts are integral to primary health care (PHC). Social inclusion and social exclusion lie at two ends of the same continuum. Along this continuum, people have varying opportunities to achieve health. Social *exclusion* leaves many members of society without the support and resources they need for health and wellbeing. Social *inclusion* creates social capital, trust, norms of reciprocity and cohesion; the essence of a healthy community. These vital elements of community life are important to any discussion of the power relations that exist in society. Gender has been identified as a separate social determinant of health, yet the gender relationships in a family and community may be intensified by the intersection of racial or ethnic issues, family conflict, societal norms of behaviour, migration experiences and gender identity. The chapter unravels the issues inherent in gender, culture and power relationships that impinge on the health and wellbeing of communities and those who live in them. The central theme of Chapter 12 is inequity and exclusion, and the need to draw health professionals' attention to the special needs of men and women respectively, and to the gendered nature of health, and its social determinants. The ultimate objective for society is to ensure equity of access to education, social supports and the environmental structures within which women and men can achieve the level of health to which they aspire.

Chapter 13 addresses the need for communities to provide the foundations for cultural safety, especially in relation to Indigenous people's health, risk and potential. International reports indicate that there has been some progress in redressing the culturally constructed inequities in societies that have left a legacy of illness, injury and disability among Indigenous people. New initiatives have been developed within the auspices of the World Health Organization's Commission on the Social Determinants of Health, and at a national level, Closing the Gap initiatives in Australia and New Zealand. Yet cultural disadvantage is socially embedded, and the barriers to equality of opportunity are well known. Redressing the social conditions that create disadvantage is a matter of urgency. We therefore focus on Indigenous people's health as a critical element of cultural inclusiveness. Our discussion revolves around the need to share both the risks and wisdom of each of our nations with one another for mutual benefit and capacity enhancement. The end-point of the chapter is a renewed call to create an ethos of community and social life built on equitable foundations. Perhaps with cross-fertilisation of good ideas, and the cautionary tales of barriers to equity, we can draw into clearer focus strategies for achieving inclusive communities and social justice.

Chapter 14 addresses strengths and weaknesses in our policy environments as a culmination of the policy discussions from previous chapters, particularly in Section 2, with recommendations for strengthening existing policies and developing new ones. The convergence of policies also informs an analysis of health care systems. We address recent initiatives in Australian health care management aimed at developing a PHC approach. This follows a similar approach implemented in New Zealand over the past decade. PHC remains an appropriate approach for focusing health planners' attention on the critical needs of a community: access, equity, empowerment, cultural sensitivity and cultural safety, and intersectoral collaboration. Our discussion culminates in a list of characteristics of an ideal health system, so that we can all strive beyond today, to create a better policy environment, more responsive systems and healthier communities for tomorrow.

Chapter 15 provides an exploration of research, its major elements and strategies and where we need to fill gaps in our knowledge base for translating evidence into practice. Evidence-based practice is outlined as important to informing community health strategies, but evidence is generated and used in many forms. Everyone working with communities has some level of obligation to be research-minded, and to embrace the trend

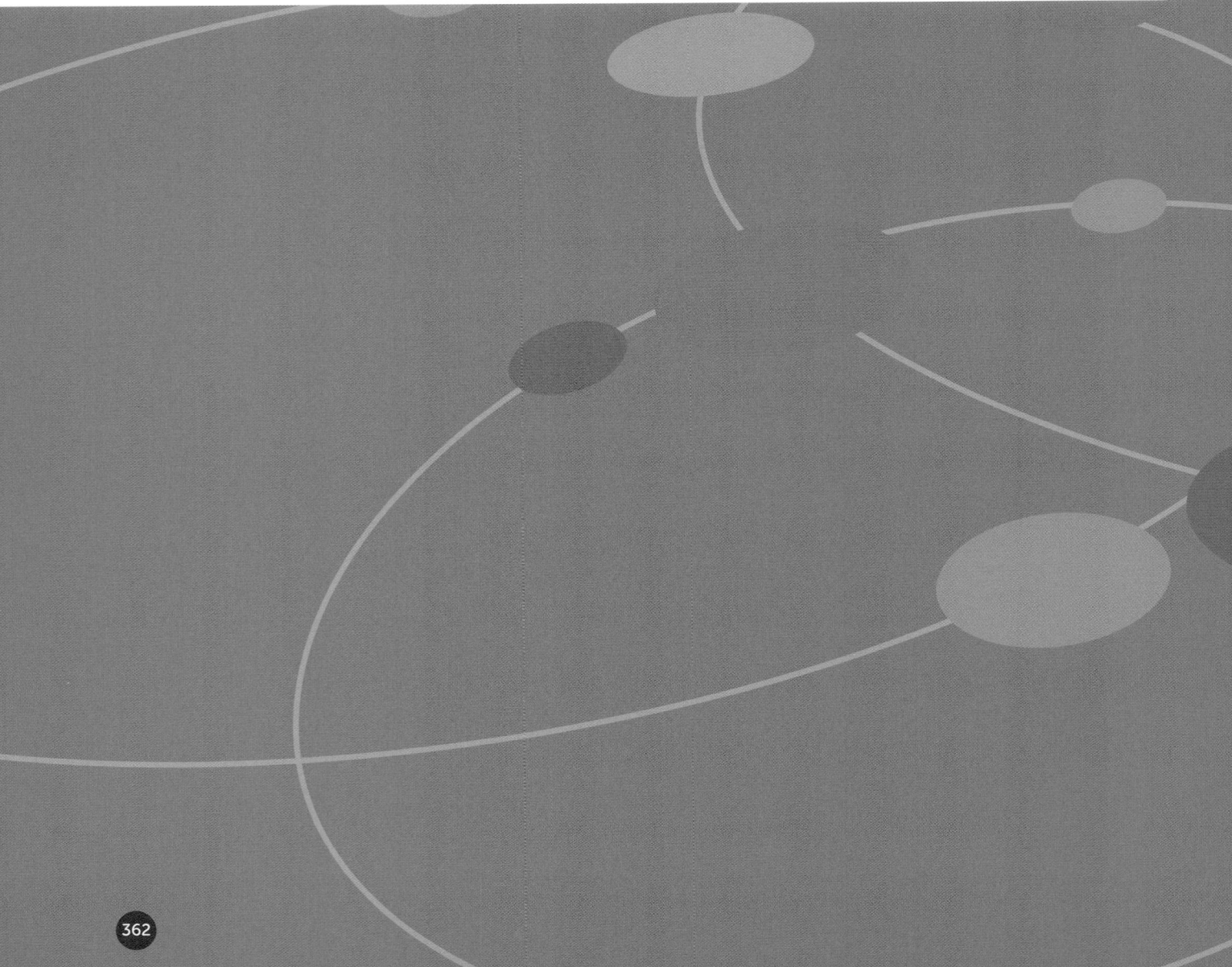

towards knowledge translation (KT), ensuring research findings are adopted in practice. We have undertaken a major scan of the nursing and midwifery publications over the past several years, to develop a sense of what gaps remain in the growing knowledge base for community practice. Reporting on this body of knowledge in Chapter 15 is intended to inspire further participation in research by practitioners as well as students. When research is integral to planning, implementing and evaluating the merits of community-level interventions, we will all be speaking in a language that helps create enthusiasm for change, and incremental development of rational, justified and defensible community health and wellbeing policies and strategies.

Inclusive communities: gender, culture and power

CHAPTER **12**

Introduction

This chapter focuses on gender, culture and power; that is, the roles of women and men in society, their membership in cultural and gender groups, and how this is linked to social inclusiveness. Attention to gender issues is important for several reasons. Gender is a pivotal social determinant of health (SDH) and instrumental to socio-economic position (SEP). A person's gender can determine the extent to which they have opportunities to achieve health and wellbeing. People are also assigned relatively different positions in society depending on their gender, particularly in being granted differential education, work opportunities or social support. Gender influences can be cumulative along the life course. As individuals develop along the critical pathways from birth to older age, gender, like other SDH, shapes not only biology, but experiences and opportunities that become reinforced over time. Because men and women occupy different social positions in the household, the workplace and in the community, they are exposed to different risks and potential. Along the pathways of women's and men's life course, gender differences are apparent at every stage, and this is the case in different countries and contexts. These gender differences interact with other life circumstances to create complex webs of factors affecting health and wellbeing.

Environmental conditions play a large part in gender relations, in determining the physical and social geographies of people's lives, and the effect of 'place' on their lives, especially their access to material resources and support. Rurality, for example, operates as a determinant of inequity, affecting men and women in different ways, limiting opportunities for women outside the home and causing considerable health risks for men. Urban life also creates different outcomes for men and women, most notably in their relative access to sufficient income, appropriate housing and employment. In any environment, parenting is enacted in different roles for women and men, and, combined with socio-economic status, tends to leave women in a more inequitable position than

their male counterparts, both within and beyond marriage. At the extreme, poverty affects men and women differentially, with more profound effects for women who are caring for children. This creates a 'feminisation of poverty', as we mentioned in Chapter 7. Women are typically those with the fewest resources, and have the least involvement in the type of health and social decision-making that would help them improve their current situation, and their potential for the future. We discuss this in relation to their roles as partners and mothers.

The community is an ideal place to address inequities that arise from social exclusion, particularly in the process of unravelling constraints and facilitating factors involved in developing capacity. Gender and cultural equity, and differential access to childhood education, health literacy, prevention, care, and economic opportunities are pivotal to community development, community competence and building social capital. Support for equity must therefore begin in the community; otherwise, in this rapidly changing global world, civilisations will grow stagnant. To flourish, societies need to address the way power and social inclusion interact with the social determinants of health, and to seek ways of creating more harmonious, socially just communities.

INEQUALITY, SOCIAL EXCLUSION, GENDER, CULTURE AND POWER

Social exclusion plays an important role in the relationship between many of the social determinants of health (SDH) and poor health. Socially excluded people are unable to access opportunities to become educated, earn a living, receive social support for their personal needs, live in safe houses and neighbourhoods with a secure food supply and a viable physical environment, raise their children in a nonviolent home, cultivate friendships, or participate in social and political life. The Australian Government defines four domains of social inclusion. These are the opportunity to:

1   participate in society through employment and access to services

2   connect with family, friends and the local community

3   deal with personal crises such as ill health

4   be heard (AIFS 2011).

Social exclusion is not the equivalent of poverty or deprivation, which can result from other circumstances. Instead, it is about connectedness and participation (AIFS 2011). When people are excluded from full participation in social life, the effects prevent societal development by inhibiting them from reaching their full potential. For example, children living in a jobless household grow up with the risk of becoming socially excluded through a lack of education, and other opportunities to change the course of their lives, which can lead to intergenerational poverty. Women confined to physical work from an early age, such as occurs in many developing countries, are socially excluded by virtue of having no opportunities to become educated or to change their status or that of their children. Men working in isolated circumstances may be socially excluded because they have few opportunities to find a partner, raise a family or gain employment in a geographic area with social amenities. Members of sexually diverse minorities such as lesbian, gay, bisexual or transgender/transsexual/intersex (LGBTI) groups are also at risk of social exclusion, especially young gay men who live in environments where there are strict norms of socially determined heterosexual gendered behaviour. Because of the dominance of our Western health and education systems cultural minorities are often socially excluded from some of the most significant aspects of social life, with profound negative impacts on their health and wellbeing. People with disabilities can also be excluded from social participation on the basis of a perceived lack of capabilities. Although social exclusion can arise

from a lack of capabilities, it is often the result of a denial of resources, rights, goods and services that are available to the majority of people in society. Clearly, there is a mandate for health and social service professionals to work towards overcoming social exclusion to promote equity and cohesion in community life.

SOCIAL EXCLUSION

Gender, culture, disability or any point of social 'difference' can lead to social exclusion, which is detrimental to health and wellbeing.

Cultural norms can play a major role in social exclusion, particularly in ascribing roles on the basis of gender. Gender differences are grounded in biology, but they are enacted within different social and cultural constructions of roles, norms, behaviours, activities and attributes that are considered appropriate for men and women (Baker 2010; Hosseinpoor et al. 2012). Gender equality refers to equal opportunities for men and women to enjoy socially-valued goods, opportunities, resources and rewards (ICN 2013). Equitable societies provide these opportunities to both. Inequitable societies place many women at risk through law, religion, or cultural norms that treat women as productive chattels to care for the household but with little decision-making over their life, health, sexuality and fertility (ICN 2013). Even in relatively equitable societies there are differences in the social expectations of masculine and feminine roles, which typically privilege men in the home and workplace (Baker 2010). The differential expectations and inequalities are manifest in power imbalances created from social pressures to conform to gender roles.

> ### GENDER
>
> Socio-culturally constructed roles and norms of behaviour for men and women.

> ## REMINDER
>
> **Inequality**—measurable outcomes in terms of opportunity
>
> **Inequity**—value-based concept of unfairness

Life experiences demonstrate patterns of gendered expectations that have changed little in terms of marriage and family life. Trends in marriage and childrearing have seen dual-earner families become the norm, with many women choosing to work part-time. However, many women are socially excluded from this mix of work-home lifestyle because of economic circumstances or lack of access to opportunities. Others have greater freedom to choose lifestyles but social norms create pressure on women to nurture, and on men to be breadwinners. Employers also shape understandings of gender by providing greater opportunities to men in the workplace, because of their role as a family provider or on the assumption that men have better management skills. This situation creates job insecurity and lower promotional opportunities for many women, who tend to work flexible schedules to meet home and workplace needs. Some women, such as those in male-dominated workplaces like mining, soon become discouraged by their exclusion from management and decision-making roles (Lord et al. 2012). As women in the workplace approach retirement, they also discover a gender gap between income and retirement savings (Pit & Byles 2012). While some women continue working to remain socially engaged or to prepare for a better lifestyle, others remain at work after retirement age because of financial necessity, often created by a fragmented career or caregiving obligations (Byles et al. 2013; Pit & Byles 2012). Marital trends that see many couples divorcing has led some women to move into new roles as family providers, but as head of single-parent households, they continue to undertake the traditional homemaker role. Within couple families, gendered and cultural norms prevail, and the division of household labour continues to be the most contentious gender issue. Globally, these gender roles are pervasive, with single-parent households headed by women creating a high risk of impoverishment (UNFPA 2000). So societies throughout the world continue to be structured in ways that disadvantage women. If they were truly inclusive, there would be no policy or social discrimination on the basis of gender, culture, sexual identity or ethnicity. Instead, members of all groups would be equally empowered to live the life to which they aspire (Sen 1999).

> ### QUICK FACT
>
> The division of household labour continues to be one of the most contentious gender issues facing families in today's society.

Gendered power imbalances can have serious consequences, especially in some cultures where women's domination by men is responsible for major traumatic events throughout their life course, and sometimes, systematic violence against them. Family violence and sexual abuse contribute to social exclusion and inequities by pushing some young people into self-exile, which can worsen their experience of being marginalised (Commonwealth of Australia 2008). Human trafficking of women is an example of extreme exploitation of women's vulnerability to ongoing systematic abuse, which can create a self-sustaining loop of social exclusion. Girls or young women who have been abducted or bonded into forced labour by poverty, war or sex trafficking become part of a cycle of social exclusion through involuntary servitude or slavery (Dovydaitis 2010). They are then subjected to social discrimination by a society that considers vulnerability undesirable, 'associated with susceptibility, debility, failure, flaw and weakness' (Jackson et al. 2012:142). For migrants and refugees, the dual vulnerabilities of gender and mental health issues that can arise from the stress of dislocation and relocation can also create cycles of ongoing vulnerability to ill health (Cross & Singh 2012).

Because gender relations are part of social structures, processes and the interactions people have in their everyday lives, gender is dynamic. This means that a person's gender is not simply a static attribute or simple assignment of a sex role. Instead, gender roles may change in the context of changing trends and events. Twenty years ago, during the post-feminist movement, many young women in Western countries were concerned with gaining a career, becoming successful in areas that had been previously inaccessible to them. In contemporary Western societies, although motherhood remains central to women's notions of femininity (Arendell 2000), women's aspirations are changing, as many place a greater emphasis on work-life balance and having choices (Johnstone & Lee 2012). Society has brought new opportunities, albeit with constraints, challenges and shifting aspirations. Respondents to recent waves of the Australian Longitudinal Study of Women's Health indicated that many 23-year-olds planned to be married and have a child by age 35 (Johnstone & Lee 2012). Yet some who have experienced traditional motherhood roles after being in the workforce have found that on their return to work they felt somewhat left out of the workforce culture. Others regret losing momentum in terms of career development after the interruption of family caregiving.

Clearly, young women's attitudes and expectations of gender roles are influenced by personal interests and goals, but these are often moderated by structural and social constraints in the home, workplace, neighbourhood and marketplace, as well as the socio-cultural norms that define their group identity. Over the past two decades, societal level changes have created what Eckersley (2012) describes as an unrelenting pressure of excessive materialism and individualism, which has a particularly important effect on adolescent girls' aspirations. Media-fuelled materialism seems to have created perverse pressures on young women to fashion their identity and meaning from personal attributes, achievements, possessions and lifestyles rather than cultural connections or accomplishments in the world of work (Eckersley 2012). The pressure to conform has, in some cases, had a detrimental effect on health by socially excluding some, who may not be part of the 'in group' or what young people call the 'TCs' (Too Cool). This type of sweeping change can lead to disempowerment as young women become disappointed, depressed or anxious about external things rather than developing a deep and enduring sense of intrinsic worth (Eckersley 2012). Box 12.1 describes Eckersley's (2012) suggestion for an alternative perspective of the world.

GROUP EXERCISE: Gender inequity

In groups of three or four discuss the following question: To what extent does gender inequity still exist in your country? What about in nursing? Identify three key points to share with the larger group—be prepared to justify your conclusions.

BOX 12.1 Redefining the self

In charting the evolution of social life over the past decades Eckersley (2012) argues that society should create the impetus for our 'cultural redefinition' from self-interested individualists to becoming more altruistic and cooperative. In this brave new world, he believes we would see one another from inside a fuzzy cloud of relational forces and fields. Some relationships would be more intimate than others, but all would build a sense of community or place; a type of national or ethnic identity. Some elements of connectedness would be subtle yet powerful, as in a spiritual connection or a love of nature. On reflection, we would start to reframe notions of change and development in a more positive way. Even marital breakdown would be seen positively, as a 'change' not the 'end' of something. Likewise, death would be envisioned as a change, rather than something to fear.

This utopian perspective of the world within a single community requires radical reforms to galvanise opinions around the things that matter: limiting or banning political donations by anyone with a vested interest; putting an extremely high price on carbon; abolishing tax deductions for advertising as a disincentive to spend on consumer goods or consume harmful foods; and creating socially needed jobs rather than those contrived by business people.

? Are these suggestions feasible? Can you see the changes creating a more equitable society? Are there any downsides to these suggestions in terms of health and wellbeing? Equity? Diversity? Cultural sensitivity? Empowerment?

EMPOWERMENT

Empowerment is a term frequently found in the literature on gender and discrimination, but often with ambiguous meanings. In some cases, empowerment is explained as advocacy, the type of actions nurses and others take to help people overcome disempowerment (Kasturirangan 2009). For example, in helping women victims of intimate partner violence (IPV), or other forms of deprivation, empowerment may be equated with safe shelter, counselling and other support services. As admirable as these measures are, the term 'empowerment' actually refers to the processes by which people gain *mastery* over *their* lives, rather than something that is done for them. From the individual's perspective empowerment may be experienced as a perceived sense of control, or an actual increase in control over resources (Rappaport 1987). To support women in becoming empowered requires a paradigm shift from a focus on illness to creating the conditions that will support women in becoming empowered to optimise their health and wellbeing across the life course (ICN 2013). Empowerment often begins with critical awareness or participating in activities to create social and political change. Some of those actions may be aimed at fostering 'distributive justice'; that is, the equitable distribution of resources (Kasturirangan 2009). The extent of empowerment that is possible depends on the situation, and the needs and values of a person who is working towards empowerment. For example, some people can be empowered by information and the development of health literacy. Others would be frustrated by such an approach, given a lack of resources or opportunities to make changes in their lives, even if they had the knowledge to do so. Powerlessness is therefore highly contextualised to a person's life. Ideally, empowerment begins with consciousness raising, understanding the oppressive social forces that are barriers to development, taking intentional action to overcome those forces, and sustaining a belief in the possibility for change (Love in Kasturirangan 2009).

> **Empowerment**—having control and mastery over one's life and resources
>
> **Advocacy**—actions a nurse may take to help a person overcome disempowerment

Disempowerment, especially disempowerment on the basis of gender, lies at the core of social exclusion. This is why the power imbalance between men and women is so important. In Western societies, men typically hold economic, political, organisational and physical power over women, and this affects many aspects of their lives. These societal-level power imbalances create multiple layers of disadvantage for women who may have begun life in vulnerable circumstances through poverty, racism or other forms of marginalisation, or whose pathway to adult life may be stymied by discrimination, and other gender-related barriers to development. In some cases, men can be disempowered relative to women; for example, through the biological power of childbirth. However, given the right circumstances and support, the quality of parenting may be equal for both a father and a mother, and current trends suggest that new fathers today have embraced a more equal role, having greater involvement in parenting than their own fathers (Dempsey & Hewitt 2012). The main issue for nurses and other health professionals working with families is that there are modifiable factors in community life that can change historical gender roles, to promote equity through equality of opportunity. To this end, the following discussion focuses on the experience of being a woman or a man in contemporary society, and how these experiences can shape health and wellbeing.

BOYS, GIRLS AND INTIMACY

Gender issues come into full focus around the time of adolescence, when young men and women become sexually active. However, this precarious time in a young person's life is traversed differently for males and females. At adolescence, sexuality and intimacy are often confused, as media images of blatant sexuality often overwhelm young people's attempts to distinguish between the two. Overt images and actions portrayed on television, music videos and the internet show young men engaged in violent acts of aggression and very young women acting out sexually explicit roles. Fuller (2013) explains that young people are not more violent than their forebears, but they are more lethal in the types of violence they perpetrate. He describes boys as part of a 'click and go' generation who play video games with controls shaped like hand guns, and witness vivid portrayals of murder vicariously in all forms of media (Fuller 2013). Some commit acts of aggression as a result of 'grievous envy' for what they believe they should have in terms of consumer goods. These images can be confusing for those on the brink of adolescence and transition into adulthood, and they are highly confronting for many pre-pubertal young children. The starkness of some of these media images overshadows the need for young people to imagine sexuality and intimacy in a way that acknowledges their sensitivity and tentativeness about relationships with one another. The 'raunch culture' of music videos and magazines that encourage a culture of sex obsession depicts promiscuity as the societal norm, which contradicts the notion of sexual health as feelings of sexual self-efficacy (Siebold 2011). Sexual self-efficacy creates a feeling that a person can act on their sexual needs and on the need to protect themself from pregnancy and STIs (Siebold 2011). As Siebold's (2011) survey of Australian nursing and midwifery students revealed, these images seem to perpetuate a double standard where young girls are pressured by boys to engage in risky and unprotected sex from an early age instead of developing intimacy and a positive progression toward sexual health.

Intimacy may be easier for girls' lives than boys', especially in the closeness of female friendships that have no parallel in the lives of young boys. Boys may become more intimate as they reach adulthood, but for many, especially those without access to a father figure, the risk of idealising a 'tough guy' image is high. Fuller (2013) explains this as a subconscious inner dialogue boys sometimes have with themselves, especially if they are the only male in the household. Their self-talk revolves around the thought that 'If I can't be with Dad, I'll try to be like what I think a real man's Dad should be' (Fuller 2013). Often the consequence of this type of thinking is a tenuous distancing from their mothers, through a combination of rage, misogyny and homophobia. At this time of their lives, young boys are in danger of developing lifelong antipathy towards women. It is crucial that they are exposed to positive male role models, such as male teachers, male coaches or others in their lives who can provide alternatives to the 'tough guy' persona, and show a more respectful, sensitive side (Fuller 2013). Big brother/big sister programs may be particularly helpful for boys who lack a male role model in the home. Research to date shows that such programs are cost effective, and have good outcomes for both boys and girls (Moodie & Fisher 2009). Parents also play an important role in helping them manoeuvre through these transitions to healthy young men who value and respect healthy young women.

WOMEN'S HEALTH ISSUES

Women's health issues are influenced by many factors: childbirth, gender-linked health conditions including unique reproductive health risks, women's health behaviours, and their longevity and social position relative to men. Women's innate constitution gives them an advantage over men in terms of life expectancy, but living longer is a double-edged sword, with older women suffering from chronic diseases for more years of their lives compared to men (Hosseinpoor et al. 2012). Data from the World Health Survey of 57 countries showed that worldwide, women's health is significantly lower than men's, with most of the inequality attributed to the social determinants of women's lives (Hosseinpoor et al. 2012). Although these inequalities span all age groups, the social conditions associated with contraception, pregnancy, childbirth and a lack of autonomy in seeking health care are major factors in women's health, as are changes in marital status. In Hosseinpoor et al.'s (2012) analysis socio-economic position (SEP), which is the culmination of education, income and occupation, was found to have a powerful influence on the type, magnitude, and distribution of health across all countries. This is also the case in other societies where women are disadvantaged by their social position.

> **REMINDER: SEP**
> - Education
> - Income
> - Occupation

Globally, the two leading mortality risks for women are similar to those of men: cardiovascular disease and stroke. Gender differences lie in the fact that women's symptoms may be different from those of men's, they tend to develop later in life, and, in some cases, suffer more post-treatment complications (Davidson et al. 2012a). Women in developing countries suffer a disproportionate burden of diseases, including those related to pregnancy, childbirth and unsafe abortions (WHO 2013). They are also more vulnerable to the effects of climate change because of their inability to relocate when their community is imperilled by weather events or disasters (WHO 2011). Many women in developing countries and some Western countries are engaged in unpaid, low-status domestic work, with no protective legislation and with only fragmented leisure time (WHO 2006; World Bank 2009). Those who enter non-traditional occupations suffer discrimination and sexual harassment more often than men, and earn less money. In their later years women also experience a higher burden of dementia and other cognitive disorders, primarily because of their longevity (AIHW 2012; ICN 2013). The older years are often a time when women are left on their own, given their longer lifespan compared to their spouses/partners. Research has shown that, compared with married women, older single women are disadvantaged, and this is linked to the fact that marriage is known to be protective of all-cause mortality in both women and men (Idler et al. 2012). Retirement income schemes can also disadvantage women who may have planned on living on their husband's retirement income, only to lose access to this financial support when their partner dies. In these cases, they may be forced to rely on a minimum pension scheme for a longer period of time than they expected. With the baby boomer generation having lower rates of marriage and higher rates of separation and divorce than previous generations, many women will be ageing alone in the future, some in disadvantaged financial situations. Loneliness can also impinge on their health, creating both physical and psychological risks. Without the protective influence of a marital partner the risk of dying within three months of a cardiac event is almost double that of married women (Idler et al. 2012).

PROTECTIVE EFFECTS OF MARRIAGE

- Spousal social control, regulating lifestyle
- Social support
- 'Warm touch' of intimacy reduces stress-sensitive biomarkers
- Practical and calming support in a crisis

(Idler et al. 2012)

Another disadvantage arises from the fact that women's medical treatments often show marked differences from the way men's health is managed. The way male medical specialists understand women's needs is sometimes based on presumption rather than scientific evidence. In some cases, sexual norms of behaviour are dictated by clinicians and sexologists on the basis of cultural expectations rather than the way women themselves interpret sexual needs (Hinchliff et al. 2009). These expectations are implicit in the pervasive and dominant heterosexual discourse of male 'need' and female 'response' (Hinchliff et al. 2009). Women's treatment for other illnesses is also different to men's. Women are also less likely to be treated according to guideline-indicated therapies, such as cardiac rehabilitation programs, despite evidence indicating the advantages of such programs (Lavie & Milani 2009; Shaw et al. 2009). When women are referred to rehabilitation programs, it is often for shorter periods of time than their male counterparts (Lavie & Milani 2009; WHO 2006). Some of these differences are evident in treating women for cardiovascular diseases. Studies have shown that women are under-treated, which has been linked to physicians' lack of awareness of risk factors in women, and options for their treatment (Oertelt-Prigione & Regitz-Zagrosek 2009). Women in rural areas can also be disadvantaged by the lack of specialist practitioners to help in dealing with family planning or pregnancy issues, particularly those that require confidential discussions of treatment or interventions.

Some medical practitioners have little understanding of the cross-cultural differences in women's experience of health. For example, a study in Western Australia found that Aboriginal women did not experience the premenopausal protective effect from cardiovascular disease that was present in non-Indigenous women (Katzenbellenogen et al. 2010). Because many Indigenous cultures tend to see 'women's business' as private they do not seek medical help for symptoms of menopause, which could place them at risk of under-diagnosis of other conditions (Jones et al. 2012). Women's mental health also suffers from the combination of lack of understanding and inability to access a range of treatments. In some cases, Indigenous women are under- diagnosed with mental ill health due to the high acuity and prevalence of conditions such as postnatal depression (PND) being considered as normal in their population. Another problem is that when women are diagnosed with mental illness such as depression, they tend to be quickly prescribed biochemical solutions, primarily antidepressants, without further investigations. Many remain on this type of medication for years, creating the impression that women's mental health problems do not warrant in-depth discussion or longer term exploration. Protracted use of medications for depressive illness can be a mind-numbing solution to a problem that may have a social cause. The most well-known of these causes is workplace stress or the unrelenting boundary-spanning roles that blur the boundaries between work and home (see Chapter 10) (Glavin et al. 2011). These multiple roles can generate considerable guilt about giving sufficient attention to either work or home, and prevent women from accessing opportunities for physical activity, or other stress-management supports (Coulter et al. 2009; Glavin et al. 2011).

Women and poverty

The cumulative effects of different lifestyles and health risks from childhood to ageing also affect women and men differently, especially in relation to their economic capabilities. Poverty is a major problem for women worldwide, and it affects women disproportionately, because of the difficulty of maintaining good nutrition for themselves and their children, and in some countries, the use of unsafe cooking fuels (ICN 2013; WHO 2011, 2013). The persistence of poverty among women of wealthy nations seems a social contradiction, given the international declarations to alleviate inequality and discrimination during the 1990s. These included the International Conference on Population and Development in Cairo (1994), the Platform for Action of the Fourth World Conference on Women in Beijing (1995), and the Convention for the Elimination of all Forms of Discrimination Against Women (CEDAW), the latter being ratified by 150 nations, excluding the US and Afghanistan (WHO 2009). Yet, discrimination against women and the lack of opportunities for them to develop their capacity is rampant around the world. Poor women are sometimes seen as responsible for their circumstances. Being a poor and dependent woman, particularly where there are children to support, attracts a societal judgement that, somehow, a woman has a choice, and has chosen badly. Some women also self-stigmatise, believing they are somehow responsible for their circumstances, which leads to further disempowerment. This kind of thinking at a personal or societal level helps justify the social exclusion of poor women, which becomes part of an endless cycle of deprivation, especially for those who may be recruited into sex trafficking, prostitution or hazardous work (Dovydaitis 2010). A woman may be too poor to refuse this type of abuse because she has no means to manage her life and that of her children, to gain education, opportunities and resources. Inequity is then transformed into a deprivation of basic capabilities (Sen 1999). The gendered nature of the problem has been known for many years, yet the socio-economic disadvantage of women in many countries, including the wealthy countries of the West, is not improving, and women remain disempowered around the world (WHO 2013). The WHO attributes the disparity to unequal power relationships; social norms that decrease women's education and employment opportunities; an exclusive focus on women's reproductive roles; and potential or actual experience of physical, sexual or emotional violence (WHO 2013).

WOMEN'S GLOBAL DISADVANTAGE

- Unequal power relationships
- Social norms impinging on their opportunities
- Focus on reproductive roles
- Physical, sexual, emotional violence

A lack of education is a major risk to women's health. In every region of the world, educating girls is the single most powerful way to promote equitable personal opportunities, and pathways to health and wellbeing. It is also good for the economy, with a flow-on effect for building social cohesion. Women with access to education tend to marry later than uneducated women. They have smaller families, make better use of antenatal and delivery care, and understand how to use family planning methods. They seek medical care sooner in the event of illness, maintain higher nutritional

standards, and raise their daughters to receive sufficient education to keep the cycle of health improvements moving in a positive direction (UNESCO 2000; UNFPA 2000). Educated women typically have the level of health literacy to retain control over their reproductive function. They understand the issues involved, the presence of risk, and the steps that need to be taken to ensure health and safety for them and their babies. It is also widely accepted that education prepares mothers in developing early, enhanced child-rearing practices, which affects their children's lifelong potential. Most educated mothers have an appreciation of the need to foster learning readiness and a good preschool foundation for subsequent stages of a child's development (AIFS 2012). However, education alone cannot completely prevent a gender gap in terms of women's professional lives, as Box 12.2 reveals.

EDUCATING GIRLS

… the single most powerful way to promote equitable personal opportunities and pathways to health and wellbeing in any country.

MIGRANT AND REFUGEE WOMEN: THE INTERSECTION OF GENDER, POWER AND CULTURE

Another area of women's vulnerability is the heightened risk of severe ill health and trauma for migrant and refugee women. Global studies conducted within the context of the WHO, the United Nations and numerous government agencies consistently show alarming outcomes for migrant, refugee and asylum seeking women. These are related to the fact that their health is not considered as important as that of men because of cultural norms, culturally determined subservient roles, and their pre- and post-migration experiences (WHO 2006; World Bank 2009). For these women, social exclusion has dire consequences. Researchers from the Australian Domestic & Family Violence Clearinghouse report estimates of pre-migration sexual abuse and rape of these women at rates as high as 80% (Zannettino 2013). In many cases, the women are raped simply because they have come from war zones where rape is a common strategy to terrorise, control, displace or eliminate the enemy. The perpetrators rape to demoralise an enemy in situations where there is a high cultural value on women's purity and men's ability to protect them, or where troops are rewarded by access to sex

BOX 12.2 **Academic women and their expectations of promotion**

The study described here shows that education per se is not a panacea for gender discrimination. A review of academic positions in New Zealand, Australia and Canada reveals that women now occupy 20% of all senior academic positions, an improvement from 5% in the 1960s. However, more men are viewed as experts and scholars, and men are more likely to be promoted to the level of professors. The gender gap is explained on the basis of several areas of disadvantage for academic women: their teaching versus research focus in the context of university research culture; humanities versus science areas of specialisation; family circumstances, and institutional practices that reward long hours and international travel (difficult for those with family responsibilities); access to professional networks; and varying career length. Baker (2010) interviewed New Zealand women academics about their experiences as university academics and found that all of these factors influenced their 'glass ceiling'. In addition, women reported that their love of scholarship and teaching was being destroyed by growing bureaucracy, high teaching loads, long hours, rapid turnover and the competitive work environment. The 'audit culture' that requires so much attention to detail in defending productivity was disheartening, along with juggling breastfeeding between classes, escorting children to and from day care, or having child care problems during research leave, with little collegial support. One of the participants summed it up succinctly: 'It's not that universities are *gender* blind, it's that they're *family* blind'. Most agreed that they are at the mercy of their husbands/partners in terms of moving to another university, and many found that the effect of low collegial recognition and esteem is a lack of confidence (Baker 2010).

So what does this tell us about education and the gender gap?

Nursing academics are vulnerable to the kinds of organisational changes that are occurring in universities in New Zealand and Australia.

? If your aspirations were to enter academic life, how might you be able to manage the gender issues? Would any of your strategies be different to managing the gender issues of women in mining or other male-dominated industries?

(Zannettino 2013). This is sexual terrorism, which blurs the boundaries between public violence and intimate violence, leaving women assaulted, victimised, demoralised and subjugated for political purposes. In situations where war and conflict may cease, women continue to suffer by being shunned by their husbands or families as symbolic of the nation's humiliation, or because they are mothering a child of the enemy. Some are forced to stay with their captors, and a life of continuing re-victimisation, sexually transmissible diseases, and ill health. Many of these women also suffer postnatal depression (PND) (Collins et al. 2011), suffering in silence and unable to enact cultural rituals after childbirth. Many are forced into 'survival sex' in detention, fearful of reprisals if they refuse, or guilt at having brought dishonour to their families (Ostapiej-Piatkowski & Allimant 2013; Pittaway & Eckert 2013).

WOMEN IN DETENTION

- Multilayered risks of abuse, torture, oppression
- Ongoing sexual assault, other traumas
- Witnessing child abuse
- PND, STIs
- PTSD, depression
- Survival sex
- Shaming

In Australia, the US, the UK and some other European countries and Asia it is established practice, and enshrined in law, to detain asylum seekers and immigrants without visas (Burchill 2012; Coffey et al. 2010). The asylum seeker debate rages continually in the Australian public media, with many expressing righteous indignation that people would act as 'queue jumpers' and seek asylum without waiting their turn to be considered for migration. Being 'warehoused' in detention centres, both male and female asylum seekers experience high levels of mental illness, including severe depression, anxiety and post-traumatic stress disorder (PTSD). A record number of asylum seekers have drowned in recent years, seeking to reach Australian shores. In detention, their family members are left to mourn, sometimes for young children who could not be rescued; sometimes for spouses or parents who accompanied them on the journey in boats supplied by indiscriminate people smugglers. Behind the walls of the detention centres, women and children are exposed to multiple suicide attempts, self-harm, child sexual abuse and other manifestations of disempowerment and alienation. These injustices are only the tip of the iceberg in terms of the lasting effects of their incarceration, which can continue for several years or for the rest of their lives (Coffey et al. 2010). Children often miss out on schooling as their mothers try to protect them from the confrontation of an alien environment. Women's lives are a constant struggle to care for their family, even the children borne of rape, while trying to avoid being viewed as prostitutes, or jeopardising their chance of gaining a visa as a genuine refugee (Collins et al. 2011; Zannettino 2013). Without visas they are not eligible for Medicare and must rely on charities for assistance. Beyond detention, both men and women who have been resettled experience insecurity and a sense of injustice, difficulties with relationships, poor self-esteem, low concentration and memory disturbances. Many women are not able to go to English language classes to help their transition into society, either because of child care or cultural norms. Researchers have found that the extent of their mental ill health is correlated to the length of time they have spent in detention, and many feel a sense of powerlessness, alienation and abandonment to the extent that they are irrevocably disabled (Coffey et al. 2010).

For women who have been sexually assaulted, the experience of being in detention creates cumulative risks. Most hesitate to seek help because of shame, embarrassment or feeling guilty, fear of losing what relationships they may still have, feeling culturally obliged to submit to sexual violence by their husbands, wanting to protect children and maintain relationships with other family members, fear of humiliation by police or others in the criminal justice system or deportation (Zannettino 2013). Once they are resettled in Australia some continue to be sexually abused by their partners, because of traditional gender roles. Culture, trauma and displacement therefore create layers of social exclusion because of traumatic histories, difficulties with language, housing, education and discrimination, and sometimes because of their feelings of difference as a member of a minority group (Mwanri et al. 2012; Zannettino 2013). Although the trauma is not usually as intense among other migrant women who are not tortured as refugees from civil war or conflict, they also experience feelings of social isolation, especially those from non-English speaking backgrounds (NESB). For those who do gain employment, their health and safety is often at the mercy of employers, who, in Australia, may not see cultural diversity as an important priority, leaving them to cope with

extra difficulties in the workplace that add to their transition stress (Syed & Murray 2009). Some also have to confront dramatic changes in lifestyles that may be common in Australia and New Zealand, in relation to food, parenting, religious observance, consumption of alcohol or exercise. In Middle Eastern cultures, for example, the dominant cultural expectation of modesty means that women must dress according to cultural norms and exercise in gender-specific locations. This can act as a deterrent to exercise, which would be a positive step in helping them cope with the stress of migration. In many cases, their health literacy may be problematic. Although they may have been health literate to a degree that they can meet their needs in their country of origin, they face additional challenges on migration, in knowing how to navigate the health care system or where to seek help.

As nurses, our obligation to these women is to work with other members of the health care team to help them through the multiple transitions, supporting the women and their families in achieving health and wellbeing at as high a standard as possible. Community nurses encounter these women in the context of home visiting, child and school health centres, neighbourhood or community groups, or in specialised community centres for victims of torture and trauma, including women who have been trafficked. Nurses must be wary of imposing Western ideals of health care, parenting and maternity on migrant mothers. Ways in which nurses traditionally provide care to the individual may paradoxically disempower migrant women whose collective ideals may differ from those of their care providers (Desouza 2013). The Centre for Refugee Research (CRR) at the University of New South Wales has a number of resources available to help those guiding refugee women. Their approach includes assessing women using the Heightened Risk Identification Tool developed by the CRR as part of the 'Women at Risk' program. Australia is one of the few countries with a 'Women at Risk' program, modelled on that of the United Nations High Commissioner for Refugees. The aim of the program is to protect vulnerable refugee women and girls, irrespective of which visa category provides the basis for their resettlement. Researchers and counsellors have used the tool successfully to date, for 500 women in the process of being resettled, and 100 of their service providers (Pittaway et al. 2013). The tool is very detailed, using a step-wise checklist to assess pre-arrival factors, current factors, risk responses and monitoring mechanisms, available on the CRR website (www.crr.unsw.edu.au).

For women victims of human trafficking the 'Campaign to Rescue and Restore Victims of Human

Trafficking' also provides a list of possible clues that someone may be a victim. These include being extra vigilant for women who may be new to the country; non-English speaking women; women without a visa or passport and with evidence of being controlled; women who are bruised or battered, or expressing fear of deportation (Dovydaitis 2010). Help for these and other women who have been detained must go beyond the assessment, to assisting them with their most pressing needs; that is, housing, English language, employment, dealing with agencies such as Centrelink and intergenerational conflicts. In some cases these are dealt with by Humanitarian Settlement Service (HSS) providers, but it is important that all health professionals work as a team, understanding one another's role and the common goal of providing timely, intersectoral and culturally appropriate services (Pittaway et al. 2013;

Zannettino 2013). HSS providers adopt a human rights approach, where specialist counsellors try to address violence against these women as both a men's and a women's issue, and work with both partners in a way that preserves the woman's safety (Parris 2013; Pittaway & Eckert 2013). For those imperilled by torture and trauma, including having spent time in detention, our obligation as health professionals lies in our expressed support for the human rights agenda, and our commitment to engage in political advocacy to restore the fundamental human right to seek asylum. In New Zealand, this has been the approach taken over some years, where a commitment to human rights means that everyone has a right to asylum, clearly indicating that refugee policies are more closely aligned than those of Australia with the UN Charter of Human Rights (see Box 12.3). As numbers of

BOX 12.3 New Zealand refugee policy

Due to its geographical remoteness, New Zealand has not faced the same migration pressures as Australia; however, there are some in New Zealand who believe this may change and policy is being altered accordingly. Annually, New Zealand resettles approximately 750 'quota' refugees. These refugees are referred by the United Nations High Commission for Refugees (UNHCR) and are considered under the following categories: women at risk; protection; and medical/disability (NZMOH 2012a). New Zealand is one of only nine countries—including Australia, who takes 20 000 UNHCR referred refugees per year— that host refugees under a quota system. New Zealand also takes refugees under a family reunification system whereby family members of refugees who have already settled in New Zealand may also emigrate. 'Asylum seeker' is the third category under which people seeking refugee status arrive in New Zealand. In 2008–09, no asylum seekers arrived via boat in New Zealand and only 23 arrived at an international airport, although 246 people did make application to the Refugee Status Branch of Immigration New Zealand for consideration as an asylum seeker—30% of these applications were approved (NZ Refugee organisation, Online. Available: www.refugee.org.nz/ stats.htm#Table%201 [accessed 30 October 2013]). Despite the small number of asylum seekers arriving in New Zealand, in 2012 the New Zealand Government introduced legislation designed to enhance New Zealand's ability to manage effectively and efficiently any mass arrival (over 11 people) of irregular or potentially illegal migrants. The bill was

passed into law in August 2013. (NZ Govt, Online. Available: www.legislation.govt.nz/act/public/2009/ 0051/latest/DLM5296635.html?search=qs_act%40bill %40regulation%40deemedreg_mass+arrivals_ resel_25_h&p=1 [accessed 30 October 2013]). The new legislation increases powers of detention and has been criticised by many as not aligning with New Zealand's previously highly regarded commitment to refugees (Frelick 2012). As we reported in Chapter 2, the New Zealand Prime Minister agreed with the Prime Minister of Australia to accept 150 'boat people' in return for access to Australia's refugee detention centres for any 'boat people' that made it to New Zealand. These agreed extra 150 asylum seekers would be taken into New Zealand under the quota scheme, meaning New Zealand will now only accept 600 UNHCR referred refugees.

Australia's refugee detention centres have been condemned as inhumane and prolonging the suffering of refugees who are among the world's most vulnerable people (Frelick 2012). Refugees experience significant trauma both mentally and physically in their journey to safety. Countries have a responsibility to work with their communities to develop refugee and asylum seeker policies that do not perpetuate the trauma of fleeing from a country of origin, but provide safe and enabling processes for supporting these people in need. In addition, Australia and New Zealand have a responsibility to work globally to address human rights issues in countries of refugee origin.

women who have been subjected to trafficking and detention in New Zealand are very small, nurses working with refugee and migrant communities must be even more vigilant to ensure these women do not slip through the gaps.

INTIMATE PARTNER VIOLENCE AND EMPOWERMENT

Although we have addressed intimate partner violence (IPV) in the context of family relations in Chapter 7, it is addressed here as one of the most gender-specific causes of women's disempowerment. IPV is usually about one partner in a relationship controlling another. Researchers have described a typology of four different versions of IPV: common couple violence, intimate terrorism, violent resistance and mutual violent control (Fortin et al. 2012). Common couple violence occurs where unresolved couple conflicts escalate to psychological or physical violence. Intimate terrorism is asymmetric violence used by one partner to control the other. Violent resistance refers to the actions of a victim who attempts to counteract the abusive partner's control, and mutual violent control is a symmetric model of violence where both partners try to control the other (Fortin et al. 2012). In young couples experiencing conflicts, women tend to perpetrate a higher number of violent acts against their partner, but with fewer injuries than they suffer from male perpetrators; however, women report more psychological suffering than men, and are more likely to seek help (Fortin et al. 2012). In some cases, violent behaviours begin with the dating experience, when young people confuse violent controlling acts with the normative behaviours associated with love, flirting and playfulness. Young girls in particular shy away from reporting disrespect or 'relationship dramas' as coercion, control or abuse (Martin et al. 2012:958). This distortion occurs because some abusive behaviours create ambiguity about whether or not they are harmful, especially those communicated using electronic technology, where social networking and text messages can seem innocuous but soon escalate to psychological aggression (Burke Draucker & Martsolf 2010). Young girls can become confused about which type of interactions are abusive and which are not. Their reluctance to seek advice when they are uncertain can be problematic in that it can establish relationship patterns that may be harmful to them and their partner in the context of marriage or long-term partnerships.

> ### TYPOLOGY OF IPV
> - Common couple violence
> - Intimate terrorism
> - Violent resistance
> - Mutual violent control

Marriage is often used to legitimise a range of sexual and familial violent acts against women, and this varies with different cultures. Serious acts of violence include practices such as the following: sex selective abortion, denial of the means to prevent pregnancy or infection, female genital mutilation, treating young girls as a commodity-in-trade by marrying them off before puberty, or offering a girl's sister to the matrimonial home as compensation for her death; providing a girl to a family to ensure an inheritance or fulfil an obligation to produce an heir; acid thrown to disfigure a woman because of dowry disputes; honour killing based on the presumption of infidelity; elder abuse; or various forms of trafficking in women and prostitution (WHO 2013). One way of conceptualising the impact of IPV is described by Tower et al. (2012) in terms of the theory of biographical disruption. The violence is a major disruptive experience, which leads a woman to re-examine her self-concept to make sense of the violence, and then re-arrange the conditions of her life to restore her sense of self. Yet women in developing countries or living in disadvantaged circumstances are not often able to rearrange the conditions of their lives. In these cases and where a woman is unable to access guidance to help her out of her confusion and self-doubt there is little likelihood of her being able to reconstruct a positive self-concept (Tower et al. 2012).

> ### ACTS OF WOMAN ABUSE
> - Sex selective abortion
> - No reproductive choices
> - Female genital mutilation
> - Child marriage
> - Selling girls for inheritance
> - Disfigurement, honour killings
> - Trafficking
> - Elder abuse

The effects of IPV also have profound harmful effects on the children witnessing abuse in any context (see Box 12.4). Young children in detention centres are often exposed to gender norms of violence that may be culturally acceptable but not appropriate in terms of the gendered behaviours they will observe in their host country post-migration, which are usually more gender balanced. Their time in detention can therefore leave them at risk of a distorted view of gender relations. In other living environments children may be caught between violent parents or partners role modelling violence on a regular basis, or intermittently at the time of transitions between staying with one or another parent. Their exposure is a serious problem in both the immediate and long term. Between seven and 10 children on average are killed each year in New Zealand by someone who is supposed to be caring for them, and in 2010, 209 children aged under 15 required hospital treatment for assault-related injuries (Bennett 2012). Of the 52 800 care and protection notifications made to the New Zealand child protection agency (Child, Youth and Family), a total of 9411 cases of neglect, physical or sexual abuse were found (Bennett 2012). These cases have widespread repercussions as children who witness abuse are more likely to be abused themselves, to have behaviour problems, and increased exposure to other adversities such as alcohol and drug abuse, crime and other antisocial coping strategies (Holt et al. 2008). The risk factors for violence against women and their children vary across cultures, and to date, there remains no definitive pattern for predicting which factors will lead a man to abuse a woman. Those factors that have been identified comprise a multi-faceted web of causation, where violence is a result of the interaction between aspects of the individual, the relationship, the community and society, as illustrated in Figure 12.1.

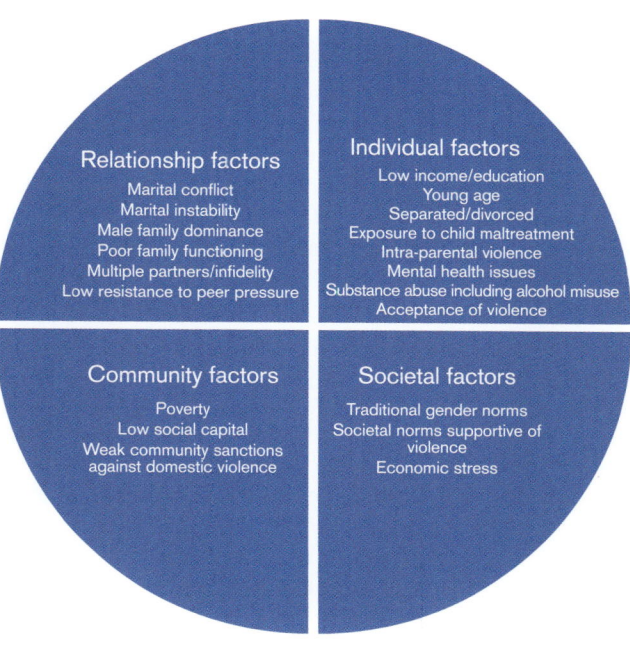

FIGURE 12.1
Factors associated with a man's risk of abusing his partner (Adapted from World Health Organization/London School of Hygiene and Tropical Medicine 2010 Preventing intimate partner and sexual violence against women: taking action and generating evidence. World Health Organization, Geneva)

PRACTICE STRATEGY

Screening for interpersonal violence is an effective means of reaching women who may be at risk of violence. It also offers the opportunity to provide support, safety and validation of the woman's experience.

Besides physical injuries the outcomes of violence against women can include stress, poor mental health, PTSD, self-harm, substance abuse, suicide or homicide (Hooker et al. 2012). The unborn children of women who are abused during pregnancy are also at risk for injury or fetal death. The threat of having the children removed from a violent home can act as a deterrent to disclosure (Postmus et al. 2009) and lead women to escape the domestic situation for the sake of their children. Some then become homeless, which starts a vicious cycle of disempowerment for them and their children. The social context of homelessness can leave them enmeshed in a network of alcohol and substance abusers as well as ongoing vulnerability to further violence on the streets. Young homeless women in particular are vulnerable to sexual coercion simply to survive. In some cases, women who have fallen into this type of cycle become further victimised by health and social services, especially where personnel have been ill-prepared to understand the depth or breadth of their distress or the physical effects of sex workers, which can include sexually transmissible diseases and other illnesses (Adams Tufts et al. 2009; Postmus et al. 2009).

The frequency of violence against women has inspired the WHO Global Campaign for Violence Prevention to implement the recommendations of the world report on violence and health. The campaign is aimed at raising awareness of what has become a major source of injury among women, highlighting the role of public health in addressing

BOX 12.4 **Intimate partner violence: the hidden victims**

Violence against an intimate partner is usually part of a gendered relationship of power and control; typically men attempting to control women. Sometimes gender-related violence is perpetrated on individuals on the basis of their gender expression as a lesbian, gay, bisexual, transgender or intersex (LGBTI) person. In the LGBTI community, violence is often perpetrated for no other reason than a person's intolerance of diversity, the inability to control others' sexual identity or expression. Gay relationships have the added difficulty of few available sources of support or assistance. Like women victimised by their partners, they need to find a way out of the situation where their life is under the control of someone else. Also like women in an IPV situation, they may be caught up in a situation from which they can see no way out. Many victims of IPV tend to direct their efforts to reducing the violence, instead of leaving. This is particularly the case for women with children who have no economic resources, and no alternative avenue of assistance. In many violent partnerships, the woman's life becomes dominated by trying to please the abuser/controller. The abuser tries to exploit the relationship, creating further dependency through little acts of treachery; creating a financial debt, or holding her to ransom by excessive neediness or a sense that she is the abusive one. During this time, the situation becomes dysfunctional for both of them, and for the children. In male-to-female violence, the male tyrant abuses his power because of an inability to control a female partner. But this may be an oversimplification of a complex set of relations, often defying disentanglement. In some societies where women have low status, men can control their wives through economic dependence, without reverting to violence. In other, more equitable societies where women have well-established economic power and a role in decision-making, violence is also less prevalent.

Violence is highest in societies where there is greater economic equality, but where sex role stereotypes prevent women from being decision-makers. Campbell's (2001) research around the world shows that the greatest danger lies in situations where women's status is changing, and in contention with men's status, challenging their control. This often occurs in situations where, after many years of domestic life, a woman chooses to develop her educational and economic capacity by undertaking formal studies, or secures a job that may be beyond her partner's expectation of her. Sometimes this dramatic change in marital expectations leads to family separation. With so many marriages in Australia and New Zealand ending in divorce, a large number of households are in upheaval, because of the change to the couple's power relations. Violence in these families often subjects young children to the conflicts related to family separation. In many cases, they are witness to, or unwitting pawns in, episodes of IPV, leading up to family separation, during protracted negotiations and following the separation. This cycle also repeats itself in many blended families. In the case of culturally sanctioned violence, women and children may also be involved in systematic, patriarchal terrorism in their own homes for a wide range of reasons, usually violating norms of obedience to the perpetrator. For adults, the gender wars of everyday life are difficult. For children, they often have lasting effects. Some child victims of violence grow up to find love and commitment elusive, and often replicate their dysfunctional upbringing with their own children. The cradle of violence in their family lives therefore becomes a cradle of societal violence (Strauss 2001).

Young children witnessing IPV are often damaged by the experience, developing no sense of a woman's experience of self-esteem. They see their mother as a whipping post, and they feel her frustration and defeat. How, then, can a child of such a household develop effective relationships of equal power, characterised by respect, support and a sense of the future? Does this occur because society labels domestic violence a woman's problem, instead of a problem of civilisation itself? If this is society's approach, we pay only lip service to social justice, and the world continues to privilege one gender over another, and prevent alternative forms of gender expression. As nurses and other health professionals we need to see gender-based violence as a human rights issue. Our obligation, like that of other members of society, is to engage in policy debates and let our voices reverberate in the chambers of those who do not appreciate that all people are deserving of a nonviolent, harmonious and optimistic future.

its causes and consequences and in fostering prevention. The campaign also provides an online platform for dissemination and exchange of evidence-based knowledge about violence prevention as well as policies, plans and experiences (WHO, Online. Available: www.who.int/violence_injury_ prevention/violence/global_campaign/en/ (accessed 26 August 2013)). Addressing all four risk factors associated with family violence (individual, relationship, community and society factors) is the ideal approach to preventing violence. Nurses and midwives throughout the world who work in communities are often best positioned to respond with assistance and support (ICN 2013). Many are leading advocates for championing the rights of women and addressing IPV, and its effects on health and wellbeing. The research agenda informing their practice is gradually expanding, albeit slowly, with a need to create evidence for best practice in assisting women and children victims of family violence (Hooker et al. 2012). Screening for violence in health settings and home visits by maternal, child and family nurses is also gaining momentum, particularly with research studies indicating that women appreciate being asked about abuse (Adams Tufts et al. 2009; Koziol-McLain et al. 2008). Women interviewed in New Zealand reported that being screened afforded them an opportunity to learn about IPV, and the resources available to them as well as giving them permission to talk about abuse in their lives (Koziol-McLain et al. 2008).

The New Zealand and Australian screening protocols are based on empowerment and safety, and ensuring that there are adequately prepared health professionals to be of primary, secondary and tertiary assistance to women. Researchers have found that the services that do have a lasting impact on women's ability to survive abuse such as IPV, rape or child abuse, are those that provide for women's and children's immediate needs through welfare benefits, food and spiritual counselling (Postmus et al. 2009, WHO 2013). Helping women gain financial independence has also been identified as the strongest predictor of a woman being able to leave the violent partner (Kim & Gray 2008). Financial support and practical services can help women become self-sufficient, and begin to develop self-efficacy and empower them to live their lives in freedom. Once their immediate needs are met, longer term empowerment can be based on providing them with the opportunity to explore the issues of power and control embedded in their relationships (ICN 2013). Support groups, advocacy, shelter, education, legal aid and collaboration between service providers are also important components of service provision (ICN 2013; WHO

2013). Equally as important is the need for mutual support friendship networks, which women often find the most accessible means of support, and the need to keep social inclusion on the research agenda.

EVIDENCE-BASED PRACTICE FOR EMPOWERMENT AND SOCIAL INCLUSION

The research agenda that would inform practice to assist victims of violence is slowly evolving, but many gaps remain. Community-based participatory research (CBPR), which we have mentioned earlier in this book, is ideal in helping give voice to vulnerable people who may find it difficult to articulate their needs. Using a partnership approach CBPR researches 'with' rather than 'on' various groups: women, children, refugees, migrants, Indigenous people, those with mental illness, people who are incarcerated, or any other group who are 'invisible' or 'voiceless' to those who can assist them. This approach to researching empowerment is strengths-based (see also Chapter 15). The participants are the unit of identity, and the research team seeks to build on their strengths and resources, collaborating with them throughout the research in generating and using knowledge and action for mutual benefit. This is a classic PHC partnership approach, where all parties become co-learners and use information to overcome their disempowerment (Nyamathi et al. 2012).

? Which group in your community that may be disadvantaged in terms of power relationships would be most likely to work with you on a CBPR project to identify their needs? What strategies would you use to recruit such a group?

What resources would you need to have in place to meet their needs once these were identified?

MEN'S HEALTH ISSUES

Like women's health, men's health is created in the context of the SDH. Sometimes these determinants go unrecognised, especially when it comes to the socially determined differences between men and women. It is far easier for most people to relate to men's and women's health in terms of biological factors, categorising health and health needs in terms of their respective reproductive systems or body parts, instead of socially constructed patterns of behaviours. Images of health and wellbeing are also socially engineered by the media. These images disguise reality, by portraying biologically perfect specimens doing exciting things or, in complete contrast, images of young people engaged in a wide range of antisocial acts. Little wonder that those on the verge of developing their gender identity are uncertain of where to find role models. Some of the most important gender issues for men are bound up in stereotypical roles ascribed by society. Some men acknowledge their androgynous selves (having both male and female characteristics) without a problem, but others experience role strain in dealing with the fact that they have multidimensional, and sometimes complex, character traits. Men are also subjected to gendered expectations that can leave them vulnerable to ill health, and this is the case for some rural men who are expected to be stoical and resigned to the hardships of being a family breadwinner. Another example of the negative outcomes of stereotyping lies is the issue of LGBTI communities who are also Indigenous, or put another way, Indigenous men who are also gay. Focusing on one stereotypical aspect of their lives negates their needs in other areas.

> ### GENDER AND MALENESS
>
> Men's behaviours are due to a combination of social and cultural expectations regarding expectations of the 'male ideal'.

Will Courtenay (2000), a leading men's health researcher, argues that social and institutional structures help to sustain and reproduce men's health risks and the social construction of men as the stronger sex. These structures reproduce a *hegemonic* view of gender. Hegemony refers to the fact that men are more culturally valued in Western society, and therefore the dominant sex. Gender, as an SDH, is one of the most significant influences on health-related behaviour for men, as well as for women, yet common perceptions of gender as a social determinant revolve around women's health. The way men negotiate gender roles actually creates *higher* health risks for many men as compared to women. Their elevated risk of some of the most prevalent conditions, such as cardiovascular disease, type 2 diabetes and mental illness, is linked to a cluster of healthy lifestyle behaviours that many men see as synonymous with masculinity. These are the deadly risks of smoking, drinking and driving, unhealthy diets, avoiding exercise and emotional help, or screening for various conditions.

Men's lifestyles and health

Besides notions of the 'male ideal', men's lifestyles are also determined by their socio-economic position (SEP) on the social gradient. Men at the lower end of the gradient especially, tend to see their bodies as a work instrument, and large body size as an indication of strength and dominance (Khlat et al. 2009). This perspective can lead to a lack of concern for the combination of diet and exercise that would reduce their risk of cardiovascular or metabolic diseases. Large body size can also be culturally mediated. Tongan men, for example, consistently prefer larger body sizes, seeing these as more attractive than slimness in both men and women (Coyne in NZMOH 2008a). Addressing culturally embedded notions of gender and body size is challenging. Efforts among Pacific communities living in New Zealand frequently revolve around church and community-based activities that focus on nutrition and exercise. Working with local communities in spaces and places that are relevant to them and guided by their needs are proving to be the most effective approaches to addressing the health and lifestyle needs of Pacific people (Tava'e & Nosa 2012). Although somewhat stereotypical, men's employment often drives their motivation for taking care of themselves, particularly in terms of exercise. For many men, strenuous manual work limits their motivation for recreational exercise. Although men at higher levels of the social gradient are more disposed towards physical exercise for recreation, this group also tends to value being physically dominant. These attitudes about body image differ dramatically from that of women, who, at higher SEP levels, see slimness as a marker of beauty and professionalism. Aspirations for body shape also differ for those at the lower end of the social gradient, who associate being overweight with femininity and maternal qualities (Khlat et al. 2009). Another distinction between men's and women's 'embodiment' is that in Western society, women's bodies are extensively defined and overexposed, whereas societal forces take men's bodies for granted and exempt them from the same type of scrutiny (Coward in Courtenay 2000).

> ### SDH, EBP AND MEN'S HEALTH
>
> Research into the interplay of the SDH and their impact on men's health will enable the development of more culturally appropriate and gender-specific health services for men, rather than blame them for their health outcomes.

To some extent, men's unhealthy behaviours are due to the greater social pressure to conform, relative to women. Conforming to the male ideal means a man sees himself as not only strong, but independent, in control, self-reliant, robust and tough (Courtenay 2000). In the process, men deny weakness and vulnerability, assume emotional and physical control, and value the appearance of strength. This construction of masculinity has been explained in terms of mastery of self and others (Brown 2009). Men respond to societal expectations by dismissing any need for help, displaying aggressive behaviour and physical dominance, and, in some people's view, a ceaseless interest in sex (Courtenay 2000). Although some behaviours are shaped by ethnicity, social class and sexuality, most men also take unnecessary risks to assert their masculine side. They brag about resisting the need for sick leave from work, boast that drinking does not impair their driving, and dismiss the need for preventative health care, all aimed at maintaining their ranking among other men (Courtenay 2000; Willott & Lyons 2012). Illness is not masculine, so they tend to ignore anything that does not seem to be life-threatening. These stereotypes of behaviour can become entrenched in a boy's life from an early age, and subsequently, in the pursuit of power and privilege in relation to women and other members of society. In Western society, boys are often systematically restricted in the amount of access they have to affectionate physical contact. The contact they do have with other boys tends to be either sexualised or furtive, and their sexual expression and intimacy is carefully scripted in terms of heterosexual behaviours (Brown 2009). They are discouraged from expressing grief, and instead encouraged to suppress all emotions except anger, and to ignore pain (Brown 2009). As a result of this cultural and institutionalised stoicism and the suppression of emotion, boys can develop defensive emotional strategies, and limited capacity for, or discomfort with, empathy (Brown 2009; Fuller 2013).

CAUTION! MEN'S RISK AND HEALTH

- Conformity
- Aggressiveness
- Dismissive of illness
- Discouraged from expressing grief
- Suppression of emotion
- Too busy for exercise
- Risky behaviours

To examine men's health issues the question must be asked: what is unique to men that compromises their health and wellbeing, and conversely, what will help men live healthy lives? Most descriptions of men's health issues are problem-based, addressing the 'problems' of being a man, or of having male-specific health hazards. An SDH approach shifts the problem-orientation, from pathologising a man's behaviour or blaming him for unhealthy behaviours to trying to identify his needs as a person and as a member of his family, cultural group and society. This shift in emphasis should be informed by research into the interplay of social determinants, including gender, social class, education, age, employment status, geographical location and community, occupation, marital status, race, ethnicity, sexual orientation and disability, and the ways these combine to cause unhealthy outcomes (Saunders & Peerson 2009).

To some extent, this approach mirrors that of women. For both women and men, low socio-economic status can cause stress, which may impinge on job opportunities, transportation difficulties, social exclusion and a range of coping behaviours used to cope with these factors. Like women, men can become stuck in dead-end jobs, trying to support a family in difficult circumstances, and be relegated to substandard housing, discrimination and racism. Their job insecurity may affect them the same way as women, provoking diminished sense of self and loss of self-esteem. Physiologically though, job insecurity affects men differently than women. For men, job insecurity results in increased blood pressure but for women, the impact is in higher rates of depression (Kalil et al. 2010). Unlike women, many men do not have personal support networks, which can further exacerbate their distress, and sometimes lead them to seek support in antisocial ways, such as overconsumption of alcohol or drugs (AIHW 2013).

Men's health risks

The social construction of masculinity does not negate biological differences, but there are several other important social and cultural determinants of men's health. Men have more intentional and non-intentional injuries than women, particularly Indigenous men. They die younger than women, with three times as many young men (four times as many young Indigenous men) dying from suicide than women (AIHW 2013). Like women, the main causes of death among Australian men are cardiovascular disease and stroke (AIHW 2013). Deaths from cancers in men are from lung cancer and prostate cancer. The prevalence of prostate cancer in men is slightly higher than the prevalence of breast cancer in women, and young men are more likely than young women to be diagnosed with cancers, especially the lymphoid leukemias (AIHW 2012). As with breast cancer, survival rates from prostate cancer are increasing, but the link between survival and screening rates is unclear. National screening guidelines do not recommend the prostate-specific-antigen test (PSA) with or without rectal examination as an appropriate screening approach (AIHW 2012), and it is unknown how this guideline, or media attention, has affected men's screening behaviours.

The cluster of major risk factors for men's ill health includes obesity, physical inactivity, alcohol and substance abuse, tobacco smoking, injuries and violence. These risk factors, combined with hereditary predisposition and social disadvantage, lead to high rates of type 2 diabetes (especially in the over 55s), cardiovascular disease, cancers and depression (AIHW 2012). Participation in sport and recreation among Australian adults is falling rather than increasing, with 25–34-year-olds exercising the least, and adolescent boys exercising the most (AIHW 2012). In New Zealand, exercise rates do not vary significantly across the age groups for men until age 75 when exercise rates fall off markedly. Men are more likely to meet the recommended daily exercise regime of 30 minutes daily for five or more days per week (57%) than women (51%). Despite this, obesity rates are similar between men and women in New Zealand (NZMOH 2012b). Because of the persistence of unprotected sexual activity men's rate of STIs, especially chlamydia (the most frequently occurring STI), are slightly higher than in women (AIHW 2013). In both Australia and New Zealand, alcohol consumption causes men's greatest burden of disease, particularly in causing motor vehicle accidents. Forty-three per cent of Australian males are at risk of injury from alcohol consumption on a single occasion. They are also at greater risk of experiencing violence, particularly while consuming alcohol or drugs (AIHW 2012; NZMOH 2008b). Men are also disproportionately represented in workplace injury statistics, especially in construction, mining and, in New Zealand, forestry.

In Australia and New Zealand, fewer male adolescents take up tobacco smoking than women, but across all age groups more men than women smoke, especially those of lower socio-economic status, unemployed, LGBTI men, Indigenous men and those living in remote locations (AIHW 2012; NZMOH 2012b). Psychological health is also a different experience for men and women. Depression is a problem for many young people, but girls tend to seek help more readily than young males. Among adolescents, males have higher rates

of substance abuse than girls, even though the rate of illicit drug use among young Australian males has decreased over the past few years (AIHW 2013). For indicators of psychological health, such as self-esteem, men tend to be favoured, but in the web of factors comprising mental health, men's risks are greater. The social pressures of masculinity, especially in socially dictated norms and roles, create conditions that see many men disadvantaged in relationships. Men hesitate to talk about sensitive issues, especially sexual problems, which are often seen as damaging to their identity (Nobis & Sanden 2008). Their hesitancy to disclose stress or other psychological problems is a major problem for rural men, who have few sources of community support (AIHW 2012). For young New Zealand men, suicide is a significant issue, claiming 80 lives in 2011–12 (NZ Govt, Online. Available: www.stuff.co.nz/national/7603221/Boy-aged-under-ten-committed-suicide-stats-reveal [accessed 7 September 2013]).

Depression is the major risk factor for suicide, and in men, it is often less likely to be diagnosed, due to health professionals' lack of recognition of male-specific symptoms (Men's Health Forum 2006). Depression can manifest in aggressive behaviour, obsession about work, substance abuse, destructive thoughts and refusal to seek help. Behind these behaviours may be vulnerabilities that are not well understood, including a predisposition to postnatal depression (PND) in cases where their partner may be suffering from PND (O'Connell-Birns 2009). This context of mental ill health has thus far been virtually ignored in the health care system. Similarly, attention to the psychological and physical health of single fathers has been overlooked, yet the same factors of low income, unemployment, social isolation, and child care affect both men and women as single heads of the household (Janzen et al. 2006). Women rely heavily on friends for support, but men's inclination when they are depressed is often to camouflage their need, especially rural-living men. This prevents them from accessing the most important elements that would help develop resilience: social support and a sense of belonging (Kutek et al. 2011; McLaren & Challis 2009). This underlines the inverse care law: those who most need help are least likely to receive it (ICN 2013; O'Connell-Birns 2009). Men's psychological health is further jeopardised by a lack of appropriate counselling services, especially those that could address the constellation of determinants that shape men's lives. Whereas women-only services have been developed to help women feel comfortable in treatment and screening, equivalent services for men have yet to emerge, and where they do exist, they are often provided to address deficiencies, such as sexual dysfunction clinics. The exception is 'Men's Sheds', which have evolved in tandem with the men's health movement to encourage safe spaces for men to interact and share emotional as well as physical issues.

MEN AND DEPRESSION

Depression may manifest itself among men in different ways to women. Health professionals need to be able to recognise male-specific symptoms and risk situations in order to be able to provide appropriate care.

MASCULINITY, BEHAVIOUR AND THE MEN'S HEALTH MOVEMENT

As most people are aware, the women's movement was successful in raising consciousness across many societies, which for many years excluded women from various aspects of everyday life, for no reason other than gender. The women's movement has not succeeded in achieving gender parity in the workplace, and stereotypical behaviours continue. However, the increased awareness has been a major step forward. A similar men's movement began in the early 1990s, and within a decade, there has been a groundswell of support to better understand men and their health needs. Like the women's movement, men themselves have mounted a grassroots effort to draw attention to the issues that affect their health and wellbeing. Their voices are joined by those of health professionals who are trying to help nurture changing perspectives, and help men become empowered to live the lives they seek.

MEN'S HEALTH MOVEMENT

The movement considers men's behaviour in light of the SDH, the circumstances of men's lives and the interactions that take place in these environments. It is aimed at informing the development of new approaches to men's health and wellbeing.

Most agree that men's distinctive characteristics involve risk and risk-taking, and they must deal with the challenges surrounding various notions of masculinity, and how these inform behaviours. In some cases, their risk-taking is scorned; attributed to men behaving badly (Courtenay 2000). In others it is reified, confronted and men become pushed to extremes. The men's movement is not about entrenching or excusing the old traditional way of using their masculinity for self-aggrandisement. Nor does it revolve around the 'sensitive new age guy' approach, which, in the guise of learning more intimate ways of relating, actually reinforces the masculine privileged power relationship to dominate the emotional agenda by eliciting support from women (Brown 2009:126). Instead, the new men's movement situates men, and their behaviours, within social space and time, and frames their health within an SDH approach, to create deep understandings of how behaviour is shaped by the environment, and the interactions that take place there.

EVIDENCE FOR PRACTICE

The Fathering Project from the University of Western Australia provides a compilation of themes demonstrating the impact of fathers on child development, social skills and relationships, mental health and self-esteem, tobacco, alcohol and drug use, school engagement and performance, bullying adolescent sexual behaviour, delinquent behaviours, overweight/obesity and physical activity (Wood & Lambin 2013).

So what?

We knew all this—but it's good to have the evidence.

The men's health movement, and the broader men's movement, has drawn attention to a number of important issues, including issues of masculinity involved in parenting. It has normalised the idea of fathering identities and practices within the heterosexual nuclear family, resulting in men being increasingly involved in parenting (Dempsey & Hewitt 2012), albeit without concomitant participation in domestic work. The effect on children is significant, particularly where children have the benefit of close relationships with both parents. Parenting provides an avenue of support for men's health by giving them an opportunity to express human warmth, and to receive positive gains from the affection of their children. This role has been the subject of research in New Zealand, where men interviewed about barriers to parenting felt that society did not recognise the importance of fathers, and that the media portrayed them in a poor light (Luketina et al. 2009). Because this negative media portrayal can affect men's relationships with their children, the researchers concluded that there is a need to ensure that men's health policies are justified, and targeted appropriately (Luketina et al. 2009). Research into fatherhood is also flourishing in Australia, through the Australian Research Alliance for Children & Youth (ARACY) Fatherhood Research Network (www.aracy.org.au/networks/australian-fatherhood-research-network) and the Fatherhood Research Network Bulletin that is disseminated through the University of Newcastle (www.newcastle.edu.au/research-centre/fac/research/fathers/afrn.html). The ARACY network acts as a forum and advocacy network to encourage father-inclusive and evidence-informed policy and practice and sustained commitment to fatherhood research. The Bulletin provides brief reports of research being conducted at several Australian universities, along with blogs and web resources, and conference reports. Study findings disseminated through the ARACY network provide empirical evidence that can be shared by the research community as well as community advocates. Other research resources are aimed at supporting the gay community to enable gay fathering identities to emerge (Power et al. 2010). These initiatives represent milestones in the men's health movement, which has not always attracted recognition of the importance of a holistic view of health, which, for men, would include their psychological and social relations as equally as important as the way they should be taking care of their bodies. The men's movement has not been inspired by the type of oppression that led women to rebel against the system, as men continue to dominate political, economic and social affairs. The campaign for men's health seems more appropriately directed toward the health of individual men, and the social conditions that will enable them to thrive, and coexist with women, in enabling communities that protect and support both in whatever lifestyle they choose.

GENDER ISSUES AMONG SEXUALLY DIVERSE POPULATIONS

The health of members of LGBTI populations is a particular challenge, because they are marginalised in many Western societies such as our own, by discrimination and social exclusion. Although women and men within these groups have distinctive needs, as a group, they have an additional illness burden related to their sexual identities and expressions. The socially patterned discrimination

that exists in many aspects of their lives leads to heightened risks of violence, social invisibility and marginalisation, isolation, self-denial, guilt and internalised homo/bi/transphobias (Mule et al. 2009). Population studies in the UK, the US, Australia and New Zealand indicate that lesbian and bisexual women have higher rates of depression, anxiety, suicidal ideation and substance use than heterosexual women (McNair et al. 2011). These conditions are exacerbated by lower levels of access to appropriate, culturally and gender sensitive health services, which leaves both homosexual women and men with unmet health needs (McNair et al. 2011; Sirota 2013). Lesbian women and gay men often fail to disclose their gender identity to avoid being stereotyped, stigmatised or treated in a prejudicial or discriminatory manner (Sirota 2013). Some lesbian women have found that even when they do disclose to medical professionals, they are often subject to the type of discrimination that leaves them without tests such as Pap smears. This type of stereotyping is based on the presumption that their sexual habits are known and they do not need testing because they haven't ever engaged in risk behaviours (McNair et al. 2011). Lack of recognition of the fluidity of their relationships can therefore create barriers to comprehensive, individualised care (Rounds et al. 2013). Worse still, in some cases, members of sexual minorities are refused care, or have their needs dismissed by health professionals, which creates a lack of trust in the health system and perpetuates the disparities that they have experienced throughout their lives (Rounds et al. 2013).

Older members of the LGBTI community also find that personal and social wellbeing depends on having a strong sense of community. Researchers tracking the HIV/AIDS epidemic have found that the past decade has seen changes in gay men's participation in gay community life in the context of HIV prevention (Zablotska et al. 2012). In Australia 85% of all new HIV diagnoses are among men who have sex with men, most of whom identify with the gay community, but more of these men socialise with the wider community than in the past. This seems to reflect a growing legal equality and a greater social acceptance of homosexuality, which have actually made HIV a lesser threat to gay men's lives than in the past. This reduced threat is due to gay and bisexual social networks, which have provided gay men with the opportunity to meet other men through the internet rather than in gay bars or sex-on-premises venues (Zablotska et al. 2012). As a result, men are better able to seek out a compatible partner without

LGBTI COMMUNITIES AND RISK

Lesbian, gay, bisexual and transgender/transsexual/intersex people are at increased risk of a range of mental and physical health manifestations due to the existence of discrimination and social exclusion practices in the wider society.

Additional health problems arise when members of minority groups adopt risky coping behaviours to counter their experiences of discrimination. For example, some women members of gender minorities have higher rates of cancer and asthma, which have been linked to tobacco or marijuana smoking or passive smoking in bars (McNair et al. 2011). Other negative health effects include high rates of drug and alcohol consumption, elevated risks of STIs from unprotected sexual activity, and high rates of depression and suicide (Mule et al. 2009). The social determinants of sexually diverse populations are intensified by the fact that their education and career opportunities may be affected by prejudice and phobic reactions experienced at school, in the workplace or in the community (Mule et al. 2009). Some become homeless as a result of social reactions, creating a plethora of health problems and the risk of gender-based violence.

Few heterosexual health professonals have a deep understanding of how difficult life can be for LGBTI groups. Prior to 1973 being gay was pathologised as a mental disorder. Since that time, the research agenda has advanced public understanding of identity development in 'coming out models' (Cox et al. 2010:1199). Like all young people, their identity formation begins during adolescence, when they become sensitised to feelings, including being attracted to another person. When these feelings are toward a person of the same sex, there is a challenge for the young person to deal with the feelings in a way that will help them 'come out' and reach a degree of comfort in and enjoyment with their sexual identity and satisfaction with membership in the LGBTI community. The expectation is that they will gain self-esteem in the context of being with like-minded people, 'acculturating' to their new group as a member of a minority ethnic culture acculturates to the dominant society (Cox et al. 2010). In many cases, this is made easier through affiliation with others in the LGBTI community, which can buffer the stress of marginalisation by the larger cultural group (Cox et al. 2010). Acculturation can be stressful, but with social support and a sense of community, young people can maintain psychological wellbeing.

TRENDING IN HOMOSEXUAL FAMILIES

- Lower risk of HIV/AIDS because of reduced promiscuity
- Equality in housework
- More opportunities to socialise
- Young men have difficulty coming out
- Some children face discrimination, bullying
- Ageist attitudes
- Overlooked in mainstream health services

having to frequent the gay networks and bars. Similar trends are evident in the global community, where there are substantially higher rates of monogamy and fewer extra-relational sexual encounters among homosexual couples than in the past (Gotta et al. 2011).

Research into contemporary same-sex relationships shows greater egalitarian attitudes than in heterosexual couples. Because same-sex couples do not rely on gender-linked divisions of household labour there is more equality in support, decision-making, communication and undertaking household tasks (Gotta et al. 2011). The researchers tracking the social trends also found that lesbians reported more equality of communication, support and decision-making than heterosexual women. Another difference is that conflict was found to occur equally in heterosexual and homosexual couples, but gay male couples and lesbian couples were better at resolving their conflicts than heterosexual couples (Gotta et al. 2011).

As with other minority groups, the theory of intersectionality provides a way of looking at the many layers of the SDH in relation to LGBTI populations. Gender inequalities and prejudice are multiplied for lesbian and bisexual women, members of racial and ethnic minorities, those with disabilities or those excluded from services and support, such as occurs in rural areas (Mule et al. 2009). Another group that suffers from several layers of prejudice is the children of sexually diverse parents. Many do not identify as gay, but spend their lives concealing the sexual orientation of their parents as a way of preventing bullying or overt discrimination. Their problems can also be exacerbated where they have a non-resident parent, and they are challenged to communicate across settings and across gender groups (Weber 2009). For many of these children, the school nurse is one of the few sources of support and empowerment to deal with other non-diverse peers, and to help them maintain perspective and mental health (Weber 2009).

Mental health issues have a major impact on the lives of sexually diverse people. Gay men aged 18–48 have been found to suffer from anger, anxiety, negative self-esteem, emotional instability and lack of emotional responsiveness, in addition to the depression and suicide tendencies found in other sexually diverse groups (Bybee et al. 2009). The effects of discrimination are also worse for gay men than sexually diverse women, who also suffer, but the relationship of sexual orientation to their emotional problems is not as clear. To some extent this is because lesbian women have been regarded as part of the 'gay' community, and invisible in their own right (MacDonnell 2009). Both males and females suffer from the identity confusion and turmoil of adolescence, and adding discrimination to the mix can be a heavy burden, particularly for gay Indigenous people. Bybee et al.'s (2009) body of research has found that chronic shame and guilt underlie many gay men's problems. As gay men age, they tend to develop greater self-acceptance. Although life gets easier as they age, ageism in some communities can add insult to a lifetime of discrimination.

The years of young, gay adulthood can be fraught with shame, guilt associated with deception, or fear of being disowned, fired from a job or physically attacked (Bybee et al. 2009). According to these researchers, the shame they may feel can be destructive. It can arise from multiple factors, parental admonishment, being preoccupied with others' negative evaluation, embarrassment, being belittled and feeling that they have gone against social norms. Guilt can then emerge from feelings of regret and remorse, as the gay person continues to conceal his sexual identity. Coming out, or another scarring event such as an HIV-related bereavement, or a personal diagnosis of HIV, can lead a gay person to experience enduring anger and ongoing guilt, which inflicts a major assault on a man's mental health (Bybee et al. 2009). These events can establish a vicious cycle of depression, stress, social exclusion and sexual dysfunction (Mao et al. 2009).

Because sexually diverse people have not been recognised as an identifiable population group for health care, their health needs are virtually ignored in mainstream service planning (Mule et al. 2009). Intersex people are visibly marginalised as soon as a person is asked to identify their gender. For those who identify as intersex, which box do they tick—male or female? Some researchers are adding 'prefer not to say' to surveys but this approach is also

problematic—it still does not identify those who identify as intersex and may skew gender analyses. As a group, sexually diverse people under-utilise health services, often because of a lack of confidence and systemic discrimination, which leaves some with sub-standard care. Because of typical patterns of medical history taking, their gender identity, sexual orientation and health-related behaviour or circumstances are often overlooked. This leaves health problems undiagnosed, misdiagnosed or untreated, especially where risky sexual practices have not been identified. Another issue is that, in treating sexually diverse people the same as others, health professionals do not develop familiarity with some of the most significant issues that may be affecting their health (Mule et al. 2009). Current attempts to redress this situation include research and practice debates to help empower members of these groups by educating PHC providers and other members of the multidisciplinary health care team, to provide a more comprehensive approach to their care (Mao et al. 2009) (see Box 12.5). Because health services are generally based on the expectation that most clients are heterosexual, it is important that nurses and others ensure that they use inclusive language, and that questions regarding sexuality and sexual orientation are included in assessment processes.

As LGBTI people age, a new risk arises. Residential care homes are frequently poorly equipped to manage heterosexual couples, but care providers must now also consider how they will cater for LGBTI individuals and couples. Many older LGBTI people have hidden their identity for many years, having grown up during a period when homosexuality was considered a pathological condition (Horner et al. 2012). As they age, many fear being 'outed' as their needs for care become known. Although LGBTI communities have more recently become accepted as part of wider society and many LGBTI people are now more open about their sexuality, both those who have hidden their sexuality and those who have been more open will have growing care needs as they age in similar ways to the heterosexual population. How residential care homes address the needs of LGBTI couples can mean the difference between ageing with dignity or ageing with discrimination. A survey of residential care facilities in Western Australia found few facilities had procedures for managing disclosure of sexual orientation or gender identity and that older LGBTI and intersex people accessing retirement and residential aged care are a hidden population (Horner et al. 2012). Others have also reported on the hidden nature of the LGBTI population in aged and residential care

BOX 12.5 A portrait of the whole family

Despite many of the negative health impacts attributable to being LGB, there have been attempts to explore why some of these occur and how they can be addressed. 'Lavender Islands: A Portrait of the Whole Family', was the first national strengths-based study of the lives of LGB people in New Zealand. The Massey University based researchers consulted widely with LGB people in New Zealand, to develop a survey that explored the everyday lives of LGB people and their families. The study explored aspects of LGB life, including identity and self-definition, families of origin, immigration and internal migration, relationships and sexuality, wellbeing, politics, education, income, community connections and challenges. In general, findings indicated that the LGB population in New Zealand are a robust, highly educated, relatively high-income, politically active community. The study found significant differences in the ways male and female respondents experienced same-sex relationships and identity. One of the key areas explored in the study was the perceptions of LGB people of PHC providers. Female participants in particular indicated that the attitude of their health care provider toward their non-heterosexuality identity was important in their selection of provider. Many health care providers assumed that women presenting for care were heterosexual, and this has major implications for their overall health care and management (Neville & Henrickson 2006). There have been a range of publications from the study and many of them can be found listed online at: http://tur-www1.massey.ac.nz/~mhenrick/Articles.html.

- Health literacy, targeting the fundamental issues related to gender equality, such as poverty and social exclusion
- Equal access to fair conditions and fair remuneration in the workplace
- Gender equality in power and decision-making in the family
- Eliminating all forms of discrimination and violation of human rights
- Heightening awareness of the gender bias inherent in globalisation
- Gendering the social and political debates on child care, gun control, crime prevention, transportation, education and other forums for intersectoral collaboration
- Heightening awareness of linkages between health, health care, cultural norms and human rights
- Promoting the health and safety of all family members, free from violence in the home
- National child care strategies accommodating the needs of different family types
- Healthy, just and equitable public policies (UNFPA 2000)

To overcome the stereotypes that are the basis of many existing health promotion campaigns in our Western societies, it is appropriate to situate health initiatives for both women and men within the broader framework of the Ottawa Charter for Health Promotion.

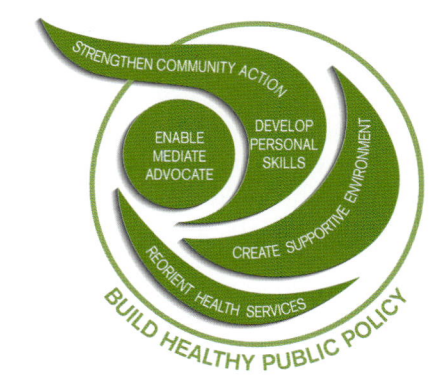

Building healthy public policies

Gender-sensitive communities emerge from conditions where everyone has an equal opportunity in their daily lives. Affirmative action policies and other policy initiatives aimed at enhancing equality are all steps in the right direction, but to have sufficient impact, gender considerations, as well as

(Peate 2013). Isolation for any older person can be an issue but for LGBTI people the isolation can be compounded by a lack of close family and the risk of discrimination from other residents and care staff (Peate 2013). Staff education and the embedding of principles and guidelines into practice in all facilities is a first step in supporting LGBTI older people (Horner et al. 2012; Peate 2013).

GENDERING SOCIETY: GOALS FOR THE HEALTH OF MEN AND WOMEN

- Eliminating all forms of gender bias
- Public awareness of the need for gender-sensitivity in health

policies that promote social participation by vulnerable groups, should be integrated across all policy developments. This is the 'health in all policies' approach. Globally we need intersectoral collaboration and public policies to reduce gender inequities and empower women across the life course, as per Millennium Development Goal 3 (Davidson et al. 2012b; Hosseinpoor et al. 2012; ICN 2013). In 2010 the United Nations General Assembly formed the UN Entity for Gender Equality and the Empowerment of Women (UN Women), which has been joined by other peak organisations such as the International Council of Nurses (ICN), the World Health Federation, and the International Council on Women's Health Issues (ICOHI) to work towards greater recognition and advocacy for women's health (Davidson et al. 2012b). ICN (2013) also argues that gender must be mainstreamed in all policies.

SOCIAL INCLUSION POLICY

- Belonging
- Inclusion
- Participation
- Recognition
- Legitimacy

Australia has been somewhat tentative in developing a social inclusion policy. In 2009, the Commonwealth Government developed a social inclusion committee, with representation from many health policy leaders throughout the country, although the group was disbanded with the change of government in 2013. State and territory health departments continue to include equity initiatives in some of their policies; however, there remains a need for a European-style national social inclusion policy that would establish specific goals and action plans based on intersectoral collaboration (Hatfield Dodds 2012). In general, healthy policies to accommodate gender disadvantage or social exclusion are those that are designed around distributive justice, redistributing wealth, opportunity and support services where they are most needed and rearranging structural conditions to create more equitable conditions for health. New Zealand's social inclusion policy is underpinned by five key dimensions to inclusion including belonging, inclusion, participation, recognition and legitimacy (Bromell & Hyland 2007). The Ministry of Social Development has a social inclusion and participation working group that includes the Office of the

Community and Voluntary Sector, the Office of Disability Issues, the Office for Senior Citizens and the LGBTI policy team. These groups have been working together since 2007 to ensure equity and inclusion across all policies. Although they have had some successes, it is a constant battle—particularly with political emphasis on economic growth rather than social growth although some politicians are starting to call for a greater balance between the two (NZ Govt, Online. Available: http://wellington.scoop.co.nz/?p=57957 [accessed 13 September 2013]).

Policy issues should be developed collaboratively and focus on education, wage parity, safety, self-respect, parental leave, eliminating discrimination among same-sex couples, providing culturally and gender sensitive choices for reproductive health, better subsidies for child care, services for supporting parents, and refuge and other supports for those escaping violence in the home. At the community level, men and women would be supported by safe neighbourhoods and adequate housing, crime prevention, and food supplementation and crisis care, especially for the homeless. The current initiatives of the Women's Health and Male Health policies (Commonwealth of Australia 2013 a, b) provide opportunities to embed gender considerations in all policies that affect people throughout the lifespan. Together, advocates for men's and women's health would be a powerful alliance; one with the potential to advocate for gender equality, and the way gender intersects with other policies that address racism, and other forms of disadvantage. These include policies for occupational health, migration, Indigenous health, mental health, criminal justice, and health and social services that are culturally and gender sensitive.

Policies governing the organisation and delivery of health promotion programs should also incorporate gender sensitivity. This includes drug and alcohol programs, smoking interventions and programs against violence and sexual assault, all of which need to be cognisant of the special needs of men and women respectively. Likewise, policies that frame preventative screening for certain diseases, such as diabetes, CVD and various types of cancer, should ensure that gender-specific initiatives are developed, funded and evaluated in terms of their applicability for women and for men. To reconceptualise men's health promotion in terms of gender relations requires interdisciplinary collaboration and synthesis of different disciplinary ideas. The combination of perspectives would help health promotion practitioners to acknowledge diversity and the wide range of influences on identity, such as sexuality, ethnicity, disability and social class.

As mentioned previously, workplace policies should be inclusive, but special emphasis may have to be placed on the needs of migrant and minority group workers, who often neglect their health needs to a greater extent than others. Policies in the workplace can be aimed at integrating health into safety training, and ensuring that occupational health and safety personnel have a broad enough brief to conduct opportunistic assessments of health problems and make appropriate recommendations or referrals. As we mentioned in Chapter 7, family-friendly workplaces should satisfy parental preferences for type and hours of care, and accommodate different family structures. Ultimately, healthy public policies also promote freedom, which is the capability to live the life one has reason to value (Sen 1999).

In civilised societies, policies to overcome violence, especially intimate partner violence (IPV), are crucial. Humanitarian, as well as economic reasons, indicate the need for renewed interest in policies to reduce violence in any setting where it occurs, including detention centres or any of the places that accommodate people fleeing from war or civil unrest. Valuing human rights includes valuing the lives and wellbeing of migrants and refugees. Some balance should be struck between zero tolerance policies that are focused exclusively on punitive measures for perpetrators of violence, and taking too lenient an approach, so there are few deterrents to committing acts of violence, especially where children are involved. A balanced, long-term solution involves government legislation designed to enforce punishment with mandatory re-training for those committing violent offences against intimate partners, children or members of the public. In addition to the punitive measures, policies to protect women need to acknowledge the structural causes of violence, including our systems of incarceration. They need the support of both men and women to mobilise resources at the community level that will enhance awareness, and provide not only refuge, but treatment and justice forums, wherein people can address the threats to community life from violence in the family (Paterson 2009). The Family Violence Intervention guidelines for health professionals developed by the New Zealand Ministry of Health provide an example of how an integrated approach to family violence can be achieved (www.moh.govt.nz/familyviolence). More recently, the *Vulnerable Children's Act 2013* has seen the introduction of a range of strategies designed to support children who have been harmed by, or are at risk from, an adult. These strategies include mandatory screening and vetting for all people who work with children (including professionals and volunteers), and a range of strategies to prevent people who have harmed children from being able to harm them again (www.legislation.govt.nz).

Creating supportive environments

Gender equity requires an *enabling,* rather than discriminatory, society (UNIFEM 2005). Men's and women's health concerns need to be equally embedded in an ecological perspective. Supportive environments are those that provide material support for those most vulnerable, such as the mentally ill, LGBTI populations, migrants, refugees, older persons and the homeless. A supportive environment may begin at birth, with accurate assessments of family need, and then extend through many variations across a child's life course. Environments supportive of early childhood and parenting are typically community-based, informal groups—parents' groups, or exercise groups that bring young families together. However, many are focused on mothers, and in today's environments, fathers may be the primary caregiver, so there is a need for gender sensitivity in those neighbourhoods where encouragement is necessary to foster the participation of all families. Many communities are starting to establish support groups aimed specifically at men, often with specific times for men and their children (Menz, Online. Available: http://menz.org.nz/support/ [accessed 3 September 2013]).

> **ACTION POINT**
>
> Support children and young people dealing with gender issues at school by undertaking gender-sensitivity training and developing socially inclusive school health policies.

Supportive schools are integral to healthy environments, and the expanded role of the school nurse provides a link between health and education that is crucial for young boys and girls. Other sectors can also be brought into the school environment, including the police, social workers and others involved in providing community support, who are often significant role models for gender-appropriate behaviours. Within the microcosm of the school, gender issues are exposed and, given the right resources, resolved. This requires strong alliances for anti-bullying programs, support for educating teenage girls who become pregnant, and sensitive counselling for children who may be caught in family conflicts over separation, divorce, blended families, child abuse or gender-identity issues. The role of the school nurse is crucial for children of sexually diverse parents. Some of these children have suffered from relationship breakdowns that are very different from that of their friends. For example, the change to family structure precipitated by a separation that leads to gender changes in parenting, such as a change to being parented by a mother and her lesbian partner. This is difficult for children to accommodate, especially if they are young adolescents on the verge of developing their own identity. A supportive school environment can make the difference between whether or not such a child becomes resilient or socially withdrawn (Fuller 2013). Research has shown that the main risk for these children is school bullying by same-age peers, especially through digital or internet media. They also experience divided loyalties, especially where they have been exposed to marital separation and custody issues. Gender-sensitivity training can help school nurses become aware of the type and extent of problems they may experience, and help them develop health literacy and relationship skills (Weber 2009).

Andrew Fuller, who is a specialist in adolescent health at the University of Melbourne, suggests 10 things we can do to at the community level to create a resilient society (Box 12.6).

BOX 12.6 Creating a resilient society

1 Increase people's sense of belonging, their friendship networks, and social capital.

2 Clarify what we mean by 'a good school', a 'clever country'.

3 Reduce social toxicity.

4 Invest in prevention.

5 Ensure that every young person receives affirmation.

6 Reduce economic inequality.

7 Use the whole village to protect childhood.

8 Base social policy on human rights.

9 Make better use of the fact that we are spiritual beings.

10 Recognise the importance of androgyny; the need for mindfulness, love and compassion. This means that males feel free to be in touch with their feminine side, and for women to see their power and personal agency to create change in society.

(Source: Fuller 2013)

Clearly there is a need to focus societal attention on the young, but older men and women also have particular needs, which they may only find in the neighbourhood. For example, with older women especially, the safety of public transport systems is an issue. For older men, there is often a danger of becoming recluse, especially older widowers, who tend to grieve for long periods after losing a spouse. In these cases, supportive environments are those in which neighbourhood residents take responsibility for checking on older residents, especially where it is known that no relatives are visiting on a regular basis. With the pace of community life, it is more important than ever for members of the neighbourhood to keep an eye out for the needs of older people, and to understand the gendered health issues that may keep them inside. This is also particularly important following a disaster or weather event. Older people may be very resilient following such events but others may be frightened and/or injured and not know where or how to seek help. Checking on neighbours and supporting them in the immediate aftermath of a challenging event can mean the difference between a person continuing to manage alone or needing to go into care. It has been observed that cognitive decline among older people can increase following disaster, and managing medications, incontinence and electrically powered oxygen supplies can be challenging (Goldstraw et al. 2012). Health services must also be aware of the needs of this vulnerable group following disasters and have in place strategies for managing both those in care already and those in their own homes.

Strengthening community action

Community action on gender issues is being implemented at the global and local levels. Global initiatives to address gender issues include a global charter for investment in girls: a ten-point action plan. This is a call for all countries of the world to reduce the disparities and social inequities confronted by women, especially in developing countries. The action plan includes 10 resolutions (see Box 12.7).

At the community level, collaborative ventures to galvanise people into action can be strengthened by formal and informal community input, whether this is at a sporting venue promoting men's or women's health or an event aimed at encouraging either women or men to participate in screening. Supportive activities range from helping community members organise themselves, to acting as a peripheral resource to community-determined activities. For example, the Ignite project was a year-long project designed to improve employment opportunities and social connectedness of former

BOX 12.7 Global gender action plan

1 No compromise on global gender equality goals and international commitments.

2 Promote the full integration of gender equality principles into national and regional economic policies.

3 Prioritise girls' education from their earliest years through to adolescence and beyond.

4 Maintain national social protection programmes and safeguard social services.

5 Scale up investment in young women's work opportunities.

6 Support young women workers and ensure they get decent pay and conditions.

7 Invest in young women's leadership.

8 Ensure equality for girls and young women in land and property ownership.

9 Count and value girls and young women's work through national and international data disaggregation.

10 Develop and promote a set of practical global guiding principles on girls and young women at work.

(Source: World Bank 2009)

refugees in Nelson, New Zealand. Although Ignite's primary focus was on improving interpretation services, driver's license training and family violence prevention, the community wanted to keep the project going. As a result, although funding has formally ended, the project leaders have continued to organise a range of courses at the request of community members. These have included cooking classes, bicycle maintenance, parenting, haircutting, legal advice, car maintenance and leadership seminars (Ignite, Online. Available: www. nelsonmulticultural.co.nz/ONGOING+PROJECTS/Ignite.html [accessed 13 September 2013]).

PARTNERSHIPS

Remember PHC—community members should be involved in all developments.

The Ignite project captures the link between health and place, supporting former refugees in a context that feels good and which can help them adjust to their new environment. In many cases, the support people require in the community is validation of their feelings and acknowledgement of their strengths and weaknesses. Providing this type of support often relies on the leadership of nurses and other health professionals working with the community, with interdisciplinary groups and with community volunteers. Supporting grassroots initiatives can then lead to national and international advocacy, helping oppressed groups have a voice where it counts. A group called 'Border Crossing Observatory', from the Faculty of Arts at Monash University, has played an important role as a virtual voice connecting national and international stakeholders to cutting-edge interdisciplinary research on border crossings. Their major goal is to bring new insights into policy debates associated with irregular migration and border control. The studies emanating from this centre also focus on trafficking and labour exploitation, peacebuilding, global conflict and gender security. Part of their campaign is to encourage community support for migrant health by drawing public attention to the issue of 'deaths in custody'. This important social issue is familiar to most Australians concerned with the ongoing problem of Aboriginal deaths in custody, but members of the observatory argue that we have thus far overlooked deaths in immigration custody, and they seek to document and make these tragedies accessible on their public website (The Border Crossing Observatory, Online. Available: http://artsonline.monash.edu.au/thebordercrossingobservatory/ [accessed 30 September 2013]).

Developing personal skills

Developing gender-sensitive personal skills begins in the family. In many communities, the vocal minority is outspoken about the need for respect and tolerance for difference. However, our national agendas strike fear into the hearts of communities, with cautiously disparaging descriptions of those who are different. This is most evident in the dialogue about terrorism, people smugglers and border protection. Personal opinions, and therefore personal behaviours, tend to mimic societal values, as portrayed in daily life and through the media. When communities are led by political notions of respect for others, respect for difference, and a healthy curiosity about the 'real story', there is greater likelihood that individuals will become more thoughtful about events in the world, and make their own decisions on how to behave. The prevailing dialogue on gender identity and gay rights, migration, styles of worship, the right to life and the right to protect oneself, the right to live in a safe home and the rights of the world's children provide numerous examples of where personal views are shaped by pre-set opinions set down in the daily newspaper or the nightly news. To break away from the pre-digested version of public opinion requires time, effort and a commitment to social justice. It is made easier when tolerance and respect are role-modelled at the highest level, from global policymakers, to national, state and local leaders. Given our knowledge of developmental pathways, it is important to develop the personal skills of mutual respect between genders at an early age, to overcome entrenched behaviours and conditions that lead to violence, discrimination, or systematic inequity and bias.

Changing people's attitudes and behaviour is challenging at any time, especially when the desired change runs counter to family attitudes or entrenched ideas about the way of the world. For boys and young men, attempts to create heightened awareness of gender issues are difficult if they are not reinforced in the home; however, there have been many boys from inequitable home environments who, through education and experience, have transformed their views dramatically. Key intervention points to heighten men's awareness of gender bias occur at primary school age; first-time fatherhood; during significant life transitions, such as when a man is separating or has separated from his partner; and after retirement, when many men stop to reflect on the world. Social relations during each of these phases are never predictable, and a sensitive approach will be able to accommodate the needs of minority groups such as same-sex parents, and others who may seem different but whose experiences may be remarkably similar to those of the dominant culture. Helping men change their risky behaviours, especially those from minorities where personal bravado often masks the need for help and support, is difficult but not impossible.

SENSITIVE TRANSITIONS

- Primary school
- First-time parenthood
- Separation
- Retirement

Nurses and other health professionals should be aware that gender is an important issue. ICN endorses a gender mainstreaming approach in all aspects of health, including research, nursing education, service planning and care delivery, in which nurses should advocate for greater awareness of the consequences of gender inequity and inequality of health for girls and women (ICN 2013). Advocacy is crucial to changing societal norms that see 'women do two thirds of the world's work, earn one tenth of the world's income, and own less than one percent of the world's property' (World Bank, in ICN 2013:32). As health professionals our advocacy extends to the workplaces in all countries that perpetuate gender inequities through jobs that generate differential incomes for men and women, compromise family commitments, carry few social security benefits or influence education and career paths through the requirements of managing pregnancy or maintaining a home (ICN 2013).

Understanding policy, legislation and planning is critical to maintaining socially inclusive practice, and overcoming inequalities (McGee 2009). To provide guidance, nurses need to know how men's and women's behaviour is socially constructed, and to understand the differences between their risks and patterns of help-seeking (McGee 2009). Programs designed to foster health literacy, or behaviour change, therefore need to evoke reconsideration of the way society has maintained unequal gender relations, and work towards social and structural change. In some cases, strategies will include helping adolescents and young adults understand the media and how it is shaping social norms. In other cases, health education strategies will focus on drawing women's attention to the vulnerability that results from being brought up to depend on males for social and personal esteem.

Women and men need to recognise the need for a balanced lifestyle, and a woman's right to develop her personal capacity in a way that may differ from her partner's. Because most women are relatively invisible in major decision-making forums, they need to be encouraged to learn how decisions are made, so they can participate in securing their preferred future. Interventions to help advance these goals may be focused on garnering support from the community for women's empowerment. It also requires community level sanctions against abuse of either girls or boys, to send a strong message, that the community values its young people. To counter domestic abuse, person-centred and problem-focused interventions are essential. These entail programs to help young people develop personal coping strategies and self-esteem, by helping them accept ownership and direction for their own lives. Programs aimed at empowering young people are based on the belief that empowerment is everyone's entitlement; that all people must be able to speak for themselves, that everyone has a right to dignity and a non-violent lifestyle.

Reorienting health services

In general, and excluding poor women living in vulnerable circumstances, women have gained on males in terms of both longevity and quality of life. Some of this advantage is biological, but there is also a major effect from the services they access. There remains a need to continue offering woman-friendly services, as these have made a major contribution to screening and reducing women's risk. However, in a multicultural context gender is only one area requiring attention from service providers. Many people, especially women from culturally and linguistically diverse (CALD) societies find service provision problematic, especially if they have suffered abuse of any kind. For those who have mental illness they are disadvantaged not only by stigma and discrimination, but difficulties in access and use of services because of language or cultural differences (Cross & Singh 2012). Those who are refugees or recently released from detention centres tend to seek assistance from community groups or ethnic networks rather than the health care system, often because of their misunderstanding or mistrust of bureaucratic services of any kind. They may also find the 'system' inadequate, alienating, culturally insensitive and difficult to navigate, given their social and cultural isolation (Cross & Singh 2012).

The health care system may be difficult for other women as well, especially if they suffer from mental ill health, are homeless or have interventions for substance abuse or violence. Researchers have found that despite one-third of women experiencing IPV at some time in their lives, few health care providers, including GPs, recognise their plight, or have risk-assessment strategies in place to identify the extent of their problems (Tan et al. 2012). A lack of consistency in nursing settings leaves many women without comprehensive assessment of their needs. Maternal and child health nurses in Victoria use practice guidelines to routinely ask women about IPV during the four-week postnatal visit and then at subsequent visits if this is warranted (Hooker et al. 2012). In New Zealand, Plunket nurses screen for family violence as a matter of course and the *Vulnerable Children's Act 2013* makes it compulsory for all health service providers to have a family violence policy. Other Australian states have instituted screening programs, but to date, approaches to screening are uneven across Australia and often internationally. Barriers to screening include time pressures, a lack of appropriate education and skills, the absence of evidence-based practice guidelines and a lack of referral resources and support, especially in seeking to help rural women (Hooker et al. 2012; Tower et al. 2012).

When women do report IPV they often feel stigmatised and judged, leaving them feeling punished and undeserving of care (Tower et al. 2012). Nurses themselves report disquiet in trying to help women victims of violence, some reacting by distancing themselves rather than validating their concerns and providing acknowledgement and support (Tower et al. 2012). Clendon's (2009) study of home visiting in New Zealand and Shepherd's (2011) study of Tasmanian child health visits indicate that maternal, child and family nurses continue to address women's health issues in the context of a home visit, because of their ability to span the personal and professional boundaries in the context of interacting with the mother and child.

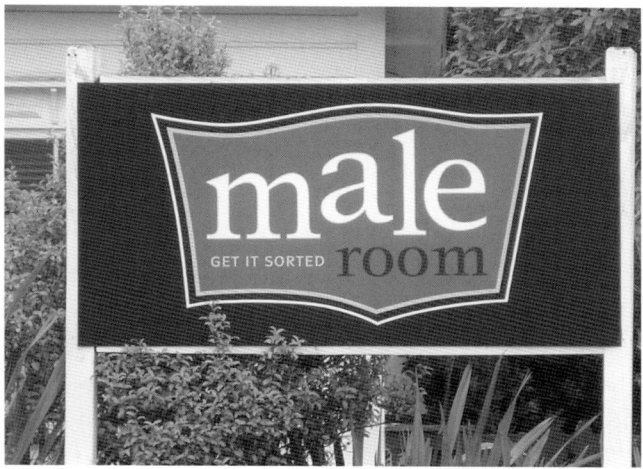

(Photo: Jill Clendon)

For men, there are few male-designated health services and continual problems attracting men to services because of scheduling difficulties. Men's help-seeking behaviour is remarkably different from women's. They are often ambivalent about seeing a health practitioner, with most seeing a GP three times a year, compared to women's attendance five times a year (Cole 2009). The reasons for their hesitance have been identified as machismo, fear, surgery opening times and a sense that any information presented will be female friendly (Cole 2009). Because of their reticence to seek help, and the difficulties most men face because of work schedules, nurse practitioners have developed outreach health promotion services to barber shops, pubs, bus depots, trade shows, service stations and truckstops (Cole 2009). In New South Wales, nurses have developed a 'Pitstop' program (Russell et al. 2006), which has been replicated in the US (Kuhns 2009).

These programs are aimed at rural men's health risks, and the nurses provide them with information and brief health screening as they wait at the grain elevator to unload the harvest (Kuhns 2009). In Nelson, New Zealand, local men's health promoter Philip Chapman has established a men's drop-in centre called The Male Room where men can stop in and discuss issues, gain support or receive counselling over a cup of fresh coffee. The Male Room also provides a location for fathers' groups to meet. Various researchers have suggested different approaches to promoting men's health. Some argue for supporting programs like 'Pitstop', which uses masculine metaphors for aspects of men's health that may resonate with men's constructions of masculinity. Others suggest circumventing this type of approach, by making the environment more amenable to healthy choices (Saunders & Peerson 2009). The National Male Health Policy emphasises the need to conduct research into men's perceptions of their health, and how diverse masculinities inform men's behaviours and risk-taking (Commonwealth of Australia 2013b). An alternative approach would seek to understand how men embody gender, experientially and pragmatically, and how men's health issues intersect with women's health issues. This 'relational' approach would incorporate individual and social-structural elements, and their interconnections.

Like women's services, responsive men's services need a man-friendly environment, and an attitude of empathy. Men's hesitancy to freely discuss health issues and their reticence to explain themselves elicits compassion, especially for men disadvantaged by being members of minority groups. Many men also shy away from any notion of counselling, seeing counsellors as there to fix a specific problem, rather than begin a process of self-discovery. Men also tend to feel uncomfortable with the language and modes of communication used in counselling, which is why counsellors specialising in men's issues will be more effective than those who cater for more general problems (O'Brien & Rich 2002). To develop a man-friendly attitude, there needs to be recognition of how society generalises on the basis of men putting on a good front. To turn this around, there needs to be a commitment to listening to men, allowing them to express themselves, their needs and preferences. To help men build a repertoire of healthy behaviours, some of the same solutions as are used for women should be used, such as assuring anonymity and privacy, and providing workplace-based services. Gender-specific clinics, especially those that accommodate the needs of LGBTI communities, can achieve positive outcomes for those who are timid or embarrassed about their

health needs, particularly if there are health issues of a sexual nature present.

One of the biggest problems for men and women in full-time employment is accessing services after working hours, and this needs to be addressed so that health and preventive care are integral to daily life. The current trend toward providing comprehensive services in PHC organisations will be helpful to both women and men, but there may be a need for satellite clinics to deal expressly with men's and women's health issues, especially mental health issues. Young and older men often hesitate to seek help for depression or anxiety early enough, and are not brought into care until they have come to the attention of criminal investigations or domestic violence programs. Community mentors and role models can help, especially through peer support programs at school. Men's helplines have also enjoyed considerable success, as men tend to view phone messages as safe and non-threatening. Where gender-sensitive services are funded by governments, and promoted as necessary, there is a greater chance of men and women availing themselves of what is offered. This also reflects the fundamental idea that gender sensitivity must begin at the top, and filter down through all aspects of society to normalise the importance of mutual respect, human rights, dignity and freedom from bias.

Inclusive health services also require considerable transformation to meet the needs of the sexually diverse in the community, establishing goals of access, cultural sensitivity and equity (Mule et al. 2009). Clearly, this requires a PHC approach to work towards equity in services and social inclusion in the community (MacDonnell 2009; Mao et al. 2009). Like other community-based services, these work best when there is a team approach, helping individuals develop a core sense of self, the ability to take action based on self-determination, a sense of control over one's life and a feeling of being connected with others. They should also include community-wide promotion of inclusive approaches and the integration of gender-sensitive materials in all community services. The LGBTI community is particularly under-serviced by health professionals and, as mentioned above, this has left many with unmet needs. In the health care system we tend to stereotype their needs instead of conducting sensitive assessment of their self-identified needs (Rounds et al. 2013). When people who are part of minority groups feel their needs are not being met they are less likely to seek health care, which has detrimental effects on their health and creates disparities in the wider community (Rounds et al. 2013). Despite having positive attitudes toward inclusive care, nurses are not educationally well prepared to help homosexual people (Sirota 2013). An American Academy of Nursing policy has been developed in the US to endorse nursing efforts to assist these groups, but there remains a dearth of curricula even in that country, or research that would help prepare nursing graduates for LGBTI-sensitive

practice (Sirota 2013). This is an issue that should be addressed in Australian and New Zealand nursing curricula so that our approaches to their care become more closely aligned with changing social norms. We now address some of the gender issues affecting the Mason and Smith families.

CASE STUDY: Women's health, men's health in the Smith and Mason families

The occupational health nurses in the mining community have instituted a prostate screening program as part of their men's health initiative. A GP from one of the rural communities has agreed to come in to the mine site and provide health education and screening on a 3 monthly basis. The men's health initiative has already addressed some of the general issues around depression and coping with stress but the nurses are now also focusing on the unhealthy coping strategies such as alcohol and substance misuse and talking about violence in the camps as well as family violence issues.

Rebecca is receiving advice from the practice nurse to help her cope with her mother's breast cancer, and has attended one self-help group for cancer family members. She is also part of a blogging forum to support FIFO wives and help them air their concerns in the privacy of their homes.

Huia has also found this blogging forum helpful, especially with the lack of other wives and mothers experiencing the FIFO lifestyle in her home community.

REFLECTING ON THE BIG ISSUES

- Social inclusion and social exclusion are two points on a continuum of social equity.
- Our society remains unequal, with pockets of systematic discrimination and oppression on the basis of gender, race, ethnicity and sexual diversity.
- Women and men have different health issues, and some common issues related to a combination of biological, behavioural and social factors.
- Women's relative longevity compared to men leaves them suffering more chronic illness and severe disability than men over their lifetime.
- Men's health is often victim to men's notions of masculinity and their need to convey strength,

robustness and good health, which leaves many hesitant to seek health care when they need it.
- Intimate partner violence is caused by one person's need to exert power and control over another.
- Migrant, refugee and LGBTI groups have multiple layers of disadvantage through discrimination and stereotyped societal responses to their needs.
- Primary health care principles can be used to guide inclusive policies for gender relations.
- A human rights perspective maintains that every member of society has a right to live in dignity in a non-violent, adequately resourced community without discrimination or fear.

REFLECTIVE QUESTIONS: How would I use this knowledge in practice?

1 What indicators of social exclusion exist in your community?

2 Analyse three gender-sensitive issues in your community in relation to principles of primary health care.

3 What are the advantages and disadvantages of having separate or integrated women's health and men's health policies?

4 What would be the most important issues affecting the men in their mining workplace?

5   Revisit the genograms of the Smith and Mason families from Chapter 7. Are there any updates you could add at this stage?

6   What are the most prevalent issues confronting women in today's workplace?

7   What should be included in a comprehensive policy to counter intimate partner violence?

8   How can pressure be brought to bear on Australia's policy of immigration detention?

References

Adams Tufts, K., Clements, P., Karlowicz, K., 2009. Integrating intimate partner violence content across curricula: developing a new generation of nurse educators. Nurse Educ. Today 29, 40–47.

Arendell, T., 2000. Conceiving and investigating motherhood: the decade's scholarship. J. Marriage Fam. 62, 1192–1207.

Australian Institute of Family Studies (AIFS), CAFCA, 2011. Social inclusion and social exclusion: resources for child and family. Online, Available: <www.aifs.gov.au/cafca/pubs/sheets/rs/rs3.html> 20 August 2013.

Australian Institute of Family Studies (AIFS), 2012. The longitudinal study of Australian children, annual statistical report 2011, AIFS, Melbourne.

Australian Institute of Health and Welfare (AIHW), 2012. Australia's Health 2012 Series no 13,Cat No AUS 156, AIHW, Canberra.

Australian Institute of Health and Welfare (AIHW), 2013. The health of Australia's males: from birth to young adulthood, AIHW Cat. No. PHE 168, Canberra.

Baker, M., 2010. Career confidence and gendered expectations of academic promotion. J. Sociol. 46 (3), 317–334.

Bennett, P., 2012. Children's action plan: Identifying, supporting and protecting vulnerable children, Ministry of Social Development, Wellington, New Zealand.

Bromell, D., Hyland, M., 2007. Social inclusion and participation: A guide for policy and planning, Ministry of Social Development, Wellington.

Brown, B., 2009. Men in nursing: Re-evaluating masculinities, re-evaluating gender. Contemp. Nurse 33 (2), 120–129.

Burchill, J., 2012. Barriers to effective practice for health visitors working with asylum seekers and refugees. Community Pract. 85 (7), 20–23.

Burke Draucker, C., Martsolf, D., 2010. The role of electronic communication technology in adolescent dating violence. J. Child Adolesc. Psychiatr. Nurs. 23 (3), 133–142.

Bybee, J., Sullivan, E., Zielonka, E., et al., 2009. Are gay men in worse mental health than heterosexual men? The role of age, shame and guilt, and coming-out. J. Adult Dev. 16, 144–154.

Byles, J., Tavener, M., Robinson, I., et al., 2013. Transforming retirement: New definitions of life after work. J. Women Aging 25, 24–44.

Campbell, J., 2001. Global perspectives of wife beating and health care. In: Martinez, M. (Ed.), Prevention and control of aggression and the impact on its victims, Kluwer Academic/Plenum Publishers, New York, pp. 215–227.

Clendon, J., 2009. Motherhood and the 'Plunket Book': A social history. PhD thesis, Massey University, Auckland.

Coffey, G., Kaplan, I., Sampson, R., et al., 2010. The meaning and mental health consequences of long-term immigration detention for people seeking asylum. Soc. Sci. Med. 70, 2070–2079.

Cole, L., 2009. A pro-active approach to men's health. Pract. Nurse 37 (11), 37–39.

Collins, C., Zimmerman, C., Howard, L., 2011. Refugee, asylum seeker, immigrant women and postnatal depression: rates and risk factors. Arch. Womens Ment. Health 14 (3), 3–11.

Commonwealth of Australia, 2008. Social Inclusion, origins, concepts and key themes. Paper prepared by the Australian Institute of Family Studies for the Social Inclusion Unit, Department of the Prime Minister and Cabinet, Canberra.

Commonwealth of Australia, 2013a. National Male Health Policy, Department of Health and Ageing, Canberra.

Commonwealth of Australia, 2013b. National Women's Health Policy, Department of Health and Ageing, Canberra.

Coulter, P., Dickman, K., Maradiegue, A., 2009. The effects of exercise on stress in working women. J. Nurse Pract. 5 (6), 408–413.

Courtenay, W., 2000. Constructions of masculinity and their influence on men's well-being: a theory of gender and health. Soc. Sci. Med. 50, 1385–1401.

Cox, N., Banden Berghe, W., Dewaele, A., et al., 2010. Acculturation strategies and mental health in gay, lesbian, and bisexual youth. J. Youth Adolesc. 39, 1199–1210.

Cross, W., Singh, C., 2012. Dual vulnerabilities: Mental illness in a culturally and linguistically diverse society. Contemp. Nurse 42 (2), 156–166.

Davidson, P., Mitchell, J., DiGiacomo, M., et al., 2012a. Cardiovascular disease in women: Implications for improving health outcomes. Collegian 19, 5–12.

Davidson, P., Sindhu, S., Meleis, A., et al., 2012b. Women's health is now core business and a global health issue. Collegian 19, 1–3.

Dempsey, D., Hewitt, B., 2012. Fatherhood in the 21st century, Editorial. Contemp. Nurse 8 (2–3), 98–102.

Desouza, R., 2013. Regulating migrant maternity: Nursing and midwifery's emancipatory aims and assimilatory practices. Nurs. Inq. doi:10.1111/nin.12020.

Dovydaitis, T., 2010. Human trafficking: The role of the health care provider. J. Midwifery Womens Health 55, 462–467.

Eckersley, R., 2012. Whatever happened to Western civilization? Futurist Nov–Dec, 16–22.

Fortin, I., Guay, S., Lavoie, V., et al., 2012. Intimate partner violence and psychological distress among young couples: Analysis of the moderating effect of social support. J. Fam. Violence 27, 63–73.

Frelick, B., 2012. Exporting Australia's Asylum Policies. Human Rights Watch. Online, Available: <www.hrw.org/news/2012/10/23/exporting-australias-asylum-policies> (accessed 30 October 2013).

Fuller, A., 2013. Valuing boys valuing girls. Online, Available: <http://www.andrewfuller.com.au/free/ValuingBoysValuingGirls.pdf> 26 August 2013.

Glavin, P., Schieman, S., Reid, S., 2011. Boundary-spanning work demands and their consequences for guilt and psychological distress. J. Health Soc. Behav. 52 (1), 43–57.

Goldstraw, P., Strivens, E., Kennett, C., et al., 2012. The care of older people during and after disasters: A review of the recent experiences in Queensland, Australia and Christchurch, New Zealand. Australas. J. Ageing 31, 69–71. doi:10.1111/j.1741-6612.2012.00613.x.

Gotta, G., Jay-Green, R., Rothblum, E., et al., 2011. Heterosexual, lesbian and gay male relationships: A comparison of couples in 1975 and 2000. Fam. Process 50 (3), 353–376.

Hatfield Dodds, L., 2012. Social inclusion: we need smarter policy. Online, Available: <www.abc.net.au/unleashed/3770172.html> 27 August, 2013.

Hinchliff, S., Gott, M., Wylie, K., 2009. Holding onto womanhood: a qualitative study of heterosexual women with sexual desire loss. Health 13 (4), 449–465.

Holt, S., Buckley, H., Whelan, S., 2008. The impact of exposure to domestic violence on children and young people: a review of the literature. Child Abuse Negl. 32, 797–810.

Hooker, L., Ward, B., Verrinder, G., 2012. Domestic violence screening in maternal and child health nursing practice: A scoping review. Contemp. Nurse 42 (2), 198–215.

Horner, B., McManus, A., Comfort, J., et al., 2012. How prepared is the retirement and residential aged care sector in Western Australia for older non-heterosexual people? Qual. Prim. Care 20 (4), 263–274.

Hosseinpoor, A., Williams, J., Amin, A., et al., 2012. Social determinants of self-reported health in women and men: Understanding the role of gender in population health. PLoS One 7 (4), e34799:1–e34799:9.

Idler, E., Boulifard, D., Contrada, R., 2012. Mending broken hearts: Marriage and survival following cardiac surgery. J. Health Soc. Behav. 53 (1), 33–49.

International Council of Nurses (ICN), 2013. Improving the health and well-being of women: A life course approach, ICN, Geneva.

Jackson, D., Hayter, M., Carter, B., et al., 2012. Revisiting the concept of vulnerability: recognising strength in the context of risk and susceptibility. Contemp. Nurse 42 (2), 142–143.

Janzen, B., Green, K., Muhajarine, N., 2006. The health of single fathers. Demographic, economic and social correlates. Can. J. Public Health 97 (6), 440–444.

Johnstone, M., Lee, C., 2012. Young Australian women and their aspirations: 'It's hard enough thinking a week or two in advance at the moment'. J. Adolesc. Res. 27, 351–376.

Jones, E., Jurgenson, J., Katzenellenbogen, M., et al., 2012. Menopause and the influence of culture: another gap for Indigenous Australian women? BMC Womens Health 12, 43–53.

Kalil, A., Ziol-Guest, K., Hawkley, L., et al., 2010. Job insecurity and change over time in health among older men and women. J. Gerontol. 65B (1), 81–90.

Kasturirangan, A., 2009. Empowerment and programs designed to address domestic violence. Violence Against Women 14 (12), 1465–1475.

Katzenellenbogen, M., Sanfilippo, F., Hobbs, M., et al., 2010. Incidence and case fatality following acute myocardial infarction in Aboriginal and non-Aboriginal Western Australians (2000–2004): A linked data study. Heart Lung Circ. 19 (12), 717–725.

Khlat, M., Jusot, F., Ville, I., 2009. Social origins, early hardship and obesity: A strong association in women, but not in men? Soc. Sci. Med. 68, 1692–1699.

Kim, J., Gray, K., 2008. Leave or stay? Battered women's decision after intimate partner violence. J. Interpers. Violence 23 (10), 1465–1482.

Koziol-McLain, J., Giddings, L., Rameka, M., et al., 2008. Intimate partner violence screening and brief intervention: Experiences of women in two New Zealand health care settings. J. Midwifery Womens Health 53, 504–510.

Kuhns, S., 2009. Men's Health Pitstop. Am. J. Nurs. 109 (7), 58–60.

Kutek, S., Turnbull, D., Fairweather-Schmidt, A., 2011. Rural men's subjective well-being and the role of social support and sense of community: Evidence for the potential benefit of enhancing informal networks. Aust. J. Rural Health 19, 20–26.

Lavie, C., Milani, R., 2009. Secondary coronary prevention in women: it starts with cardiac rehabilitation, exercise, and fitness. J. Womens Health 18 (8), 1115–1117.

Lord, L., Jefferson, T., Eastham, J., 2012. Women's participation in mining: What can we learn from EOWA reports? ABL 38 (1), 68–95.

Luketina, F., Davidson, C., Palmer, P., 2009. Supporting kiwi dads: role and needs of New Zealand fathers. A Families Commission report. Families Commission, Wellington.

MacDonnell, J., 2009. Fostering nurses' political knowledges and practices. Education and political activation in relation to lesbian health. Adv. Nurs. Sci. 32 (2), 158–172.

Mao, L., Kidd, M., Rogers, G., et al., 2009. Social factors associated with Major Depressive Disorder in homosexually active, gay men attending general practices in urban Australia. Aust. N. Z. J. Public Health 33 (1), 83–86.

Martin, C., Houston, A., Mmari, K., et al., 2012. Urban teens and young adults describe drama, disrespect, dating violence and help-seeking preferences. Matern Child Health J. 16, 957–966.

McGee, P., 2009. Who says we're all equal? Gender as an issue for nurses and nursing care. Contemp. Nurse 33 (2), 98–102.

McLaren, S., Challis, C., 2009. Resilience among men farmers: the protective roles of social support and sense of belonging in the depression-suicidal ideation relation. Death Stud. 33, 262–276.

McNair, R., Szalacha, L., Hughes, T., 2011. Health status, health service use, and satisfaction according to sexual identity of young Australian women. Women's Health Issues 21 (1), 40–47.

Men's Health Forum, 2006. Mind your head. Men, boys and mental wellbeing. National Men's Health Week 2006 Policy Report, MHF, London.

Moodie, M., Fisher, J., 2009. Are youth mentoring programs good value-for-money? An evaluation of the Big Brothers Big Sisters Melbourne Program. BMC Public Health 9, 41.

Mule, N., Ross, L., Deeprose, B., et al., 2009. Promoting LGBT health and wellbeing through inclusive policy development. Int. J. Equity Health 8 (18), doi:10.1186/1475-9276-8-18.

Mwanri, L., Hiruy, K., Masika, J., 2012. Empowerment as a tool for a healthy resettlement: a case of new African settlers in South Australia. Int. J. Migrat. Health Soc. Care 8 (2), 86–97.

Neville, S., Henrickson, M., 2006. Perceptions of lesbian, gay and bisexual people of primary health care services. J. Adv. Nurs. 55 (4), 407–415.

New Zealand Ministry of Health (NZMOH), 2008a. Improving quality of care for Pacific peoples, NZMOH, Wellington.

New Zealand Ministry of Health (NZMOH), 2008b. A Portrait of Health. Key Results of the 2006/07 New Zealand Health Survey, NZMOH, Wellington.

New Zealand Ministry of Health (NZMOH), 2012a. Refugee Health Care: A handbook for health professionals, Ministry of Health, Wellington.

New Zealand Ministry of Health (NZMOH), 2012b. The Health of New Zealand Adults 2011/12: Key findings of the New Zealand Health Survey, Ministry of Health, Wellington.

Nobis, R., Sanden, I., 2008. Young men's health: A balance between self-reliance and vulnerability in the light of hegemonic masculinity. Contemp. Nurse 29 (2), 205–217.

Nyamathi, A., Jackson, D., Carter, B., et al., 2012. Creating culturally relevant and sustainable research strategies to meet the needs of vulnerable populations. Contemp. Nurse 42 (2), 243–246.

O'Brien, C., Rich, K., 2002. Evaluation of the Men and Family Relationships Initiative, Commonwealth Department of Family and Community Services, Canberra.

O'Connell-Birns, K., 2009. Men's mental health during the first year postpartum. J. Community Nurs. 23 (7), 4–8.

Oertelt-Prigione, S., Regitz-Zagrosek, V., 2009. Women's cardiovascular health. Editorial. Arch. Intern. Med. 169 (19), 1740–1741.

Ostapiej-Piatkowski, B., Allimant, A., 2013. Best practice considerations when responding to people from CALD backgrounds, including refugees, with mental health issues and experiences of domestic and sexual violence. In: Improving responses to refugees with backgrounds of multiple trauma, University of New South Wales, pp. 14–19.

Parris, J., 2013. Responding to refugees affected by domestic and sexual violence: working with men. In: Improving responses to refugees with backgrounds of multiple trauma, University of New South Wales, pp. 19–26.

Paterson, S., 2009. (Re)constructing women's resistance to woman abuse: Resources, strategy choice and implications of and for public policy in Canada. Crit. Soc. Policy 29 (1), 121–145.

Peate, I., 2013. Caring for older lesbian, gay and bisexual people. Br. J. Community Nurs. 18 (8), 372–374.

Pit, S., Byles, J., 2012. The association of health and employment in mature women: A longitudinal study. J. Womens Health 21 (3), 273–280.

Pittaway, E., Eckert, R., 2013. Domestic violence, refugees and prior experiences of sexual violence: factors affecting therapeutic and support service provision. In: Improving responses to refugees with backgrounds of multiple trauma, University of New South Wales, pp. 10–13.

Pittaway, E., Eckert, R., Bartolomel, L, 2013. The Women at Risk Assessment Tool. Improving responses to refugees with backgrounds of multiple trauma, University of New South Wales, pp. 27–30.

Postmus, J., Severson, M., Berry, M., et al., 2009. Women's experiences of violence and seeking help. Violence Against Women 15 (7), 852–868.

Power, J., Perlesz, A., Brown, R., et al., 2010. Diversity, tradition and family: Australian same-sex attracted parents and their families. Gay Lesb. Issues Psychol. Rev. 6 (2), 66–81.

Rappaport, J., 1987. Terms of empowerment/exemplars of prevention: Towards a theory for community psychology. Am. J. Community Psychol. 15, 121–148.

Rounds, K., Burns McGrath, B., Walsh, E., 2013. Perspectives on provider behaviors: A qualitative study of sexual and gender minorities regarding quality of care. Contemp. Nurse 44 (1), 99–110.

Russell, N., Harding, C., Chamberlain, C., et al., 2006. Implementing 'Men's Health Pitstop' in the Riverina, South-west New South Wales. Aust. J. Rural Health 14, 129–131.

Saunders, M., Peerson, A., 2009. Australia's National Men's Health Policy: masculinity matters. Health Promot. J. Austr. 20 (2), 92–97.

Sen, A., 1999. Development as freedom, Alfred A. Knopf, New York.

Shaw, L., Bugiardini, R., Bairey Merz, C., 2009. Women and ischemic heart disease. J. Am. Coll. Cardiol. 54 (17), 1561–1575.

OBJECTIVES

By the end of this chapter you will be able to:

1 explain the influence of culture on health and social justice

2 discuss Indigenous health within the context of primary health care

3 identify risk factors for Indigenous health at the family, neighbourhood and community level

4 explain the importance of historical and cultural knowledge in promoting the health of Indigenous people

5 describe strategies for promoting health literacy in an Indigenous community

6 explain the importance of place-based initiatives in helping Indigenous people maintain health and wellbeing

7 devise a comprehensive strategy for working with Indigenous families to improve individual, family and community health

8 define cultural safety as a concept and explain its relevance and importance in the provision of health care.

always achieve this. The challenge is to advance this knowledge as a basis for informing community awareness, then providing a rationale for policy and practice with the ultimate goal of social justice. Questions for members of our professions revolve around how we can enact our role as advocates to support political enthusiasm for change, and how we can use Indigenous knowledge and skills to inform the direction of change. These questions lie at the basis of sustaining health improvements for all people so that they become entrenched in good and best practice.

We are both members of the non-Indigenous cultures of our respective countries, and we write this chapter drawing on a wide range of Indigenous and non-Indigenous literature, in consultation with members of Indigenous cultures, and on our respective experiences of the health and political environments in which we live and work. We begin this chapter by delving into some of the successes and failures in Indigenous health in Australia and New Zealand. This is explained within a framework that addresses the influences of the historical, social, economic and situational factors that have prevented Indigenous people from achieving good health. From this base of knowledge, we can work together, seeking common solutions that redress past and current barriers to health and wellness. Then we can work toward helping Indigenous people negotiate retention of their culture, and promote equitable, inclusive environments for health and wellbeing.

CULTURE AND HEALTH

Cultural groups are bound together by a tapestry of historically inherited ideas, beliefs, values, knowledge and traditions, art, customs, habits, language, roles, rules and shared meanings about the world. *Culture* is therefore multidimensional. Cultural influences are often tacit in people's behaviours, as unconscious, shared predispositions, rather than deliberate attempts to be distinctive. Despite the commonalities that bind members of a cultural group, behaviours, cultural traits, and predispositions are not always expressed in the same way by all who claim membership in the group. Individual expressions of attitudes, beliefs and behaviours vary according to age, gender, personal histories and situational factors, and these are, in turn, influenced by family, group and community influences.

CULTURAL HETEROGENEITY

Although there are many commonalities that bind members of a particular cultural group, individual expressions of culture vary according to a person's characteristics and experiences.

Diversity in expressions of culture is also a product of how people relate to their environments. Culture is integral to a person's social life, part of his or her ecological relationship with the world, which is dynamic and adaptive. In ecological terms, as people in any cultural group interact with their environments, there is a reciprocal effect on the environments and the people themselves (Eckermann et al. 2010). The way people respond to, initiate and adapt to changes is therefore a reflection of the natural, economic, historic, social and political environments; the traditions of their culture, including acquired knowledge, guides to action, language, thoughts and lifestyles; and the way their socialisation has led them to interpret experience and shape behaviour. Culture is also experienced differently at different ages and stages of life, as people self-reflect, develop their own identities, and respond to circumstances and self-reflection. Their cultural behaviours are therefore shaped by a range of experiences besides the cultural norms of language, lifestyle habits and family expectations. Although cultural traditions can bind people together, it is inappropriate to consider members of one or another culture as homogeneous, as within cultural groups there is often wide variability.

A critical view of culture seeks to overcome the *monolithic* view that all members are relatively similar. Instead, understanding individuals comes from exploring their history, behaviour and particular view of the world as it is embedded in their culture, but distinctive in their patterns of attitude and behaviour. Conducting nursing assessments of a person's needs therefore has to include both unique and common strengths and needs. Like other cultural groups, Indigenous 'culture' is not something that can be made explicit, as a formula from which to develop culturally appropriate guidelines and culturally competent care (McMurray & Param 2008). Trying to define a certain culture as a cultural outsider is difficult, and can lead to stereotyping. To be authentically inclusive, health professionals have to understand the history and structural factors that have been part of a person's experience, in the context of diversity within, and external to the group (Gerlach 2012; Williamson &

Harrison 2010). This non-stereotypical approach provides insight into people's worldview and their history, their declaration of what they value, and the barriers and strengths that can lead to empowerment and self-determined decision-making. Ultimately, accommodating multiple views of culture grants the members of a group the freedom to articulate their lives, and their expectations in the voices of their own language and values (Sen 2000). These choices are embedded in family and community and the human right to achieve social and cultural capital (see Figure 13.1). We have previously defined social capital in terms of trust, civic engagement, participation and belonging. Cultural capital refers to the source of power and resources that can help people maintain social capital in a way that will be beneficial and validate their ways of knowing and understanding.

> ### Social capital
> Trust, reciprocity, participation, belonging.
>
> ### Cultural capital
> The power and resources that help people maintain social capital in a way that values cultural understandings.

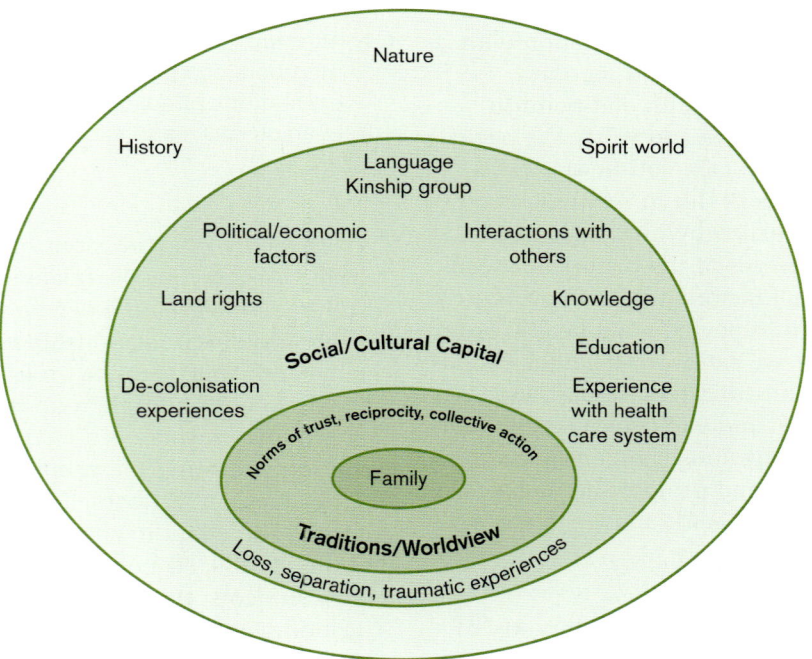

FIGURE 13.1
Family, culture and social capital

CULTURE CONFLICT

In some cases, the ecological interactions between people, their culture and other cultural groups is mutually beneficial. People of different cultures settling together in a new land often learn from one another, enjoying each other's foods and ways of cooking, lifestyles and folkways, such as festivals and celebrations. Over time, their long-term contact with one another can result in the type of *acculturation* where two cultural groups become integrated; or relatively similar (Beiser 2005). However, attempts at acculturating two groups can also be fraught with conflict. Berry (1995) describes four different reactions to acculturation. The first is *assimilation*, where one culture abandons their culture in favour of the new or host culture. *Integration* is the creative blending of the two cultures. *Rejection* is a reaction in which the new culture replaces the heritage culture, and *marginalisation* occurs where neither the new nor the old culture are accepted. Clearly, the most desirable option is integration, with marginalisation the least desirable.

> **Assimilation**—abandoning culture
> **Integration**—blending cultures
> **Rejection**—replacing culture
> **Marginalisation**—non-acceptance of culture

Culture conflict typically occurs where people are not committed to similar goals or ambitions, and where societal decision-making is based on dissimilar principles and philosophies. In its extreme form, culture conflict can be enacted within racialised social structures, such as occurs when all groups are defined and their behaviours measured according to white Western beliefs. Racialised social structures often pervade Indigenous cultures in countries like Australia, Canada, New Zealand and the US, where discriminatory and often racist attitudes promulgated by media stereotypes portray Indigenous people as a 'problem' rather than showing balanced, positive images of successful Indigenous people and families. Problematising their lives can subjugate Indigenous knowledge, beliefs and values in a way that disempowers members of Indigenous cultures by establishing standards and expectations against which differences, or deviations from the norm, are measured, valued and often demeaned (Durey & Thompson 2012). Even in the health care system, we tend to purvey the impression that non-white populations need to be benchmarked and reconciled within white, Eurocentric models of care, and their behaviours corrected, to conform with disembodied, purified, scientific solutions (Puzan 2003). The impact of this attitude can be that racism is internalised by Indigenous people, who then self-stigmatise, believing that they are, in fact, inferior (Durey & Thompson 2012; Oda & Rameka 2012). This lack of self-belief and self-valuing then perpetuates unresolved issues that continue to plague the lives of Indigenous peoples, adding cumulatively to their unresolved burden of inter-generational trauma and grief (Menzies 2008).

At the community level, culture conflict erodes social and cultural capital by causing disharmony. When this occurs, members of the conflicting groups close ranks, and withdraw from each other, rather than cooperating to build a system of mutual community support. On the other hand, when people from different cultures live with realistic possibilities for the future, they are more likely to work within a type of *cultural relativism*; acceptance of one another's culture as the legitimate adaptation of different peoples to various historical, natural, socio-economic and political environments (Eckermann et al. 2010). Cultural relativism lies at the centre of tolerance and social inclusiveness. For two cultures to work together, no one culture needs to abandon its traditions or philosophies, but each suspends judgement of the other's beliefs and practices. In this process, each makes a conscious decision to proceed on the basis of their willingness to recognise and respect the beliefs and practices of others, and to continually question their own views and presumptions (Eckermann et al. 2010). This is also the first step in maintaining cultural safety.

CULTURAL SAFETY

Cultural safety is a term that grew out of the colonial history of Aotearoa (New Zealand). It was first described in 1988 by Māori nursing students expressing their concern about safeguarding their culture as they were socialised into the world of nursing education, and ensuring the safety of Māori culture among those they would be helping in practice (Eckermann et al. 2010). Their concerns were recorded by Ramsden, a Māori nurse who spearheaded the cultural safety movement in Aotearoa, ensuring that cultural safety found its way into curricula and nursing practice (Eckermann et al. 2010). As we mentioned in Chapter 1 cultural safety is a concept that refers to exploring, reflecting on, and understanding one's own culture and how it relates to other cultures with a view toward promoting partnership, participation and cultural protection. By the 1990s cultural safety had been refined beyond Māori culture to be inclusive of all cultures and all health care recipients whose culture differs from their health care provider in any way (Gerlach 2012). Cultural safety is a form of cultural relativism, which is concerned with how culture shapes power relations within the social world of the community. It is designed to enable safe spaces for the interaction of all cultural groups, and their understanding of cultural identity. It is absent in the face of actions that assault, diminish, demean or disempower the cultural identity and wellbeing of any individual (NCNZ 2012).

protection of others' cultures. Cultural safety is therefore a type of advocacy informed by a recognition of self, the rights of others and the legitimacy of difference (NCNZ 2011). It is aimed at unveiling the unconscious and unspoken assumptions of power of health professionals with a view toward transferring some of this power to those seeking care by using an inclusive approach, receptive to new ways of knowing and understanding (Gerlach 2012). Nurses in New Zealand are required to demonstrate how they practise in a culturally safe manner as part of maintaining their nursing registration (NCNZ 2012). In the process of being inclusive of others' voices, they gain an authentic understanding of health issues as a basis for planning care, or *cultural competence* (Duke et al. 2009; Gerlach 2012). Culturally competent care shifts the balance of power to the recipient of care, which is more closely aligned with the partnership approach of primary health care (PHC) (Hamlin & Anderson 2011). Equally as important is the need for culturally competent health care systems to value diversity and demonstrate reciprocity between and among cultures (Farmer et al. 2012).

CULTURALLY SAFE PRACTICE

1   Acknowledge that the health care relationship is power-laden, with the health care professional holding the majority of power.

2   Develop cultural sensitivity by reflecting on your impact on the 'other'.

3   Make a commitment to preserve and protect all cultures.

CULTURALLY COMPETENT HEALTH SYSTEMS

• Acknowledge diversity.

• Provide culturally appropriate care.

• Enable self-determination and reciprocity.

• Hold governments and health planners accountable for meeting needs of all cultures.

• Manage from culturally competent evidence base.

• Recognise need for culturally competent training.

The first step in achieving cultural safety is *cultural awareness*. This includes recognising the fact that any health care relationship is unique, power-laden and culturally dyadic. In other words, there is always the potential for one person (the health provider) to hold power over the other person (someone seeking to access services). When the health care relationship is built on a foundation of *cultural sensitivity*, there is a greater recognition of, and respect for, cultural differences. People develop cultural sensitivity when they begin to engage in self-exploration of their own life experience and realities, and the impact this may have on others. The final stage in developing cultural safety is a conscious commitment to ensuring preservation and

MULTICULTURALISM

Multiculturalism is a value-laden term that has sometimes been used as a panacea for intolerance. The term has been used to camouflage feelings of superiority of one culture over another. It has also been used to salve the consciences of many people, believing that because they live in a community containing many cultures, the community must be inclusive, when this may be disputed by the realities of daily life. In its truest sense, multiculturalism means 'that people are in fact linked in many more ways than their birthplace divides them' (Wilding & Tilbury 2004:3). Globalisation has brought multiculturalism under close scrutiny because of the spurious arguments used by the most dominant cultures to maintain their position of power over those who are economically dependent on them for survival. In advancing the global economic development agenda, Indigenous people have often been ruthlessly ignored or dismissed, which is discriminatory and adds to their level of disadvantage. Languages have disappeared and cultural characteristics have gradually withered, as people try to minimise feelings of 'difference', and find ways of coping with feeling excluded from mainstream society. These psychosocial outcomes have been accompanied by widening gaps in health, favouring the dominant culture and disempowering those already disadvantaged. Cross-border or multinational decisions take little account of local needs and local voices with little negotiating power, and this exacerbates the cycle of disempowerment by invalidating cultural traditions, eroding the cultural scaffolding that supports health and wellbeing. When this occurs there is a polarised society; one group dominates and the other is left to feel like the 'other'.

Although small steps have been made towards heightening public awareness of the role of culture in health, these have been only marginally effective in improving health outcomes. To advance multiculturalism, societies need to institutionalise understanding and tolerance of one another's cultural beliefs and practices in the context of daily living as well as in the health care system, and in planning for a future in which all cultures will be sustained. Not many societies achieve this level of equity, but it is seen to be an aspiration worthy of just and civil societies. Canada is the only country in the world to have a national multiculturalism law, which was devised in 1971 as an attempt to legitimise the need for harmony among Indigenous and non-Indigenous groups and those who migrated to Canada from other countries (Kulig 2000). This law enshrined equality, diversity and dignity for all people, and confirmed the rights of Canada's Indigenous peoples and the status of the country's two official languages: French and English. The Canadian policy initiative is somewhat similar to the 'biculturalism' that exists in New Zealand, where the use of both Māori and Pakeha languages is seen as integral to cultural safety (Williamson & Harrison 2010) (see Box 13.1). However, the important test of these initiatives is how all members of society interpret one another's right to social inclusion and mutual empowerment.

BOX 13.1 Biculturalism in New Zealand: struggles and successes

Biculturalism can be understood as two distinct cultures in some form of co-existence. In New Zealand, this can be understood and enacted as a Māori-Pakeha (non-Māori New Zealander) partnership (Jones & Creed 2011). This partnership is considered equal, not a case of majority membership—thus although Māori may constitute 15% of the population of New Zealand, a true bicultural partnership does not see 15% of governance held by Māori, but 50%. In essence, a bicultural organisation is one that recognises the ideal of equal partnership in governance. The Treaty of Waitangi provides the foundation for biculturalism in New Zealand and sets the parameters around partnership, participation and protection for Māori at all levels. New Zealand government policy has called for organisations to develop bicultural policies as a means of demonstrating commitment to the Treaty but many organisations have still to develop true bicultural policies and the road to biculturalism can be challenging. Many organisations reject the notion of biculturalism, but health sector organisations have embraced the idea as a means of acknowledging and improving the health status of Māori, addressing existing disparities in health status between Māori and other New Zealanders, and enacting their commitment to the Treaty of Waitangi. Organisations such as the New Zealand Nurses Organisation (NZNO) and the College of Nurses (Aotearoa) operate under bicultural constitutions, although each organisation's path to, and practice of, biculturalism has been different. Biculturalism in practice includes not only an equal voice at the governance level but a commitment to consultation, discussion and equitable resourcing and outcomes for Māori.

? What is your understanding of biculturalism? How would this work in the organisation you work for? In what way would truly bicultural organisations improve the health and wellbeing of Indigenous people in your country?

ETHNOCENTRISM, RACISM AND DIFFERENTIAL HEALTH CARE

Ethnocentrism is the tendency to view the world through one's own cultural filters, perceiving and interpreting others' behaviours according to a personal belief system and set of behaviours (Durey

& Thompson 2012; Farmer et al. 2012). Each of us views the world through the cultural lens with which we have been socialised, and this is why it takes a conscious effort to really 'see' other cultures. When people develop an aversion to the very notion of tolerating other cultures, they are described as *xenophobic*: fearing and despising those who differ. Xenophobia is often used synonymously with *racism*, which is a belief in the distinctiveness of human races, usually involving the idea that one's birth-ascribed race or skin colour is superior to another (Durey & Thompson 2012). Maintaining feelings of superiority about another race, or another group, is called *stereotyping*. These feelings can lead to *prejudicial attitudes,* which, when acted upon, result in *discrimination*. Discrimination is shown by speaking against the other person or group, excluding or segregating them, committing acts of violence against them, or, at its extreme, exterminating them as has occurred in World War II and other wars and conflicts.

> ## WHAT IS … RACISM?
> Prejudice + power

Today, because of numerous inquiries into historical examples of aggression against one culture by another, we have come to recognise *ethnic cleansing* as an offensive, prejudicial act of violent discrimination. This is also *racist*. When offensive behaviours are entrenched in socio-legal structures or scientific research, the notion of biological inferiority can lead to *scientific racism*. This occurs when one group is attributed with inferiority on the basis of race, often justified by comparative studies that seek to investigate differences, rather than commonalities (Durey & Thompson 2012; Eckermann et al. 2010; Puzan 2003). It is important that students, academics and practitioners who either generate or use scientific evidence recognise this type of racism as embedded in research approaches that are conducted from a 'white' standpoint and focus on risky individual behaviours rather than the structural and social determinants of people's health (Durey & Thompson 2012). Systemic bias occurs where research is conducted 'on' instead of 'with' Indigenous people. This research approach perpetuates inequality and imbalanced power relations, and we discuss this further in Chapter 15 in relation to Indigenous research. *Institutional racism* operates at the level of legal, political and economic organisation in a society, and it creates the impression that, because power dominance is exerted by essential and respected forces in society, it is somehow tacitly acceptable (Eckermann et al. 2010). *Systemic bias* allows one group to dominate another through the predominant social order, where organisational and communication skills, financial resources and commitment of those involved in running a system are able to exclude others, making them dependent on the powerful group rather than allowing them full participation (Eckermann et al. 2010). In some cases, this type of power imbalance occurs because of a lack of knowledge and awareness rather than an intention to dominate. For example, *culture blindness*, where, inadvertently, someone who believes they are working within an ethos of social justice develops universalism, or an approach to health and social care where an individual proclaims to 'treat everyone the same' (Durey & Thompson 2012:160). The issue here is that some people have greater needs than others, so a universal approach will not help achieve equal opportunities, and therefore may perpetuate disparities for disadvantaged cultural groups (Theunissan 2011).

> ## SYSTEMIC BIAS
> - Benchmarking Indigenous health against non-Indigenous population norms
> - Using a universal or 'one-size-fits-all' approach to health care
> - Attributing needs to culture instead of structural and social determinants of health

The other manifestations of systemic bias are evident when the health of Indigenous people is analysed according to benchmarks established for non-Indigenous populations, or when the blame for social and health problems is attributed to cultural characteristics instead of inequities in the health care system (Durey & Thompson 2012). There is now a body of evidence showing that Indigenous people in Australia and New Zealand have inadequate access to health services and lower rates of medical interventions when they are hospitalised (Durey & Thompson 2012; Oda & Rameka 2012). New Zealand Māori have experienced barriers to access such as fewer referrals to specialists, slower treatment, lengthy waiting times, and economic deprivation that impacts on their ability to afford and access services, particularly for those who must take time off work to attend service providers (Theunissan 2011). In Australia, breast cancer screening among Indigenous women is roughly half the rate of non-Indigenous women (AIHW 2012a). There is no definitive cultural explanation for these disparities, however, the desire to keep 'women's business' private may explain some women's hesitancy to be tested. What seems to be the case is that differential treatment may be because of a lack of access to services, or women do not understand their options or the potential impact of various services on their health and wellbeing. In some cases, health professionals have been insensitive to Indigenous people's needs, treating them in a discriminating way, which creates the impression that their cultural needs and their cultural safety is being undermined (Astin et al. 2012; Theunissan 2011). Stereotyping anyone's health needs can be detrimental to health. For example, there are cases where a person's refusal of treatment is described as a lack of adherence, when it could be due to communication difficulties. Other examples include treating an Indigenous patient as if they were intoxicated when their symptoms may be related to conditions such as stroke or diabetes, or refusing a child treatment because of a lack of consent from her/his parent, in a case where the child may be in the custody of relatives (Astin et al. 2012). Clearly, culturally insensitive communication is a major problem in health care, especially when health professionals are unable or unwilling to help them with health literacy, which can affect not only the person seeking help, but the transmission of knowledge from one generation to another (Astin et al. 2012).

Although we have outlined a number of disparities in health outcomes for Indigenous people we recognise that focusing on the disparities instead of the conditions that create the disparities can accelerate the marginalising process of 'othering' (Giddings, in Oda & Rameka 2012). We present comparisons to draw attention to the disproportionate needs of Indigenous peoples and to explain how discrimination can create re-victimisation. A common stereotypical pattern of re-victimisation lies in the way women victims of violence and child victims of sexual abuse are dealt with in the health care system. In many cases, the injuries and need for ongoing therapy and emotional support are dismissed by broad-brushing the problem as a cultural one, when the victim's needs for protection and care are personal and intense. When victims of violence are differentiated on the basis of Indigenous versus non-Indigenous, there is a conflation of culture and race (Anderson et al. 2003). This socially exclusive differentiation leads to *alienation* of the victim and her people. Another group of Indigenous people are then disempowered and disengaged from society, leading to disorientation, helplessness, powerlessness and

normlessness (Anderson et al. 2011; Durie 2004; Eckermann et al. 2010). Similarly, the high prevalence of low birth weight (LBW) babies born to Indigenous women living in remote locations on traditional lands is often attributed to culture. Unpacking the layers of a pregnant woman's life in those environments reveals a high incidence of tobacco smoking, which increases the risk of a LBW baby and a number of concomitant risks to the mother's health.

Few researchers have closely examined the circumstances of smoking among young pregnant girls, or the differences in smoking patterns between rural, remote or urban mothers. However, studies show that in remote communities, smoking is a social act, a way of sharing a yarn, gaining status with their peer group (Passey et al. 2011). The girls begin to smoke as teenagers, and they smoke to stay connected, to assert their group membership and their Aboriginal identity as a way of belonging, not as any form of rebellion or to cause any harm. They are at a distance from any activity that would replace smoking, such as a sporting or recreational event, which might be available to urban dwellers. Living remotely, they place a higher value on reciprocity and sharing, and cultural obligations in relation to smoking ('your mob does it, so it's in your blood to do it') (Passey et al. 2011:62). They are also exposed to considerable smoke because of overcrowding in homes where everyone else smokes, and under-exposed to peers who do not smoke (Passey et al. 2011). The conclusions anyone planning a health promotion intervention would draw from this knowledge is that strategies to help these women reduce smoking would be ineffective without introducing structural and cultural changes that were mindful of the context and the social determinants of their health.

ABORIGINALITY, CULTURE AND HEALTH

The term *Aboriginal* refers to the initial, or earliest, inhabitants of a place. They are also described as *First Nations,* or *Indigenous,* people. Nelson et al. (2010) explain that the definition of an Australian Aboriginal person is social rather than racial: a person who has descended from an original inhabitant, who identifies as an Aboriginal person and is recognised as Aboriginal by his or her community. Despite this commonality, Indigenous people have diverse subcultures and worldviews. Members of different groups also have different influences on their lives, many as a result of their environment. Like non-Indigenous people, those who live in a remote area have substantially different experiences of health from their kin in urban or other rural settings. Likewise, those who live inland have different health opportunities from those who live close to the sea. The influences on their health are shaped by different determinants beyond biology, age, gender, education, socio-economic status, family membership or neighbourhood. In some groups, cultural knowledge may prescribe diet and eating habits, child-rearing practices, reactions to pain, stress and death, a sense of past, present and future, community and economic structures, responses to health care services and practitioners, and which behaviours are considered a violation of social norms.

> ## INDIGENOUS UNDERSTANDINGS
>
> Health and wellbeing are manifest within holistic, symbolic, spiritual and ecological perspectives.

The most distinctive feature of Indigenous cultures is a holistic, ecological, spiritual view of health and wellbeing. This perspective encompasses physical, mental, cultural and spiritual dimensions of health, and the harmonised inter-relationships between these and environmental, ideological, political, social and economic conditions (Eckermann et al. 2010). At the centre of Indigenous people's relationship with each dimension of health is a fundamental spiritual connection with land, symbolising their responsibility as inhabitants of the land, to take care of it and preserve it for the next generations (Anderson et al. 2011). This is integral to their ecological connection between health and place.

INDIGENOUS PEOPLE'S RELATIONSHIPS BETWEEN HEALTH AND PLACE

The spiritual relationship with land is a metaphysical connection, governing all other inter-relationships. The land is typically described by Indigenous Australians as 'Country', which is the place that gives and receives life and is part of the support cycle of life-death-life (AIHW 2012a; Kingsley et al. 2009). Indigenous Australians 'talk about Country in the same way that they would talk about a person, they speak to Country, visit Country, worry about Country, feel sorry for Country and long for Country' (Australian Heritage Commission, in Kingsley et al. 2009:291). For Indigenous people, the spiritual connotation of caring for Country links people with their

ancestors. This is a different concept of land from the non-Indigenous understanding, where land is considered an empty space to be 'tamed' or worked (Kingsley et al. 2009). New Zealand Māori articulate a similar connection with the land. The land historically provided the sustenance necessary for life, but it is also the spiritual, cultural and ancestral home for Māori. This relationship is based on the worldview that Ranginui (Sky Father), and Papatuanuku (Earth Mother), are the primal parents from whom all Māori descend. Māori refer to themselves as Tangata Whenua (people of the land), which captures the spirit of this kin relationship making the people and the land inseparable (NZ Govt, Online. Available: www.teara.govt.nz/en/Māori/page-1 [accessed 13 September 2013]). Platforms for Māori health are considered to be '... constructed from land, language, and whānau; from marae and hapu; from Rangi and Papa; from the 'ashes of colonisation; from adequate opportunity for cultural expression; and from being able to participate fully within society' (Durie 2004:35–36).

What Indigenous and non-Indigenous people have in common is the concept of 'biophilia', a construct that reflects how human beings are innately connected and attracted to the natural environment (Kingsley et al. 2009). Biophilia is integral to our ecological view of health and wellbeing, reflecting the understanding that ecological connections give meaning and purpose to life, as well as influencing health and wellbeing. Kingsley et al.'s (2009) interviews with traditional custodians of their lands revealed the importance of this connection in fostering mental and spiritual health. One of the custodians reported that the land 'speaks to you ... allowing you time to look within yourself ... to be grounded ... to hear'. Others described the land as being intrinsic to identity, a way of connecting with culture with a sense of pride, a sense of belonging, and engendering a sense of responsibility to preserve traditional lands. Importantly, this group of people advocated a return to Country for young people having difficulties in urban living. They felt that working on Country was good therapy for those who were 'numb from the city', dislocated from society or needing empowerment (Kingsley et al. 2009:296), a view that is shared by many advocates for Indigenous youth.

The close connection with land is what distinguishes the Indigenous 'holistic' view from other common perceptions of holism (Anderson et al. 2011). The biomedical literature and its scientific foundations typically refer to an all-encompassing, comprehensive set of factors that contribute to health, describing these in terms of holism. An Indigenous worldview with its connection to Country and land is holistic in a more mind-spirit-body sense, and includes the way an Indigenous person's life is steeped in the events and stories of their lives (Anderson et al. 2011; Munford & Sanders 2011). The uncritical way non-Indigenous policymakers and health planners understand Indigenous 'holism' is problematic when it is seen as a biomedical concept, and translated into strategies for health and health services without deeper understandings of this holistic worldview (Durey & Thompson 2012). Locally relevant interventions need to reflect local knowledge from place-based communities whose members have developed the skills to articulate their needs from the holistic interpretations that resonate with the community (Anderson et al. 2011; McDonald et al. 2010; Munford & Sanders 2011). Yet these holistic understandings represent a gap in the research literature. Studying the issues surrounding environmental dispossession would help illuminate how removing Indigenous people from their lands has undermined their potential for health and wellbeing, particularly by disconnecting this important aspect of their life and the other social determinants of health (SDH) (Ford 2012).

COLONISATION AND DISCONNECTION BETWEEN HEALTH AND PLACE

In many nations, including Australia, New Zealand, Canada and the US, Indigenous people were displaced from their lands by colonising invaders. Colonisation, and the subsequent political decisions that followed, have disrupted Indigenous people's connection between health and place, leaving generations of Indigenous people feeling dispossessed of their place, symbolically, geographically and politically (Eckermann et al. 2010; Pomaika'i Cook et al. 2005; Richmond & Ross 2009). Breaking the bond that connected Indigenous people to their traditional lands and environments eroded their identity, their culture and ultimately, their health and wellbeing. This disconnection has created an imbalance that threatened the health of the community (Richmond & Ross 2009). A further level of disconnection was experienced by those who were subjected to intensive missionary activity and taken to residential schools to enforce assimilation into the dominant culture. Part of this assimilation was to extinguish cultural practices by punishing certain behaviours, including dances, ceremonies, language and songs, many of which tied Indigenous people to features of their lands, and the symbolic importance of water, animals and plants (Richmond

& Ross 2009). Where once they had been self-governed, colonial laws forced them to abandon their traditions and self-determination, and become subservient to colonial institutions (Richmond & Ross 2009). Dispossession from land and Country is therefore one of the most critical issues that must be dealt with meaningfully if Indigenous people are to develop and enhance their capacity for health, especially in this era where climate change is adding another layer of displacement from the land (Ford 2012).

COLONISATION

Displacement from the land by colonising invaders has disconnected Indigenous people from their environment, creating spiritual disharmony and ill health.

The colonisation history of Africa, Australia, New Zealand, Canada and the US reveals a belief by their white European conquerors in their superiority over the native people. In most cases, this view was so extreme that the early explorers dismissed the very presence of Aboriginal people as irrelevant, because they failed to use the land in a way that would be expected in a civilised country. The colonisers thus declared the respective countries *Terra Nullius*—an empty, uninhabited land, belonging to no one (Australian Government 2013a). In Australia, this belief represented institutionalised racism, given the colonisers' view that land not cultivated represented a failure of Indigenous people to use the land, a mark of 'civilisation' according to British/European culture. Their colonisers were therefore able to claim the land without having to conquer Indigenous people or negotiate a treaty with them (Eckermann et al. 2010). To the present time there remains no treaty in place between Indigenous and non-Indigenous Australians.

The Australian situation differs markedly from North America and New Zealand, where treaties have been established as a mark of socio-legal commitment between Indigenous and non-Indigenous people. Treaties established in Canada and the US have enshrined mutual obligations between Indigenous people and the governments, although these were originally developed as a foundation for assimilation and colonial control (Richmond & Ross 2009). In New Zealand, the Treaty of Waitangi, signed in 1840 but not honoured and recognised until the 1970s, was established to protect Māori cultural beliefs, practices and intellectual life and provide equitable access to the benefits of modern life through granting full citizenship rights (NCNZ 2011; Williamson & Harrison 2010). The Māori Land Court holds much of the written information on Māori land ownership and the historical connections that exist between iwi, hapu, whānau and the land. It was established as the Native Land Court in 1865 in order to define the land rights of Māori and to translate those rights into land titles recognisable under European law (NZ Justice Department, Online. Available: www.justice.govt.nz/courts/Māori-land-court [accessed 16 September 2013]). The functions of the Māori Land Court today are to promote the management of Māori land by its owners by maintaining the records of title and ownership information, to contribute to the administration of Māori land, and to preserve taonga Māori. Approximately 1.47 million hectares is now designated as Māori freehold land (NZ Justice Department, Online. Available: www.justice.govt.nz/courts/Māori-land-court [accessed 16 September 2013]).

LAND RIGHTS

The issue of land rights for Indigenous people is addressed in different ways by different countries; but there is a persistent attempt by non-Indigenous cultures to limit the rights of Indigenous cultures to make claim to the land.

The land rights issues in Australia are substantially different from the New Zealand situation. Australian Aboriginal people were not granted citizenship until a referendum in 1967, 179 years after Australia was colonised by the British (Williamson & Harrison 2010). Native title—that is, acknowledgement that Indigenous people were the original owners and custodians of various lands in Australia—was granted in the *Native Title Act* of 1993 after a ten year legal battle led by Eddie Mabo. Mabo's legal challenge disputed the doctrine of *Terra Nullius*: that the country was unsettled prior to the Europeans' arrival (Australian Government 2013a). As a result of the native title acknowledgement, many things have changed. Native title holders and claimants are able to negotiate Indigenous Land Use Agreements about the management of land and water. Indigenous people's spiritual connection to land remains *inalienable*, which means the land cannot be sold. By 2012 the Australian Government had declared 36 million hectares of the country

Indigenous Protected Areas and, by 2013 Indigenous people owned or controlled 20% of Australia's land under various titles (Australian Government 2013a). However, some disputes remain over Land Use Agreements, primarily in having to work through tortuous government red tape. Box 13.2 below illustrates one of the few cases where an intergenerational group of Indigenous people have persevered over many years to claim their rightful place in the land.

CLIMATE CHANGE EVIDENCE

- Document Indigenous knowledge
- Collect baseline data on vulnerability
- Improve surveillance and monitoring
- Evaluate opportunities for policy
- Interdisciplinary research

The case study in Box 13.2 exemplifies the struggle of people who were first on the land to simply gain it back from intruders. The early years of colonisation brought environmental destruction from over-grazing, and the destruction of grasslands and forest, with its edible seeds, roots and fauna, all of which have been a personal affront to Indigenous people. The destruction of Indigenous habitats destroyed the metaphysical connections between people, their Country and their family. As in ancient history, Indigenous systems of resource ownership and exchange were intended to provide the opportunity to develop autonomy and mastery over life, and to help young men especially with culturally appropriate identity formation and social integration. Destroying their ability to accomplish these connections, and to manage natural resources in an Indigenous way, has disrupted cultural continuity for young people and adolescents, and the very essence of Aboriginality. Today's threat of climate change intensifies the problem of their adaptive capacity. Climate change will continue to affect Indigenous people disproportionately because of their habitation in regions undergoing changes and their sensitivity to climate-related health risks such as infectious diseases, water and food insecurity, natural disasters and population displacement (Ford 2012). The climate change discourses of scientists also tend to dismiss Indigenous ways of knowing about the land, and instead of drawing on Indigenous people's accumulated wisdom they construct the problem in terms of their powerlessness (Ford 2012). There is widespread acknowledgement that temperature

BOX 13.2 Gunyangara and the Yolngu journey

Nicolas Rothwell is an Australian journalist who has been mapping the journeys of many Indigenous people over the past decades, demonstrating an extraordinary commitment to ensuring that all Australians understand the multilayered nature of their lives, and the barriers they encounter along the way. He tells a remarkable story of the strength and perseverance of the Yolngu people of Gunyangara. Many Australians know of the Yunupingu family who belong to the Gumatj clan, Yolngu people, particularly through their music. Galarrwuy Yunupingu, a former Australian of the Year, is perhaps the most well known. However, few people are familiar with the extent of their struggles to empower their people with land, jobs and the kind of conditions that will help sustain the next generations. In the 1970s the clan witnessed destruction of their land and sacred sites by a large multinational mining company. They fought and lost the battle to protect their land in the courts, and once the strip mining began, the extra money that flowed to their communities created only intense rivalry, dissent and other social problems such as alcohol abuse, which destroyed the health of several family members and led to the suicide of others, eventually destroying families through violence and child abuse. The Gumatj families built a new settlement to escape the troubles and live out their dream to have peace, full employment and autonomy to preserve their traditions. From their land on the Gulf they watched the ships remove boatloads of money bound for overseas markets. Despite their disempowerment they formed a strategy based on political, economic and financial plans, which had been a dream of their forefathers. Time marched on, and as the new century progressed, the mining lease was about to expire. Rio Tinto, a multinational with a strong commitment to Indigenous people, took over the lease, which presented a window of opportunity to negotiate for their own mining rights. They assembled a team of advisors and developed a business model that would see them receive assets, a property portfolio, and a bauxite mining sub-lease. Through long, drawn-out negotiations and careful planning the clan developed a corporation to supplement welfare income among their 600-odd members. They redesigned their world, and by 2011 they had invested in a 'future fund' for their people, building profitable businesses with well-paid, real-world jobs for locals. Now they have diversified into several different businesses, all of which add value to the community and some of which are run by women. Each business dovetails with another and the overarching plan is adaptive in that they are finally able to engage with mainstream Australia on equal terms. The clan has achieved the dream of their elders in a way that has helped them become educated and experienced in the skills that give them the freedom to preserve their traditions. As Rothwell recounts (2012:30) 'The bushfires are burning into the sky, and the new energies are alive in the minds of men'.

increases, droughts, storms, flooding and uncertainty about the viability of many lands for growing food are a problem for Australian people. The effects of these changes will impact on traditional food systems, and therefore Indigenous people, to a greater extent than those who are not impoverished, living in crowded conditions or suffering from poor health. To avoid the dire consequences of environmental destruction for future generations requires a roadmap for future research that can inform conservation strategies. The roadmap includes articulating Indigenous conceptualisations of the land–health connections; collecting baseline data on the SDH and levels of vulnerability; develop and improve surveillance and environmental monitoring; evaluate opportunities for policy intervention and adopt interdisciplinary approaches to research (Ford 2012).

CULTURE BLINDNESS AND THE STOLEN GENERATIONS

Dismissing Indigenous ways of knowing or failing to generate sufficient Indigenous knowledge has led to profound social problems. One of these is the 'cultural trauma syndrome', a violation of selfhood where disenfranchised individuals take on the role of perpetrator, inflicting cultural wounds on others, leading to intergenerational transference of their grief rather than resolving it in culturally appropriate healing (Pomaika'I Cook et al. 2005:119). History shows that Indigenous groups who hold collective experiences and memories of abuse, dispossession and insensitivity are typically those who experience discrimination in housing, education, employment and the justice system and least likely to be offered help and support for capacity building (Durey & Thompson 2012). In 1997 the Human Rights and Equal Opportunity Commission published a report of the National Inquiry into Separation of Aboriginal and Torres Strait Islander Children from their Families (HREOC 1997). The Inquiry found that approximately 8% of Indigenous Australians aged 15 or over had been forcibly removed from their natural family. The result was mass undermining of Indigenous social organisation, dispersal of geographic groupings and the capture of Indigenous women (Eckermann et al. 2010). Their displacement was accompanied by sexual abuse, the introduction of alcohol, and economic and environmental exploitation, which was further demoralising. Then, ludicrously, Indigenous people were blamed for being demoralised and living in squalor—a classic case of what health educators now call 'victim blaming'. The dislocation of the 'Stolen Generation' has been linked to a range of negative outcomes, including higher rates of emotional distress, depression, anxiety, heart disease and diabetes, as well as cultural detachment (Trewin & Madden 2005). Many have had contact with mental health services, or lived in households where there were problems caused by gambling or overuse of alcohol. An inter-generational effect is evident in the fact that the children of those who had been forcibly removed from their homes were more than twice as likely to be at high risk of clinically significant emotional or behavioural difficulties, and approximately twice as likely to use alcohol and other drugs compared with those who had not been forcibly separated from their family (Zubrick et al. 2005).

STEALING CHILDHOOD

Approximately 8% of Indigenous Australians over the age of 15 years were forcibly removed from their natural families.

The separation of Indigenous children from their families has also perpetuated racism and culture-blindness. Removing young Indigenous children from their parents and sending them to white schools to gain what was considered to be 'appropriate' educational preparation was a culture-blind policy that traumatised Indigenous people and the place of family as the epicentre of life. When this occurred in the last century, Australian Indigenous children who were light-skinned were

primary targets for removal, conceivably to protect them from abuse by their family members and other Indigenous people who rejected them as being neither black nor white. The children who were removed grew up in white missions and schools presuming that no such family existed, and often were subjected to inter-racial aggression. Women and children became victims of exploitation and sexual abuse, and most suffered the emotional cost of being confined for prolonged periods, whether in institutionalised housing or hospitals. The parallel situation with refugees being held in detention is remarkable. Both groups suffer ongoing, severe, intergenerational traumatisation. The consequent loss of freedom and space has a lasting effect that is not easily resolved. Another series of events that has had major consequences for Indigenous families has arisen from what is known as 'The intervention' as outlined in Box 13.3.

THE HEALTH OF INDIGENOUS PEOPLE THROUGHOUT THE WORLD

There are approximately 370 million Indigenous people in the world, representing more than 5000 cultures in 72 countries (Ford 2012). For all of these groups, life expectancy at birth is approximately 10–20 years less than for the rest of the population; infant mortality is 1.5–3 times greater than the national average and a large proportion suffer from malnutrition and communicable diseases (WHO 1999). In most regions of the world, the health of Indigenous people is also threatened by damage to their habitat and resource base (Ford 2012). Indigenous people's burden of illness, injury and disability is so disparate from that of non-Indigenous people, that in 1999, the WHO convened a meeting with Indigenous representatives from many countries, to develop the Geneva Declaration on the Health and Survival of Indigenous Peoples (WHO 1999). The objective of the declaration was for Indigenous people throughout the world to reaffirm their right of self-determination, and to remind states of their responsibilities and obligations under international law to help address these. Their statement placed responsibility for Indigenous ill health on colonial negation of their way of life and worldview, the destruction of their habitat, the decrease of biodiversity, imposition of sub-standard living and working conditions, dispossession of traditional lands and the relocation and transfer of populations (WHO 1999). The Geneva Declaration was followed by the United Nations Declaration on the Rights of Indigenous Peoples (UN 2007). The UN Declaration drew together existing rights from international laws and conventions such as the

BOX 13.3 'The intervention'

In 2007 the Australian Government instituted the Northern Territory Emergency Response (NTER), commonly known as 'the intervention' as a reaction to the *Little Children are Sacred* report, highlighting significant child sexual abuse in Aboriginal settlements. The intervention became government policy with no public discussion and marginalisation of Indigenous leadership. It was intended to protect children, make communities safe and build a better future for those living in Indigenous communities through seven specific measures:

1 restricting alcohol on Aboriginal lands

2 compulsory income management wherein welfare money would be used only for approved items

3 enforcing school attendance by linking income support and family assistance to attendance

4 compulsory health checks for all Aboriginal children

5 acquiring townships through five-year leases to streamline redevelopment

6 increasing policing levels in prescribed communities

7 improving housing and reforming living arrangements in prescribed communities.

The intervention inflamed public debate throughout the country, fuelled by the popular press. From one perspective the measures sounded like an ideal solution to the problem of child protection; another view saw them as a form of paternalism and a breach of human rights for failing to engage constructively with Aboriginal people (Evans 2012). Those in favour of the intervention believed it addressed the core issue of disadvantage. The others felt the manner in which the new measures were implemented was too heavy handed and politically motivated, representing a kind of social engineering

where Canberra micro-managed remote Aboriginal Australia (Rothwell 2013b). Numerous pilot projects were run, reports were filed and managers hired, all without local control. Once the measures were instituted, government reports outlined the new services that had been provided in the prescribed communities, and 1300 Indigenous people were surveyed to ascertain their views on these services. Results indicated that 41% felt their community was safer since the intervention and 32% thought this was 'a bit' safer, because of new police stations, night patrols and safe houses. In terms of providing a better future 47% thought the community was improving, but 42% saw no difference from pre-intervention. School attendance remained static with academic standards well below the minimum. The cost of the intervention was $1.3 billion, deemed to have been spent ineffectively, mostly on administration. The child health checks were undertaken and substantiated cases of child abuse rose, presumably because of better reporting.

Human rights advocates argue that the intervention has violated the principles of self-determination by mainstreaming Aboriginal people, trying to assimilate them into non-Indigenous culture and negating their right to choose between cultural maintenance and engagement with the mainstream economy. In some ways the intervention has been effective, but in a way that has inflamed cultural debate and polarised opinions. The top-down, centralised structure attracted the greatest criticism for being demoralising and disempowering, eroding trust between Indigenous and non-Indigenous residents (Evans 2012).

? What do you think could be done to maintain the momentum in improving child safety while empowering Indigenous communities to determine their own future?

Universal Declaration of Human Rights, explaining how these rights applied to Indigenous people. The statement represented the culmination of 20 years of research and discussion on how to develop a framework that would resonate with countries having different histories and circumstances experienced by their Indigenous people. Surprisingly, Canada, the US, Australia and New Zealand voted against the Declaration over concerns about national unity. However, our countries acknowledged the need to include Indigenous people's participation in decisions affecting their rights, and now

support the Declaration (Reconciliation Australia 2013).

One of the most common outcomes of the dispossession and demoralisation of Indigenous people is incarceration. Indigenous people in Canada, the US, Australia and New Zealand are over-represented in prisons, and often suffer from mental illnesses and/or substance abuse, all of which results in compounding their risk of racial discrimination in the prison situation (Durey & Thompson 2012). In addition, the destructive effect of confinement on the balance of Indigenous family and community life has always been underestimated, and only recently has become recognised as a powerful and enduring influence on Indigenous people's sense of alienation from their land and erosion of their spiritual identity (Kingsley et al. 2009; Richmond & Ross 2009). Until colonial powers established prisons, Indigenous people enacted their own form of tribal justice. Imprisoning people to try to deal with violence, and fighting violence with violence, have had a backlash effect. They have failed to reduce crime or conflict, and instead have left many families fatherless (Cripps & McGlade 2008). Attempts at assimilation have also failed. Trying to force non-Indigenous culture on Indigenous people in the guise of protecting them has been utterly destructive around the world, and has led to dispossession and displacement (Eckermann et al. 2010). As a result, Indigenous people continue to be the most disadvantaged and marginalised members of the community. Although we have just drawn attention to the fact that these groups are widely diverse, it is important to draw the attention of health planners and policymakers to the extraordinary constraints on their capacity to become empowered and achieve the health status to which they are entitled.

THE HEALTH OF AUSTRALIAN INDIGENOUS PEOPLE

Of the nearly 23 million people in Australia, around half a million (2.5%) are Indigenous: Aboriginal or Torres Strait Islanders, one-quarter of whom live in remote or very remote areas (AIHW 2012a). Compared to non-Indigenous Australians, Indigenous Australians are less healthy, die at a much younger age and have more injuries, disability and lower quality of life (AIHW 2012a). As a population group they are younger than non-Indigenous Australians, with 57% under age 25, and only 3% over age 65. This is attributed to relatively higher fertility rates and earlier mortality than non-Indigenous Australians (AIHW 2012a). More than twice as many Indigenous infants die at birth, or are born with low birth weights. Morbidity and mortality rates for Indigenous people are imprecise, because of the potential to misclassify or under-report Indigenous status, but existing data show twice the all-cause rates of death for both men and women, with many more deaths occurring before age 65 (AIHW 2012a). Chronic diseases are responsible for 80% of the mortality gap between Indigenous and non-Indigenous Australians. There are complex causal relationships between the chronic conditions of cardiovascular disease, diabetes and chronic kidney diseases, each of which may be a complication of

one or both of the others (AIHW 2012b). Many illnesses are directly linked to poverty and for some conditions, such as end-stage kidney disease, Indigenous adults suffer enormously: up to six times the rate of non-Indigenous Australians (AIHW 2012a). Children also have disproportionate rates of communicable diseases, particularly eye diseases and hearing problems (AIHW 2012a). The gap in life expectancy between Indigenous and non-Indigenous Australians has drawn considerable attention from the Commonwealth Government, with 'closing the gap' becoming a centrepiece of policy development, and a stimulus for health planners. The gap in life expectancy is estimated at around 11.5 years for males and 9.7 years for females, but these figures may also be inaccurate because of classification issues, and variability in the way they are calculated (Durey & Thompson 2012).

INDIGENOUS ILLNESSES

Similar illnesses plague Indigenous and non-Indigenous people, but the burden of illness is worse for Indigenous people because of an unhealthy start to life, social disadvantage, greater exposure to diseases and lack of access to services.

The main causes of illness and disability for Indigenous Australians are similar to those of non-Indigenous people, but the incidence of acute and chronic illnesses is higher not only because of the difficulties of accessing health services, but because of the lack of a healthy start to life. Many Indigenous people who are middle aged were low birth weight infants, and therefore have lived their lives with both biological and social disadvantage. Indigenous people who live in remote or very remote areas of the country are also disadvantaged because of a lack of health services and exposure to communicable diseases prevalent in those communities (AIHW 2012a). Remoteness also affects older people. Indigenous Australians enter aged care at a younger age than non-Indigenous Australians because of their poorer health status and do not always have options for hospital or palliative care services. Where they do have access to hospital care, the most common reasons for hospitalisation are dialysis treatment, endocrine diseases such as diabetes, respiratory and digestive diseases, treatment for injuries and mental health issues (AIHW 2012b).

As a group, Indigenous people have lower incomes, higher rates of unemployment, lower educational attainment and lower rates of home ownership than non-Indigenous Australians. However, we have tried to explain some of the structural and social reasons for these disparities, and current government initiatives suggest there are reasons to be optimistic about the future. There has been considerable progress in Australia in educational attainment, with 53.9% of Indigenous young people aged 20–24 achieving Year 12 or equivalent by 2011 (Australian Government 2013a). Those who do not complete school often remain in situations of socio-economic disadvantage with greater exposure to risk factors such as smoking, alcohol misuse, violence or other forms of abuse and relatively high rates of suicide, especially for young males (AIHW 2012a). These factors are also linked to overcrowded housing conditions, particularly in remote areas, where crowding and poorly maintained homes prevent people from engaging in the fundamental elements of hygiene that would help prevent infections (McDonald et al. 2009). Indigenous people in Australia, as in other countries, place a high value on 'family' as the heart of community life. Because many people live in extended families, substandard living conditions can affect many family members and it is often a barrier to developing parenting practices that would help reduce some of the eye and ear infections, poor growth and low cognitive outcomes that have plagued Indigenous children in many remote areas (Australian Government 2013a; McDonald et al. 2009). Living closely with others also makes it difficult for parents to go against traditional social norms and parenting practices. Consequently, families living in these conditions have neither the freedom to protect their living space from others, or appropriate role models to secure even the basic healthy living practices.

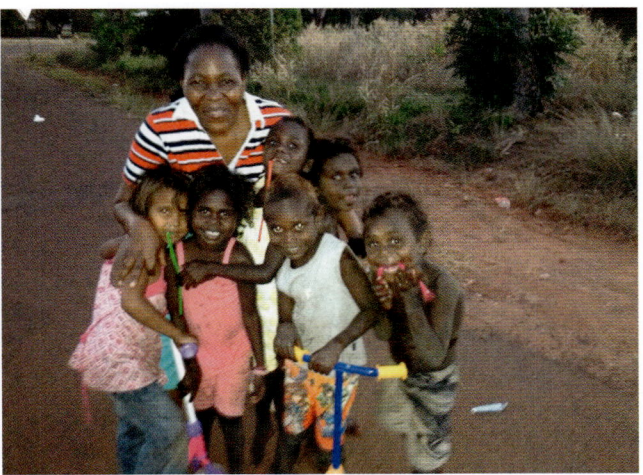

Tshepiso Mojapelo (Daisy), child health nurse in Wurrrimiyanga (Bathurst Island),Tiwi Islands, Northern Territory (photo courtesy of Tshepiso Mojapelo)

THE HEALTH OF NEW ZEALAND MĀORI

At the 2006 New Zealand Census (Statistics New Zealand 2006), people identifying with the Māori ethnic group comprised 15% of the total population—up 7% since the previous census in 2001. Māori are a youthful population, with a median age of 23 years, compared to 36 years for the total population. Māori predominantly live in urban areas of the North Island, although are more likely to live in minor urban areas with a population between 1000 and 9999 than non-Māori. Māori life expectancy also varies substantially from non-Māori. Māori women have a life expectancy of 77.6 years compared to 84.4 years for non-Māori, and Māori men have a life expectancy of 73.3 years, compared with 79.9 years for non-Māori men. The gap in life expectancy is not as marked as the gap between Australian Indigenous and non-Indigenous people, and it does continue to improve, from 9.8 years a decade ago to 6.7 years in 2011 (NZMOH 2013a). Despite these improvements in life expectancy, on average, Indigenous Māori have the poorest health status of any ethnic group in New Zealand; with age-standardised mortality for some conditions being worse than non-Māori by margins larger than 100% (Oda & Rameka 2012; NZMOH 2012a). For example, Māori rates of rheumatic fever are six times greater than non-Māori, and rates of diabetes mellitus are five times greater (NZMOH 2012a). In a 'land of plenty', food security remains a problem for 20–22% of New Zealand households with children, with higher rates among Māori and Pacific peoples (Signal et al. 2012).

CLOSING THE GAP

Māori have a life expectancy of 6.7 years less and suffer significantly higher mortality rates than non-Māori.

QUICK FACTS

Australian Indigenous people comprise 2.5% of the population, while 15% of the New Zealand population is Māori. Both populations are younger than non-Indigenous people, with lower socio-economic position, lower educational attainment, housing, food security and life expectancy, more disability, lower quality of life, a higher burden of chronic illness and communicable diseases, and inadequate health care.

Compared to non-Māori, inequalities in health status and mortality are large and increasing. The death rate for Māori men is 81.8% higher than non-Māori men, and the death rate for Māori females is 94.6% higher than for non-Māori females and is also higher than the death rate for non-Māori men (NZMOH 2012a). In 2009, Māori had a total mortality rate that was 1.9 times the non-Māori rate. The two largest differences between Māori and non-Māori age-standardised mortality rates as mentioned above were chronic rheumatic heart disease, where the Māori rate was more than six times that of the non-Māori rate, and diabetes mellitus, where the Māori rate was five times higher than the non-Māori rate.

Māori and Pacific people are twice as likely as the European population to be hospitalised with serious infectious disease, and this has increased substantially in the past 20 years, particularly for the poorest (Baker et al. 2012). The major causes of mortality for Māori, however, are largely lifestyle diseases including cancer, ischaemic heart disease and chronic lower respiratory disease followed by chronic obstructive pulmonary disease (COPD), diabetes mellitus and cerebrovascular disease in that order. Māori have at least double the non-Māori age-standardised death rate for lung cancer, stomach cancer, cervical cancer, chronic lower respiratory diseases (COPD), other forms of heart disease, transport accidents (including motor vehicle accidents), hypertensive disease and assault (NZMOH 2012a). In spite of this data, approximately 84% of Māori adults report they are in excellent, very good or good health, and parents report nearly all Māori children as in excellent health. The percentage of children who were fed solid foods prior to four months of age has decreased from 22% in 2006 to 16% in 2012, and Māori adults have similar rates of exercise and vegetable intake to non-Māori (NZMOH 2013b). However, smoking rates for Māori have remained static since 2006 and remain substantially higher than non-Māori rates, the obesity rate for Māori boys has increased, and Māori have higher unmet need for health care than non-Māori. Most of this unmet health need was related to the cost of attending a general practice or after-hours clinic and was 1.5 times higher than unmet need for non-Māori (NZMOH 2013b).

In terms of the SDH, large disparities exist between Māori and non-Māori. Approximately 48% of Māori secondary school students gain a qualification prior to leaving school compared with 69% of non-Māori (New Zealand Ministry of Education 2010). Unemployment rates are twice as high as those of non-Māori (NZMOE, Online.

Available: www.stats.govt.nz/browse_for_stats/income-and-work/employment_and_unemployment/HouseholdLabourForceSurvey_HOTPJun13qtr.aspx [accessed 18 September 2013]), and the median annual income for Māori in 2013 was $25 948 compared with $29 588 for the total population (NZMOE, Online. Available: www.stats.govt.nz/browse_for_stats/income-and-work/Income/NZIncomeSurvey_HOTPJun12qtr.aspx [accessed 18 September 2013]). In a study of the health and wellbeing of older Māori, researchers found Māori are more likely to be divorced or widowed, have less education and be less physically active, and are more likely to smoke than their non-Māori counterparts (Dulin et al. 2011). In the same study, Dulin et al. found the lower scores for Māori on all physical and mental health markers were partially explained by lower living standards (Dulin et al. 2011). Māori are also more likely to be living in overcrowded housing environments than non-Māori (Robson et al. 2007) and are less likely to own their own home (Te Puni Kokiri 2010). Young Māori men are more likely to be arrested for minor offences than non-Māori, and are more likely to be referred to the courts, rather than directly for family group conferences (Robson et al. 2007). Māori account for 49% of the prison population despite making up only 15% of the population (NZ Human Rights Commission 2012). These factors, along with evidence of the existence of differential access to health care, and of racial discrimination in health care (Reid & Robson 2007; NZ Human Rights Commission 2012), serve to further disadvantage Māori as they attempt to redress the factors that contribute to poor health.

Māori are 10 times more likely than others to experience discrimination in New Zealand (Oda & Rameka 2012). Discrimination has been linked to poor health, including mental illness, cardiovascular disease, hypertension, cancer, mortality and risky behaviours such as tobacco and alcohol consumption (Oda & Rameka 2012). Like Australian Indigenous people Māori are also exposed to institutional racism. They are less likely than non-Māori to access a GP, some have been denied access to cardiac and cancer interventions, and are subjected to mainstream media that portray their people as needy, passive and dependent (Oda & Rameka 2012). These images create internalised thinking similar to the self-stigma mentioned earlier, which demoralises people by making them think they should not have similar aspirations to non-Māori. In 2012, the auditor-general called on DHBs to improve their reporting on health disparities among Māori as a means of identifying gaps and addressing these (Provost 2012).

The Treaty of Waitangi provides the basis from which Māori can contest disparities and enjoy self-determination (Oda & Rameka 2012; Theunissen 2011). The treaty also grants them the right to name themselves as tangata whenua (people of the land), to live as Māori, to claim their rightful territory and their prestige (Oda & Rameka 2012; Reid & Robson 2007). This should mandate equal opportunities and equal outcomes for Māori and non-Māori (Theunissen 2011), but as mentioned previously, it was not until the 1970s that the New Zealand Government acknowledged that significant breaches to the Treaty of Waitangi had occurred. As a result, the Crown began to implement a number of policies that sought to address the legacy of inequities suffered by Māori since the arrival of European settlers in the early 1800s. These included revamping the Māori Land Court and establishing the Waitangi Tribunal. The Waitangi Tribunal was established in 1975 to make recommendations on claims brought by Māori relating to actions or omissions of the Crown that breach the promises made in the Treaty of Waitangi (NZ Govt, Online. Available: www.waitangi-tribunal.govt.nz [accessed 20 September 2013]). Claims against the Crown continue, and although the Waitangi Tribunal does not have final authority to decide points of law, it has made recommendations in over 120 reports on claims and a range of settlements have been made (NZ Govt, Online. Available: www.waitangi-tribunal.govt.nz/reports [accessed 20 September 2013]).

Efforts to address the inequities that exist for Māori also extend into the health care sector. Although New Zealand, like Australia, provides equal access to health care services, access is not equitable when it does not go the distance in providing culturally appropriate care for those who start their journey from a position of greater disadvantage (Theunissen 2011). There has been some progress in redressing the disparities in access, in the significant growth in health service provision since the mid-1980s of 'by Māori for Māori' health services. Such Māori health services recognise and implement a Māori-centred approach to health care (Kaupapa Māori services), which has been demonstrated as effective in reaching Māori whānau (Hamerton et al. 2012; NZMOH 2006; Oda & Rameka 2012). These services also address the need for holistic approaches based on Māori ways of knowing. They are also responsive to the PHC principle of intersectoral collaboration, providing access to a breadth of services that span housing, research, crime prevention, education, welfare and health (Oda & Rameka 2012).

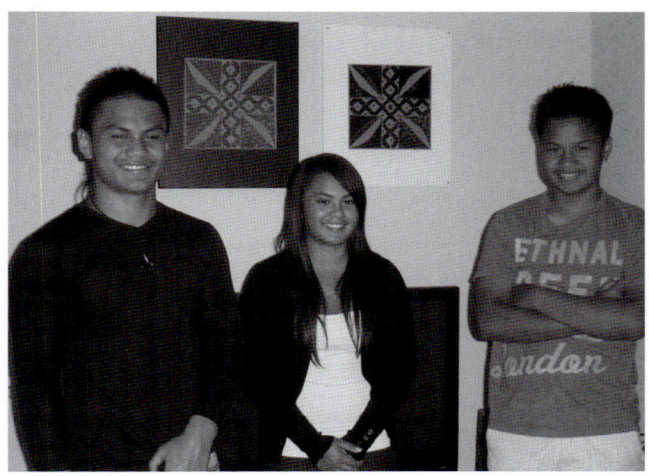

Young Māori thriving (photo courtesy of the Powell whānau)

There are more than 283 Kaupapa Māori health providers spread throughout New Zealand (NZ Govt, Online. Available: http://www.health.govt.nz/our-work/populations/Māori-health/Māori-health-providers/ka-tika-ka-ora-Māori-health-provider-work-programme [accessed 20 September 2013]). Kaupapa Māori health providers not only improve access to affordable and accessible health care for Māori, they contribute to the economic wellbeing of Māori communities and the Māori workforce (NZMOH 2009). Many of the services provided through Kaupapa Māori health providers are also provided by nurses (Theunissen 2011). Although numbers of Māori nurses are still not representative of the number of Māori living in New Zealand, many Māori nurses are working with Māori models of care providing effective and appropriate care for Māori individuals and families/whānau. As discussed in Chapter 7, the family or whānau is seen as the principal source of strength, support, security and identity for Māori and plays a central role in Māori wellbeing individually and collectively (Boulton et al. 2013). Nurses working with Kaupapa Māori models of care draw on this knowledge to provide culturally appropriate care (see Box 13.4).

BEHAVIOURAL RISK FACTORS

SMOKING

Forty-five per cent of Australian Indigenous people and 41% of Māori engage in smoking—the greatest preventable cause of death.

BOX 13.4 Kaupapa Māori health services

Te Hauora O Ngāti Rārua was established as a Māori health provider in 1996 and is located in Marlborough in the South Island of New Zealand. In 2005, a Māori diabetes nurse educator was appointed to provide a mix of one-on-one nursing care with a six-week education program to Māori clients and their whānau living with diabetes. Nursing care is provided to approximately 18 clients per week in both clinic and home environments and is supported by two other staff members in health support roles. Not only is care provided in a Māori-centred way, the nurse works intersectorally to ensure that clients and their whānau receive coordinated care from the variety of health providers with whom they interact. Evaluation of the nurse-led diabetes program demonstrated that clients maintained short-term improvements in physiological status, but most were unable to maintain this once the program ended. However, it was clearly demonstrated that using a Māori-centred approach to nursing care served to keep clients engaged with the service. As the service moves to including long-term family/whānau support meetings, it is anticipated that clients may be able to maintain the improvements seen in physiological status during the shorter program of care currently offered (Janssen 2009).

Some health risks among Indigenous people emanate from behavioural factors, and these have seen marked improvements over the past decade. There are fewer deaths, a decrease in infant mortality, reductions in diseases such as trachoma, tuberculosis and other communicable diseases, fewer respiratory conditions, stroke and kidney problems, and a decrease in smoking (Australian Indigenous HealthInfoNet 2013). Despite the improvements in health, disadvantaged circumstances have continued to plague Indigenous communities and these help perpetuate a range of behavioural risk factors. Approximately 45% of Australian Indigenous men and women smoke tobacco daily, primarily those living in disadvantaged circumstances, overall, roughly twice the number compared to non-Indigenous people (ABS 2013). In New Zealand, 41% of Māori smoke. Of greatest concern is the fact that Māori women are three times as likely to smoke as non-Māori women, which is one of the highest rates of smoking among any Indigenous group in the world. Māori men are 2.1 times more likely to smoke

than non-Māori men (NZMOH 2012b). Social disadvantage clearly constrains individual choices in terms of beginning or quitting smoking, including the disadvantage experienced by young children and adolescents who live in homes where others smoke. These factors and the difficulties of quitting contribute to disproportionate rates of cancer deaths among Indigenous people in North America, New Zealand, and Australia (Shahid & Thompson 2009). Box 13.5 outlines Kaupapa Māori programs for smoking cessation initiatives.

In relation to alcohol consumption, overall, Indigenous Australians are less likely to consume alcohol than non-Indigenous Australians. For those who do, their consumption tends to be at high risk levels, and this type of drinking can lead to injuries (Australian Indigenous HealthInfoNet 2013). In New Zealand, Māori women are 2.3 times more likely than non-Māori women to have potentially hazardous drinking patterns. Māori men are 1.65 times more likely to have a hazardous drinking pattern than their non-Māori counterparts (NZMOH 2013c). Illicit drug use has been reported as approximately twice the rate of that of non-Indigenous people (AIHW 2012a). Obesity is also a problem for many Indigenous people in Australia and New Zealand. Indigenous Australian women are more likely to be overweight or obese than non-Indigenous women, whereas among males the rates are similar. One in six Māori children in New Zealand are obese (NZMOH 2012c), and Māori adults, both men and women, are almost twice as likely to be obese than non-Māori adults (NZMOH 2012b).

STRUCTURAL IMPEDIMENTS TO HEALTHY LIFESTYLES

- Overcrowding
- Lack of access to healthy foods
- Few facilities for exercise, recreation
- Few culturally appropriate support systems, sources of guidance
- Judgemental attitudes
- Low social capital

Overcrowding is a challenge for those who wish to refrain from smoking or alcohol use, when others are engaging in these behaviours (AIHW 2011; Passey et al. 2011). Overcrowding can be especially difficult for adolescents, who may find the influence of peers and other family members difficult to

BOX 13.5 Kaupapa Māori smoking cessation initiatives

Rates of smoking among Māori remain high when compared with non-Māori—particularly among Māori women, 44% of whom smoke (NZMOH 2012b). Failure of smoking cessation programs for Māori have been attributed to their focus on the individual (Barnett et al. 2009) and a lack of relevance (Fernandez & Wilson 2008). Research indicates smoking cessation programs that are whānau-centred and underpinned by Māori values are more likely to support Māori women to quit (Grigg et al. 2008). Gifford (2011) and Glover (2000) both stress the need for Kaupapa Māori interventions.

Providing smoking cessation is an important role for all nurses—particularly for Māori nurses who work in Kaupapa Māori health services and often act as role models for other Māori women. But rates of smoking among Māori nurses are also high at 21.5% (Gifford et al. 2013) when compared to non-Māori nurses at 16.5% (Edwards et al. 2008). Nurses who smoke are at risk of poorer health, suffer the disapproval and misunderstanding of other non-smoking health professionals (Ponniah & Blomfield 2008) and find giving smoking prevention and cessation information to their clients harder than their non-smoking colleagues (Radsma & Bortloff 2009; O'Donovan 2009). Nurses who smoke also see themselves as inadequate role models, and their sense of hypocrisy reduces their ability to work with patients who smoke (Radsma & Bortloff 2009).

In 2012, a group of researchers started working together to develop a program to support Māori nurses to quit smoking so that they may be better able to support the whānau they work with to quit smoking. Using a Kaupapa Māori research methodology, the group firstly consulted with Māori nurses to develop an appropriate methodology for the study. They then surveyed Māori nurses to determine smoking prevalence, perceptions and experiences (Gifford et al. 2013). Finally they began talking with Māori nurses to develop an appropriate program of intervention that will increase the number of quit attempts and support the nurses to become smoke free.

? How do you think being a smoker impacts on a nurse's ability to provide smoking cessation advice? What other examples of Indigenous-led research are you aware of? How does this approach support Indigenous people to become self-determining?

overcome in their struggle for independence, especially when others are engaging in harmful behaviours (AIHW 2011). Most remote-living Indigenous girls have few outside influences and little access to reproductive advice or culturally appropriate health service providers. This situation may explain the teenage birth rate, which is five times that of non-Indigenous teenagers (AIHW 2011). Housing and the health needs of these young people are important elements of the Australian Government's 'closing the gap' initiatives as well as the policies of state governments (AIHW 2011; Australian Government 2013a; VCOSS 2013). Plans have been outlined to provide decent homes for Indigenous people wherever they live. Housing is being addressed by building new homes in areas where crowding is worst, improving the condition of existing houses, making sure new houses are designed and built for their locations, and ensuring arrangements for maintaining homes (Australian Government 2013a). Programs are also being developed to strengthen primary health care services and cultural supports for the SDH of Indigenous people of all ages. These programs have attracted considerable funding to focus on children and adolescents, their education, health, recreation and employment needs in the context of maintaining Indigenous identities while developing and sustaining health and wellbeing (Australian Government 2013a, b; VCOSS 2013).

In New Zealand, around 13% of Māori households are overcrowded. Although overcrowding rates have been decreasing for Māori, the disparity between European and Māori rates of overcrowding has remained the same with six times as many Māori people living in overcrowded situations than non-Māori (Flynn et al. 2010). Housing has also become less affordable for Māori with 29% now paying more than 30% of their income on housing compared with 8% in 1988. Home ownership rates have also been declining—by 13.4% for Māori, but by only 9% for European (Flynn et al. 2010). In a literature review on Māori housing experiences, Waldegrave et al. (2006) noted that Māori conceptualisation of housing may be different to that of non-Māori and this needs to be considered in relation to housing stock. For example, although European people may consider a house as a material resource, this is not always the case for Māori who may view housing in a similar way to how they view land—as something they hold guardianship over for the next generation. Remaining cognisant of these differing views is important for nurses working with families to obtain safe and appropriate housing.

The combination of physical activity and good nutrition is a key factor in overcoming the risks of chronic illness. However, over half of Indigenous people who live in urban or regional communities in Australia do little or no physical exercise, many of whom also report no usual daily fruit or vegetable consumption (AIHW 2012b). Māori do similar levels of activity to European New Zealanders, but are less likely to eat the recommended levels of fruit (NZMOH 2012b). Poor nutrition has been attributed to a lack of access to local produce, inappropriate storage facilities and the prohibitive costs of transportation (Australian Government 2013a). Inadequate access to nutritious food and low levels of physical activity can also be linked to a lack of Indigenous community initiated and managed programs, based on local resources and cultural supports. Supporting lifestyle changes depends on the interplay between the physical environment, human behaviour and social policy (McDonald et al. 2010). So instead of developing either individual or wide-sweeping policies and programs aimed at all Indigenous people, it is important to identify local systems that could support a portfolio of interventions that are relevant and sustainable for the local environment (Signal et al. 2012). The community environment must be enabling, and ready to support and nurture culturally appropriate change. In addition, there must be a commitment to developing knowledge and skills in a way that will empower local people to help one another (McDonald et al. 2010). Where external advice is needed, there must be mutual trust. Where outsiders 'parachute in' to help initiate change in any community, there is always the possibility that those receiving the expert advice may feel excluded, which can erode social capital (Biddle 2012). The tenuous relationship between health promotion personnel and community residents can be strengthened through collaborative processes. For example, in helping a community manage nutrition/food security and physical activity, community input is necessary to solve the problems of affordability of healthy foods, understand families' needs for nutrition literacy, and identify which environmental features could be modified to support culturally appropriate physical activities (see Box 13.6). Signal et al. (2012) also advocate Health Impact Assessments on all interventions so that any unseen risks to sustainability may be identified.

Some culturally appropriate programs have been successful in helping family and local groups increase their participation in sports and improve levels of physical activity, but most have been short-term and lack rigorous evaluation data that would indicate how they can be sustained (AIHW 2012b). External advisors have to guard against stereotypical attitudes, such as conveying the notion that physical activity is morally 'right', which can disempower those who, for whatever reason, decline to participate (Nelson et al. 2010:504). A more subtle attitude that exists in Australia and New Zealand is that Indigenous people, especially young men, are esteemed as having innate sporting abilities, while simultaneously being portrayed as being unreliable or ill-disciplined (Nelson et al. 2010). At a superficial level, appreciating the strength and ability of young Indigenous people may sound acceptable, but it can also produce racial stereotypes that negate other dimensions of their cultural wealth, including academic and employment contributions to society (Nelson et al. 2010). Some of these stereotypical views are a legacy of the past, when young Indigenous men were encouraged to participate in sports to become 'civilised'. Clearly, this view is dismissive of and devalues the cultural and social context of sport (Nelson et al. 2010:501). Perpetuating this type of image can also place pressure on young Indigenous men to perform in sports, which is discouraging if aspirations cannot be met. Once again, the structural inadequacies in remote areas are a barrier to participation because of the lack of appropriate equipment, trainers and activities as well as the hot climate. In the final analysis it is the combination of structural disadvantage, disempowerment, low social capital and a lack of peer support that can create a propensity towards unhealthy lifestyles that last throughout the life course (Biddle 2012; Dulin et al. 2011).

INJURY AND FAMILY VIOLENCE

Indigenous Australians and Māori also suffer from a greater intentional and non-intentional burden of injury than non-Indigenous citizens, some from habitual subsistence activities, and for those in remote areas, injuries from road trauma, because of unchecked safety automobile standards and poor road conditions (Plani & Carson 2008). Injury-related deaths among Indigenous people are nearly three times as high as non-Indigenous deaths, and account for twice the amount of hospitalisations. Most are injuries inflicted by another person, at a rate 12 times that of non-Indigenous people (AIHW 2012a). In New Zealand the rate of injury is 1.5 times higher among Māori. One of the most significant causes of injuries is domestic and family violence, with Indigenous Australian women and Māori women in New Zealand being several times more likely to be victims of intimate partner violence (IPV) than non-Māori women (Families Commission 2009). As mentioned in Chapter 7, for Māori, family violence is considered to be at epidemic levels (Te Puni Kokiri

BOX 13.6 Project REPLACE

The New Zealand Healthy Eating Healthy Action (HEHA) Strategy is an initiative of the New Zealand Health Strategy aimed at reducing health disparities by improving the health of Māori communities. As part of HEHA, project REPLACE was devised as a program to promote healthy environments and practices tailored to the particular needs of each of six Māori communities (Hamerton et al. 2012). It was planned around the principles of the Ottawa Charter; that is, to create supportive environments; develop personal skills; strengthen community action, and reorient existing health services. A Kaupapa Māori approach required face-to-face engagement with community members to create trusting relationships and develop a 'by Māori for Māori' approach to helping people change based on their conceptions, responses and experiences of what would be appropriate for their community. The project team provided the communities with different tools depending on their self-identified needs. These tools included education, and individual plans to help improve nutritional knowledge, increase physical activity and reduce obesity, all based on the physical, mental, spiritual and family/social dimensions of health. What each project had in common was a set of goals as follows:

Regular exercise   Replace 1 short drive in the car with a walk.

Eat healthy food   Replace 1 pie normally eaten with fruit.

Participate   Replace 1 TV program to go out and exercise.

Lose weight   Replace 1 takeaway meal with a home cooked one.

Alcohol reduction   Replace 1 alcoholic drink with juice.

Cut out smoking   Replace 1 cigarette with a glass of water.

Educate   Replace 1 negative thought with a positive one.

Some communities shared recipes, discussed portion sizes and other dietary information; others established community gardens. Increased activities included dancing, tai chi or different types of fitness initiatives combining cultural music with the activity. Some groups combined physical activities with gathering food, planning unique walking adventures or discussing traditional food practices, including planned changes to school menus. In the context of evaluating the outcomes the project team found a 'ripple effect', where small lifestyle changes made from the 'bottom-up' led to broader changes that filtered through to the community. Focus groups with participants indicated that the program was appreciated and effective, especially in having reinforced the cultural focus that made it acceptable and appropriate in the community context. They concluded that because the program was grounded in cultural and community-based initiatives, there is a greater likelihood that it will be sustainable.

2010). There are numerous violence programs to counter this type of violence, including those that focus specifically on Indigenous people. These provide support, counselling and advocacy. Some focus on strengthening identity, behavioural reform, community policing and monitoring, and many provide shelter, protection and legal support (Plani & Carson 2008). As we reported in Chapter 7, many assaults against women and children are fuelled by alcohol and have variable levels of follow-up. There is also a lack of appropriate preparation for those providing emergency care and support, and inconsistent screening for violence. Because many Indigenous victims of violence live in remote areas, they are also disadvantaged by distance from services, especially where specialist intervention is required. The onus is often on ambulance paramedics and police to provide emergency

life-saving treatment, to manage their trauma and minimise transfer problems. These tasks are frequently undertaken in collaboration with local elders, who can help ease the tension between family members or family groups.

IPV AND INJURY

Indigenous Australian and New Zealand Māori women are significantly more likely to be victims of intimate partner violence than non-Indigenous women.

Health professionals and nurses working in remote areas of Australia have also attempted to contend with the problem of child sexual assaults, which inspired 'the intervention' mentioned previously. It is a serious issue, as is any case of oppression against children, but solutions are often masked by the media hysteria that has not recognised the effective interventions that have been quietly taking place in communities confronting sexual violence (Cripps & McGlade 2008). Part of the problem is the lack of evaluative data that would provide benchmarks for successful interventions. The other aspect of the problem that has not been widely publicised is the context in which violence is regularly occurring. Cripps and McGlade (2008) categorise the contextual realities of violence in Indigenous communities in two groups. Group 1 factors include colonisation: policies and practices, dispossession and cultural dislocation, including removal of families. Group 2 factors include marginalisation as a minority, direct and indirect racism, unemployment and welfare dependency, previous history of abuse, poverty, destructive coping behaviours, addictions, physical and mental health issues, and low self-esteem and a sense of powerlessness. Research findings have shown that a disproportionate number of victims of violence are people who have been removed from their families, those with disabilities and people who are living in low-income households or are unemployed (Cripps & McGlade 2008). In New Zealand the Te Rito New Zealand Family Violence Prevention Strategy is aimed at reducing the incidence of family violence among both Māori and non-Māori families through a variety of approaches, including the development of practice guidelines, extensive training for health professionals, and the appointment of family violence intervention coordinators in all District Health Boards.

EMPOWERMENT AND SELF-DETERMINATION

To date, programs to tackle violence in Indigenous communities have not yielded positive results, although there are some improvements. The problems surround 'law and order' interventions, which have left women fearful of retribution if their oppressor is released from custody. Restorative justice programs are considered a positive step towards resolution. These include holding offenders responsible for their behaviour, without stigmatising them; giving victims a greater voice in the criminal justice process, with a say in how the offender is treated; devising punishments aimed at repairing the harm done; and restoring community safety (Cripps & McGlade 2008). Cripps and McGlade describe a 'best practice' example of this type of approach from Canada, where a Community Holistic Circle Healing process has been developed on the basis of the

healing power of both the law and the community. The program focuses as much on the abuser as the victim, and requires a long-term commitment to spiritual healing and restoration. Its success rate has been widely acknowledged, with a low recidivism rate of offending, cost effectiveness and community empowerment. The Community Holistic Circle Healing program is an example of culturally sensitive, community self-determination. It is a model adopted by other Indigenous groups, particularly in North America where the healing circles have been used to help people with the intergenerational trauma of having been removed from their families (Menzies 2008). A similar program has been implemented in South Australia, where a multidimensional community healing project has been successful in developing community capacity to deal with violence (Kowanko et al. 2009).

BEST PRACTICE IN HEALING
- Cultural, spiritual approaches
- Self-determination
- Restorative justice

These models are a response to the disempowerment that occurs when diagnostic approaches to mental health issues tend to re-traumatise the victims, excluding meaningful discussions of culture that might help them move forward (Menzies 2008). However, critics of this approach argue that it is not consistent with Indigenous tradition or culture, which would severely punish offenders for such crimes as sexual assault. Other criticisms include the risk of powerful members of the community being able to interfere with the healing processes, which could potentially have a negative impact on the victim, especially if these were previous perpetrators of abuse. Cripps and McGlade (2008) contend that the restorative justice approach has a better chance of being effective than the current adversarial legal system, which often subjects sexual assault victims to further abuse from the Australian justice system. They recommend adapting the healing model in culturally appropriate contexts in Australia, in a way that does not cause further discrimination on the basis of gender or race (Cripps & McGlade 2008). This intersection of gender and race that was mentioned in Chapter 10 is a major problem for Indigenous women who have been subjected to institutional racism. For many, identifying with the Indigenous community rather than with other women exposes them to a different kind of pressure than that experienced by non-Indigenous women (Kowanko et al. 2009). In some cases, the way they have been treated in refuges and health services has been re-traumatising, creating new cycles of victimisation (Vincent & Eveline 2008). Clearly, the solutions lie in refraining from discussing family violence as an Indigenous problem, and ensuring that it is included in policies and practices that recognise the gendered power relations between men and women, and the structural factors that perpetuate inequalities in the roles of men and women.

MENTAL HEALTH AND HEALING

A large proportion of Indigenous Australians and New Zealand Māori of every age group report high levels of psychological distress (AIHW 2012a; NZMOH 2013b). However, like members of other cultures, the experience of distress is often linked to the way individuals manage their embeddedness in their culture, how they preserve the social order, and their relationship to the social and natural environment (Fisher 2006). In Australia, remote-living Indigenous people tend to have higher levels of social participation with other Indigenous people than their urban counterparts, and sometimes this can intensify their feelings of sadness and distress to a greater extent than those who have diverse social networks (Biddle 2012). Mental illness is prevalent in some of these communities; it is the leading cause of disease burden after cardiovascular disease (ABS AIHW 2008). For many Indigenous people, seeking outside help for psychological distress or mental illness is a source of shame and embarrassment, and may be seen as culturally inappropriate (Anderson 2008). These feelings can lead some people to self-stigmatise, feeling ashamed of their difficulties, and mistrust mainstream services (Isaacs et al. 2012). For Māori, if psychological distress is perceived by the family to be associated with makatu (a penalty for the infringement of tapu or sacredness), regardless of the severity of the illness, all effort will be made to avoid medical intervention (Durie 2001). Counselling those who are in distress must therefore be cognisant of the person's worldview. Whereas Western medical approaches to counselling tend to revolve around crisis management, counselling Indigenous people moves through a circular process of holistic, spiritual and cultural understandings of the contextual realities of a person's life, family context and past experiences (Stewart 2008). Local cultural understandings are typically different from a non-Indigenous perspective where mental illness may be seen as a parallel concept to physical illness.

Assessing an Indigenous person's mental health must be done in a way that is sensitive to the way mental health is conceptualised, whether this embodies makatu as mentioned above, or alternative views. For example, some Indigenous Australian groups may believe they are being 'sung' by an aggrieved party, married the 'wrong way', 'caught out' by the law or 'crying for Country'. The latter example illustrates the interrelatedness of health and place, acknowledging Indigenous people's close connection to Country. The other major aspect of holistic, spiritual perspectives lies in the profound effect on many Indigenous people from a history of loss, separation, traumatic experiences and previous experiences with mental health services, all of which frame the way new events are experienced (AIHW 2012f; Isaacs et al. 2012). Therapeutic approaches therefore must be based on understanding of the cultural meanings of kinship, the land, spirituality and heritage (O'Brien 2006). The Whare Tapa Wha Māori Model of Health developed by Mason Durie in New Zealand articulates a concept of holism that has been adopted by many Māori and non-Māori, as a means of understanding the way in which Māori conceptualise health. The four cornerstones of the Whare Tapa Wha model are Hinengaro (mental wellbeing), Tinana (physical wellbeing), Whānau (family wellbeing) and Wairua (spiritual wellbeing). Each cornerstone is interlinked, and health may not be achieved without a balance between all four cornerstones (Durie 1994).

As a spiritual journey, healing requires time and a culturally safe, capacity-strengthening approach to assist in the recovery from past traumas, addictions or other problems. The journey is aimed at cultural renewal and strengthening identity, often through language, dance and song, all of which can help a person reconnect with family, community and culture (AIHW 2012f). The 'by Māori for Māori' health services in New Zealand, as outlined previously, has been one approach to addressing many of the cultural needs of Māori as they seek to address their health needs. These services are based in both traditional settings, such as hospitals, and in non-traditional settings, such as on Marae (Māori meeting ground). Importantly, past traumas, such as those experienced by the Stolen Generations, cannot be resolved until there is government and societal acknowledgement of the source of these problems. Left unresolved, the history of trauma can lead people to internalise shame and guilt, and whole communities can begin to think that pain and chaos is normal (AIHW 2012f). Long-term grief and trauma can become transgenerational, and can lead to dysfunctional family life, including violence, self-harm and suicide. In Australia, Indigenous suicide rates are estimated to be twice that of non-Indigenous people; in some cases up to 70% higher, particularly for males (AIHW 2012f). A study by Vicary and Bishop (2005) revealed that some Indigenous people can fall into a depressed and anxious mood state, needing to go to Country, restless to connect with their land in a way that a depressed non-Indigenous person would not experience. This unique need may explain why so many Indigenous men who suffer from mental illness or the combination of mental illness and substance use problems do not find traditional services helpful (Isaacs et al. 2012). In Vicary and Bishop's (2005) study, male research participants explained that Indigenous men were more likely to be predisposed to mental ill health, because of the weakening of their traditional role as a provider. This caused the men to have low self-esteem, depression and an inability to see practical alternatives, whereas the women felt they could not afford to become ill, because they had taken over the key family functions (Vicary & Bishop 2005). One of the implications of this study is that healing should take place 'on Country' in the context of gender-sensitive, culturally appropriate conversations, rather than in the type of health facilities or therapeutic approaches used by non-Indigenous people.

WHARE TAPA WHA

- Mental wellbeing
- Physical wellbeing
- Family wellbeing
- Spiritual wellbeing

A number of health promotion programs have been developed to respond to the problem of young men's mental health, all of which include cultural healing and counselling. The Indigenous Hip Hop program and an Indigenous adaptation of the Resourceful Adolescent Program, MindMatters have been helpful. The Aboriginal and Torres Strait Islander Healing Foundation was instituted to help prevent suicide and self-harm and improve emotional wellbeing, particularly among members of the Stolen Generation (AIHW 2012f). Various Indigenous groups and initiatives have also used motivational interviewing and planning (see Chapter 4), but in the absence of formal evaluations it is difficult to measure their impact. The most effective approaches to suicide prevention and emotional wellbeing seem to be those that restore culturally and economically sustainable homelands

as place-based initiatives for strengthening the cultural transmission of values, language and a sense of the future (Pearson 2009). Stronger bonds with the land provide a grassroots opportunity to foster confidence and help Indigenous people develop resilience and cultural identity, which can act as protective factors against mental ill health. Suicide rates have also been found to be lower in communities that have achieved self-determination through title to and governance over traditional lands and services (AIHW 2012f).

Identity is integral to all of these approaches (AIHW 2012e). Kickett-Tucker (2009) explains that Australian literature confuses racial identity with cultural identity, group identity, collective identity, ethnic identity and self-concept. Racial identity can be a source of confusion and conflict, especially in the context of racism in society, and this can, in turn, compromise an individual's self-esteem (Kickett-Tucker 2009). Kickett-Tucker's (2009) interviews with young Aboriginal children were designed to investigate racial identity as a social construct, shaped by their interactions with others, and with social structures surrounding their lives. The children revealed that a strong sense of self, connection to family and kin, Aboriginal language, culture, inheritance, appearance and friends, all were important contributors to their racial identity, which was the centre of their health and wellbeing. This sense of identity has a protective function, helping children learn to deal with stressors such as racism in their environment, and providing them with a circle of strength, love and support (Kickett-Tucker 2009). Clearly, primary prevention for mental health in Indigenous people requires major interdisciplinary initiatives by child care, education, health and social service professionals, to ensure the secure development of identity formation.

One approach to Indigenous mental health is to support communities to 'flourish'. 'Flourishing' is a term used to describe a sustainable state of mental wellbeing or positive mental health. People who are flourishing in their mental health have happier, more meaningful lives, better physical health, and better social outcomes (Norris 2011). The ability to flourish is linked to the values, practice and communities in which individuals and collectives interact (Blisset 2011). Where a community is faced with multiple challenges to self-determination—such as many indigenous communities—the ability to flourish may be limited. In order to identify what factors may support Māori to flourish, Blisset (2011) interviewed nine Māori informants for their perspectives and definitions of flourishing. Together, he and the nine informants identified five elements that are considered essential for Māori mental wellbeing to flourish. First, having a strong connection with the land was required to ensure a positive identity and to be proud to be Māori. Second, flourishing was seen as a platform for future generations to build on, an important element of intergenerational continuity. Third, Māori participants noted that there was no point in only individuals flourishing, it had to be the collective—if one member of a whānau was not flourishing, then the whānau could not flourish. Fourth, ensuring health was essential. This included having access to traditional healing techniques such as rongoā Māori and mirimiri, having warm, smoke-free houses, and taking part in kapa haka for physical activity. Finally, choice and self-determination were key requirements (Blisset 2011). Embedding these elements into mental health programs may support communities to flourish, enabling indigenous communities to build self-esteem and maintain mental wellbeing.

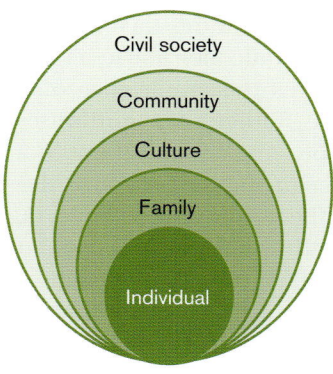

FIGURE 13.2
Protecting, preserving, empowering self, family, culture, society

---

FLOURISHING

- Connection to land
- Intergenerational connections
- Group must flourish
- Access to supports for health
- Choice and self-determination

STRENGTHENING CAPACITY AND SOCIAL CAPITAL

The oppression of Indigenous people is indisputable, and it creates enormous challenges for medical practitioners, nurses, midwives, paramedics, health workers, teachers, police and other professionals working in Indigenous communities. For all of these health advocates the objective is to work out ways of helping people retrieve their sense of self, family, culture, community and society (see Figure 13.2). This can begin through delving into the root causes of a set of behaviours such as alcohol or substance misuse that create cycles of risk, then working with individuals and families to see what can be done to reset the pattern for a more optimistic future. Noel Pearson (2004) and members of the Cape York Institute in Australia's Cape York Peninsula have devoted considerable effort to studying risk and potential in Indigenous people. For example, they address the problem of drug and alcohol abuse, criticising some of the ways it has been addressed in the past. They reject most of the common approaches used by those seeking to change behaviour. For

example, the 'symptom theory', which sees addiction as a symptom of societal problems, is seen as unhelpful. The theory argues that symptoms can be redressed by understanding social and historical wrongs, and rearranging the person's environment. Likewise, they reject the 'voluntary rehabilitation' perspective. This approach holds the expectation that addicts will eventually seek help for their addiction. Another perspective, the 'normalisation' or 'responsible drinking' view is based on the notion that promoting responsible drinking will effect behaviour change, while the 'harm minimisation' approach is aimed at dealing with the consequences of abuse by trying to minimise harm to self and others. According to Pearson (2004) and Rothwell (2013b) none of these is as effective as intolerance of abuse. Pearson (2004) equates the problems of substance abuse with other risky conditions—tobacco smoking, poor environmental health and poor nutrition—as all of these have a major impact on families and communities. He argues that the responsibility lies in the following five social conditions: availability of the addictive or harmful substance; easily accessible money to acquire the substance; spare time to use it; others in the immediate environment who are engaged in the behaviour; and a permissive social ideology that reinforces the behaviour (Pearson 2004:8).

PREVENTING SUBSTANCE ABUSE

Develop community-determined and community-managed strategies that build on family and community strengths to create a place where young people can develop identity, capacity and self-esteem.

Pearson's (2004) solution to the problem is to reduce these precipitating factors, charging that an over-emphasis on alcohol abuse as a health problem obscures the importance of political and social ideology. Rather than minimise the harm by reducing supply or demand, there is a need to deal with the consequences, to manage the situation from within the community, conveying basic convictions and establishing a sense of the future. Instead of focusing on disadvantage as an outcome of colonial history, he suggests that a community-determined, community-managed strategy would be a better focus to help put hope into people's hearts, and improve governance in their communities. This involves rebuilding tolerance, controlling the supply, managing money and time, instituting treatment and rehabilitation programs, and fixing up homes and the community to restore social and cultural capital (Cape York Institute 2013). It also involves making the family and community viable, as places where young people can develop their capacity and personal self-esteem. A parallel approach could be applied to violence against women and children. Ideally, this would involve empowering the community from within, modifying environmental conditions so that they are not conducive to violence and abuse, ensuring there is available, viable employment, appropriate role models, strong cultural identity and a sense of self-worth.

The Cape York agenda for change is framed in the language of the Nobel Prize winning economist Amartya Sen. Sen's philosophy, as mentioned earlier in this book, revolves around *substantive freedom*. Indigenous people require a range of choices and having the capabilities to choose a life that they have reason to value (Pearson 2005). This means that resources cannot simply be allocated to people with an expectation that they will improve their lives. Networks of families, communities and businesses do not emerge from bureaucratic power, but from a combination of public order and safety, and the motivation to develop skill, self-confidence and personal responsibility. This argument posits that Indigenous people need support and resources, but these must be accessed by members of the community seeking to enhance and revitalise their capacity and that of their community in a way that is mutually responsive and accountable. A stable, functioning family is the moral core of a community, the repository of the seeds of social capital. Any resources given to the community are thus *socially invested* and help the community build its own capacity through individuals bonding with one another, bridging together with other communities, and establishing linkages within

interactions with institutions. Mignone and O'Neil (2005:S53) explain that this is a 'culture where families can help each other due to strong norms of reciprocity, where different community sectors and leadership offer support to families in need, where youth sense that they can trust adults before or during moments of crisis'. It is also a well-resourced environment where governments ensure land title, where Indigenous language and culture are seen as national priorities (Pearson, 2005:10).

GOALS FOR INDIGENOUS HEALTH

- Eliminate racism and all forms of discrimination against Indigenous people.
- Address the social determinants of disadvantage and inequity for Indigenous people.
- Improve child and youth health and wellbeing through perinatal and early childhood intervention and prevention strategies.
- Recognise the uniqueness and importance of Indigenous family and extended family networks.
- Promote public acceptance of the unique needs and sensitivities of Indigenous people.
- Improve the cultural responsiveness of mainstream services through better transparency and accountability, and develop specific services tailored to cultural needs.
- Develop a well-resourced evidence base for best practice in Indigenous health.
- Recognise the impact of environmental degradation on Indigenous people, and create genuine opportunities for affected communities to participate in decision-making for environmental restoration.
- Acknowledge the uniqueness of Indigenous systems of knowledge in caring for Country.
- Maintain the health of Indigenous people as the highest priority for health planning.
- Support the development of economic, social and cultural capital to foster self-determinism, and strategies for culturally appropriate, sufficiently resourced education and skill development.
- Adopt strategies for intersectoral collaboration in all policies and planning strategies at all levels.
- Ensure cultural safety in all service provision for all people.
- Enshrine diversity and culture in the laws and social processes of the country.

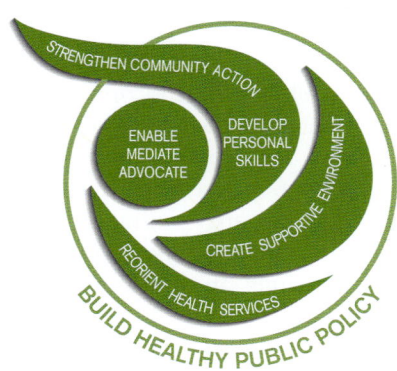

Building healthy public policy

Healthy public policies are those that ensure access and equity of different cultural groups, and that guide action on inequalities. They are based on the understanding that social inclusion is a social determinant of health equity (Baum et al. 2010). Achieving equity and, therefore, social justice begins with acknowledging the inter-relatedness of health, place and economic viability. At the international level, the Geneva Declaration on the Health and Survival of Indigenous People (WHO 1999) has not yet been successful in encouraging all countries to address Indigenous inequities. This reflects the failure of non-Indigenous governments to enshrine their obligations to Indigenous people in law or policy. Adequate policy development requires national initiatives around five major areas: evidence-based decision-making on Indigenous health issues; incorporating traditional health knowledge in health promotion systems; improving health systems' capacity to identify, and meet the needs of marginalised, ethnic populations; poverty-reduction strategies; and political will to better meet the health and development needs of all marginalised populations (WHO 1999).

SOCIAL INCLUSION

A social determinant of health equity.

The rhetoric of health policy in Australia and New Zealand reflects a commitment to each of these international recommendations. However, much remains to be done to develop policies that will bring about change. The 'closing the gap' initiatives established by the Australian government demonstrate a commitment to improving the policy environment that would affect Indigenous people

across the lifespan (Australian Government 2013 a, b). Some of the most important policy initiatives are aimed at mental health reform, especially the 2013 National Aboriginal and Torres Strait Islander Suicide Prevention Strategy, which focuses on early intervention and the need for stronger community supports (Australian Govt, Online. Available: www.health.gov.au/internet/ministers/publishing.nsf/Content/mr-yr13-mb-mb052.htm [accessed 25 June 2013]). The strategy was produced by an interdisciplinary Indigenous and non-Indigenous group who have identified social and emotional wellbeing as the centrepiece of the policy. The policy focus on community is crucial, and is an attempt to respond to reports by community leaders that many of their Aboriginal communities have become dysfunctional as well as disadvantaged in relation to the social order that exists in mainstream communities (Cape York Institute 2013). Organisations like the Cape York Institute argue that there is a need to rebuild from the ground up with a social, cultural, spiritual and legal intolerance of substance abuse rather than harm minimisation, and to develop food security policies to help control both obesity and hunger in remote territories (Cape York Institute 2013). Indigenous-specific elements of the National Drug Strategy have been developed to guide actions on substance misuse and petrol sniffing in remote areas, and some of these initiatives have yielded results, particularly in reducing petrol sniffing (Australian Government 2013b).

ACTION POINT

Use tools such as Health Impact Assessment with input from Indigenous people to determine the potential impact of any policy on Indigenous people's health.

Other 'closing the gap' policies have been aimed at creating a stronger sense of identity among Indigenous Australians, especially among young people. The policies also include support for culture and language expression, antenatal care, pre-pregnancy and teenage sexual and reproductive health, mothers and babies care, early childhood and adolescent education (Australian Government 2013b), but the outcomes of these policies are unclear in terms of health improvements. It will be important to track the impact of these new policies on closing the disadvantage gap as well as the gap in life expectancy, and this will require substantial research funding to generate the appropriate evidence base. In the past, there has been inadequate data from which to evaluate the effectiveness of government initiatives, especially with multi-level state-Commonwealth collaborations. Previous barriers to health improvement have also included a lack of local consultation in implementing many programs for Indigenous people. Some of the worst examples include programs for violence and/or suicide prevention implemented in communities that have not had the greatest need. For example, because funding is allocated to violence prevention, and because there have been reports of violence among some Indigenous communities, numerous grant applications from Indigenous communities have been successful, whether their community has a violence problem or not. This type of untargeted funding does not ensure that programs will be effective where they are most needed. Another barrier lies in the complexity of funding arrangements from different layers of government bureaucracy, and a mixture of private, public and Aboriginal Medical Services (AMS). There is no over-arching policy about the need for accountability, which means that funding is not always linked with health outcomes. Instead, 'bucket funding', where program money is allocated from specific buckets of money, creates duplication in some places, and service gaps in others (Hudson 2009).

Despite New Zealand's ongoing commitment to Māori health articulated in policy documents such as the New Zealand Health Strategy (NZMOH 2000), the New Zealand Primary Health Care Strategy (King 2001), He Korowai Oranga: the Māori Health Strategy (NZMOH 2002a), the Māori Mental Health Strategic Framework (NZMOH 2002b), and the Māori Health Action Plan (NZMOH 2006), the fact remains that, as outlined above, the health status of New Zealand Māori remains poor and ethnic inequalities persist. The most recent policy imperative designed to address Māori health is the Whānau Ora approach to social service provision. As mentioned in Chapter 7, Whānau Ora, which is defined as 'families supported to achieve their maximum health and well-being' (NZMOH 2002a), is designed to reduce health and social wellbeing disparities among vulnerable families. The Whānau Ora approach has been a key policy platform of the Māori Party. The Māori Party was formed in 2004 and supported the National-led government at the 2008 election. Following the election, the two co-leaders of the Māori party became ministers outside of Cabinet from where they were able to push through the Whānau Ora policy. Whānau Ora is now well-embedded in New Zealand health and social policy and has developed into a philosophy, a distinct model of practice, and an outcome (Boulton

et al. 2013). The core principles of a Whānau Ora approach are derived from both Māori cultural beliefs and values, and from best practice in public policy (Boulton et al. 2013). Appropriate resourcing, intersectoral practice, competent and culturally safe practitioners, and a focus on whānau capacity are common elements of successful Whānau Ora approaches. Challenges are associated with the differing understandings of what Whānau Ora is across different settings, and the importance of ensuring communities are involved in identifying and addressing priorities (Boulton et al. 2013). Whānau Ora has been described as a formalisation of what Kaupapa Māori health providers have been doing for many years (Boulton et al. 2013) and there have been some initial successes as the policy is rolled out across mainstream providers as well (NZMOH 2013d). Longitudinal evaluation of the wide variety of Whānau Ora initiatives will be required to determine if the policy is successful in the long term.

In Australia, criticisms of the existing arrangements for Indigenous health continue. Some argue that, despite the failures, there are no new policies, simply old policies recycled (Hudson 2009). Most of the old, recycled policies simply thrust money at an undefined target called 'Indigenous health', aimed at 'closing the gap' in life expectancy. Continually highlighting the 'gap' instead of lifestyle factors, or gender issues, perpetuates the notion that every problem is related to race (Hudson 2009). This can be damaging not only as a racist approach, but in developing inappropriate health plans. For example, when maternal smoking and Indigenous status are disentangled and shown as separate risk factors, the difference between non-Indigenous and Indigenous low birth weight infants disappears (Hudson 2009). Similarly, failing to identify violence against women as a gender issue masks it as an Indigenous problem. The focus of health promotion policies to deal with these issues should therefore be maternal smoking and gender, rather than Indigenous status. Likewise, the appalling state of housing of remote-living Indigenous people should be seen as the main cause of rheumatic fever and infectious diseases, rather than attributing these to Indigenous status (Hudson 2009; McDonald et al. 2009). Acknowledging the source of the problems is crucial to developing appropriate solutions.

ACTION POINT

First acknowledge the source of problems.

justice system. Youth programs, community policing and night patrols can help convey the impression that the community, not the legal or corrections systems, is accountable for behavioural outcomes. When these pro-social reinforcements of community self-determination are established in the community, there is a higher likelihood of developing local leaders and cohesive structures for harmony (Ryan et al. 2006). For example, the Māori warden program operating in many towns and cities in New Zealand provides a culturally safe community patrol to assist young Māori and others who may be on the streets. School-based programs also help strengthen the environment, especially when programs are thoughtfully conceived, and based on in-depth knowledge of the community. The National Children's Nutrition Survey in New Zealand, for example, found that Māori children and Pacific island children were significantly more likely to skip meals and to purchase food items from school tuckshops than non-Indigenous New Zealand children (Utter et al. 2006). Despite the fact that these children were generally physically active, many skipped breakfast and had a low intake of fresh fruits and vegetables, whereas their snack foods contained high sugar and carbohydrate content. Numerous research studies have shown that there is a direct relationship between a diet low in fruit and vegetables and poverty. Therefore programs to improve nutritional health should begin by lobbying for food subsidies in schools to help children in the setting where they spend the largest part of their day. The New Zealand study showed that obesity among the children was more closely linked to food rather than a lack of exercise, which provides a basis for this type of advocacy (Utter et al. 2006). Since the nutrition study was completed, many New Zealand schools have begun providing food for children in schools as we outlined in Chapter 2. The Milk in Schools program and the Fruit in Schools program are two examples. Some schools also provide a breakfast in schools program to ensure children start the day ready to learn (NZMOH, Online. Available: https://kickstartbreakfast.co.nz/ [accessed 22 September 2013]).

Strengthening community action

Community action means getting involved in the community's self-defined priorities for health and wellbeing. Our general understandings of Indigenous cultures are often limited due to the widespread confusion over land rights, native title, the various levels of regulation, and how laws are interpreted in various areas. Because of the way these issues are presented in the public media, often with densely worded legal arguments, understandings can be open to misinterpretation. Advocacy is an important role for nurses, midwives and other health professionals working with Indigenous people. To be effective, it is important to maintain current knowledge of the decisions that are being taken at the political level. The most important input to our deliberations will come from seeking the views of local Indigenous people on how that may affect their capacity for self-determination. For example, addressing the social ecology within which cultural traditions are preserved also has the potential to reinvigorate Indigenous authority, and retain the transference of land for the next generations. This can create a self-perpetuating cycle of cultural empowerment.

Community action is also locally determined. Actions that are focused on developing and sustaining human capacity must include full participation, a strengths-based approach, long time frames, and intersectoral collaboration (Hunt 2012). As the researchers from the Australian Centre for Independent Studies reported, programs such as those targeting family violence are being developed according to racist policies (Hudson 2009). This is a contradiction of the primary health care (PHC) approach, where community-determined priorities should govern the allocation of resources. A more culturally appropriate program is exemplified by the South Australian Healing program for family violence which is based on a whole-of-community approach, as shown in Box 13.7.

Other strategies to strengthen community action are aimed at developing different types of responses according to self-defined need and preference. The care of children and pregnant women should be a priority in all communities. Initiatives should be developed at the community level, especially in caring for urban-dwelling Indigenous children who may not have the elders and adults available to buffer their experiences of poverty or other types of disadvantage (Milroy 2013). Similarly, mentoring programs from within cultural groups can ensure that young girls receive reproductive advice in a way that is responsive to culture, especially if there are inputs from local health professionals for both mentors and mentees. Birthing on Country programs can be developed for those wanting to access midwifery services in a place where they feel supported by family. This is challenging for high-risk pregnancies, but efforts should be made where possible to try and accommodate cultural needs at the time of childbirth. The most enduring birthing program in the Northern Territory has been the 'Strong Women, Strong Babies, Strong Culture' initiative, which has had a significant effect on improving the birth weight of Indigenous mothers (D'Espaignet et al. 2003).

1   Build community capacity to support safe families. This includes physical as well as cultural safety.

2   Equip Indigenous people with the skills for effective communication and conflict resolution. This includes appropriate counselling and guidance strategies that are aimed at men's and women's styles of communication and confidence building.

3   Support families in crisis. Multidimensional programs focus on both prevention and interventions, which includes helping women find accommodation, support, legal and financial assistance.

4   Build capacity of mainstream agencies and services within the region. This requires intersectoral collaboration and partnerships. In the South Australian program women worked with crafts while learning to manage stress and develop new communication skills. A range of programs can be offered that reinforce existing strengths and help build new ones such as anger management or mutual support networks.

5   Workforce development: support groups require training programs that help build a healing culture. In many cases, staff members suffer burnout and stress, and they require healing support to help them cope.

6   Data and evaluation: systematic evaluation of program effectiveness provides a foundation for change, expansion and sharing knowledge in other programs and centres.

(Source: Kowanko et al. 2009)

will be shaped by introspection on our thoughts, feelings and attitudes. For Indigenous communities, health outcomes will only be improved by solutions that are conjointly developed within authentic partnerships between community members and others they choose to include in their decision-making. This will ensure that planning is closely aligned with the culturally embedded knowledge of the community, as transmitted by the guardians of their culture. If our knowledge lies outside the culture of those we seek to assist, our role is to listen, to reflect on both our culture and theirs, then to see whether we can respond to their needs in a way that adds value to their self-determined solutions. This first step is the most important. Each of us needs to build our own personal understanding and tolerance from a studious approach to Indigenous health. Literally, this means that we first assume the role of learner, having the humility to realise that non-Indigenous voices do not speak for Indigenous people. Second, we need to better understand their perspectives and worldviews, through the lens of culturally appropriate ways of knowing (Nelson et al. 2010). This requires a respectful and receptive attitude, to learn, to build trust, credibility and ultimately, to share intellectual, cultural and social capital. Once these steps have been taken, personal skills can be developed and strengthened in a spirit of mutual capacity building.

STRATEGY FOR ACTION

Implement skills training in health literacy for all people involved in Indigenous health. Practitioners, parents, grandparents, elders, Indigenous health workers and children can then work together to undertake culturally appropriate planning.

Developing personal skills

CULTURAL SAFETY

Personal reflections first: What is my culture and how does it help me understand other cultures?

What do I value in culture and how does it help me understand others' cultural values?

Being culturally safe in our approach to helping people develop personal skills begins with self-development. How we personally approach the problems of inequitable ill health for Indigenous people and others disadvantaged by race or ethnicity

In many Indigenous communities, particularly in rural and remote areas, healthy literacy is the most pressing problem. Education programs in a person's native tongue are helpful in fostering Indigenous identity and providing resources written or presented in the appropriate language is also helpful. Where it is not appropriate or impossible to provide resources in their own language, there will also be a need to support English language comprehension, in order to help Indigenous people develop the ability to read, and understand issues related to health. Some Indigenous adults lack the functional health literacy that would help them read medication labels or understand the instructions given by a medical practitioner, nurse or Aboriginal or Māori health worker (Hudson 2009). Aboriginal health workers (AHW) practise in stressful conditions, sometimes torn between their obligations as a health service employee, and the obligations to their family and community. They are often the only health worker in their remote community, and like the people they are caring for, may also have low literacy and numeracy skills (Hudson 2009). Implementing skills training for health literacy has to be an inclusive strategy, where everyone, including Aboriginal and Māori health workers, parents, grandparents, elders, and health professionals working in a particular community, can come together for culturally appropriate planning. Making health literacy a priority begins with good schooling and connecting schools to the community. In this context, there can be mutual learning opportunities and meaningful input into some of the barriers to learning, such as chronic otitis media, which affects many young children in remote areas. Collaborative learning can also help identify the best way to change such things as hygiene, child development, education and parenting skills. A further step towards developing health literacy is to ensure that health education materials are framed in culturally appropriate, and symbolic language and images that can be linked to the realities of a person's life. This would help counteract some of the problems that have existed in remote communities to date. In some cases, non-English speaking Indigenous people have been provided with written materials with no recognisable message in the local language. This is most evident in diabetes self-management programs, some of which have been given to groups with a lack of both literacy and numeracy, and little understanding of terms like 'elevated blood sugar', 'healthy weight range' or the skills to calculate medications (Hudson 2009:14–15).

One of the findings of Zubrick et al.'s (2005) study of Australian Indigenous children was that there is a 20% loss of Indigenous languages in areas of moderate to extreme geographic isolation. Cultural isolation is also a major problem, often causing emotional difficulties for those especially who have been removed from their natural families in childhood, leaving them unsure of their cultural roots and identities (Eckermann et al. 2010; Kickett-Tucker 2009). Continued efforts must therefore be made to preserve, document, teach and encourage identity and the use of local languages and culture. Cultural heritage is also critical to survival of any particular group, which is the basis for the Whānau Ora approach in New Zealand as outlined earlier in the chapter, where health promotion programs based on community cultural frameworks have been shown to be more effective than any imposed from outside (Hamerton et al. 2012). In both countries, culturally appropriate programs are based on pride, strength, determination and survival, not inadequacies, impairment or hopelessness, which can demonise and disconnect people from their cultural identity. Identifying and building on strengths, instead of deficiencies, is therefore the appropriate approach for intervention. Education programs at the University of Adelaide are currently teaching education students from Indigenous communities to teach in their native language. New graduates of this unique program should be both congratulated and celebrated, as should those who have instigated such an important program, as they provide a more optimistic outlook for the future of Indigenous language retention.

The other major issue for education is to address the reasons for high failure rates among young Indigenous children and plan authentic solutions to invest in their lives. Researchers from the Centre for Independent Studies argue that the government has been overly concentrated on individual performance and overlooked the need for high-performing schools to support Indigenous children and to help raise the expectations and aspirations of their parents (Hughes & Hughes 2012). Even in the rhetoric of 'closing or reducing the gap', the commitment to children's education is not targeted appropriately to solutions that lie in structural conditions. In urban schools as well as those in regional and remote areas, Indigenous children with the same capabilities as non-Indigenous children are prevented from achieving better results by poor schooling. This is also one of the most important priorities of the Cape York Institute which has been lobbying for better instruction methods and stronger teaching programs, both based on research evidence (Hughes & Hughes 2012). Concomitant with better early years education is the need to eliminate welfare dependency through training reform; that is, preparing young people and adults for real employment rather than simply teaching skills that have no job at the end of the training (Hughes & Hughes 2012). The 'Generation One' initiative established by Andrew and Nicola Forrest and other wealthy Australians represents another step in this training reform agenda. As an organisation with several national partners and employers throughout Australia, Generation One provides education, training, mentoring and employment for Indigenous people to help end the disparities between Indigenous and non-Indigenous people (Generation One 2013). A number of successful mentoring programs have been developed for Indigenous youth at risk for problem behaviours. Evaluation data show that the strong connection to culture is foremost among the influences on success, but continuity of at least 12–18 months is another factor. Successful programs are those that begin mentoring before young people exhibit antisocial behaviour. They involve elders, and rely on consistent peer mentoring from other young people who have 'been there, done that', who can inspire strength and convey the importance of taking small steps toward personal empowerment (AIHW 2013).

Education programs in Te Reo Māori are now available in most New Zealand cities and many rural areas as well. Building language skills empowers communities to identify more closely with their communities of origin and the Māori language movement has made important steps toward saving Te Reo Māori, a language that was considered almost dead as recently as 1979 (Ka'ai-Mahuta 2011). The kohanga reo movement was the first to provide Māori language immersion preschool education in the early 1980s and this now extends to Te Reo Māori immersion schools (Te Kura Kaupapa Māori) at primary, intermediate and secondary school levels. The New Zealand Government also provides greater funding for tertiary institutions when doctoral theses are completed in Te Reo Māori. New Zealand is a bilingual country with Te Reo Māori, English, and New Zealand Sign Language recognised as official languages. These initiatives have helped embed Māori language into everyday use although as noted above, this has not always been the case. By the late 1970s there was a belief that the language would die as colonisation and assimilation policies had led to few people willing or able to speak the language publicly. Despite the efforts to save the language, numbers of people speaking Te Reo Māori fluently are still relatively few, and there remains a risk that the language could die (Ka'ai-Mahuta 2011). Government still needs to commit to improving the educational achievement of young Māori through resourcing, policy and support at all levels. Young people achieve well in Te Kura Kaupapa Māori and there is hope that this approach will serve to transform New Zealand society and culture in appropriate and meaningful ways (Takao et al. 2010).

Adopting the WHO Health Promoting Schools approach to enhancing Indigenous capacity is another way to develop personal skills (AIHW 2012e). However, the school approach is reliant on having committed teachers and well-resourced schools who can help children develop health literacy as they are learning other subjects. Schools that are effective in promoting health are those with an Indigenous presence through role models, teachers and mentors. The curriculum must have the flexibility for students to acknowledge and maintain their Indigenous identity, and include family and community members as partners in their education

(AIHW 2012e). This is congruent with the Cape York Partnerships Initiative, based on a family empowerment program for isolated families. Educators in this program used the school setting with young people living in a remote area, and engaged in a step-by-step development of self-knowledge and understanding, in terms of how they fit into the immediate and broader social environment. The young people had an opportunity to explore relationships, issues typical of school attendance, such as bullying, emotions, beliefs and attitudes, and their own needs and aspirations. They were then offered opportunities to connect these with the needs and aspirations of others. The mutual understanding and self-confidence they gained helped reinforce connections between people, and developed the leadership skills for networking and problem-solving (Tsey et al. 2005).

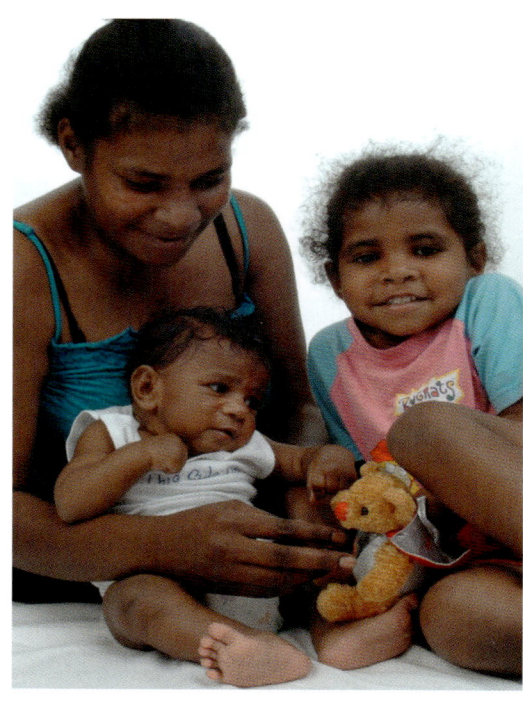

Rita, Freedom and AJ (photo courtesy of Professor Jeanine Young, with permission)

Besides the school connection the core element in helping young children develop cultural identity, health and wellbeing lies in supporting their families. Effective parenting support programs are those that use cultural consultants as well as parent educators and health professionals who can conduct home visiting. This mix of expertise can help provide the dual focus on both the children and their parents, and draw from family strengths as well as the extended cultural group (AIHW 2012c).

Some initiatives to support parenting have also used groups tailored to cultural needs (AIHW 2012c). One such group is the Boomerangs Aboriginal Circle of Security Parenting Camp Program, which is based on attachment theory and aims to improve parent caregiving behaviours and promote child safety. Another is the Group Triple P Positive Parenting Program, modified for Indigenous families to promote effective child behaviour management strategies for behaviour problems and developmental issues. A third program is the Exploring Together program for preschool children and their parents to help with social and emotional development. Each of these programs have been conducted in specific locations for small groups of parents, and each has been evaluated by the parents as improving their parenting confidence. However, these programs require rigorous evaluation to determine their long-term viability across different settings (AIHW 2012c). Although they are successful for those who attend, longer time frames are necessary for all programs to judge the extent to which they are effective for the parents; build trusting relationships with Indigenous families and the community; promote Indigenous understandings and foreshadow long-term change (Lohoar 2012). Importantly, these programs must be delivered in a way that conveys cultural, and multicultural, competence to participants, which is integral to helping with healing past traumas instead of focusing on any deficits in parenting skills (Olavarria et al. 2009). As we outlined in Chapter 6, the Halls Creek Community Families program has been one of the most effective in providing a multidimensional, culturally competent approach by targeting the greatest needs in that area, including language, education, social, emotional and cognitive skills, and addressing issues related to nutrition and health (Munns 2010).

Reorienting health services

STRATEGY FOR ACTION

To reorient health services to effectively meet Indigenous health needs, health practitioners must make use of all opportunities for training and education in Indigenous health.

It is an irrefutable fact that health services for Indigenous people around the world are woefully inadequate. As our national and international gaze turns from problems to solutions, another indisputable fact is reiterated over and over. The health of Indigenous people will not be improved until there is culturally appropriate, community-controlled but accountable, community-based health services, supported with adequate financial resources linked to health outcomes. These services need to be collaborative; joined-up, wraparound services aimed at promoting cohesive and strengths-based community support (Robinson et al. 2012). Improving health services also depends on building Indigenous workforce capacity through national training plans and ongoing skills and capacity development (AIHW 2011; Astin et al. 2012). For Indigenous health professionals who are already working with their communities, the focus is on 'capacity strengthening', acknowledging their need for support (AIHW 2012d). In Australia, the need for Indigenous health professionals is acute. There is also a need to respond to the recommendations of the National Health and Hospitals Reform Committee (NHHRC) to better manage and coordinate funding for Indigenous programs. The 'closing the gap' initiatives are a good start, but oversight by a national authority that is accountable for funding and administration will help ensure that patient outcomes are linked to the quality, cost and appropriateness of services. Throughout Australia, there is wide variability in models of service delivery, with some areas having small clinics operating out of regional hospitals, others having PHC centres, and others having only intermittent services. As we have underlined, remoteness is a health hazard, and this varies depending on which state and under whose control health services are administered. Unless there is transparency and accountability in services, health service-community partnerships pay only lip service to genuine collaboration (Hudson 2009). To strengthen the capacity of those who are involved in service delivery it is critical to have transparent, highly organised governance, leadership, income generation, collaboration, evaluation, advocacy and evidence-based planning (AIHW 2012d). To purvey the strengths-based approach, organisations need to provide both tangible and intangible support. Interventions should foreshadow continuity of care and continuity of providers, and structural supports such as education and transportation to bring people together for culturally connected peer support (Baker et al. 2011). For health professionals themselves, their needs are similar to those working with other population groups. They need technical skills, equipment, infrastructure, financial resources and support for their engagement, motivation, cultural understanding and wellbeing so that they have the confidence and self-belief to transfer skills and knowledge to the local community wherever possible (AIHW 2012c).

Existing health service arrangements for Indigenous people are funded on a basis of per capita allocations, through a number of agencies. This one-size-fits-all model is unfair for those whose communities have few health professionals and many needs. To reduce service inequities it would be necessary to change the funding structure to meet health needs, rather than on the basis of Indigenous status. The other problem with health funding is the fee-for-service model, where wastage occurs because of top-down planning where health services are only considered viable if they stay within budgets. This can lead to overservicing to meet quotas, and can disadvantage individual patients. Regional allocation of funds for health services with accountable oversight would potentially be more responsive to locally determined needs and result in better coordination of care (Hudson 2009). New Zealand is working toward this approach.

One important area requiring attention for health services effectiveness is the training, and continuing education, for health professionals servicing rural and remote areas. The professional, cultural and personal isolation experienced by health professionals in remote areas is profound, and many have little preparation and training for the cultural or geographic context (Kildea et al. 2009). Health professionals working in these non-urban areas need an expanded repertoire of skills and attributes, including advocacy skills and in-depth cultural understanding of an Indigenous world view of health and wellbeing (Durie et al. 2008). This includes understanding the relative importance placed on cultural, rather than clinical, proficiency. The PHC agenda dictates that cultural safety and cultural competence guide the practice of all health professionals, including nurses (Gerlach 2012; Theunissen 2011; VCOSS 2013). This means that the first step is to develop and articulate Indigenous capacity for change by building Indigenous people's skills to organise their services and provide cultural awareness training for others according to Indigenous ways of knowing (VCOSS 2013). Our research agenda should also foster a philosophical stance of critical inquiry (Gerlach 2012). Cultural competence is particularly essential for helping people with mental health problems (Isaacs et al. 2012). Where they are available, mental health professionals often have the skills to help most people, but the needs of Indigenous men and women may differ, and there are few specialists in men's health and women's health accessible to those living at a distance from mainstream services.

For those educated in other countries, there may be little understanding of the cultural domains and layers of identity that frame Indigenous people's experiences of health and ill health, particularly in their relationship with health and place (Durie et al. 2008). In addition to adopting culturally safe approaches, it is important, to act as advocate and convey a willingness to help eliminate discriminatory barriers to service to improve Māori outcomes (Theunissan 2011). To work effectively with diverse groups requires reflexive self-awareness. Reflexive practices can be nurtured in pre-service preparation or as an ongoing expectation of the professional role. Adopting a reflexive approach to community engagement helps connect practice with a more inclusive, culturally competent, caring approach that does not ignore, override, discount, reject or violate the integrity of any group of people (Puzan 2003). Importantly, socially inclusive practices recognise the negative feedback loop between social exclusion and poor health (Baum et al. 2010).

The Australian Government has instituted a National Aboriginal and Torres Strait Islander Health Workforce Training Package with the express purpose of funding a range of organisations preparing the future health workforce. These include the Australian Indigenous Doctors Association; the National Aboriginal and Torres Strait Islander Health Worker Association; Indigenous Allied Health Australia; the Congress of Aboriginal and Torres Strait Islander Nurses; the Workforce Information Policy Officers Network; the Aboriginal and Torres Strait Islander Health Registered Training Organisation National Network, and the Leaders in Indigenous Medical Education Network (Australian Government 2013b). Many of these organisations also grant scholarships and provide mentors to assist Indigenous health professionals with their studies. The nursing profession has yet to educate adequate Indigenous nurses, who would be able to promote culturally appropriate models of care. In addition to shortages, current programs in Australia have only minimal Indigenous curriculum components, although both curricula and the proportion of Indigenous nurses are improving with the advocacy of organisations like the Congress of Aboriginal and Torres Strait Islander Nurses (CATSIN). In New Zealand, efforts to encourage Māori into health careers are also taking place. There are a number of undergraduate nursing degree programs that offer Bachelor degrees designed specifically to focus on the health needs of Māori. These programs are targeted specifically to Māori students and use a Kaupapa Māori approach to teaching and learning. The programs aim to produce graduates with both mainstream nursing skills and culturally specific skills. Like Canada and Australia, New Zealand has also built in a plan for workforce development (scholarships and training opportunities) as part of service quality. Coordinated strategies adopted in New Zealand include increasing the number of Māori health care providers and health workers, increasing resources where there are higher levels of deprivation and higher proportions of minority residents, requiring agencies to implement Māori-specific strategies for health, and, as noted earlier in the chapter, increasing Māori representation in health sector governance (Bramley et al. 2005). There has also been a website set up to encourage Māori young people to consider careers in health (www.kiaorahauora.org.nz). However, Māori working in the health sector remain underpaid when compared with non-Māori, and the government has failed to collect data on the Māori workforce to enable effective workforce planning (Manson 2013).

Despite these challenges, New Zealand does seem to be as far advanced as any country in establishing self-governance for Māori communities. Based on the Treaty of Waitangi, the New Zealand Government has adopted a PHC approach to help Māori and non-Māori society have control over the direction and shape of their own institutions, their communities and their development as people (King 2001). The government strategy makes visible its commitment to people accessing support and health care in consideration of their language preference, and participation in decision-making in regards to health and healing.

In a socially just, and thus healthy environment, the relationship between health professionals and the community has to be one of mutual respect, partnership and genuine exploration of need. People from all cultures should be free to choose the pathways to health that best suit their needs and customs, and be assured that the over-arching principles of cultural safety pave the way to their self-governance over health (Eckermann et al. 2010). This will help ensure system-level cultural competency. When we value diversity, help people develop their capacity for cultural self-assessment, and understand the dynamics of interacting cultures in a health care situation, cultural knowledge becomes institutionalised in service delivery and workforce development. Our case study now examines some of the most pertinent cultural issues affecting the Smith and Mason families.

CASE STUDY: Cultural issues for the Smith and Mason families

The mining site has encouraged the employment of Indigenous men through the Australia One initiative. The Indigenous mining training program has proven successful in creating employment for local Indigenous people. The management group and health and safety group have done some public awareness work on the company's social inclusion agenda in all aspects of the mining operations.

Huia is very connected to her Māori culture and is determined that her children remain engaged in Māori culture, so she makes the effort to send them to the nearest Māori immersion school (Te Kura Kaupapa Māori) and preschool (Kohanga Reo). While having her mum come to live in the family home is challenging, Huia finds the relationship and connections between her mother and her children rewarding.

REFLECTING ON THE BIG ISSUES

- The reasons for the lower health status and shorter lifespan of Indigenous people compared with non-Indigenous people include socio-economic disparities, deprivation, unequal treatment, racism and discrimination, and unhealthy environments.

- Societies cannot be inclusive until historical traumas against Indigenous people are dealt with by the wider society.

- Reducing health risk factors for Indigenous people should be planned according to the specific risk rather than Indigenous status.

- Community engagement must be undertaken from a perspective of cultural safety and respect for Indigenous culture.

- Solutions to Indigenous socio-economic disadvantage have to extend beyond increasing funding to strengthening long-term capacity.

- Intersectoral and interagency collaboration is a major element in ensuring continuity of Indigenous capacity development.

- Developing a base of research evidence is essential to providing a foundation for change in Indigenous communities.

REFLECTIVE QUESTIONS: How would I use this knowledge in practice?

1   Identify the chain of factors related to colonisation that predispose Indigenous people to ill health.

2   Develop a web of causation for the disproportionate burden of chronic illness among Indigenous people.

3   Outline a strategy for promoting health literacy among middle-aged Indigenous residents of a rural or remote community with a view toward managing chronic illness.

4   Explain how you would develop a plan for a domestic violence prevention session to include Indigenous and non-Indigenous workers at the mining site.

5   What primary health care initiatives would you include in a program to develop a socially inclusive Health Promoting School in either Maddington or Papakura?

6   Construct a set of guidelines or prompts that you might use to ensure your interactions are culturally safe irrespective of your client group.

References

Anderson, J., 2008. Cultural liaison workers. Learnings from the mensline Australia Cultural X Change Project. AIFS, Family Relationships Quarterly 12, 3–6.

Anderson, J., Perry, J., Blue, C., et al., 2003. "Rewriting" cultural safety within the postcolonial and postnational feminist project. Adv. Nurs. Sci. 26 (3), 196–214.

Anderson, J., Pakula, B., Smye, V., et al., 2011. Strengthening Aboriginal health through a place-based learning community. J. Aborig. Health March, 42–53.

Astin, C., Brown, N., Jowsey, T., et al., 2012. Strategic approaches to enhanced service delivery for Aboriginal and Torres Strait Islander people with chronic illness: a qualitative study. BMC Health Serv. Res. 12, 143–152.

Australian Bureau of Statistics (ABS) and Australian Institute of Health and Welfare (AIHW), 2008. The Health and Welfare of Australia's Aboriginal and Torres Strait Islander Peoples, ABS, AIHW, Canberra.

Australian Bureau of Statistics (ABS), 2013. Indigenous Smoking. Online, Available: <www.abs.gov.au/AUSSTATS/abs@.nsf/lookup/4704.OChapter755Oct+2010> 3 September 2013.

Australian Government, 2013a. Closing the Gap Prime Minister's Report, AGPS, Canberra.

Australian Government, 2013b. National Aboriginal and Torres Strait Islander Health Plan—Companion Document on Commonwealth Government Strategies & Reforms. Online, Available: <www.ATSIgapreport2013natishp-companion.pdf> 9 July 2013.

Australian Indigenous HealthInfoNet, 2013. Online, Available: <www.healthinfonet.ecu.edu.au/health-facts/summary> June 25 2013.

Australian Institute of Health and Welfare (AIHW), 2011. Young Australians, their health and wellbeing, AIHW Cat no PHE 140, Canberra.

Australian Institute of Health and Welfare (AIHW), 2012a. Australia's Health 2012 Series no 13, Cat No AUS 156, AIHW, Canberra.

Australian Institute of Health and Welfare (AIHW), 2012b. Healthy lifestyle programs for physical activity and nutrition, Closing the Gap Clearinghouse, Resource Sheet No. 9, AIHW, Canberra.

Australian Institute of Health and Welfare (AIHW), 2012c. Parenting in the early years: effectiveness of parenting support programs for Indigenous families, Closing the Gap Clearinghouse, Resource Sheet No. 16, AIHW, Canberra.

Australian Institute of Health and Welfare (AIHW), 2012d. Improving Indigenous community governance through strengthening Indigenous and government organizational capacity, Closing the Gap Clearinghouse, Resource Sheet No. 10, AIHW, Canberra.

Australian Institute of Health and Welfare (AIHW), 2012e. Engaging Indigenous students through school-based health education, Closing the Gap Clearinghouse, Resource Sheet No. 12, AIHW, Canberra.

Australian Institute of Health and Welfare (AIHW), 2012f. Strategies to minimize the incidence of suicide and suicidal behavior, Closing the Gap Clearinghouse, Resource Sheet No. 18, AIHW, Canberra.

Australian Institute of Health and Welfare (AIHW), 2013. Mentoring programs for Indigenous youth at risk. Closing the Gap Clearinghouse, Resource Sheet No. 22, AIHW, Canberra.

Baker, P., Shipp, J., Wellings, S., et al., 2011. Assessment of applicability and transferability of evidence-based antenatal interventions to the Australian indigenous setting. Health Promot. Int. 27 (2), 208–219.

Baker, M., Telfar Barnard, L., Kvalsvig, A., et al., 2012. Increasing incidence of serious infectious diseases and inequalities in New Zealand: a national epidemiological study. Lancet 379 (9821), 1112–1119.

Barnett, R., Pearce, J., Moon, G., 2009. Community inequality and smoking cessation in New Zealand, 1981-2006. Soc. Sci. Med. 68 (5), 876–884.

Baum, F., Newman, L., Biedrzycki, K., et al., 2010. Can a regional government's social inclusion initiative contribute to the quest for health equity? Health Promot. Int. 25 (4), 474–482.

Beiser, M., 2005. The health of immigrants and refugees in Canada Canadian. J. Public Health (Bangkok) 96 (S2), S30–S44.

Berry, J., 1995. Psychology of Acculturation. In: Goldberg, N., Veroff, J. (Eds.), The culture and psychology reader, New York University Press, New York, pp. 457–488.

Biddle, N., 2011. CAEPR Indigenous population project 2011 Paper 3, Indigenous housing need, Centre for Aboriginal Economic Policy Research, Research School of Social Sciences, ANU College of Arts and Social Sciences, Canberra.

Biddle, N., 2012. Measures of Indigenous social capital and their relationship with well-being. Aust. J. Rural Health 20, 298–304.

Blisset, W., 2011. Flourishing for all in Aotearoa. A creative inquiry through meaningful conversation to explore a Māori world view of flourishing. Mental Health Foundation of New Zealand, Wellington.

Boulton, A., Tamehana, J., Brannelly, T., 2013. Whānau-centred health and social service delivery in New Zealand. Mai J. 2 (1), 18–32.

Bramley, D., Hebert, P., Tuzzio, L., et al., 2005. Disparities in Indigenous health: A cross-country comparison between New Zealand and the United States. Am. J. Public Health 95 (5), 844–850.

Cape York Institute, 2013. Empowered communities principles for reform. Online, Available: <www.cyi/org.au> 12 October 2013.

Cripps, K., McGlade, H., 2008. Indigenous family violence and sexual abuse: Considering pathways forward. J. Fam. Stud. 14 (2–3), 240–253.

D'Espaignet, E., Measey, M., Carnegie, M., et al., 2003. Monitoring the 'Strong Women Strong Babies, Strong Culture' Program: The first eight years. J. Paediatr. Child Health 39, 668–672.

Duke, J., Connor, M., McEldowney, R., 2009. Becoming a culturally competent health practitioner in the delivery of culturally safe care: A process oriented approach. J. Cult. Divers. 16 (2), 40–49.

Dulin, P., Stephens, C., Alpass, F., et al., 2011. The impact of socio-contextual, physical and lifestyle variables on measures of physical and psychological wellbeing among Māori and non-Māori: the New Zealand health, Work, and Retirement Study. Ageing Soc. 31, 1406–1424.

Durie, M., 1994. Whaiora: Māori health development, Oxford University Press, Auckland.

Durie, M., 2001. Mauri Ora: The dynamics of Māori health, Oxford University Press, Auckland.

Durie, M., 2004. An Indigenous model of health promotion. Health Promot. J. Austr. 15 (3), 181–185.

Durie, A., Hill, P., Arkles, R., et al., 2008. Overseas-trained doctors in Indigenous rural health services: negotiating professional relationships across cultural domains. Aust. N. Z. J. Public Health 32 (6), 512–518.

Durey, A., Thompson, S., 2012. Reducing the health disparities of Indigenous Australians: time to change focus. BMC Health Serv. Res. 12, 151–162.

Eckermann, A., Dowd, T., Chong, E., et al., 2010. Binan Goonj: Bridging Cultures in Aboriginal Health, third ed. Elsevier, Sydney.

Edwards, R., Bowler, T., Atkinson, J., et al., 2008. Low and declining cigarette smoking rates among doctors and nurses: 2006 New Zealand census data. N. Z. Med. J. 121, 43–51.

Evans, B., 2012. Northern Territory emergency response: Criticism, support and redesign. Aust. J. Rural Health 20, 103–107.

Families Commission, 2009. Family Violence Statistics Report, Families Commission, Wellington.

Farmer, J., Bourke, L., Taylor, J., et al., 2012. Culture and rural health. Aust. J. Rural Health 20, 243–247.

Fernandez, C., Wilson, D., 2008. Māori women's views on smoking cessation initiatives. Nurs. Prax. N. Z. 24 (2), 27–40.

Fisher, R., 2006. Congruence and functions of personal and cultural values: Do my values reflect my culture's values. Pers. Soc. Psychol. 32 (11), 1419–1431.

Flynn, M., Carne, S., Mai'anaima, S., 2010. Māori housing trends 2010, Housing New Zealand Corporation, Wellington.

Ford, J., 2012. Indigenous health and climate change. Am. J. Public Health 102 (7), 1260–1266.

Generation One, 2013. Online, Available: <www.indigenousjobsaustralia.com.au> 2 September 2013.

Gerlach, A., 2012. A critical reflection on the concept of cultural safety. Can. J. Occup. Ther. 79 (3), 151–158.

Gifford, H., 2011. Using Kaupapa Māori approaches to reduce smoking. Kai Tiaki Nurs. N. Z. 17 (1), 25.

Gifford, H., Walker, L., Clendon, J., et al., 2013. Māori nurses and smoking; conflicted identities and motivations for smoking cessation. Kai Tiaki Nursing Research 4 (1), 33–38.

Glover, M., 2000. The Effectiveness of a Māori Noho Marae smoking cessation intervention: utilising a kaupapa Māori methodology, The University of Auckland, Auckland.

Grigg, M., Waa, A., Bradbrook, S., 2008. Response to an indigenous smoking cessation media campaign—It's about whānau. Aust. N. Z. J. Public Health 32 (6), 559–564.

Hamerton, H., Mercer, C., Riini, D., et al., 2012. Evaluating Māori community initiatives to promote Healthy Eating, Healthy Action. Health Promot. Int. doi:10.1093/heapro/das048.

Hamlin, L., Anderson, L., 2011. Cultural competence and perioperative nursing practice in New Zealand. AORN Journal 93 (2), 291–295l.

Hudson, S., 2009. Closing the accountability gap: The first step towards better Indigenous health, Centre for Independent Policy Studies CIS Monograph 105, Melbourne.

Hughes, H., Hughes, M., 2012. Indigenous Education 2012, Centre for Independent Studies Monograph 129, Canberra.

Human Rights and Equal Opportunity Commission, 1997. Bringing Them Home: Report of the National Inquiry into the Separation of Aboriginal and Torres Strait Islander Children from their Families, HREOC, Sydney.

Hunt, J., 2012. Community development for sustainable early childhood care and development programs: A World Vision Australia and Central Land Council partnership. Working Paper 86/2012 Centre for Aboriginal Economic Policy Research, ANU College of Arts & Social Sciences, Online, Available: <http://caepr.anu.edu.au/> 3 July 2013.

Isaacs, A., Maybery, D., Gruis, H., 2012. Mental health services for Aboriginal men: Mismatches and solutions. Int. J. Ment. Health Nurs. 21, 400–408.

Janssen, J., 2009. Meeting the needs of Māori with diabetes: an evaluation of a nurse-led service. Masters thesis, Victoria University, Wellington.

Jones, D., Creed, D., 2011. Your basket and my basket: teaching and learning about Māori-Pakeha bicultural organizing. J. Manag. Educ. 35 (1), 84–101.

Ka'ai-Mahuta, R., 2011. The impact of colonisation on te reo Māori: a critical review of the state education system. Te Kaharoa 4, 195–225.

Kickett-Tucker, C., 2009. Moorn [Black]? Djardak [White]? How come I don't fit in mum? Exploring the racial identity of Australian Aboriginal children and youth. Health Sociol. Rev. 18 (1), 119–136.

Kildea, S., Barclay, L., Wardaguga, M., et al., 2009. Participative research in a remote Australian Aboriginal setting. Action Res. 7 (2), 143–163.

King, A., 2001. Primary Health Care Strategy, Ministry of Health, Wellington.

Kingsley, J., Townsend, M., Phillips, R., et al., 2009. 'If the land is healthy ... it makes the people healthy'. The relationship between caring for Country and health for the Yorta Yorta Nation, Boonwurrung and Bangerang Tribes. Health Place 15, 291–299.

Kowanko, I., Stewart, T., Power, C., et al., 2009. An Aboriginal family and community healing program in metropolitan Adelaide: description and evaluation. Australian Indigenous Health Bulletin 9 (4), 1–12.

Kulig, J., 2000. Culturally diverse communities: The impact on the role of community health nurses. In: Stewart, M. (Ed.), Community Nursing: Promoting Canadians' Health, second ed. WB Saunders, Toronto, pp. 194–210.

Lohoar, S., 2012. Safe and supportive Indigenous families and communities for children, Child, Family Community Australia Paper No 7, AIFS, Melbourne.

Manson, L., 2013. New Zealand Nurses Organisation submission on the 18th session of the Human Rights Council—Universal Periodic Review New Zealand 2013. Online, Available: <http://www.nzno.org.nz/Portals/0/Files/20130617%20NZNO%20UPR%20submission.pdf> 23 September 2013.

McDonald, E., Bailie, R., Grace, J., et al., 2009. A case study of physical and social barriers to hygiene and child growth in Australian Aboriginal communities. BMC Public Health 9, 346. doi:10.1186/1471-2458-9-346.

McDonald, E., Bailie, R., Grace, J., et al., 2010. An ecological approach to health promotion in remote Australian Aboriginal communities. Health Promot. Int. 25 (1), 42–53.

McMurray, A., Param, R., 2008. Culture-specific care for Indigenous people: A primary health care approach. Contemp. Nurse 28 (1/2), 165–172.

Menzies, P., 2008. Developing an Aboriginal healing model for intergenerational trauma. Int. J. Health Promot. Educ. 46 (2), 41–49.

Mignone, J., O'Neil J., 2005. Social capital and youth suicide risk factors in First Nations Communities. Can. J. Public Health 96 (S1), S51–S54.

Milroy, H., 2013. Beyond cultural security: towards sanctuary. Editorial. Med. J. Aust. 199 (1), 14.

Munford, R., Sanders, J., 2011. Embracing the diversity of practice: indigenous knowledge and mainstream social work practice. J Soc. Work Pract. 25 (1), 63–77.

Munns, A., 2010. Yanan Ngurra-ngu Walalja, Halls Creek Community Families Programme. npchn 13 (1), 18–21.

Nelson, A., Abbott. R., Macdonald, D., 2010. Indigenous Australians and physical activity: using a social-ecological model to review the literature. Health Educ. Res. 25 (3), 498–509.

New Zealand Human Rights Commission, 2012. A fair go for all? Addressing structural discrimination in public services, Human Rights Commission, Wellington.

New Zealand Ministry of Education, 2010. Education statistics of New Zealand 2009, Ministry of Education, Wellington.

New Zealand Ministry of Health (NZMOH), 2000. New Zealand Health Strategy, Ministry of Health, Wellington.

New Zealand Ministry of Health (NZMOH), 2002a. He Korowai Oranga, Māori Health Strategy, MOHNZ, Wellington.

New Zealand Ministry of Health (NZMOH), 2002b. Māori mental health strategic framework, MOHNZ, Wellington.

New Zealand Ministry of Health (NZMOH), 2006. Whakatataka Tuarua: Māori health action plan 2006–2011, MOHNZ, Wellington.

New Zealand Ministry of Health (NZMOH), 2007. Whānau Ora Health Impact Assessment, Ministry of Health, Wellington.

New Zealand Ministry of Health (NZMOH), 2009. Māori provider work programme, NZMOH, Wellington.

New Zealand Ministry of Health (NZMOH), 2012a. Mortality and Demographic Data 2009, NZMOH, Wellington.

New Zealand Ministry of Health (NZMOH), 2012b. The health of New Zealand adults 2011/12, NZMOH, Wellington.

New Zealand Ministry of Health (NZMOH), 2012c. The health of New Zealand children 2011/12, NZMOH, Wellington.

New Zealand Ministry of Health (NZMOH), 2013a. Health loss in New Zealand: A report from the New Zealand burden of diseases, injuries and risk factors study, 2006–2016, NZMOH, Wellington.

New Zealand Ministry of Health (NZMOH), 2013b. The health of Māori adults and children, NZMOH, Wellington.

New Zealand Ministry of Health (NZMOH), 2013c. Hazardous drinking in 2011/12: Findings from the New Zealand health survey, NZMOH, Wellington.

New Zealand Ministry of Health (NZMOH), 2013d. Report on the performance of general practices in whānau ora collectives as at March 2013, NZMOH, Wellington.

Norris, H., 2011. Flourishing, positive mental health and wellbeing, Mental Health Foundation, Wellington. Online. Available: <http://www.mentalhealth.org.nz/newsletters/view/article/22/312/2011/> 21 September 2013.

Nursing Council of New Zealand, 2011. Guidelines for Cultural Safety in Nursing and Midwifery Education, NCNZ, Wellington. Online. Available: <www.nursingcouncil.org.nz/Publications/Standards-and-guidelines-for-nurses> 30 September 2013 Online.

Nursing Council of New Zealand, 2012. Code of conduct for nurses, NCNZ, Wellington. Online. Available: <www.nursingcouncil.org.nz/Publications/Standards-and-guidelines-for-nurses> 13 September 2013.

Oda, K., Rameka, M., 2012. Racism and cultural safety in nursing. Contemp. Nurse 43 (1), 107–112.

O'Brien, A., 2006. Moving toward culturally sensitive services for Indigenous people: A non-Indigenous mental health nursing perspective. Contemp. Nurse 21 (1), 22–31.

O'Donovan, G., 2009. Smoking prevalence among qualified nurses in the Republic of Ireland and their role in smoking cessation. Int. Nurs. Rev. 56 (2), 230–236.

Olavarria, N., Beaulac, J., Belanger, A., et al., 2009. Organizational cultural competence in community health and social services. J. Cult. Divers. 16 (4), 140–150.

Passey, M., Gale, J., Sanson-Fisher, R., 2011. 'It's almost expected': rural Australian Aboriginal women's reflections on smoking initiation and maintenance: a qualitative study. BMC Womens Health 11, 55–67.

Pearson, N., 2004. The Cape York Substance Abuse Strategy, Griffith University Centre for Governance and Public Policy, Sept. 3, Brisbane.

Pearson, N., 2005. The Cape York Agenda. Address to the National Press Club, Canberra, Nov. 30.

Pearson, N., 2009. A people's survival. The Weekend Australian Oct 3–4, Inquirer: 1–2.

Peiris, D., Brown, A., Cass, A., 2008. Addressing inequities in access to quality health care for indigenous people. Can. Med. Assoc. J. 179 (10), 985–986.

Plani, F., Carson, P., 2008. The challenges of developing a trauma system for Indigenous people. Injury. 3955, S43–S53.

Pomaika'I Cook, B., Tarallo-Jensen, L., Withy, K., et al., 2005. Changes in Kanaka maoli Men's Roles and Health: Healing the Warrior Self. Int. J. Mens Health 4 (2), 115–130.

Ponniah, S., Blomfield, A., 2008. An update on tobacco smoking among New Zealand health care workers, the current picture, 2006. N. Z. Med. J. 121 (1272), 104.

Provost, L., 2012. Health sector: Reports of the 2010/11audits, Office of the Auditor General, Wellington.

Puzan, E., 2003. The unbearable whiteness of being (in nursing). Nurs. Inq. 10 (3), 193–200.

Radsma, J., Bortloff, J., 2009. Counteracting ambivalence: Nurses who smoke and their health promotion role with patients who smoke. Res. Nurs. Health 32 (4), 443–452.

Reconciliation Australia, 2013. Reconciliation Australia UN declaration on the Rights of Indigenous Peoples. Online, Available: <www.reconciliation.org.au/home/resources/factsheets/un-declaration-on-the-rights-of-indigenous-peoples>; 2 September 2013.

Reid, P., Robson, B., 2007. Understanding health inequities. In: Robson, B., Harris, R. (Eds.), Hauora: Māori Standards of Health IV. A study of the years 2000-2005, Te Ropu Rangahau Hauora a Eru Pomare, Wellington, pp. 3–10.

Richmond, C., Ross, N., 2009. The determinants of First Nation and Inuit health: A critical population health approach. Health Place 15, 403–411.

Robinson, E., Scott, D., Meredith, V., et al., 2012. Good and innovative practice in service delivery to vulnerable and disadvantaged families and children, Child Family Community Australia Paper No. 9, AIHW, Melbourne.

Robson, B., Cormack, D., Cram, F., 2007. Social and Economic Indicators. In: Robson, B., Harris, R. (Eds.), Hauora: Māori Standards of Health IV. A study of the years 2000-2005, Te Ropu Rangahau Hauora a Eru Pomare, Wellington, pp. 63–102.

Rothwell, N., 2012. New Horizons, The Weekend Australian Dec 15–16, Sydney.

Rothwell, N., 2013a. Place, not race, is key to the gap. The Weekend Australian, March 23-24, Sydney.

Rothwell, N., 2013b. The great unmentionables of remote life. The Weekend Australian, Feb 2–3, Sydney.

Ryan, N., Head, B., Keast, R., et al., 2006. Engaging Indigenous communities: Towards a policy framework for Indigenous community justice programmes. Soc. Policy Adm. 40 (3), 304–321.

Sen, A., 2000. Development as Freedom, Knopf, New York.

Shahid, S., Thompson, S., 2009. An overview of cancer and beliefs about the disease in Indigenous people of Australia, Canada, New Zealand and the US. Aust. N. Z. J. Public Health 33 (2), 109–118.

Signal, L., Walton, M., Ni Mhurchu, N., et al., 2012. Tackling 'wicked' health promotion problems: a New Zealand case study. Health Promot. Int. 28 (1), 84–94.

Statistics New Zealand, 2006. 2006 Census. Online. Available: <www.stats.govt.nz/Census/2006CensusHomePage.aspx> 21 July 2014.

Stewart, S., 2008. Promoting indigenous mental health: cultural perspectives on healing from Native counsellors in Canada. Int. J. Health Promot. Educ. 46 (2), 49–57.

Takao, N., Grennell, D., McKegg, K., et al., 2010. Te Piko o te Mahuri. The key attributes of successful Kura Kaupapa Māori, Ministry of Education, Wellington.

Te Puni Kokiri, 2010. Arotake tukino whānau literature review on family violence, Te Puni Kokiri, Wellington, New Zealand.

Theunissan, K., 2011. The nurse's role in improving health disparities. Contemp. Nurse 39 (2), 281–286.

Thompson, S., Greville, H., Param, R., 2008. Beyond policy and planning to practice: getting sexual health on the agenda in Aboriginal communities in Western Australia. Aust. New Zealand Health Policy 5 (3), doi:10.1186/1743-8462-5-3.

Trewin, D., Madden, R., 2005. The Health and Welfare of Australia's Aboriginal and Torres Strait Islander Peoples ABS Cat. No. 4704.0, AIHW Cat. No.IHW14, Canberra.

Tsey, K., Whiteside, M., Daly, S., et al., 2005. Adapting the 'Family Wellbeing' empowerment program to the needs of remote Indigenous school children. Aust. N. Z. J. Public Health 29 (2), 112–116.

United Nations (UN), 2007. Report of the Human Rights Council: United Nations Declaration on the Rights of Indigenous Peoples, UN, Geneva.

Utter, J., Scragg, R., Schaaf, D., et al., 2006. Nutrition and physical activity behaviours among Māori, Pacific and NZ European children: identifying opportunities for population-based interventions. Aust. N. Z. J. Public Health 30 (1), 50–56.

Vicary, D., Bishop, B., 2005. Western psychotherapeutic practice: Engaging Aboriginal people in culturally appropriate and respectful ways. Aust. Psychol. 40 (1), 8–19.

Victorian Council of Social Services, Youth Affairs Council of Victoria, 2013. Building the Scaffolding, strengthening support for young people in Victoria, VCSS, Melbourne.

Vincent, K., Eveline, J., 2008. The invisibility of gendered power relations in domestic violence policy. J. Fam. Stud. 14 (2–3), 322–333.

Waldegrave, C., King, P., Walker, T., et al., 2006. Māori housing experiences: Emerging trends and issues, Te Puni Kokiri, Wellington.

Wilding, R., Tilbury, F., 2004. Constructing a changing people. In: Wilding, R., Tilbury, F. (Eds.), A changing people: diverse contributions to the state of Western Australia, Department of the Premier and Cabinet, Office of Multicultural Interests, Perth, pp. 1–7.

Williamson, M., Harrison, L., 2010. Providing culturally appropriate care: A literature review. Int. J. Nurs. Stud. 47, 761–769.

World Health Organization (WHO), 1999. Indigenous and Tribal Peoples: Legal Frameworks and Indigenous Rights, WHO, Geneva.

Zubrick, S., Silburn, S., Lawrence, D., et al., 2005. The Western Australian Aboriginal Child Health Survey: The Social and Emotional Wellbeing of Aboriginal Children and Young People, Curtin University of Technology and Telethon Institute for Child Health Research, Perth.

Useful websites

www.abs.gov.au—Australian Bureau of Statistics

www.aihw.gov.au—Australian Institute of Health and Welfare

www.Maorihealth.govt.nz—New Zealand Ministry of Health, Māori Health

www.health.gov.au/internet/main/publishing.nsf/Content/Aboriginal+and+Torres+Strait+Islander+Health-1lp—Aboriginal and Torres Strait Islander Health

www.health.gov.au/internet/main/publishing.nsf/Content/mental-stratNational—Mental Health Strategy

www.humanrights.gov.au/publications/bringing-them-home-report-1997—Bringing Them Home Report (Stolen Generations)

cyi.org.au—Cape York Institute for Policy & Leadership (Noel Pearson)

www.thehealthyaboriginal.net/—Healthy Aboriginal Network (creating comic books on Aboriginal youth health issues)

www.hreoc.gov.au—Indigenous Native Title, Australian Human Rights website

www.reconciliation.org.au—Reconciliation Australia

www.nrha.org.au—National Rural Health Alliance

www.waitangi-tribunal.govt.nz—The Waitangi Tribunal

www.justice.govt.nz/courts/maori-land-court—The Māori Land Court

Inclusive policies, equitable health care systems

CHAPTER **14**

Introduction

Policymaking for community health is basically a political process in which those in positions of power make decisions on how best to allocate resources. As health professionals, it is our responsibility to become aware of how these decisions are made, and to advocate for equity in allocations to the communities we assist. This can take us into unfamiliar territory, carefully examining the needs and priorities of the community, while, at the same time, understanding the constraints on services and resources. Policymaking is an important step in health promotion. Without policies, decisions for resource allocation could be made on the basis of the loudest voices, the highest population or the desires of those best able to articulate their requests. To work towards equitable distribution of resources requires policies that are fair. Fairness means that there is advocacy for those who are most in need, whose voices are often silent. Fairness also means that those born to privilege are not overlooked, but their needs are carefully considered alongside those of the wider population. Guided by the principles of primary health care, we consider how policies and systems of health service are able to balance needs and services on the basis of social justice at the global, national, regional and local level.

> ### WHAT ARE ... POLICIES?
> Plans for equitable resource allocation.

National health policies are usually informed by, and responsive to global priorities and conditions. Ideally, state or regional priorities would also be designed to follow or complement the directions of national policies. However, where political agendas differ, this may not always be the case. So, for example, it is possible that in one Australian state or territory, policymakers could place a high priority on environmental issues in its health planning, whereas another might see child health as its greatest priority.

Both states would be governed by the goal of better health, but they may change the distribution of resources according to their respective priorities. In countries such as New Zealand, where there is a single health department (the New Zealand Ministry of Health), policymaking is more consistent across the country, even though there may be some differences in the way different District Health Boards implement policies. Yet, even in this environment, there is a need for constant vigilance, to ensure that policymaking is inclusive, and results in all members of the community having equity of access to what they need to maintain good health.

Because of the complexity of health policymaking, it is important to understand how decisions are made. Optimally, decisions would be bi-directional, bottom-up and top-down. Local citizens' groups, health professionals, town councils and city planners would convey the needs of local communities upward, to the regional, state and national levels, where they would participate in informed debates about health and health care. Policymakers would hear their voices and preferences, and attempt to accommodate multiple perspectives in the way they allocate resources for health. In this context, debates and decisions would be approached on the basis of equal partnerships, and expedient information systems, so that all policy decisions would also be evidence-based; or informed by the latest research and demographic data. Once considerations were aired and consensus was achieved, the policymaking group would communicate with the wider community, gathering further data and/or responses, which would instigate further cycles of input for decision-making. As a result, the policy would achieve three main outcomes. First, it would have a significant effect in improving the health of the population. Second, it would be fair. Third, it would be administered through efficient governance structures, with transparent goals, expectations, financial accountability and evaluation strategies. Yet, impediments to achieving this type of system remain for reasons that are often political and financial. Too often, political positions dictate the

OBJECTIVES

By the end of this chapter you will be able to:

1 identify the factors influencing the development of policies that affect the health of the population

2 explain the global issues that have an impact on national and regional policy development

3 analyse the successes, failures and policy gaps that have occurred in your national health policies

4 discuss the issues that must be considered in planning health services to be responsive to the needs of different population groups

5 describe the features of a primary health care system that contribute to better health and wellbeing

6 discuss the role of nurses and other health professionals in policy planning and implementation.

---

terms or targets of health decisions, especially if there are vested interests involved. The discussion to follow outlines some of the most important issues in policymaking in this twenty-first century, with implications for the sustained involvement of all health professionals.

POLICY BEST PRACTICE

- Improve population health
- Fair, equitable resource allocation
- Efficient, transparent governance

POLITICS, POLICYMAKING AND HEALTH CARE

The main goal of health policymaking should be to improve and enhance health. This requires a strong health care system, and decisive leadership to guide the way policies are developed. The ideal health care system is ethical, fair and strategic in its endeavour to meet the needs of current and future communities; transparent in communicating its goals and capabilities; oriented toward community empowerment for informed choices;, and resourced to the extent that it can support those choices. But the health system alone cannot create or sustain health. This is why there has been an urgent call from global health policymakers to incorporate health in all policies. Health in all policies (HiAP) is an approach to public policymaking that systematically takes into account the implications of public policy decisions on health and determinants of health and health systems, identifies synergies across policy sectors, and seeks to avoid the harmful health effects of poor policies (Leppo et al. 2013). HiAP also aims to improve the accountability of policymakers for health impacts at all levels of policymaking, and is based on the fundamental

health-related human rights of populations, social justice and on the obligations of governments to uphold those rights (Leppo et al. 2013). If health was included in all policies our governments would ensure health and safety in education, transportation, media advertising, food services and the environment. Community planning would include health considerations in their plans for housing, infrastructure and public works. Health planners would participate in policies for safe neighbourhoods, community policing and disaster planning. There would be health considerations in decisions made by departments of immigration and multicultural affairs, and health plans for primary industry development and innovation, workplace and industrial relations. Health issues are embedded in each of these aspects of daily life, and affect people at all stages of the life course from family planning, safe maternity care, child protection and care, illness and injury prevention and management at all ages, healthy ageing and end of life care.

HEALTH IN ALL POLICIES

The health system alone cannot create or sustain health. Health must be considered in *all* policy development activities.

As mentioned above, the defining purpose of a health care system lies in the provision of accessible, appropriate, equitable health care that is responsive to people's expectations. When equity is achieved, the health care system, its policies, and the policies of other government departments are inclusive, and aligned with the social determinants of health (SDH). The fact that we live in conditions of *inequity* indicates that equity continues to be elusive, yet it is a worthy goal for our actions. To some extent, this may be due to the complexity of policymaking and all the competing interests that influence the outcome. However, some inequities persist because of events in the global and/or local environment. When global markets decline, there is a profound impact on countries that depend on these markets to sustain their population. If trade declines, unemployment increases, and there is a major effect on family health and wellbeing. When families are unable to purchase goods and services, domestic trade suffers, and more people become unemployed. When unemployment is high, there is a dramatic drain on public resources and supports for those most in need are unavailable. This is a classic 'butterfly effect' where we can see the inherently complex and ecological perspective of policymaking. Everything is connected to everything else.

ACTING ON THE BUTTERFLY EFFECT

Everything affects everything else, so 'think global, act local'.

Politics was once defined by Sax as the art of the possible in satisfying 'a strife of interests' (in Kamien 2009:65). In health policymaking there has always been a strife of interests, between rich and poor, urban and rural, young and old, sick and well, and those with competing biomedical or health promotion needs. Health care decisions revolve around distributive justice: who gets what. Ethically, the poor and disadvantaged should receive the lion's share of resources, as this would bring them up to the same level of opportunity as the rest of the population. However, no country in the world has achieved equity in resource allocation, leaving many people living impoverished lives. At the global level, the United Nation's Report on the World Social Situation indicates a need for all governments to take into account the social implications of their economic policies, especially the consequences for poverty, employment, nutrition, health and education. Each of these aspects of social life affect long-term sustainable development (UN 2011). The report argues that the disruptions to economic growth caused by the global financial crisis of 2008–09 have caused significant setbacks in achieving the Millennium Development Goals and spiked a dramatic increase in unemployment. The loss of jobs has devastated many economies, but for those in the developing world, their vulnerability is magnified many times over by the lack of income protection. As a result, over a billion people worldwide now live in hunger, the highest rate on record (UN 2011). Poverty therefore remains the central issue for global policymakers.

WHAT IS ... POLITICS?

The art of the possible in satisfying 'a strife of interests'.

ALLEVIATING GLOBAL POVERTY

Poverty remains the central issue for policymakers with an urgent need to integrate economic and social policies to achieve health.

The global financial crisis (GFC), and the neoliberal policies that led up to the crisis, represented a global over-reliance on market forces, where government efforts were focused on economic development, to the detriment of health and social services for the world's poor. The effects of the GFC have been sharp, widespread, and deep (UN 2011). Some countries have not recovered, and with shrinking markets their outlook is bleak. The UN suggests that the most important policy implication for the future is for governments to play a developmental role, integrating economic and social policies to support productivity and employment growth in all nations, while attacking inequality and promoting social justice. This is a balanced approach to alleviating poverty, urging governments to work towards equitable, sustainable employment opportunities and public social expenditures on primary health care (PHC), universal education and the provision of social security that would include insurance, pensions, disability and child benefits (UN 2011). Where workplace policies are unfair or insufficient to support the labour force, there are implications across all of the SDH. Maternal health suffers. Parents are unable to care for their children. History has shown that family relationships can be eroded, with the possibility of gender-based violence, alcohol and substance misuse, crime, depression and suicide (UN 2011). The lack of financial resources can prohibit children's educational opportunities. Cultural and family connections can be disrupted. People may have to work into older age and consequently suffer illness, injury and disability. These are only a few of the factors that cascade through family life when people cannot be gainfully employed. Together, these factors reinforce the central role of employment policies in global and national policymaking (Bambra et al. 2007). In each country, inclusive policies for better health should measure and understand local problems in the context of these global issues (CSDH 2008). From this foundation, policymakers can then assess the impact of action and inaction on community health in terms of the principles of PHC: accessible health care, appropriate technology, health promotion and health education, cultural sensitivity and cultural safety, intersectoral collaboration and community participation.

REMINDER: PHC

- Accessible health care
- Appropriate technology
- Health promotion
- Cultural sensitivity, safety
- Intersectoral collaboration
- Community participation

GROUP EXERCISE: Policymaking and nurses

Break into groups of two or three and consider the following questions:

- What is policy and why is it important for nurses to have a good understanding of this?
- What role do nurses have in the policymaking process?

Share your thoughts with the wider group.

POLICY ACTION AT THE NATIONAL LEVEL: THINK GLOBAL, ACT LOCAL

As health professionals, we can be conscious and concerned about global issues and the failure of the global community to create equity. For those who wish to become global advocates there are many lobby groups that welcome our participation. For others, becoming involved at the global level may not be possible; however, acting at a local level can encourage community participation in the policy arena, and ensure that professional knowledge and skills are used to the community's advantage. To prepare for this type of advocacy it is important to be aware of global policies. Human rights policies such as the UN Convention on the Rights of the Child, their Declarations on the Elimination of Violence Against Women and the Rights of Indigenous Peoples, and WHO policies on women's and men's health, workplace equity and health, and environmental protection can translate to local

actions. Each of these policies bring together the main issues surrounding equity, cultural inclusion, and family life. These policy areas therefore rely heavily on input from nurses and other health professionals who are present, visible and working with people where they live, work and play (Kickbusch 2012). By working towards connecting the global policy agenda vertically (at different levels) and horizontally (through different services) we can promote better care across the life course from pregnancy to the end of life, incorporating maternity care, early childhood education, adolescent and adult physical and mental health, care of the homeless and vulnerable, and healthy ageing.

ACTION POINT

Professional input is necessary in all policy areas from consultation and development to evaluation.

When community nurses coordinate the implementation of policies, they undertake an invaluable part of policymaking, particularly if they are able to send evaluative information and practitioner-informed evidence back to political decision-makers (Judd & Keleher 2013; Martin et al. 2013). Policies governing adult health such as the anti-tobacco strategies, women and men's health, family-friendly workplaces, climate change adaptation, food security, national chronic disease strategies, falls prevention, healthy ageing, rural health, social inclusion and mental health have been developed this way, with input from nurses in Australia and New Zealand. Where there are difficulties generating research evidence for change, nurses can provide informal information to policymakers in the context of community advocacy. The Australian Research Alliance for Children & Youth Declaration and Call to Action (see Appendix I) is a classic example of advocacy for family policies governing a good start to life, with significant input from many health and education professionals (ARACY 2009). The Te Rito Family Violence Intervention Strategy in New Zealand is another example of an important family policy initiative that has relied heavily on input from nurses and other health professionals prior to and during development. In these and other policy areas we are often seen as guardians of the community, ensuring health, protection from harm and cultural safety. Each of these policy areas continue to offer important opportunities to enact our social contract with society to promote health and social justice (Fawcett & Russell 2001). Equally as important is the need for us to ensure that policies are framed within a caring discourse, especially those that have been developed with an emphasis on economics and the market. The central policy theme is equity, and the strategies for achieving equity must revolve around the social determinants of health (SDH).

Connecting policies with the social determinants of health

Poverty is pervasive and persistent in some countries of the world, but it is social injustice that kills people: a toxic combination of poor policies, unfair economic arrangements and bad politics (CSDH 2008). As the UN reports, equitable social policies emanate from outside the health care system, in the economic environments of a nation or region (UN 2011). However, health care systems play three important roles in maintaining equity, by ensuring universal access to high-quality care, by advocating for health in all policies and actions related to the SDH, and by creating, managing and evaluating the evidence on health equity and the SDH in other policies (Marmot et al. 2012).

Australia and New Zealand boast universal access to high-quality care for most people, but we do not achieve the other two criteria to the extent that we could. The somewhat sporadic mention of health in the context of developing social policies may be due to the fact that our policy research is still at an early stage of development, without the longevity or level of evidence to mount cogent arguments for changes. Translating existing evidence into practice is challenging, given that ideas must be defended on the basis of expert opinion, political sensitivities, organisational constraints, and the possibility that policy development processes can become eroded by the time the evidence is presented (Dwan & McInnes 2013). The other problems lie in bureaucratic systems and the cultural divide between researchers and policymakers. Policymakers tend to rotate through government positions before evidence becomes accepted, and those who generate evidence are not always privy to policy discussions. A recent exploration of how evidence is incorporated into policymaking in New Zealand found an inconsistent range of practices and attitudes across government agencies (Gluckman 2013). These problems could be partially solved with the use of knowledge brokers or science advisors, who have the time, resources and position to build positive relationships between producers and users of research knowledge (Dwan & McInnes 2013; Gluckman 2013).

> ### EQUITY AND HEALTH CARE SYSTEMS
> * Ensuring universal access
> * Advocating for health in all policies
> * Generating evidence for equity and the SDH in all policies

Another issue concerns the type of evidence that is acceptable by government decision-makers who may be unaware of the impact of local case studies that could provide exemplars for good and best policies elsewhere. Process evaluations, for example, provide evidence of what works well, where and why (Tham et al. 2010), yet funding for this essential element of the policy process is frequently trimmed or diverted (Gluckman 2013). Australian researchers conducted a 'first estimate' of the extent and direct costs of community nursing to support diabetic patients in their homes. They found that community nursing cost an additional A$53 million annually to the health service, which, extrapolated nationally, adds an additional 5% to the total direct health care costs of diabetes (Davis et al. 2013). This type of data is important to policymakers, but it also suggests that without concurrently demonstrating the preventative value added by community nursing services, decision-makers may consider the costs prohibitive. To date, health service managers have been quick to adopt biomedical evidence, and, because the political power rests with the medical, technological and pharmaceutical industries, this is where the greatest level of funding is allocated. Public demand for scientific information also plays a role in maintaining the dominance of biomedical, technological and pharmaceutical services. Health care is not responsive to the business principles of supply and demand because cost-effectiveness is not something people generally seek. When a person is ill, they want the best, rather than the most economical health care. As a result, politicians and decision-makers find it easier to provide expensive medical care in urban environments, where demand is greatest. However, privileging hospital services over preventative, PHC programs and concentrating health care in urban environments, deprives many segments of the population from access to appropriate care and prevention of illness and injury.

POLICYMAKING AND PRIMARY HEALTH CARE

An inclusive approach to policy development resonates with a careful balance of comprehensive and selective PHC. Equitable services can be provided from comprehensive PHC systems that also accommodate selective care based on prioritised needs. Yet the logic of this type of policy environment has yet to be acknowledged by the 'strife of interests' among those competing for limited resources. Marginalised communities remain unable to control key processes that control their lives and their health or to select what they need. They are subjected to inadequate services, and difficult living conditions that prevent them from being able to challenge power brokers, or work towards building local capacity. A classic example is seen in the context of mental illness, where a 'catastrophic' reduction in acute psychiatric beds has seen many people homeless or living with family members struggling to cope with their care (Cunningham 2012). Another barrier to PHC lies in policy decisions that see staff appointed to rural and remote areas for short periods of time, which are insufficient for community engagement and, ultimately, problem solving. In some cases, they arrive in the community to find that they are expected to live in substandard, sometimes unsafe housing. As we mentioned in Chapter 5, they have few opportunities for professional interaction or continuing education. In addition, with so many regional, state and national employers making decisions about their role in health and community development, there are mixed messages and variable expectations of their role. An example is seen in the policies governing the schedule of child health assessments, which can vary according to whether the child health nurse is employed by local, regional, state, national or Aboriginal services. These factors make it difficult to maintain the focus on PHC. When communities and the people who care for them live in disadvantaged or unpredictable situations, their predominant focus is on day-to-day survival, which not only causes substandard health, but erodes social capital. Without political leadership that is committed to addressing the inequities of disadvantage, this situation will remain unchanged. The policy 'problem' is that, rather than try to mitigate the consequences of powerless groups, policymakers tend to shy away from restructuring health care, redefining labour relations or unemployment arrangements, or imposing regulations on environmental pollution, or taxes on alcohol or junk food that affect the poor disproportionately. Instead, spurred on by economic goals, social and health policies have continued to concentrate wealth in the hands of the powerful, which has left the poor and voiceless with a disproportionate amount of health-damaging experiences (CSDH 2008; Marmot et al. 2012).

> ### WHAT'S THE PROBLEM?
> - Focusing on creating wealth rather than fair distribution of wealth
> - Inadequate evidence for local policy implementation
> - Dominance of biomedical rather than social evaluations
> - Poor and disadvantaged are voiceless

Clearly, change is necessary, but it does not occur spontaneously. What is needed is an overt process of inviting community input, then an ongoing level of support. This would produce a combination of perspectives from the public, health professionals, health planners, and intersectoral policymakers to encourage multilevel, multidimensional approaches for better health. The key to success in accommodating such a breadth of opinions is authentic communication between all participants (Hawe 2009). But first, those in charge of health care have to extend the invitations, then practitioners need to become active and persistent advocates for communities, engaging with people to gain their support and input. In this era there is room for optimism, as the centrality of community engagement is being acknowledged in the contemporary policy environments of both Australia and New Zealand.

We have mentioned New Zealand's strong commitment to PHC in previous chapters, and New Zealand Government policy reflects this commitment more than a decade after the PHC strategy was introduced by devolving some hospital services to the community (Marinelli-Poole et al. 2011). Australia has now begun to follow suit, at least in the rhetoric surrounding PHC. The National Health Reform Agreement of 2011 was developed to commit the Commonwealth and the states and territories to work together on preventative health strategies and system-wide policy and state-wide planning for general practice and PHC. The objectives of the National PHC Strategic Framework of 2013 identified future policy directions and priorities including:

1 building a consumer-focused integrated PHC system

2 improving access and reducing inequity

3 increasing the focus on prevention, screening and early intervention

4 improving quality, safety, performance and accountability (Australian Government 2013a).

Critics of the government policy argue that there is too much emphasis on general practice and Medicare, rather than investing in comprehensive PHC (Donato & Segal 2013; Humphreys & Gregory 2012; Rushton & Kendall 2011). This is a legitimate criticism, given that government documents confuse primary care with primary health care, which has diluted the PHC agenda somewhat. General practitioners are also well recognised as being treatment focused rather than oriented towards health promotion (Rushton & Kendall 2011). The area of reform that has attracted strongest support is the focus on greater community engagement, particularly in the context of the Medicare Locals. The Medicare Locals are a nationwide network of organisations with the aim of coordinating primary care and addressing service gaps, ensuring that community and hospital services provide patient-centred care, where consumers have a voice in service planning and delivery (Australian Commission on Safety and Quality in Health Care [ACSQHC] 2013; Humphreys & Gregory 2012). As admirable as this initiative sounds, Medicare Locals do not have the incentive structure or mechanisms to promote integration, continuity of care or multidisciplinary care (Donato & Segal 2013). With the change of government in 2013 there is also a suggestion that the Medicare Locals may be replaced by alternative structures. The commitment to patient-centredness is, however, evident and continuing through the ACSQHC's mandate to embed health literacy into systems and organisational policies, providing focused and usable health information, and educating both health care providers and the recipients of health care to help build effective partnerships.

In New Zealand, attempts to devolve services traditionally provided in hospital settings to community settings have had mixed results. One of the primary issues has been the introduction of charges for services that were provided for free in hospitals. For example, the treatment of cellulitis (a common bacterial infection) usually requires intravenous antibiotics. In the past, a person was admitted to hospital for two to three days for treatment. Now, the person is treated in the community either at home or at their general practice. Although funding for the service was devolved to general practice, because general practice is run as a business, a consultation fee is often charged to the person in addition to the government funding. This can have major implications for low-income individuals and families and actually contribute to a delay in seeking treatment rather than improve access. It is essential that policy development in relation to devolution of services ensures equitable access to services is maintained. As in Australia, primary health care provision in New Zealand is frequently confused with primary care or general practice service provision.

HEALTH LITERACY

The key to community participation in policy development.

Empowering people with knowledge is good for their health. In the past, a lack of health literacy has prevented many people from being full participants in planning health services. Some have been reluctant to participate in technical policy discussions, feeling that their views have not been considered, or that an invitation is simply tokenism (Bruni et al. 2008). This reinforces the important role of community nurses in helping people become aware of the issues involved, and assisting them in putting forward their views (ACSQHC 2013). Participation by well-informed community members can help identify the need for services for the disadvantaged and vulnerable: those with the best understanding of the most urgent needs (Judd & Keleher 2013). Community input can also provide a basis for developing what is feasible and realistic in both developing and using policies in the local context and identifying ongoing needs. The Australian Health Literacy policy initiative demonstrates this commitment. It is based on a belief that enhancing health literacy can improve health care outcomes across the lifespan, and create a more culturally competent human-rights oriented approach to services (ACSQHC 2013). New Zealand policy also contains a commitment to building health literacy and sees this as a means of enabling people to interact with the health system more effectively and make better decisions about their health (NZMOH 2013a). These policy directions follow a strong commitment to health literacy in the US through the Institute of Medicine, and the European Health Literacy Project, both aimed at strengthening patient-centredness in the policy and service environments (HLS-EU 2012; IOM 2004).

The section to follow outlines a number of designated health policies, all of which need to be based on the principles of PHC and empowered participation by health literate community members. There is considerable overlap between policies that govern the health of people defined by age, gender, geography, history, health status and/or risk. The overlap should be recognised in policy development to promote consideration of how everything is connected to everything else in the policy arena. With this ecological mindset, policy development in one area can be used to leverage policy development in other areas, thereby maximising the use of scarce resources.

Health promotion policies

Because budgeting for health tends to be a zero sum exercise, policies that allocate disproportionate monies to acute care can impinge on the ability to fund preventative programs, including health promotion to the general community. The other barrier to health promotion policymaking is that for many years, policies have been developed on the basis of exhorting individuals to change their behaviour, rather than focus on the upstream causes of ill health, or the needs of the poor or those with disabling conditions. As a result, those with the worst health status, many of whom cannot afford health care, receive the fewest health services, and the cycle of inequities continues (Baum et al. 2009). This does not mean that policies focusing on behaviours have been entirely ineffective, because there have been some remarkable successes from a combination of behavioural and policy approaches, such as the introduction of legislation governing tobacco advertising and pricing, mandatory seatbelt legislation, devolving land to local councils to create green spaces for exercise, and a number of other initiatives designed to improve health. However, much remains to be done in promoting the health of populations, especially those disadvantaged by combinations of the SDH.

Rural health policies

As mentioned above, equity lies at the heart of good policies. Rural health policies in many countries, including Australia, remain inadequate to redress inequities that perpetuate the gradient in health status between urban, regional, rural and remote areas (Humphreys & Gregory 2012). Inequities between urban and rural dwellers are seen across the continuum from obstetric care, care for older people and the distribution of health professionals (Farmer et al. 2012; Hoang & Le 2013; Kamien 2009). The major issue in policymaking for rural communities is resource allocation and access to services that would enable PHC, but this issue seems only well articulated in rural health circles rather than the political arena. Research gaps also act as a barrier to translating policy knowledge to better rural health practice. Although the rural research to policy agenda is gaining momentum, there are few

longitudinal studies of rural health, a paucity of rigorous evaluations of what works, and a political preference for short-term outputs rather than more definitive long-term data from which sustainable PHC policy decisions could be made (Tham et al. 2010). Policies to address the needs of those disadvantaged by distance should be based on studies of a health service's ability to provide accessible, appropriate and responsive care with efficient continuity to rural residents. In addition, community-based participatory research (CBPR) can provide the essential input from the rural community (Judd & Keleher 2013). To promote sustainability, rural health services should be based on data indicating specific workforce needs, linkages between services, infrastructure, funding sources, governance, management and leadership. Research that informs these policy areas should investigate the primary, secondary and tertiary spectrum of care and how well it services rural people (Tham et al. 2010).

> ### RURAL HEALTH POLICY DATA
> - What works in the long term
> - How services can provide accessible, appropriate, responsive, continuous care
> - Workforce needs
> - Joined up services
> - Infrastructure and funding
> - Governance, management
> - Leadership

Current barriers to developing this type of comprehensive data in Australia include the complexity of Commonwealth-state-territory relations and the 'silo' mentality in all levels of government. Structural problems in the system that preclude collaborative problem-solving include jurisdictional confusion, the lack of investment in PHC, existing funding arrangements for services, the widely held view that health is a consumption rather than an investment, the metropolitan mindset, the role of the media and political expediency (Donato & Segal 2013; Humphreys & Gregory 2012). These problems have led to fragmented services, cost-shifting and an overt focus on workforce shortages rather than a comprehensive PHC and population approach (Humphreys & Gregory 2012). Even where there are health professionals available,

LEADERSHIP AT ALL LEVELS

- Organisational
- Policymaking
- Management
- Health promotion

the constraints on policymaking and implementation often include a lack of technical expertise, and the need for existing staff with varying skills to engage with many agencies, including fly-in fly-out staff, to maintain oversight of services (Bish et al. 2012). Clearly, there is a need for good stewardship in the health care system. To guide a more effective system requires leadership at four different levels: organisational, policymaking, management and health promotion (Judd & Keleher 2013).

Rural health is also disadvantaged in relation to urban health care in New Zealand. A recent health workforce policy has seen the introduction of bonding for health professionals who choose to work in areas difficult to staff, including some rural locations. As an incentive to work there, medical doctors and midwives who stay in a rural location for three to five years can have up to $10 000 per year written off their student loans (Health Workforce New Zealand, Online. Available: http://healthworkforce.govt.nz/our-work/voluntary-bonding-scheme [accessed 5 October 2013]). Interestingly, nurses who are in an ideal position to provide essential PHC to rural communities are not eligible for bonding in rural communities.

The issue of providing an adequate health workforce is a major challenge in New Zealand, which is identified as the country with the greatest inflow and outflow of health professionals among OECD countries (Buchan et al. 2011). In the 2011–12 year, the Nursing Council registered 1444 New Zealand-educated nurses (new graduates) and 1232 internationally qualified nurses (Nursing Council of New Zealand 2012). The previous two years had seen greater numbers of internationally qualified nurses registered than locally qualified nurses. By 2035, New Zealand is predicted to have a nursing workforce shortfall of 15 000 nurses (Nana et al. 2013). Like Australia, health professional education, including nursing, is costly, and less economical than international recruitment. New Zealand is also a 'source' country for Australian nursing recruitment (Buchan et al. 2011). Given the large number of unfilled vacancies in Australian rural

health the net outflow looks certain to continue, effectively further eroding the workforce capability. This will have significant ramifications for the sustainability of the New Zealand nursing workforce into the future, particularly if countries such as Australia and the US increase wages and salaries as a mechanism for meeting their own workforce demands.

Recent recommendations designed to ameliorate the impact of nurse migration to and from New Zealand include increasing funding for nurse education (to increase the number of clinical placements for nursing students and develop other models of clinical learning), developing strategies to improve recruitment of Māori and Pacific students into nursing, and considering means of increasing retention of older nurses in the workplace (Clendon & Walker 2013; Nana et al. 2013). One initiative to help redress the shortage of nurses and other health professionals has seen the New Zealand Institute of Management collaborate with University partners to develop the 'Aspiring Leaders Programme' for Māori, Pacific and Asian health professionals working for two District Health Boards (Canterbury and Manukau). Although each program is delivered in a way that is unique to local needs, the result for both is that there is a greater focus on culturally appropriate leadership for quality and patient safety throughout primary and secondary care (Marinelli-Poole et al. 2011). The program has been actively supported by Health Workforce NZ and will be expanded in future to create a mentoring program for new leaders who can develop both capabilities and system capacity through clinical leadership in all sectors of the health workforce. This type of development is an excellent example of developing workforce solutions by building local capacity.

Indigenous health policies

Indigenous health is of major concern to rural policy planners, given the proportion of Indigenous people residing in rural and remote areas. Structural features of rural health services are also differentially structured to meet the needs of Aboriginal and Torres Strait Islander people. Unlike many urban health services, Australian rural health services include Aboriginal Community Controlled Health Organisations (NACCHO) as well as the hospital, general practice and local community health centres (Bourke et al. 2012). Aboriginal Controlled Community Health Services (ACCHS) are therefore the only example of comprehensive PHC in Australia. Yet there remains a lack of integration of funding and policy responsibilities (Donato & Segal

2013). The rhetoric of national policies revolves around inclusive services that promote equity between services aimed specifically at Aboriginal and Torres Strait Islander people and those aimed at other Australians (Australian Government 2013b). A major priority is to work towards achieving positive health outcomes for those most vulnerable to ill health. The National Indigenous Reform Agreement (NIRA) was endorsed by the Council of Australian Governments in 2008, and commits all governments to six ambitious targets for Indigenous health relating to life expectancy, infant mortality, education and employment. The NIRA encompasses a National Partnership Agreement on Closing the Gap, which is the major policy initiative for Indigenous health, early childhood, education, economic participation and remote service delivery (Australian Government 2013 a, b). The agreement has been renewed until 2016 in the expectation of substantial returns on the investment in the SDH for Aboriginal and Torres Strait Islander people. The key policy targets are to close the gap in life expectancy within a generation (by 2031), and to halve the gap in mortality rates for Indigenous children under five by 2018. The partnership approach to policymaking is enacted through the National Congress of Australia's First Peoples working with the Commonwealth Government. The National Congress is intended to give Aboriginal and Torres Strait Islander people a strong voice on issues affecting them through NACCHO, the national peak body for Aboriginal and Torres Strait Islander controlled health organisations. In the interests of building a culturally competent health system the government also funds the National Anti-Racism Strategy and Reconciliation Australia to support constitutional recognition of Aboriginal and Torres Strait Islander Peoples (Australian Government 2013b).

CLOSING THE GAP

All levels of government working in partnership with the National Congress of Australia's First Peoples to improve life expectancy, infant mortality, education and employment.

Besides the overarching national policies to help achieve equity, other policy directives that influence Aboriginal and Torres Strait Islander people's health are the National PHC Strategic Framework of 2013, the National Aboriginal and Torres Strait Islander Suicide Prevention Strategy, the Roadmap for National Mental Health Reform 2012–2022, the Early

Childhood Education National Partnership and the National Strategy for Young Australians (aged 12–14) (AIHW 2012; Australian Government 2013 a, b). These reforms include a number of state, territory and Commonwealth programs that revolve around the social justice agenda of creating a fair and equitable Australia (Australian Government 2013a). At a regional and local level, policies that provide the foundation for parenting, especially in rural and remote areas, are crucial for ensuring a good start to life. Many of these programs are now being evaluated in a way that provides a stronger evidence base for policymaking, particularly within a national project to analyse the interplay between health, wellbeing, education and employment (Nguyen & Cairney 2013). The project will produce longitudinal monitoring of these relationships and study the effectiveness of interventions to inform policy and practice for the future. One of the most crucial system features to resolve is the need for greater self-determination of Aboriginal-controlled services, which has been shown to have a major impact on health in countries like the US and Canada. Future Australian health reforms must therefore address this issue as central to advancing the agenda for closing the gap (Donato & Segal 2013).

Māori health has been embedded in New Zealand health policy for many years. Chapter 13 outlines a range of policy strategies that are either specific to, or directed toward addressing the particular health needs of Māori and in particular, inequities in Māori health. These strategies include the New Zealand Health Strategy (NZMOH 2000), the New Zealand Primary Health Care Strategy (King 2001), He Korowai Oranga: the Māori Health Strategy (NZMOH 2002a), the Māori Mental Health Strategic Framework (NZMOH 2002b), the Māori Health Action Plan (NZMOH 2006a) and Whānau Ora (NZMOH 2002a). In addition, the New Zealand Government has allocated $12 million toward increasing the capacity and capability of the Māori health workforce (NZMOH, Online. Available: www.health.govt.nz/our-work/nursing/nursing-initiatives/Māori-nursing-and-workforce-initiatives [accessed 5 October 2013]), further underlining their commitment to addressing Indigenous health through policy frameworks. The health of Pacific people in New Zealand is also an area where the New Zealand Government has undertaken significant policy work and this is discussed later in the chapter.

Men's and women's health policies

Gender is an important determinant of health, closely intertwined with family and other SDH. Policies aimed at gender equity are therefore, in effect, family policies. Like other social policies, they should embody PHC principles to be effective in creating fairness and equity. In both Australia and New Zealand, the men's movements and the policies that flowed from men's lobby groups have created greater social awareness of the connection between healthy men, healthy families and a healthy and productive society. The first Australian Male Health Policy was developed in 2010 on the basis of six foundation principles: optimal health outcomes for males; health equity between population groups of males; improved health for males at different life stages; a focus on preventative health, especially chronic disease and injury; building a strong evidence base on male health as a basis for policies, programs and initiatives; and improved access to health care through initiatives and tailored health care services, particularly for groups at high risk of ill health (Commonwealth of Australia, Online. Available: www.health.gov.au/internet/main/publishing.nsf/Content/male-policy [accessed 26 August 2013]). The principles present a framework for policy planners to ensure that men's health continues to improve throughout the life course, from childhood to the older years.

> ## MEN'S HEALTH POLICY
> * Optimal health
> * Equity between groups
> * Life course focus
> * Preventative health
> * Evidence-based planning
> * Improved access to care

Similarly, the National Women's Health policy—which has been redeveloped 20 years after the first version of an Australian women's health policy—established priorities for women's health that are also useful for promoting fairness and equity in the family and society (Commonwealth of Australia 2010 a, b). The main priorities for the women's health policy are to continue to promote equitable structures and processes to support the health and wellbeing of Australian women, through selective PHC for those most at risk of ill health (Commonwealth of Australia 2010b). The women's health policy mirrors the policy for men, in adopting a life course approach, a focus on health promotion and illness prevention, in addressing equity on the basis of gender, and in relation to disadvantaged population groups, and the need for an appropriate evidence base for planning. Both policies are framed within a social inclusion agenda, and each addresses Indigenous disadvantage, as well as issues related to gender, vulnerability among migrants (see Box 14.1) and those living in rural areas.

> ## WOMEN'S HEALTH POLICY
> * Equitable structures, processes
> * Life course focus
> * Health promotion
> * Evidence-based planning
> * Sexual, reproductive health

The Australian Women's Health policy also addresses sexual and reproductive health as a priority, which is significant, given that current models of maternity care have failed to support the most vulnerable families (Sutherland et al. 2012). Research has shown that women disadvantaged by socio-economic position (SEP), social exclusion or ethnicity are the ones who have delayed presentation for pregnancy care, less contact with care providers, fewer positive experiences of care and poorer maternal and infant health outcomes (Sutherland et al. 2012). To some extent, this differential in care is due to the structural constraints of a two-tiered health system with public and private provision of services. Pregnant women with private health insurance have choices, whereas those who cannot afford private care have access only to those public services that are readily available to them. Given the unevenness in services across urban, rural and regional areas, some do not have access to midwifery models of care, which Australian women have identified as their preferred option for antenatal care (Sutherland et al. 2012). What this suggests is that in an environment of universal services, meaningful policy development must follow through with a distribution of services that will meet the needs and preferences of those they are designed to serve. Midwifery models also have a strong focus on coordination and continuity of care, which is often missing from public services in Australia. New Zealand's universal provision of maternity care based on a lead maternity care model (a model that is largely midwife-led) means that all women in New Zealand have access to free antenatal, birth and postnatal midwife-led services if they choose. Despite universal provision and increased funding for maternity services over recent years, vulnerable groups such as women on low incomes, teen

BOX 14.1 Gender, the environment, migration and refugee policies

Among the most significant changes to contemporary life is the recognition that climate change is affecting health and policymaking throughout the world. This is a gender issue in that natural disasters such as droughts, floods and storms cause higher mortality for women, especially young women of low SEP (WHO 2011). Men are also at risk from climate change, especially farmers whose livelihoods are imperilled by drought, which has, in some cases, been responsible for their depression and ultimate suicide (WHO 2011). However, particularly in developing countries, climate-sensitive impacts show significant gender differences because of women's under-nutrition, disproportionate vulnerability to diseases and social isolation, leaving them with food insecurity, caring responsibilities, and an inability to travel for clean water and food. Many of these women are already exposed to higher levels of environmental pollution, primarily through inefficient burning of biomass in unventilated homes (WHO 2011). In Western countries, women's social isolation can also leave them vulnerable, especially if they are unable to migrate elsewhere or they do not have access to information that could help them reduce their exposure to harmful substances. In our part of the world many women in Island communities face a similar fate as they watch their lands slowly fall victim to rising sea levels, and some look for ways to migrate to either New Zealand or Australia to provide for their families in future.

The influences of gender, the environment and migration also have a profound effect on children.

Besides civil wars, environmental destruction is one of the most important reasons for people migrating across borders to seek a healthier life for their families. Cassrels (2013) explains an abominable situation that has arisen in Indonesia where mixed-race children who are the progeny of teenage Indonesian women and asylum-seeking men who have left them are abandoned by both parents to fend for themselves on the street or be institutionalised in orphanages. Their fathers have set out on boats for Australia, and the mothers have left them because of the stigma over their husbands' desertion, which has left them bereft and ashamed. Many of these couples have engaged in a 'traveller's marriage'; a short-term relationship which contracts impoverished young women to serve the asylum-seeker's needs. The women tend to enter these marital contracts to avoid being labelled a prostitute, but when children are born, some of the mothers have no alternative but to turn to prostitution to support themselves. Many do not register the child's birth, which leaves the child in limbo, homeless, stateless and destitute. In some cases the authorities turn a blind eye to their plight, and they become part of a new generation of exploited girls who are sold into slavery or confined at someone's pleasure. The morality of this situation is something that evokes a range of emotions from politicians, parents, health and social welfare advocates and the general public, but the solutions lie in activating policies that protect human rights globally and locally. The United National High Commission for Refugees can only do so much. Border protection or human protection?

---

mothers, migrant mothers and women living in rural areas remain at risk of poorer birth outcomes (NZMOH 2012a). Without deliberate service coordination the childbirth experience can compound the vulnerability of some women and their children.

UNIQUE ISSUES FOR WOMEN

- Access to midwifery models of care
- Career interruptions
- Lower SEP
- Impoverished by separation
- Child care responsibilities

The other issue related to childbearing women is that because Australian women spend longer out of the workforce after giving birth than those in other countries (Johnstone & Lee 2012), there is a need to ensure that their needs for career development are recognised by employers, especially in the context of a planned expansion of parental leave. The linkages between employment and family life are relevant to both women's and men's policy development, whether the family is relatively stable, or in the context of post-separation needs. For separating families, advocacy from health professionals as well as socio-legal experts and community members can help ensure that fairness is high on the agenda for policymaking (Family & Relationship Services Australia 2012). The family issues involved in marriage and its dissolution clearly indicate the need for intersectoral collaboration to embed health in all policies in the socio-legal and health areas.

THE NEED FOR POLICY INTEGRATION: LESSONS FROM MENTAL HEALTH

Mental health is among the most significant policy areas for all countries of the world because it is pervasive and overlaps with all other aspects of health and wellbeing. In most countries, the incidence of mental illness has steadily increased over the past thirty years, while government funding for those who suffer from these illnesses has continued to decline (WHO 2010). In 2008 the WHO launched a global action program, the 'Mental Health Gap Action Programme' (mhGAP) to forge strategic partnerships that would enhance countries' efforts to combat stigma, reduce the burden of mental disorders, and promote mental health (WHO, Online. Available: www.who.int/ mental_health/mhgap/en/ [accessed 11 September 2013]). The impetus for the program was evidence that although the burden of mental illness is modest compared with other diseases, 75% of the world's people, especially in poor countries, do not have access to the treatment they need. Mental health is therefore a human rights issue. The other major WHO initiative is a program to promote mental health and treatment for substance abuse called WHO MIND. The MIND program covers four thematic areas: mental health policy, planning and integrated service development; mental health, human rights and legislation for denied citizens, including those excluded because of intellectual disabilities; mental health, poverty and development; and action in countries, a support program to help improve the lives of those with mental disorders. The overarching mission in all four areas is called the QualityRightsProject, which guides people to act, unite and empower people to improve service delivery and human rights conditions in mental health facilities and social care homes (WHO, Online Available: www.int/ mental_health/policy/legislation/en/index.html [accessed 11 September 2013]). Nurses are pivotal to helping achieve these goals, and the International Council of Nurses (ICN) has given its full support to the MIND project, urging nurses to become engaged in mental health policy development, advocate for those with mental health issues and ensure that their health assessments are inclusive of mental disorders (WHO, Nursing Matters, Online. Available: www.int/mental_health/ policy/legislation/en/index.html [accessed 11 September 2013]).

WHO QualityRights
- Act
- Unite
- Empower those hospitalised for mental illness

Nursing actions
- Assess mental health
- Engage in policy development
- Help people build coping skills

These global initiatives are relevant to community nurses, primarily because of the large number of people living with mental health problems in their home and community. From the 1970s, mentally ill patients were shifted from psychiatric hospitals to be treated in their communities. Since this change occurred, the onus has been placed on families and community support systems to care for those with mental illness (Cunningham 2012). However, without the provision of sufficient support services, many families caring for their loved ones have experienced enormous difficulties in the burden of care. In Australia and New Zealand, services are provided by a range of agencies, with heavy reliance on community mental health nurses or psychiatric nurses working as part of a team (see Chapter 5). This system is intended to provide families with specialist services and emergency responses when there are mental health crises, but major shortages of mental health specialists have meant that these services are unreliable, especially in rural areas. The shortage is compounded by the lack of positions available from the various health systems. In some cases, there is little understanding of the culturally appropriate mental health needs of Indigenous people, and instead of providing community services, the person affected may be flown out to a central service. These people are often in crisis, and further alienated when they are treated at a distance from family and community supports. Even those without the need for crisis care suffer from a lack of guidance and support services in the community.

Another important aspect of mental health policy is the need for guidance on preventative strategies. The mental health policy environment has thus far been directed towards mental illness, but the need for health promotion policies that respond to the SDH is acute. Raphael (2009) explains that, compared with other kinds of health promotion, there is less infiltration of mental health promotion into government and public health-related documents. Although his comments refer to the Canadian situation, the situation is similar in the policy environments of Australia and New Zealand. The omission of mental health in the SDH discourse is important, as mental health is seen as a mediating force between the SDH and physical health. This primarily involves mental states associated with exposure to adverse living conditions and psychosocial stress, which can cause maladaptive biological responses, weaken immune systems, and create a greater likelihood of metabolic disorders (Raphael 2009). Responses to inequalities, such as feelings of shame, worthlessness and envy, also have psycho-biological effects on health, precipitating coping behaviours such as overspending, overeating, use of alcohol and tobacco, or a range of other social behaviours that threaten health (Raphael 2009).

Good mental health policies should guide appropriate service provision for those needing help, but they should also work towards decreasing vulnerability by helping people develop coping skills. In response to the SDH, such policies should be prioritised on the basis of reducing people's exposure to negative conditions; for example, by providing educational and recreational opportunities as community entitlements. Mental health policies should also provide employment and job security, social assistance for those in need, and balance universal and identified needs, again, through comprehensive and selective PHC (Raphael 2009). This illustrates the integrated nature of mental health and other policies.

MENTAL HEALTH POLICIES AND FAMILY LIFE

As we mentioned earlier in the chapter many policies have a cascade effect that can permeate family and community life, including policies governing child care, the workplace and income security. For parents who are both in the workplace, child care is a major source of stress. Family leave policies that provide income replacement and incentives for parents to take leave can help alleviate the stress of parenting. Both New Zealand and Australia have paid parental leave, but as we discussed in Chapter 8, there is variability in the workplace in terms of supporting breastfeeding or leave to attend to children when they are ill. Gendered workplace norms also see the male partner spending longer hours at work, sometimes because of his greater earning capacity, to cover family expenses when a mother chooses to stay at home. This leaves the child deprived of the father's time, and the mother having to be the constant parent. For some women, the lack of respite can undermine their mental health, adding to the vulnerability of new parenthood. Those with existing mental health issues often fail to reveal when their health is compromised, fearing victimisation or job loss, which leads to cycles of worsening mental health.

The Global Financial Crisis has also had residual effects on mental health for residents of both countries, increasing unemployment or downsizing jobs to part-time or casual employment. Declining financial resources or economic hardship can compromise parents' mental health, and sometimes has an effect on physical health. In combination, these factors can also be a difficult challenge for the relationship, especially when parents are also physically tired from caring for the child and/or other children. These factors are all linked to a family's capacity to raise children, and they underline the need for a big-picture, intergenerational, ecological perspective in policymaking. The interrelatedness of policy decisions is also seen in government policies to encourage child bearing, fair employment, productivity, retirement and superannuation simultaneously.

Among the grandparent generation, retirees continue to have an uncertain future given losses in their superannuation investments, and they are often warned that with the long-term trend towards low fertility there will be a lower tax base to fund their pensions. Some have been persuaded to remain in the workforce into their 70s rather than drain their existing resources with no guarantee of the adequacy of government pensions should they live longer than expected. Older people are therefore watching the policy debates closely, including political arguments for increasing the population through migration to maintain productivity once they have retired. In Australia, opinions have become polarised, with one side supporting an increase in the number of migrants, and the other side worrying about sustainability of the environment and its infrastructure with a larger population.

In 2010, Australian policymakers realised that, after a decade of policy-driven cash incentives for young Australian couples to boost the fertility rate, there was a virtual baby boom occurring throughout the country. Increasing the fertility rate through the cash grants was based on the expectation that the children would become active in the workplace just when their tax contributions were most needed; that is, when they could support the growing number of retirees, who would be withdrawing their superannuation investments. Some of these parents then separated, and became single supporting parents. Then in 2012 the Australian Government scrapped the Parenting Payment for single parents with children aged 8 and over, in an attempt to get more women into the workforce and try to recoup lost revenue from several years of government overspending and a gradual decline in the resource boom, reducing national productivity. As a result, 65 000 Australian single mothers were moved onto the NewStart Allowance which dramatically reduced their level of financial support. Many single mothers suffered emotionally and financially, and the child poverty rate has increased year by year (Kleinman 2013). These young mothers are watching policy development closely. With the change of government in 2013 there is a recommendation for an extended Paid Parental Scheme, presumably funded by employers. If the policy proposal is approved by the government and the new scheme is adopted what remains to be seen is whether or not employers will reduce jobs to retain their productivity, or exert some type of subtle discrimination against single mothers in the workplace. This is a classic policy debate illustrating, again, that everything is indeed connected to everything else.

WHAT'S YOUR OPINION?

Will increasing the fertility rate now have the intended consequences? What are some of the advantages and disadvantages of this policy?

New Zealand has also introduced policies designed to encourage single mothers and other beneficiaries into work by adjusting benefit entitlements. Three reforms of the welfare system have taken place since 2012. In summary, beneficiaries are required to meet certain obligations in order to continue to receive a benefit. The types

of obligations include being in part-time work of up to 15 hours per week for parents of children aged between 5 and 13 and in full-time work if they are over 13; ensuring the child is enrolled with a general practice, in early childhood education and up-to-date with well-child checks; in education, training or work; and completing parenting and budgeting courses if they are on a youth benefit. In addition, unemployment benefit recipients must be able to pass a pre-employment drug test if required. If these obligations are not met, benefits will initially be cut and then removed entirely if a situation is not addressed (NZ Ministry of Social Development, Online. Available: www.msd.govt.nz/about-msd-and-our-work/work-programmes/welfare-reform/index.html [accessed 6 October 2013]). The primary people affected by these changes are young people and single women with or without children. While the policies are designed to encourage people into work, the punitive outcomes of not meeting the required obligations may inadvertently serve to further disadvantage vulnerable children, women and young people. There is little outlined in the new policies regarding provision of support to people who may need help in achieving the requirements. Evaluation of the policy changes will be essential to ensure that appropriate and accessible support is offered to people and that the policy has not further disadvantaged already vulnerable individuals and families.

AUSTRALIAN MENTAL HEALTH POLICY

Since its inception in the 1970s Australia's Mental Health Strategy has undergone numerous transformations. At that time, government authorities had assumed responsibility for those with mental illness, but with deinstitutionalisation, this responsibility was devolved to families. The expectation of deinstitutionalisation was that by integrating those with mental illness into the community, they would receive more humane, individualised and culturally appropriate care. This was seen to be more empowering, and equated mental ill health with physical ill health in terms of treatment options (Henderson 2005). However, the need for mental health reform continued, and the National Mental Health Policy was developed in 2008. The policy vision was to enable recovery from mental illness, prevent and detect mental illness early, and ensure effective and appropriate treatment and support. The policy revolves around mental illness prevention, reducing its impact and promoting recovery to where all people can participate meaningfully in society (Commonwealth of Australia 2009, 2010c). Evaluation of progress indicates that a strength of the policy is its focus on partnerships and workforce issues, the latter being encompassed in National Standards for Mental Health Services and Practice Standards for Workforce. The policy continues to evolve, recognising the importance of collaboration between many state, territory and Commonwealth departments in planning mental health changes, and in developing a strong workforce to support people's mental health needs. Government planners have also acknowledged the need for evidence-based initiatives and equitable arrangements that can best meet the needs of vulnerable groups such as Aboriginal and Torres Strait Islander people. As we mentioned in Chapter 13, this commitment is evident in the National Aboriginal and Torres Strait Islander Suicide Prevention Strategy and a number of initiatives to address the mental health needs of adolescents across all cultures. The importance placed on mental health is also evident in the National Women's and National Male Policies, which have a strong focus on relationships.

AUSTRALIAN MENTAL HEALTH POLICY

- Prevention
- Detection
- Recovery
- Partnerships
- Workforce
- Collaboration
- Cultural considerations

NEW ZEALAND MENTAL HEALTH POLICY

New Zealand's history of mental health policy is not dissimilar to that of Australia. Deinstitutionalisation, responsibility for care placed on family members, and commodification of health care with business models and language, have all been similar features. In 1994, the first New Zealand Mental Health Strategy was released. This was followed in 1998, by publication of the *Blueprint for Mental Health Services in New Zealand* (NZ Mental Health Commission 1998). The Blueprint described the mental health service developments required for implementation of the 1994 Mental Health Strategy, setting the scene for incorporation of mental health as a priority area in health policy. Mental health as a priority health area for the government was subsequently reflected in the New Zealand Health

Strategy (NZMOH 2000), New Zealand Disability Strategy (NZMOH 2001) and New Zealand Primary Health Care Strategy (King, 2001). In 2012, *Blueprint II: Improving Mental Health and Wellbeing for all New Zealanders: How Things Need to Be* (NZ Mental Health Commission 2012a) was published. Concurrently, the Mental Health Commission also published *Blueprint II: Improving Mental Health and Wellbeing for all New Zealanders: Making Change Happen* (NZ Mental Health Commission 2012b). This second document outlined how the proposed changes were to be achieved. Where Blueprint I focused on the 3% of people with the most severe mental illness and implementing a recovery approach, Blueprint II widened that mandate to incorporate those with lower level need but whose lives are still profoundly impacted by mental illness or addiction (NZ Mental Health Commission 2012a).

NZ MENTAL HEALTH POLICY

Focus is on promoting the mental health of all New Zealanders, not just those experiencing severe illness.

None of the Blueprint documents are government policy but all have been designed to inform the development of policy and in particular service development plans. In 2005, *Te Tahuhu— Improving Mental Health 2005–2015: The Second New Zealand Mental Health and Addiction Plan* (NZMOH 2005) was published. This was followed in 2006, by *Te Kokiri: The Mental Health and Addiction Action Plan* (NZMOH 2006b), in 2008 by *Te Puāwaiwhero: The Second Māori Mental Health and Addiction National Strategic Framework 2008–2015* (NZMOH 2008), and in 2012 by *Rising to the Challenge: The Mental Health and Addiction Service Development Plan 2012–2017* (NZMOH 2012b). This series of plans demonstrates the constant process of policy development as new information and research feeds into the policy process. The new plan sets goals that have extended the previous policy focus from care for those most seriously affected by mental illness, to promoting the mental health of all New Zealanders. Four priority goals have been identified: effective use of existing resources; building infrastructure for greater integration between primary and secondary services; building on gains in resiliency and recovery among people with low-prevalence disorders and/or high needs, Māori, Pacific, refugee people and people with disability; and delivering increased access for children and youth, those with high prevalence conditions, and the growing older population (NZMOH 2012b). The broadening of focus from identifying and treating more serious mental ill health to promoting mental wellbeing in PHC is intended to promote social equity. Care, and access to care, has already been improved for those experiencing lifestyle-related stress and anxiety (Dowell et al. 2009). The onus is now on health professionals to work closely with their communities to ensure primary mental health care is provided in an appropriate, accessible, affordable and culturally safe manner.

Of particular concern in New Zealand is the very high youth suicide rate, as mentioned in Chapter 9. In 2013 the New Zealand Government published a suicide prevention action plan with a strong focus on supporting families and communities to prevent suicide and reduce the impact of suicide, improve the range, coverage and targeting of suicide prevention services, and lift the quality of information and evidence for effective suicide prevention (NZMOH 2013b). The action plan has a particular focus on suicide prevention among Māori youth whose suicide rates are two and a half times greater than non-Māori youth. The initiatives outlined in the plan and in other mental and general health policy documents do not stand alone but are designed to run in parallel with a range of other policy initiatives designed to improve the social circumstances of all New Zealanders. These include reducing long-term welfare dependence, supporting vulnerable children, boosting skills and employment, reducing crime, and improving interaction with government (NZ Ministry of Social Development, Online. Available: www.msd.govt.nz/about-msd-and-our-work/work-programmes/better-public-services/index.html [accessed 6 July 2013]; NZMOH 2013b). As outlined earlier in the chapter, policy should be an integrated process with consideration of the impact of a policy on other policies and processes and ultimately, their impact on people.

POLICY AND HEALTH SYSTEM FEATURES

The New Zealand health care system

Health and disability services in New Zealand are delivered by a complex network of people and organisations. Overall responsibility for the delivery of health services lies with the Minister of Health, who is elected through the democratic process to government, and appointed to the role of Minister. The Minister of Health, in conjunction with the Ministry of Health, provides overall leadership and direction for the numerous providers of health care

in New Zealand. Box 14.2 provides an example of the public consultation process undertaken by the New Zealand Government. The New Zealand Health Strategy (NZMOH 2000) provides the direction for the current system of health care in New Zealand. The Strategy identified seven fundamental principles that were to be reflected across the health sector. These were:

- acknowledgement of the special relationship that exists between the Crown and Māori under the Treaty of Waitangi
- good health and wellbeing for all New Zealanders throughout their lives
- an improvement in health status of those currently disadvantaged
- collaborative health promotion and disease and injury prevention by all sectors
- timely and equitable access for all New Zealanders to a comprehensive range of health and disability services, regardless of ability to pay
- a high-performing system in which people have confidence
- active involvement of consumers and communities at all levels (NZMOH 2000).

> ## HEALTH SYSTEM STRUCTURES
>
> District Health Boards (DHBs) have responsibility for planning, managing, providing and purchasing health services for New Zealanders.

For the first time, the 2000 New Zealand Health Strategy signalled the importance of health inequalities, the SDH, and active participation by communities as key contributors to the health of the New Zealand population. The Strategy provided a framework and context for District Health Boards as the majority providers of public health services to develop services for their identified populations. There are currently 20 District Health Boards (DHBs) in New Zealand. DHBs plan, manage, provide and purchase services for the population of their district. This includes funding for public health services, primary health care services (through PHOs), aged care, and services provided by other non-government health providers including Māori and Pacific providers (NZMOH, Online. Available: www.health.govt.nz/new-zealand-health-system/overview-health-system [accessed 6 October 2013]). DHBs employ a range of health professionals to provide services including medical doctors, nurses

BOX 14.2 Engaging with the political system and policy formation

New Zealand's political system is set up to ensure that all groups have the opportunity to submit feedback on proposed policies and legislation. The development of the Green and White Papers for Vulnerable Children and the subsequent enactment of the *Vulnerable Children's Act* provide excellent examples of how the government undertook a comprehensive consultation process with the New Zealand public during the development of the policies and legislation. The Green Paper was the initial consultation paper that outlined the issues facing vulnerable children and the services that are supposed to protect them. Over 10 000 public submissions were received on the Green Paper with many submissions made by nurses, children and other members of the public (NZ Ministry of Social Development, Online. Available: www.childrensactionplan.govt.nz/home [11 October 2013]). This feedback was used to inform development of the White Paper and Children's Action Plan which provide the framework for development of new and improved services for vulnerable children and the legislative changes that were needed to improve aspects of care and protection. The Vulnerable Children's Bill went through the standard political process that included the opportunity for the public and interested agencies to provide submissions on aspects of the legislation.

Having a say in the political process and the formation of policy is an essential role for nurses.

The practice experience of nurses can help inform the development of robust policy and there are many different levels and ways in which nurses can be involved in the process. Some simple ways to engage in the process are as follows:

- contributing to or commenting on a proposed policy in your workplace or community
- commenting on or contributing to a guideline or publication written by your professional organisation
- joining a working group developing new policies or practices
- writing or contributing to a submission during a policy consultation process
- making an oral submission to a workplace committee or a parliamentary select committee
- by signing a petition, participating in a campaign or even going on strike
- by simply sending an email with your thoughts on it to a manager, policy analyst, or member of parliament (Clendon 2013).

Using examples from everyday practice that reflect the knowledge, skill and impact nurses have on patient care is a useful approach to take in writing or speaking to a submission. These real-life examples are helpful in informing policymakers of the reality of clinical practice and the potential impact of a proposed policy change.

---

and allied health staff, such as physiotherapists and occupational therapists. However, long waiting lists to receive care from public health services have seen the development of a robust private health care sector in New Zealand, particularly for the provision of surgical care. Many individual New Zealanders who can afford it choose to purchase their own health insurance policies, in order to ensure they have access to surgical care quickly if they need it. However, for those people who cannot afford health insurance, poor access to surgical care can mean prolonged suffering and disability that is easily preventable. Many medical specialists work in both private and public health systems, potentially increasing the risk of long public health waiting lists and the inequities this creates. Improving access to elective surgery is one of six government targets designed to improve efficiency and care across the health sector although strategies designed to achieve this target are not addressing the discrepancies in private/public surgical provision. The other five targets are: shorter stays in emergency departments (six hour target), shorter waits for cancer treatment, increased immunisation, better help for smokers to quit, and more heart and diabetes checks (NZ National Health Board 2011). While these targets are worthy goals, a focus on targets can divert attention from other, equally important areas of health, sometimes with severe consequences (Francis 2013). Targets such as the above also fail to address factors such as the SDH. New Zealand is ranked close to the bottom among OECD countries in terms of health inequality (Wilkinson & Pickett 2009) and as we have mentioned in previous chapters, child poverty is a significant concern in New Zealand. Until concerted political action is taken on the SDH, these factors are unlikely to improve.

DHBs also have responsibility for funding PHC, and this is done primarily through Primary Health Organisations (PHOs). The Primary Health Care Strategy (King 2001) provided a framework for the development of PHC services in New Zealand. PHOs were mooted as the vehicles through which services would be funded and provided. There are currently 31 PHOs throughout New Zealand, funded by DHBs to provide PHC services to an enrolled population. PHOs vary in size and structure, are not-for-profit, and either provide services directly by employing staff or through provider members. Most general practices are members of PHOs and provide the bulk of primary care services in New Zealand (NZMOH, Online. Available: www.health.govt.nz/our-work/primary-health-care/about-primary-health-organisations [accessed 6 October 2013]).

General practices charge a fee-for-service on top of the funding they receive through the PHO. Most general practices are run as businesses by the general practitioner, who then employs staff such as nurses within the business. This business model creates difficulties for practice nurses seeking to extend their practice, due to power imbalances inherent in employee and employer relationships, and traditional models of practice. It was hoped that population-based funding and the advent of PHOs would go some way toward addressing this issue, but to date there has been limited progress. With the business model being the predominant model of care in PHC settings, nurses' ability to develop more effective models of care for patients has been stymied, although some are now challenging this. Growing population demands and the retirement of older GPs from rural areas have seen nurses stepping up to offer nurse-led clinics and, in some cases, buying into general practices. The government has also recently improved access for nurses to direct funding for services provided to high-need populations rather than requiring GP sign-off as has traditionally been the case.

TRENDING NOW

Nurse-led clinics and nurses buying into general practices as business owners.

Aged and residential care in New Zealand is provided through a mix of privately and publicly funded services. Large business conglomerates have bought out many of the aged and residential care providers in New Zealand that were traditionally run by charitable trusts. The New Zealand Government funds providers to deliver services to those in need, yet standards of care in aged and residential care are frequently poor with a lack of appropriately skilled staff identified as one of the primary contributors to this (NZ Human Rights Commission 2012; New Zealand Labour Party, Greens & Grey Power 2010). Low pay rates in the sector make it difficult to attract and retain nursing staff and while significant lobbying has been underway for some years by union groups and the Human Rights Commission to increase pay, little action has been taken by aged and residential care providers to improve pay rates or conditions of employment (NZ Human Rights Commission 2012). Given the significant levels of funding provided by government, further work is required to improve standards of care across the sector.

A unique feature of the New Zealand health system is the Accident Compensation Corporation (ACC). The ACC was established in 1974 and is in effect an insurance scheme that provides personal injury cover for all New Zealanders and some visitors. The ACC is funded through a mixture of levies from people's earnings, businesses, petrol and vehicle licensing fees and government funding. This means that if a person has an accident in New Zealand, the majority of costs associated with this will be covered by the ACC at no cost to the person. In return for this injury cover, an individual is unable to sue another person or company for personal injury except for exemplary damages (ACC, Online. Available: www.acc.co.nz/about-acc/overview-of-acc/introduction-to-acc/index.htm [accessed 6 October 2013]). There are inequities associated with ACC funding. For example, if an accident results in a person becoming permanently disabled, the ACC will fund all the care and equipment that person requires on an ongoing basis. On the other hand, if a person is permanently disabled due to a congenital abnormality or a medical condition, all costs associated with the disability are borne by the individual with limited financial support.

A further unique element of the New Zealand health system is the Pharmaceutical Management Agency or PHARMAC. PHARMAC is an agency of the New Zealand Government that decides, on behalf of District Health Boards, which medicines and related products are subsidised for use in the community and, in some cases, funded in public hospitals (Pharmaceutical Management Agency 2013). PHARMAC was established in 1973 as an attempt to control the spiralling costs of medicines in New Zealand. Its role was to get better value and better health outcomes for New Zealanders for the money spent on medicines. Today, PHARMAC's main roles are to:

- manage the Pharmaceutical Schedule of about 1800 government-subsidised community pharmaceuticals
- promote the responsible use of medicines
- manage the funding of medicines and some medical devices used in public hospitals
- manage the Named Patient Pharmaceutical Assessment policy and other special access programs.

Since its establishment in 1993, PHARMAC's annual drug budget has increased at only 2% per annum compared to 15% in the 1980s, and by 2007, drug spending as a proportion of health expenditure was much lower than in other OECD countries (Cumming et al. 2010). Since 2000, PHARMAC has saved more than $5 billion against 1999 costs (PHARMAC, Online. Available: www.pharmac.health.nz/about/our-history [accessed 10 October 2013]). Despite these encouraging outcomes, PHARMAC still struggles to balance the needs of individuals with the needs of the population, and inevitably, some people miss out on funding for medicines that may save their lives.

Paramedic care is provided largely by the St Johns Ambulance Service. Exceptions include the Wellington Free Ambulance Service covering the greater Wellington area, and air ambulance and rescue helicopter services, which are provided privately through a mix of government funding and corporate sponsorship. The St Johns Ambulance Service has a significant volunteer base with volunteers providing the majority of paramedic services in rural areas. This has both advantages and disadvantages. Volunteerism is known to increase social capital in a community; however, increasing demands on volunteer ambulance officers and limited funding to employ full-time officers is increasing health risks for rural populations.

Primary maternity care in New Zealand is provided by Lead Maternity Carers (LMCs). A woman selects an LMC to provide her maternity care throughout the duration of the pregnancy, birth and first weeks following birth. An LMC may be a general practitioner with a Diploma in Obstetrics, an obstetrician or a midwife. Midwifery as a profession in New Zealand has its own distinct body of knowledge, scope of practice, standards of practice and code of ethics. The 1990 *Nurses Amendment Act* enabled a registered midwife to undertake full responsibility for the care of women throughout their pregnancy. It also made provision for direct-entry midwifery education. Where previously, nurses would complete a year-long postgraduate education

program to become a midwife, now midwifery qualifications are only offered through a three-year Bachelor of Midwifery program. *The Nurses Act* was superseded by the *Health Practitioners Competence Assurance (HPCA) Act* in 2003, which acts to regulate all health professionals in New Zealand.

MATERNITY CARE IN NEW ZEALAND

Lead Maternity Carers (LMCs) are funded to provide maternity care in New Zealand. Most LMCs are midwives.

POINT TO PONDER

The *Health Practitioner Competency Assurance Act* governs the competency of health professionals to practice in New Zealand.

The *HPCA Act* is designed to protect public safety, by providing mechanisms to ensure the lifelong competency of health practitioners. A number of titles are protected under the Act, and only health practitioners who are registered under the Act are entitled to use such titles. Professions regulated include nursing, midwifery, medicine, pharmacy, physiotherapy and a range of other allied health professions. The Act separates health practitioner registration activities from competence and disciplinary processes. Registration activities are undertaken by the respective health profession's council or board. For example, the Nursing Council of New Zealand is the statutory body that governs the practice of nurses, monitors and sets standards for practice, and maintains the register of nurses. The Health Practitioner Disciplinary Tribunal, however, is responsible for hearing and determining disciplinary proceedings brought against registered nurses under the *HPCA Act*.

Despite a number of inequities in the system, at present all New Zealanders have access to universal health care. New Zealand spends approximately $14.6 billion dollars on health every year, representing approximately 10% of GDP (New Zealand Treasury 2012). Current thinking suggests that this expenditure is unsustainable, and that consolidation of spending, reducing demand for health services and developing new models of health care provision need to be considered (New Zealand Treasury 2012). The election of a National conservative government in 2008 and again in 2011 saw a dramatic shift in thinking around health expenditure, as well as a reconsideration of the priorities around primary health care and social equity. Although the New Zealand Health Strategy and Primary Health Care Strategy have not been superseded, there has been a clear refocusing on efficiencies in provision of care and more emphasis on acute care and targets as outlined above. The 'Better, Sooner, More Convenient Primary Health Care' document (Ryall 2009) called for the development of a 'single system personalised care' approach to primary health care along with the development of Integrated Family Health Centres— clinics that provide a full range of medical, nursing and allied health services including minor surgery, chronic care and walk-in access. Many of the current government goals for primary health care sit around devolution of secondary services to primary health care as a means to achieve cost savings. However, as noted earlier, significant challenges have arisen with the devolution of services from secondary to primary care, and there is still significant work to be done in terms of upskilling the primary health care workforce to take on devolving services.

Also in 2009, a Ministerial Review Group led by Murray Horn was established to consider the challenges faced by the New Zealand health care sector, and to develop recommendations to help meet these challenges (NZ Ministerial Review Group 2009). Recommendations in the 'Horn Report' were structured around nine key themes:

- new models of care which see the patient rather than the institution at the centre of service delivery
- stronger clinical and management partnerships
- a sharper focus on patient safety and quality of care
- identifying the services people need
- putting the right services in the right place
- ensuring the right capacity is in place
- building a sustainable workforce
- shifting resources to the front-line
- improving hospital productivity (NZ Ministerial Review Group 2009).

FISCAL RESTRAINT OR SUSTAINABILITY?

The 'Horn Report' provided a new direction for New Zealand health care focusing on fiscal restraint.

The New Zealand Government has enacted a number of strategies designed to meet the recommendations of the 'Horn Report', and for the most part, these were focused specifically on the need for fiscal restraint. For example, a National Health Board was established in early 2010 to provide a better national focus on health spending. PHOs with a population of less than 40 000 had their funding cut and were required to merge with larger PHOs. In 2010 there were 81 PHOs and by 2013 this had reduced to 31. The risk of focusing on fiscal savings, however, is that those most disadvantaged are likely to continue to miss out on vital health care. A study of Capital and Coast DHB's decision-making around equity and primary health care following the implementation of 'Better, Sooner, More Convenient Health Care' and increased focus on fiscal restraint found that hospital expenditure grew relative to primary health care expenditure, inequitable access to primary care persisted, and unplanned hospital admissions increased (Matheson 2013). Further evidence of the risks associated with focusing on fiscal restraint is to be found in the UK. An inquiry into reports of poor care and increased mortality rates at the Mid Staffordshire Foundation Trust found that a focus on targets and fiscal restraint were among the primary causes (Francis 2013).

There are important lessons to be learnt from these reports and both underline the importance of the role health professionals have in advocating for a continued focus on social equity, the impact of the SDH and community participation in future policy— aspects that were noticeably missing from the 'Horn Report'. While health policy documents still have a secondary focus on improving outcomes for some of the most disadvantaged groups in New Zealand, and provide some direction for health professionals as they seek to address some of the glaring inequities in health, at real risk is the progress the New Zealand Ministry of Health had made in recognising the importance of PHC as a means of improving the health of populations. In particular, He Korowai Oranga: Māori Health Strategy (NZMOH 2002a), and the Pacific Health and Disability Action Plan (NZMOH 2002c) both provide strategic direction and actions to improve health outcomes for Māori and Pacific people in New Zealand. Māori health has been covered in detail in previous chapters, but we reiterate that significant disparities exist in the health of Pacific people in New Zealand compared with non-Pacific people, despite the fact that New Zealand has demonstrated its commitment to Pacific health in a number of ways (see Box 14.3). It can only be hoped that the progress thus far achieved will continue.

BOX 14.3 New Zealand's commitment to Pacific health

Pacific people comprise close to 7% of the New Zealand population and come from over 22 different Pacific nations. Each Pacific community has its own distinctive culture, language, history and health status. The largest Pacific groups are the Samoan, Cook Island, Tongan and Niuean communities. Over 67% of Pacific people live in the Auckland area (NZMOH, Online. Available: www.health.govt.nz/our-work/populations/pacific-health/tagata-pasifika-new-zealand [accessed 7 October 2013]). Pacific people in New Zealand experience poorer health outcomes than other New Zealanders across a range of health and disability indicators. Life expectancy for Pacific people is lower than all other groups except Māori, and Pacific people have higher rates of morbidity and mortality in a range of chronic diseases. For example, Pacific men and women have 3.4 times the prevalence of diagnosed diabetes than other New Zealanders (NZMOH 2012c). Pacific children also experience poorer health outcomes than non-Pacific children and are more likely to live in areas of higher neighbourhood deprivation (NZMOH 2012d), placing them at even greater risk of poor health outcomes than their non-Pacific counterparts.

New Zealand has made a significant commitment to addressing the inequities experienced by Pacific people, working closely with the Pacific community to develop a range of policies designed to improve health. This started with the Pacific Health and Disability Action Plan, which provided the initial framework and strategic direction for improving Pacific people's health and participation, and reducing inequalities (NZMOH 2002c). This was followed up in 2004 by release of the Pacific Health and Disability Workforce Development Plan, which provided a framework for health and education organisations to positively influence pathways for participation by Pacific people in the health workforce (NZMOH 2004). In 2010, both these policy documents were replaced by 'Ala Mo'ui: Pathways to Pacific Health and Wellbeing 2010–2014' (NZ Minister of Health and Minister of Pacific Island Affairs 2010). The new document identifies six outcomes to be achieved for Pacific people. These include ensuring that: the Pacific workforce supply meets service demand, systems and services meet the needs of Pacific people, every dollar is spent in the best way possible to improve health outcomes, there are more locally delivered services in the community

and in primary care, Pacific people are better supported to be healthy, and Pacific people experience improved broader determinants of health (NZ Minister of Health and Minister of Pacific Island Affairs 2010). Ala Mo'ui was developed in collaboration with a range of clinical and community leaders and built on the Pacific Health and Disability Plan Review series that arose following development of the original Pacific Health and Disability Action Plan in 2002. Wide consultation with Pacific communities has been a feature of all policy development activities, ensuring social equity and participation goals remain at the forefront of policy development.

Significant work has also been done on developing policy for supporting Pacific people with disability through the Faiva Ora National Pasifika Disability Plan 2010–2013 (NZ National Health Board 2010) and on identifying evidence to support improvements in primary care delivery to Pacific people (Southwick et al. 2012). Drawing on a culturally appropriate methodology, Southwick and colleagues interviewed Pacific people and primary care providers to determine the most effective ways of improving access to and use of primary care by Pacific people. Barriers to seeking care included transport problems, the cost of health care and a gap between participants' expectations of health services and their actual experiences. Language barriers, difficulties in making appointments and other communication problems partly attributed to cultural insensitivity and racist behavior on the part of health workers were also identified as significant issues for participants (Southwick et al. 2012). Clinical providers were focused on appointment systems, contacting people and payments. Many had developed approaches that met the needs of Pacific people but these were not 'built in' to the health system and so were contingent on the goodwill of individual providers. There appeared to be a significant mismatch between the '... hopes, expectations and aspirations of Pacific peoples in accessing and utilising primary care services and the aims, understandings and services delivered by primary care staff and systems' (Southwick et al. 2013:14). Clearly, further work still needs to be done to address the gap between the health of Pacific people and other New Zealanders; however, evidence-informed policy development is a good start in addressing many of the disparities that exist.

THE AUSTRALIAN HEALTH CARE SYSTEM

The system of health care in Australia is built on the principle of universal care for all citizens paid for by their taxes, which involves a total annual expenditure on health of 9.3% of Australia's gross domestic product (GDP) (AIHW, Online. Available www.aihw.gov.au/publication-detail/?id=10737423009 [accessed 10 September 2013]). Health services are funded through Medicare, the national insurance scheme that provides each member of society with the ability to attend any one of a number of services at no cost, or, where the service provider charges an extra fee, at an affordable cost. Most Australians use the services of medical practitioners, who charge a fee-for-services provided, and then are subsidised through the Medicare system to a standard rate. Most medical specialists, and a large number of general practitioners, charge their patients a fee above the subsidised rate. Many people also have private health insurance, which covers them, and their family, for a wider range of services than are paid for by Medicare, including dental health care, massage, optometry and other services. Private health cover can be used for care in a public or private hospital, which is a benefit to insurance companies when patients choose to be treated in public hospitals. In these cases, the insurance company is only charged one-third of the $1000 a day they would pay in private hospitals (Seah et al. 2013). The reduction in cost to the private insurance company is, in effect, inequitable, given that the true costs of hospitalisation are borne by the public system and the revenue they do not receive could be better used to support those who cannot afford timely care. Because insurance costs are high, especially for families, having additional coverage advantages the most affluent, again leaving the poor further disadvantaged.

> ### MEDICARE
>
> Australia's national insurance scheme that provides all Australians with the ability to attend many health care services at no cost or at an affordable cost.

The Commonwealth Department of Health and Ageing (DoHA) (2010) has the overall responsibility for quality and safety in health care, working through a number of statutory agencies and commissions, such as the Australian Commission on Quality and Safety in Health Care. DoHA is responsible for national health policy and subsidisation of public hospitals through the Medical Benefits Scheme, the Pharmaceutical Benefits Scheme and the Therapeutic Goods Administration, which monitors and regulates medicines, blood and tissue (Francis et al. 2008; Smith 2012). The DoHA also oversees the National Aged and Community Care Program (which includes care and support for those with a disability) the National Mental Health Program, Aboriginal and Torres Strait Islander Health, primary and ambulatory care and health protection. Health protection includes public health surveillance, emergency preparedness and responses, food policy, chronic and communicable disease control, health promotion and harm reduction related to substance abuse (Francis et al. 2008).

> ### HEALTH PRIORITIES
>
> - Cancer control
> - Injury prevention, control
> - Cardiovascular health
> - Diabetes
> - Mental health
> - Asthma
> - Arthritis, musculoskeletal
> - Health literacy

The Australian system is monitored through the National Health Performance Framework (NHPF), which measures health status, determinants of health and health system performance. The performance of a health system is rated on the basis of seven criteria: effectiveness, continuity of care, safety, accessibility, client responsiveness, efficiency and sustainability (AIHW 2012). State and territory governments are responsible for hospital and community care, including private hospitals, even though the funding for these services is provided jointly, through cooperative arrangements between Commonwealth, state and territory governments. In some state-based health and hospital services, restructuring is a regular occurrence. Various administrative bodies take responsibility for individual hospitals, or district-level services. In most cases, a health service district will include both general and specialist hospitals, some specialising in certain populations (women and children) and others specialising in certain types of treatment (cancer care, various surgical specialties).

PERFORMANCE CRITERIA

- Effectiveness
- Continuity of care
- Safety
- Accessibility
- Client responsiveness
- Efficiency
- Sustainability

Certain hospitals are designated as state trauma centres, able to accommodate a wide range of emergencies, while others have the capacity for only minor emergency treatments, and are usually bypassed in emergencies of any substance. In addition to hospital services, patients in most health service districts have access to specialised drug and alcohol treatment services, state-based ambulance services, aged care, mental health hostels, the Australian Red Cross Blood service and the Royal Flying Doctor Service, which provides air transportation for health professionals to attend to people in remote areas. Although comparisons between different health systems are difficult because of variable reporting, among OECD countries, Australia compares well on such indicators as tobacco smoking, life expectancy and all-cause mortality. Where we compare less favourably is on national indicators of infant mortality, COPD mortality, obesity, alcohol consumption, and diphtheria, tetanus and pertussis (DTP) vaccination (AIHW 2012). Most of these less favourable indicators are improving, but there remains a need to continue addressing inequities between different population groups to improve the overall health indicators. In the areas of alcohol consumption, obesity and vaccination, the country is among the worst third among OECD countries (AIHW 2012).

The Commonwealth Government establishes national health priorities for the people of Australia, and these are based on data provided by the Australian Institute of Health and Welfare (AIHW). Although priorities can change according to a particular political agenda, the priorities for population health are generally non-partisan, and based on strong research evidence. Priorities for the public's health have been relatively stable throughout the past decade, and include cancer control, injury prevention and control, cardiovascular health, diabetes mellitus, mental health, asthma, and arthritis and musculoskeletal conditions (AIHW

2012). In recent years, the government has also been working towards equitable distribution of digitally mediated communication and information exchange that would consolidate the health literacy agenda (Newman et al. 2012). Access to digital technologies is an important equity issue, with those living in disadvantaged circumstances having the least access to health information. The National e-Health Strategy is intended to help people become empowered partners in care, and to assist health professionals interact with them and with one another (Newman et al. 2012).

One of the most challenging aspects of the Australian health system is that responsibility for health services is distributed through Commonwealth, state, territory and local jurisdictions, and this causes some duplication of effort, and a lack of clarity in reporting mechanisms as well as cost-shifting (Smith 2012; van Loon 2011). Competition between acute and community services adds another layer of complexity. Community nursing services such as district nursing services are funded either directly through Regional Health Services, or through contracts with public hospitals to provide specified services, or through state or territory health departments. A large proportion of aged care services are provided through a joint Commonwealth–state funded Home and Community Care (HACC) program, or, in the case of veterans, through the Commonwealth Department of Veterans' Affairs (DVA) (van Loon 2011).

Community nurses can be employed by any of these agencies, attached to Commonwealth programs such as the HACC or DVA programs, state or territory public health or education departments, district community services such as Silver Chain Nursing, Blue Care, Royal District Nursing Services, or a range of agencies responsible for specific population groups or those with a unique focus, such as the not-for-profit centres to help victims of violence, or torture and trauma survivors. In any context, nurses' registration to practise is governed by the National Registration and Accreditation Scheme, which has oversight for accreditation, regulation and monitoring of all health professionals. Professions included in the scheme include chiropractors, dental practitioners, medical practitioners, nurses and midwives, optometrists, osteopaths, pharmacists, physiotherapists, podiatrists, psychologists, Aboriginal and Torres Strait Islander health practitioners, Chinese medicine practitioners and medical radiation practitioners, each with their own accrediting body, such as the Australian Nursing and Midwifery Accreditation Council.

NURSING PRACTICE REGULATION

Australian nurses are registered with the Australian Nursing and Midwifery Accreditation Council (ANMAC) and regulated through the Australian Health Practitioners Registration Authority (AHPRA).

Most Australian medical practitioners are self-employed general practitioners (GPs) or consultants, who practise on a contractual basis in public, and sometimes private, hospitals. Allied health professionals and paramedics are typically employed by hospitals or health districts, and some can charge a fee-for-service, including acupuncturists, podiatrists and naturopaths (Francis et al. 2008). Nurses and midwives can be employed in hospitals or health agencies, with many being appointed to government agencies either at the state, territory, regional or local level. As we mentioned in Chapter 5, some nurse practitioners and other nurse entrepreneurs have established public clinics, and there are also midwives who work privately or in group practices to provide home-birthing services, or other consultations. Based on their insights into both the 'business' of health and many dimensions in terms of achieving better health for the population, these nurses can be expected to play an expanding role in policy development in the future (Wilson et al. 2012).

HEALTH SECTOR REFORM IN AUSTRALIA

In 2009, the Commonwealth Government embarked on a program of dramatic reform for the health system. The reforms were based on a need to upgrade a health system designed in the last century, with little understanding of the widening gap between those with good and poor health.

The need for improvements was evident in a number of areas:

- poor access to care for many Australians
- consumer frustration with an overly complex system
- the health gap between Indigenous and non-Indigenous Australians
- increasing out-of-pocket costs for services
- a severe shortage of doctors, nurses and other health professionals
- insufficient focus on prevention and primary care

- inefficient allocation of resources because of tensions between the state/Commonwealth funding structures (Australian Health Care Reform Alliance (HCRA), Online. Available: www.healthreform.org.au [accessed 10 September 2013]).

The National Health and Hospitals Reform Committee (NHHRC) (Commonwealth of Australia 2009) strongly recommended three immediate and crucial responses:

1 tackling major access and equity issues that affect health outcomes

2 redesigning the health system to better respond to emerging challenges, and

3 creating an agile and self-improving health system for long-term sustainability.

The major access and equity issues revolve around improving outcomes for Indigenous people, those with serious mental illness, people living in rural and remote areas, those without access to dental care, or timely care in public hospitals. Emerging challenges include embedding prevention and early intervention for a healthy start to life, and the need to create youth-friendly community-based services, to promote adolescent mental health. The Council of Australian Governments (COAG) identified seven building blocks for reform, including early childhood, schooling, health, economic participation, healthy homes, safe communities, governance and leadership (Donato & Segal 2013). In addition to strengthening these areas, the redesigned health system is intended to better integrate health and aged-care services, so that many older persons presenting to hospitals for acute or sub-acute care can be treated in their home or community through programs such as Hospital in the Home (HITH), or designated palliative care services. Of course, these changes would have to be structured so that family caregivers and community-based health professionals would have extra support and infrastructure to meet their needs.

The Commission also recommended reshaping hospitals to separate elective and emergency care, with outpatient services organised around the needs of patients and their communities. One of the most important recommendations of the NHHRC is for strengthened PHC services. This would involve integration of PHC services so that they would be multidisciplinary, and provided in comprehensive centres and primary health care organisations, which would rely on input from the community and make better use of community specialists. The main objective is to work towards continuous improvement and a fair, accessible, democratic health system with vertical and horizontal integration, where primary care providers (mainly GPs) change from operating relatively independently of the rest of the health system to becoming more collaborative (Wakerman 2009). However, in reality there is inadequate vertical integration of policies between state and Commonwealth governments, particularly those governing the distribution of nursing and other health professional positions where they are most needed. These recommendations resonate with international trends, which include a move away from the fee-for-service model which relies on referral to specialists, to one that brings primary care closer to other services, and encourages interdisciplinary collaboration and community participation (Wakerman 2009).

> ### PRIMARY HEALTH CARE
>
> Despite the recommendation of the National Health and Hospitals Reform Committee (NHHRC) report in 2009 Australia still does not have an adequate PHC system.

The National Health Reform Agreement increased the funding for state and territory health services from a common funding pool to improve patient services in hospitals and reduce emergency department and elective surgery waiting times, expand hospital capacity in sub-acute care for rehabilitation, palliative care, mental health, psychogeriatric services, evaluation and management. The Medicare Locals began in 2011, with the intention of shifting services toward PHC, albeit focusing on general practice rather than community health promotion. In addition, the reforms have included multiple entry points to the aged-care system for the expanding older population, which are intended to provide better linkages between services for these people (Australian Government, Online. Available: www.yourhealth.gov.au/internet/yourhealth/publishing.nsf/content/nhra-agreement-fs#what [accessed 10 September 2013]).

> ### HEALTH SYSTEM EFFICIENCY
>
> Evaluation data will indicate the extent to which policy planners have achieved equitable, effective, client-centred health care in Australia.

Creating an agile and self-improving system was to be achieved with a stronger voice from the community, and focus on building health literacy, fostering community participation, and empowering people to make fully informed health care decisions. The health reforms are also intended to foster clinical leadership and governance, new frameworks for education and training for health professionals, governed by a National Clinical Education and Training Agency to support a modern workforce. Other recommendations include the smart use of data, information and communication; well-designed funding and strategic purchasing models; and knowledge-led, continuous improvement, innovation and research. The Health Literacy and Digital *e*-Health projects mentioned previously represent the culmination of several years of deliberation on these recommendations. In future, evaluative data will indicate whether these new initiatives have in fact achieved the agility and self-improvements recommended.

HEALTH CARE: BUILDING A BETTER SYSTEM

Three decades ago, few health care planners were concerned with the SDH. Yet gradually, as more evidence came to light, policymakers throughout the world came to realise that good health evolves from equity and the social aspects of people's lives, supported by an accessible health care system. Resources and good management practices play an important role, but there are other critical elements of a health system that contribute to the health of any given population. These are listed as health system features below in Box 14.4.

BEST PRACTICE IN HEALTH CARE SYSTEMS

The Scandinavian countries are often held up as exemplars of best practice in health care systems; however, even in these countries, the health systems are changing. The cost of technology and pharmaceuticals, population ageing, community awareness of new treatment, and all of the other factors that we experience in our countries, have also created financial pressures and a gradual centralisation of services in these countries (Magnussen 2013). The Nordic systems, designed to be socially democratic, are well positioned for capacity building, improving health through a 'nuanced balance of leadership', and by facilitating intersectoral collaborations for health promoting environments, which include education, infrastructure, urban planning and trade (Baum et al.

BOX 14.4 Health system features

- Health care systems should be fair, not focused on privileging hospital care in its funding at the expense of prevention or community care.

- Universal care, along with universal systems of health insurance can help reduce the disadvantage experienced by those already disadvantaged by socio-economic status and health status.

- A health system should provide appropriate, adequate and culturally acceptable care for the most vulnerable.

- The majority of health care needs are in chronic disease and disability management and these must be met with continuity of care between acute and home and community settings.

- Service decisions should be made in partnership with health-literate end users of the system.

- Efficiencies in the system should carefully balance technological and biomedical care with community care.

- Health information systems are integral to efficient and effective services.

- Effective systems are client-oriented, so they deal with waiting lists and the patient journey through hospital to home and community from a client, rather than a service provider perspective.

- A self-regulating system monitors and addresses threats to patient quality and safety.

- Adequate service provision relies on sufficient health professionals, educated appropriately for their scope of practice and employed across all settings to practice at their level of competence.

- A robust health care system is based on research evidence as a basis for good and best practice.

- A health care system should include best practice in health promotion to strengthen capacity.

2009:1967). Although each country's political and economic context differs, all health care systems should continue to work towards equity, and equalising the social gradient. This is described as good stewardship in health care, and it includes organisational cultural competence and critical examination of the areas where inequities persist (Olavarria et al. 2009). The outcome of good stewardship should be achieving the goals for a healthy society as listed in Box 14.5.

BEST PRACTICE

Scandinavian health care systems are considered some of the best in the world, particularly in their approach toward equity and equalising the social gradient in society.

HEALTH CARE SYSTEMS AND THE SOCIAL DETERMINANTS OF HEALTH

Since the health communities of the world began to focus on the SDH, we have had a closer global connection to those things that help, and those that hinder our quest for health and wellness. Rapid communication brings into our consciousness the cold, hard reality of health inequalities. We are responding to a wider breadth of knowledge on the

quality as well as the quantity of life, and as a backlash against the failures of the market to improve health in the population. As Katz (2009) suggests, we need to work toward replacing the invisible hand of the market with the visible hand of social justice. To foster vibrant, cohesive, healthy and safe communities requires leadership and advocacy (Ridde 2007). Given the financial, demographic, environmental and epidemiological threats of modern society, it will take great leadership to nurture our communities and render our health care systems safe, effective and efficient. As health professionals, we must remain in our imperfect health care systems to improve, rather than abandon our roles as purveyors of health. Every nurse and every health professional has a certain sphere of influence, which can be used to build the capacity of a human community to shape its culture and its future (Gray 2009). This is leadership. It grows from a dialogue between people, between those of us in the health care professions, and those who need us. We must use our leadership and our ability to generate evidence for practice to advance the goals of PHC with a common language and the wisdom gleaned from community engagement. The chapter to follow outlines some of the most pressing research questions and areas of interest to guide these activities. Below we return to the case study to consider policies affecting the lives of the Smith and Mason families.

BOX 14.5 Goals for healthy societies

1 Inclusivity and fairness—through a values-based commitment to equity, freedom, social inclusion and capacity development

2 Equality—where men and women and members of minority groups are treated equally for common needs

3 Cultural safety—through culturally competent management and clinical systems to ensure that all care processes acknowledge diversity, difference and ability, with an ultimate aim of empowerment

4 Responsive health systems—with timely, affordable, safe, coordinated care

5 Support for healthy behaviours—by arranging structural features of the environment to support people in achieving and maintaining health

6 Sustainable eco-systems—through public awareness and action on preserving the environment

7 Evidence-based, evidence-informed management of health and health care, where research, interventions and policy analysis are interlinked and translated into better health

8 Democratic citizen participation—where all voices are heard

9 Social capital is valued—human, spiritual, cultural and social capital is seen as equal to economic capital

10 Adequate and appropriate resources—there is congruence between needs and resources

11 Well-managed for best processes, best practices—good stewardship and strong community leadership is rewarded and supported

12 Development of goals and strategies on the basis of multiple levels of influence by an appropriate, well-educated and satisfied workforce

CASE STUDY: Policy implications for the Smith and Mason families

The occupational health nurses at the Pilbara mine where Colin and Jason are employed work within the national Occupational Health and Safety Policies which are meant to protect the workers. There are few discrepancies in workplace practices given the high-risk environment of the mine.

All families in both countries are affected by global economic policies. National government policies that affect the families include those addressing financial matters including government spending on early childhood education social service provision, women's health policy, men's health policy and children's policies such as the Healthy Schools policy. Global policy affects the Smith and Mason families' lives in terms of generating wealth from the resources of Western Australia, but the uncertainty of the resources boom and the demise of the mining tax may have unexpected results on the men's employment.

Better coordination of health services in the context of the Australian national health reform agenda will have policy implications for both families.

In New Zealand, Huia helped Jake's teachers at Kohanga Reo (Māori language kindergarten) provide feedback on the Green Paper for Vulnerable Children and is now pleased to see that some of their feedback has been included in the White Paper and subsequent *Vulnerable Children's Act*. The Whānau Ora policy has enabled new wrap-around services to be offered in the Papakura community as well, and this appears to be making a difference for some of the families in the community. Aroha, who is 8, had been complaining of a sore throat and was able to get this checked out at the sore throat clinic offered by the school nurse, which is funded by the government to prevent rheumatic fever.

REFLECTING ON THE BIG ISSUES

- Policymaking is a political process of deciding how resources are allocated.

- Many local policies are linked to global and regional goals.

- All policies influence health, and most policies are linked with one another, which means there is a need for health to be considered in all policymaking.

- Community members should have a voice in policymaking.

- Nurses and midwives can help communities develop a level of health literacy that would facilitate their participation in policy development.

- Health care systems continue to privilege hospital and high tech care over community care.

- Some inequities persist in access to care, with the most disadvantaged often excluded from the services they need.

- Primary health care can provide the fairest systems of health care.

- An ideal health care system is based on the social determinants of health.

REFLECTIVE QUESTIONS: How would I use this knowledge in practice?

1 Identify the factors influencing policy development in your health service district or primary health organisation

2 Explain why policy development is guided by the mantra 'think global, act local'.

3 What strategies would you use to ensure Rebecca's level of health literacy is adequate for caring for her family?

4 How does the New Zealand primary health care system promote access and equity in services?

5 What steps could you take to support the proposals to develop a primary health care system in Australia?

6 Update the family genogram for both families.

7 Policy action exercise: Australian and New Zealand successes and gaps:

Some consider the following policies a success, others a work in progress and still others consider some of the policies a failure or even a complete gap. Search out these policy areas and reflect on how successful they are and why.

Success?	Gaps	Work in progress
Employment policies		
Food safety, security		
Tobacco legislation		
Affordable child care		
Mandatory seatbelts		
Healthy schools, workplaces		
Healthy ageing		
Disability insurance policies		
Drug and alcohol policies		
Social inclusion		
Distribution of health professionals		
Migration policy		
Mental health policy		
Rural health policy		
Women's, men's health policies		
Indigenous health policies		
Climate change policies		

References

Australian Commission on Safety and Quality in Health Care (ACSQHC), 2013. Consumers, the healthy system and health literacy: Taking action to improve safety and quality. Consultation Paper, ACSQHC, Sydney.

Australian Government, 2013a. Closing the Gap Prime Minister's Report. AGPS, Canberra.

Australian Government, 2013b. National Aboriginal and Torres Strait Islander Health Plan—Companion Document on Commonwealth Government Strategies & Reforms. Online. Available: <www.ATSIgapreport2013natishp-companion.pdf> 9 July 2013.

Australian Institute of Health and Welfare, 2012. Australia's Health 2012 Series no 13, Cat No AUS 156. AIHW, Canberra.

Australian Research Alliance for Children and Youth (ARACY), 2009. Transforming Australia for our children's future. ARACY National Conference, Sept 4. Melbourne.

Bambra, C., Fox, D., Scott-Samuel, A., 2007. A politics of health glossary. J. Epidemiol. Community Health 61, 571–574.

Baum, F., Begin, M., Houweling, T., et al., 2009. Changes not for the fainthearted: Reorienting health care systems toward health equity through action on the social determinants of health. Am. J. Public Health 99 (11), 1967–1974.

Bish, M., Kenny, A., Nay, R., 2012. Perceptions of structural empowerment: nurse leaders in rural health services. J. Nurs. Manag. doi:10.1111/jonm/12029.

Bourke, L., Humphreys, J., Wakerman, J., et al., 2012. Understanding drivers of rural and remote health outcomes: A conceptual framework in action. Aust. J. Rural Health 20, 318–323.

Bruni, R., Laupacis, A., Martin, D., 2008. Public engagement in setting priorities in health care. Can. Med. Assoc. J. 179 (1), 15–18.

Buchan, J., Naccarella, L., Brooks, P., 2011. Is health workforce sustainability in Australia and New Zealand a realistic policy goal? Aust. Health Rev. 35, 152–155.

Cassrels, D., 2013. Desperate and born stateless. The Weekend Australian April 13–14.

Clendon, J., 2013. The value of engaging with the political process. New Zealand Nurses Organisation, Wellington.

Clendon, J., Walker, L., 2013. Nurses aged over 50 and their experiences of shiftwork. J. Nurs. Manag. doi:10.1111/jonm.12157.

CSDH, 2008. Closing the gap in a generation. Health equity through action on the social determinants of health, Final report of the Commission on the social determinants of health. WHO, Geneva.

Commonwealth of Australia, 2009. National Mental Health Policy 2008. Online. Available: <www.health.gov.au/internet/main/publishing.nsf> 11 September 2013.

Commonwealth of Australia, 2010a. National Women's Health Policy. Department of Health and Ageing, Canberra.

Commonwealth of Australia, 2010b. National Male Health Policy. Department of Health and Ageing, Canberra.

Commonwealth of Australia, 2010c. Department of Health and Aging Mental Health Information Development: National Information Priorities and strategies under the Second Mental Health Plan 1998–2003. Online. Available: <http://www.health.gov.au/> 1 February 2010.

Commonwealth of Australia Department of Health and Ageing, 2010. The National Health Priority Areas. Online Available: <http://www.safetyandquality.gov.au/internet/safety/publishing.nsf/Content/strategies> 1 February, 2010.

Cumming, J., Mays, N., Daube, J., 2010. How New Zealand has contained expenditure on drugs. BMJ 340, c2441.

Cunningham, P, 2012. The future of community-centred health services in Australia—an alternative view. Aust. Health Rev. 36, 121–124.

Davis, W., Lewin, G., Davis, T., et al., 2013. Determinants and costs of community nursing in patients with type 2 diabetes from a community-based observational study: The Fremantle Diabetes Study. Int. J. Nurs. Stud. 50, 1166–1171.

Donato, R., Segal, L., 2013. Does Australia have the appropriate health reform agenda to close the gap in Indigenous health? Aust. Health Rev. 37, 232–238.

Dowell, A.C., Garrett, S., Collings, S., et al., 2009. Evaluation of the Primary Mental Health Initiatives: Summary report 2008. University of Otago and Ministry of Health, Wellington.

Dwan, K., McInnes, P., 2013. Increasing the influence of one's research on policy. Aust. Health Rev. 37, 194–198.

Family & Relationships Australia, 2012. Community engagement in post-separation services: An exploratory study. FRSA, Canberra.

Farmer, J., Bourke, L., Taylor, J., et al., 2012. Culture and rural health. Aust. J. Rural Health 20, 243–247.

Fawcett, J., Russell, G., 2001. A conceptual model of nursing and health policy. Policy Polit. Nurs. Pract. 2 (2), 108–116.

Francis, K., Chapman, Y., Hoare, K., et al., 2008. Australia and New Zealand community as partner: theory and practice in nursing. Wolters Kluwer/Lippincott Williams & Wilkins, Philadelphia.

Francis, R., 2013. Report of the Mid Staffordshire NHS Foundation Trust public inquiry. Executive summary. Mid Staffordshire NHS Foundation Trust Public Inquiry, United Kingdom.

Gluckman, P., 2013. The role of evidence in policy formation and implementation: A report from the Prime Minister's Chief Science Advisor. Office of the Prime Minister's Science Advisory Committee, Auckland.

Gray, M., 2009. Public health leadership: creating the culture for the twenty-first century. J. Public Health (Bangkok) 31 (2), 208–209.

Hawe, P., 2009. The social determinants of health: how can a radical idea be mainstreamed? Can. J. Public Health 100 (4), 291–293.

Henderson, J., 2005. Neo-liberalism, community care and Australian mental health policy. Health Sociol. Rev. 14 (3), 242–254.

HLS-EU, 2012. The European Health Literacy Project Executive Summary, Final Report. HLS Consortium. Online. Available: <www.health-literacy.eu> 25 June 2013.

Hoang, H., Le, Q., 2013. Comprehensive picture of rural women's needs in maternity care in Tasmania, Australia. Aust. J. Rural Health 21, 197–202.

Humphreys, J., Gregory, G., 2012. Celebrating another decade of progress in rural health: What is the current state of play? Aust. J. Rural Health 20, 156–163.

Institute of Medicine (IOM), 2004. Health Literacy. A Prescription to End Confusion. The National Academies Press, Washington.

Johnstone, M., Lee, C., 2012. Young Australian women and their aspirations: 'It's hard enough thinking a week or two in advance at the moment'. J. Adolesc. Res. 27, 351–376.

Judd, J., Keleher, H., 2013. Reorienting health services in the Northern Territory of Australia: a conceptual model for building health promotion capacity in the workforce. Glob. Health Promot. 20 (2), 53–63.

Kamien, M., 2009. Evidence-based policy versus evidence-based rural health care reality checks. Aust. J. Rural Health 17, 65–67.

Katz, A., 2009. Prospects for a genuine revival of primary health care—through the visible hand of social justice rather than the invisible hand of the market: Part 1. Int. J. Health Serv. 39 (3), 567–585.

Kickbusch, I., 2012. Addressing the interface of the political and commercial determinants of health, Editorial. Health Promot. Int. 27 (4), 427–428.

King, A., 2001. Primary Health Care Strategy. Ministry of Health, Wellington.

Kleinman, R., 2013. A single-minded struggle to get by. The Age. Online. Available: <www.theage.com.au/federal-politics/federal-election-2013/a-singleminded-struggle-to-get-by-20130822-2se9f.html> 11 September 2013.

Leppo, K., Ollila, E., Pena, S., et al., 2013. Health in all policies. Seizing opportunities, implementing policies. Ministry of Social Affairs and Health, Finland.

Magnussen, J., 2013. The Scandinavian Health Care System. Online. Available: <www.siemens.com/healthcare-magazine> 15 September 2013.

Marinelli-Poole, A., McGilvray, A., Lynes, D., 2011. New Zealand health leadership. Leadersh. Health Serv. 24 (4), 255–267.

Marmot, M., Allen, J., Bell, R., et al., 2012. Building of the global movement for health equity: from Santiago to Rio and beyond. Lancet 379, 181–188.

Martin, P., Duffy, T., Johnston, B., et al., 2013. Family health nursing: A response to the global health challenges. J. Fam. Nurs. 19 (1), 99–118.

Matheson, D., 2013. From great to good: How a leading New Zealand DHB lost its ability to focus on equity during a period of economic restraint. Online. Available: <http://www.google.co.nz/url?sa=t&rct=j&q=&esrc=s&frm=1&source=web&cd=1&ved=0CCsQFjAA&url=http%3A%2F%2F publichealth.massey.ac.nz%2Fassets%2FUploads%2FFrom-Great-to-Good-Final.pdf&ei=UxFRUtKDK4qpkgWe54D4Aw&usg=AFQjCNEAuwpP_roF1ruzFdKc45RU6NLYIQ&sig2=0KTA4v5q4kModZaFVt2VOA&bvm=bv.53537100,d.dGI> 6 October 2013.

Nana, G., Stokes, F., Molano, W., et al., 2013. New Zealand nurses: workforce planning 2010–2035. BERL, Wellington.

Newman, L., Biedrzycki, K., Baum, F., 2012. Digital technology use among disadvantaged Australians: implications for equitable consumer participation in digitally-mediated communication and information exchange with health services. Aust. Health Rev. 36, 125–129.

New Zealand Human Rights Commission, 2012. Caring counts: Report of the inquiry into the aged care workforce. Human Rights Commission, Auckland.

New Zealand Labour Party, Greens and Grey Power, 2010. A report into aged care: What does the future hold for older New Zealanders. New Zealand Labour Party, Greens and Grey Power, Wellington. Online. Available: <https://www.greens.org.nz/agedcare> 4 September 2013.

New Zealand Mental Health Commission, 1998. Blueprint for Mental Health Services in New Zealand: How things need to be. Mental Health Commission, Wellington.

New Zealand Mental Health Commission, 2012a. Blueprint II: Improving mental health and wellbeing for all New Zealanders: How things need to be. Mental Health Commission, Wellington.

New Zealand Mental Health Commission, 2012b. Blueprint II: Improving mental health and wellbeing for all New Zealanders: Making change happen. Mental Health Commission, Wellington.

New Zealand Minister of Health and Minister of Pacific Island Affairs, 2010. 'Ala Mo'ui: Pathways to Pacific Health and Wellbeing 2010–2014. Ministry of Health, Wellington.

New Zealand Ministerial Review Group, 2009. Meeting the Challenge: Enhancing Sustainability and the Patient and Consumer Experience within the Current Legislative Framework for Health and Disability Services in New Zealand. Report of the Ministerial Review Group. New Zealand Government, Wellington.

New Zealand Ministry of Health (NZMOH), 2000. New Zealand Health Strategy. Ministry of Health, Wellington.

New Zealand Ministry of Health (NZMOH), 2001. New Zealand Disability Strategy: Making a World of Difference Whakanui Oranga. Ministry of Health, Wellington.

New Zealand Ministry of Health (NZMOH), 2002a. He Korowai Oranga, Māori Health Strategy. MOHNZ, Wellington.

New Zealand Ministry of Health (NZMOH), 2002b. Māori mental health strategic framework. MOHNZ, Wellington.

New Zealand Ministry of Health (NZMOH), 2002c. Pacific Health and Disability Action Plan. Ministry of Health, Wellington.

New Zealand Ministry of Health (NZMOH), 2004. Pacific Health and Workforce Development Plan. Ministry of Health, Wellington.

New Zealand Ministry of Health (NZMOH), 2005. Te Tahuhu—Improving Mental Health 2005–2015: The Second New Zealand Mental Health and Addiction Plan. Ministry of Health, Wellington.

New Zealand Ministry of Health (NZMOH), 2006a. Whakatataka Tuarua: Māori health action plan 2006–2011. Ministry of Health, Wellington.

New Zealand Ministry of Health (NZMOH), 2006b. Te Kōkiri: The Mental Health and Addiction. Action Plan 2006–2015. Ministry of Health, Wellington.

New Zealand Ministry of Health (NZMOH), 2008. Te Puāwaiwhero: The Second Māori Mental Health and Addiction National Strategic Framework 2008–2015. Ministry of Health, Wellington.

New Zealand Ministry of Health (NZMOH), 2012a. Report on Maternity, 2010. Ministry of Health, Wellington.

New Zealand Ministry of Health (NZMOH), 2012b. Rising to the Challenge: The Mental Health and Addiction Service Development Plan 2012–2017. Ministry of Health, Wellington.

New Zealand Ministry of Health (NZMOH), 2012c. The Health of New Zealand Adults 2011/12: Key findings of the New Zealand Health Survey. Ministry of Health, Wellington.

New Zealand Ministry of Health (NZMOH), 2012d. Tupu Ola Moui Pacific Health Chart Book 2012. Ministry of Health, Wellington.

New Zealand Ministry of Health (NZMOH), 2013a. Statement of Intent 2013 to 2016. Ministry of Health, Wellington.

New Zealand Ministry of Health (NZMOH), 2013b. New Zealand Suicide Prevention Action Plan 2013–2016. Ministry of Health, Wellington.

New Zealand National Health Board, 2010. Faiva Ora National Pasifika Disability Plan 2010–2013. Ministry of Health, Wellington.

New Zealand National Health Board, 2011. We are Targeting Better Health Services. Ministry of Health, Wellington.

New Zealand Treasury, 2012. Health Projections and Policy Options for the 2013 Long-term Fiscal Statement. New Zealand Treasury, Wellington.

Nguyen, O., Cairney, S., 2013. Literature review of the interplay between education, employment, health and wellbeing for Aboriginal and Torres Strait Islander people in remote areas. CRC-REP Working Paper CW13. Ninti One Limited, Alice Springs.

Nursing Council of New Zealand, 2012. Annual report 2012. Nursing Council of New Zealand, Wellington.

Olavarria, N., Beaulac, J., Belanger, A., et al., 2009. Organizational cultural competence in community health and social services. J. Cult. Divers. 16 (4), 140–150.

Pharmaceutical Management Agency, 2013. Introduction to PHARMAC. Online. Available: <http://www.pharmac.health.nz/about/your-guide-to-pharmac> 10 October 2013.

Raphael, D., 2009. Restructuring society in the service of mental health promotion: are we willing to address the social determinants of mental health? Int. J. Ment. Health Promot. 11 (3), 18–31.

Ridde, V., 2007. Reducing social inequalities in health: public health, community health or health promotion? Promot. Educ. 2, 63–67.

Rushton, C., Kendall, E., 2011. Can health partnerships re-orientate health care toward prevention? Aust. N. Z. J. Public Health 35 (5), 492–493.

Ryall, T., 2009. Better, Sooner, More Convenient: Health Discussion Paper. National Party, Wellington.

Seah, D., Cheong, T., Anstey, M., 2013. The hidden cost of private health insurance in Australia. Aust. Health Rev. 37, 1–3.

Smith, T., 2012. Overhauling health care down under. Can. Med. Assoc. J. 184 (4), E205–E206.

Southwick, M., Kenealy, T., Ryan, D., 2012. Primary Care for Pacific People: A Pacific and Health Systems Approach. Pacific Perspectives, Wellington.

Sutherland, G., Yelland, J., Brown, S., 2012. Social inequalities in the organization of pregnancy care in a universally funded public health care system. Matern. Child Health J. 16, 288–296.

Tham, R., Humphreys, J., Kinsman, L., et al., 2010. Evaluating the impact of sustainable comprehensive primary health care on rural health. Aust. J. Rural Health 18, 166–172.

United Nations, 2011. The Global Social Crisis. Report on the World Social Situation 2011. UN Department of Economic and Social Affairs, New York.

Van Loon, A., 2011. Contexts of community nursing. In: Kralik, D., van Loon, A. (Eds.), Community Nursing in Australia, second ed. John Wiley & sons, Milton, Qld, pp. 46–84.

Wakerman, J., 2009. Innovative rural and remote primary health care models: What do we know and what are the research priorities? Aust. J. Rural Health 17, 21–26.

Wilkinson, R., Pickett, K., 2009. The spirit level: why equality is better for everyone. Penguin, United Kingdom.

Wilson, A., Whitaker, N., Whitford, D., 2012. Rising to the challenge of health care reform with entrepreneurial and intrapreneurial nursing initiatives. Online J. Issues in Nurs. doi:10.3912/OJIN.Vol17No02Man05.

World Health Organization (WHO), 2010. Mental health. Online. Available: <http://www.who.int/mental_health/en> 1 February, 2010.

World Health Organization (WHO), 2011. Gender, climate change and health. Online. Available: <www.who.int/phe/en/> 9 September 2013.

Useful websites

www.who.int/social_determinants/knowledge_networks/en—WHO SDOH network

www.who.int/social_determinants/themes/prioritypublichealthconditions/background/en—WHO priority public health conditions www.health.gov.au—Australian Health policies

www.safetyandquality.gov.au/—Safety and Quality in Health Care

www.nrha.org.au—National Rural Health Alliance

www.health.gov.au/internet/main/Publishing.nsf/Content/mental-strat—National Mental Health Strategy

www.healthdirect.gov.au/—Australian health topics

http://padv.org/—Partnerships Against Domestic Violence

www.health.gov.au—Department of Health

www.aihw.gov.au—Australian Institute of Health and Welfare

www.hwa.gov.au—Health Workforce Australia

www.foodstandards.gov.au—Food standards, Australia and New Zealand

http://mhca.org.au—Mental Health Council of Australia

www.nhmrc.gov.au—National Health and Medical Research Council

www.midwives.org.au—Australian College of Midwives

www.anmc.org.au—Australian Nursing and Midwifery Accreditation Council

http://catsin.org.au—Congress of Aboriginal and Torres Strait Islander Nurses and Midwives

www.acn.edu.au—Australian College of Nursing

www.health.act.gov.au/c/health—ACT Health

www.health.nt.gov.au—Department of Health Northern Territory

www.dhhs.tas.gov.au—Department of Health and Human Services Tasmania

www.health.sa.gov.au—Department of Health South Australia

www.health.wa.gov.au/home—Department of Health Western Australia

www.health.vic.gov.au—Department of Health Victoria

www.health.nsw.gov.au—New South Wales Health

www.health.qld.gov.au—Queensland Health

http://acc.cochrane.org/cipher—Centre for Informing Policy in Health with Evidence from Research

www.health.govt.nz—New Zealand Ministry of Health website

www.acc.co.nz—Accident Compensation Corporation of New Zealand

www.hrc.co.nz—Human Rights Commission (New Zealand)

www.childrensactionplan.govt.nz—Children's Action Plan, Green Paper on Vulnerable Children, White Paper on Vulnerable Children

www.healthworkforce.govt.nz—Health Workforce New Zealand

www.hdc.org.nz—Health & Disability Commissioner New Zealand

www.nzno.org.nz—New Zealand Nurses Organisation

www.nursingcouncil.org.nz—Nursing Council of New Zealand

www.nurse.org.nz—College of Nurses Aotearoa

15

Building the evidence base: research to practice

Introduction

Rational planning for the health of individuals, families and communities relies on a base of information as to what is effective, efficient in terms of resource use, and appropriate to the people whose lives will be affected. Effectiveness, efficiency and appropriateness are important variables to study in relation to health care systems, national intersectoral initiatives that affect health, and how health services and programs are implemented in communities. What is effective, efficient or appropriate can vary for particular individuals and groups across different settings and circumstances. Because of this variability, and the fact that people's lives are constantly changing, the research agenda is constantly evolving. It will always be necessary to gather information on community needs, strengths and resources to identify what is transferable across settings, and what is unique to a particular community. For example, we know that a multidimensional health promotion strategy that is inclusive of environmental as well as behavioural factors will be more effective in helping people quit smoking than a single-factor intervention. However, the way a quit-smoking intervention is introduced, planned and received by various members of the community can vary widely.

> ### WHY RESEARCH?
> - Advance knowledge.
> - Practise effectively, from an understanding of what works, for whom, in what context, why, with what costs and outcomes.
> - Compare or 'benchmark' knowledge with others to develop guidelines for best practice.

Planning an effective intervention for smoking cessation, or any other initiative, depends not only on aggregated, population-level information from programs that have worked, but on the strengths of the community and characteristics of the group for

whom the intervention is intended. These characteristics can be demographic features such as age, stage or gender, or clinical factors, such as whether or not the impetus for smoking cessation has come from an illness, impairment or, in some cases, the influence of a significant other. Other important issues lie in situational factors such as people's preferences, their receptiveness or readiness to make a change, how they view the constraints and/or facilitating factors that affect their health choices, and what supports are available to them to sustain the change. So although the findings from a body of research can sometimes be translated into practice across settings, there remains a need for contextual information, to study effectiveness and acceptability at the local level. This is the essence of most community health research. It is often evaluative; focusing on gathering and analysing data from within and external to the community, to identify what works, for whom, where, why, with what costs and outcomes, including acceptability by local residents. However, research data also needs to advance knowledge, one increment at a time, to the evolving theoretical and practical foundations of practice by nurses and other health professionals.

Primary studies that collect evidence on the effect of certain interventions can be useful in studying population-level outcomes as a basis for benchmarking. This is a process of comparing outcomes across populations to forecast the likelihood of success in other populations. However, research is also needed on the differential needs and effects for various groups, and how certain interventions were experienced by people whose lives were changed. Although scientific evidence is important to indicate what works from a statistical point of view, community health research also requires explanations of why it did, or did not. This type of contextual information can help health planners understand what structural features of the community contributed to the health outcomes, and whether certain initiatives or processes could be tried in other contexts and with other people.

OBJECTIVES

By the end of this chapter you will be able to:

1 identify the major issues that are critical to translating research evidence into better community health and wellbeing

2 explain the importance of comprehensive, multifactor studies

3 explain the relative advantage of mixed-method research studies for researching the social determinants of community health

4 outline the most important ethical issues involved in community-based research

5 explain the major issues in undertaking culturally safe research studies

6 develop a research question grounded in the conceptual foundations of primary health care to respond to a specific community health issue

7 identify a set of research questions that correspond to the community health and wellbeing indicators for healthy safe and inclusive communities.

STRUCTURES, PROCESSES OR OUTCOMES?

Community health research needs both scientific evidence to support outcomes *and* explanations of why an intervention may or may not have worked.

Besides identifying needs, structures, processes and outcomes, the research agenda also needs to include the type of studies that are aimed at developing conceptual frameworks for community health. These studies advance the field of community health by building a scaffold for knowledge development that can attract scholars and researchers to investigate the broader dimensions of community health. To date, there has been a dearth of studies that provide a framework for researchers to advance knowledge, particularly in the nursing and midwifery evidence base, although this is gradually changing. In addition, there is a need to study examples of good and best practice by nurses and others who promote the health of a community through health education, advocacy or specific interventions. The research agenda should also include studies that link community health practice outcomes with the level or type of practitioners' educational preparation, experience, expertise and scope of practice. Attention to these issues is fundamental to informing our professional knowledge development, mapping our progress in developing and adapting new understandings.

Undertaking research should be a partnership, where information is seen to be the property of those providing it, often in the spirit of generating mutual understanding and benefits. Despite different methods, designs and philosophical approaches, the common goal of research is to inform improvements to the health of the population or the community itself, either through small incremental contributions to knowledge, or studies of such magnitude as to create system change. This chapter provides an overview of issues and progress related to community health research, and suggests a number of research challenges and strategies that could be used to inform the creation and maintenance of community health.

GLOBAL COMMUNITY HEALTH RESEARCH

Research-based practice is the hallmark of professional nursing (ICN 2012). Researching community health issues is a challenge for nurses and other health professionals throughout the world, as communities are part of a global network working toward the common goal of social justice. Ideally, research studies that underpin the social justice agenda would build a body of knowledge to inform health promotion strategies, policies and practices to respond to global problems that also have implications at the local level. These problems include poverty, inequity in resource allocation, disparities in health and education, discrimination and disadvantage on the basis of gender, culture, race, age or geography, infectious diseases among those without access to treatment, and environmental issues such as climate change and its impact on communities. However, the global research agenda continues to be disadvantaged by the lack of large, interlinked databases, inadequate funding and, in some cases, the lack of political will to secure effective mechanisms for research collaborations.

GLOBAL RESEARCH AGENDA

- Poverty
- Resource inequities
- Disparities in health, education
- Discrimination, social exclusion
- Lack of access to treatments
- Environmental issues

Research studies are expensive. They require funding for researchers, investment in support structures (including the type of databases that could help integrate findings), personnel, and in many cases, specialised equipment. Clinicians, academics, policymakers and technical staff with research skills often have work demands other than research, which means that without financial support, their research becomes relegated to a low priority. Funding can help ensure that data are gathered and analysed appropriately, and that researchers have time and resources to promote collegial deliberation and dissemination of findings. Like other activities that have resource implications, research is inherently political. This means that at the national, regional and institutional levels, there are competing agendas for budget allocations. Decisions about funding research can be made on the basis of local issues, researcher interests, or the needs of policymakers and politicians to demonstrate a short-term impact. When short-term, local goals are the focus, the broader global social justice agenda is likely to be given little attention. As health professionals, it is important to advance local agendas and be responsive to the need for local research, but at the same time, maintain a commitment to the wider agenda of collecting data and translating findings into better health care for the global population.

GLOBAL RESEARCH ACTION

Think global in translating local findings into better health care for the global population, especially those investigating the SDH.

The most salient global community issues are generally those related to the social determinants of health (SDH). Among the issues that are as yet under-researched are questions that investigate equity of access to health services, models of empowerment for various groups differentiated by gender, culture and ethnicity, mechanisms for education and health literacy, and environmental supports for healthy childhoods and lifelong wellbeing, including healthy ageing. These are complex issues, and research addressing these social determinants involves long-term, multidisciplinary studies of multiple factors across various settings and groups. The multidimensional nature of community problems is the central reason why so few research studies have been conducted into the SDH. There are limited opportunities for large-scale, comprehensive, longitudinal studies that would gather data from diverse groups in different countries over sufficient time to provide definitive answers to research questions. Such an ambitious research agenda requires multinational, intersectoral support and resources (WHO 2011). Therein lies the dilemma for well-intentioned researchers who accept the ethical and moral obligation to conduct studies into the SDH to motivate social action (Venkatapuram & Marmot 2009). In-country and national studies are important, but the findings may be less effective unless data can be linked internationally. As a result, there has been only slight progress in advancing the equity research agenda. The most pressing need is for in-depth examination of the factors that support or inhibit achievement of the Millennium Development Goals (MDGs), those that bring to light the issues compromising the health of disadvantaged groups, and strategies for narrowing the health gap between advantaged and disadvantaged groups, nationally and internationally (WHO 2011).

Another constraint on the global evidence-based agenda is the lack of coherence in the topics studied in different countries and between different cultures. To drive major change, research studies need to be collaborative, right from the stage of establishing the research agenda, to identifying and evaluating solutions. The logistics of international or cross-institutional collaboration is sometimes prohibitive in terms of time or commitment of individual researchers, or when collaborators have different organisational pressures. Some of these pressures revolve around the lack of understanding by policymakers and research-granting agencies of the need for different perspectives in investigating a problem. Funding bodies often favour studies that are highly scientific, such as systematic reviews of existing research, especially clinical trials, rather than evaluative studies based on community perspectives.

RESEARCHING EQUITY

Community-based research studies must be collaborative—locally with community members, and nationally and internationally with those committed to generating the evidence to address equity.

The current trend toward translational research, which we discuss in depth later in the chapter, involves generating evidence, combining findings from multiple studies in a systematic review, and translating the collective findings into clinical guidelines and change management strategies. This process is one of the most powerful uses of research evidence and is applauded by researchers worldwide, but thus far, knowledge transfer (KT) or knowledge translational studies have focused predominantly on institutional rather than community care, often from the perspective of service providers. Scientific, quantifiable data can be extremely useful, for example, in mapping the epidemiology of risks as a basis for planning, as we mentioned in Chapter 3. However, to inform practice, it is necessary to gather *social epidemiological* information that includes contextual details about the community, information on power relations in terms of social stratification or inequitable structures and circumstances, and participation from community members to identify the dimensions of social capital and how it can be used to foster change (Wallerstein et al. 2011). It is often difficult to persuade funding bodies of the need for this type of research, which underlines the importance of developing the 'art of argument' as part of the research repertoire. The argument must focus on the central purpose of social epidemiological research, which is to help inform measures to promote community empowerment, reduce social exclusion and develop local capacity based on cultural strengths and local systems. This is PHC research, aimed at social justice.

SOCIAL EPIDEMIOLOGICAL STUDIES

- Scientific, epidemiological data
- Contextual information
- Power relations
- Social exclusion
- Social capital
- Cultural assets
- Local capacity
- Local policies
- Differential pathways to health

GROUP EXERCISE: Making the argument for nursing research

There are innumerable topics that nurses can and do research. Working in pairs, identify a topic area that interests you. Why is it important that nurses undertake research in this area? Argue your case for undertaking nursing research in this area to the wider group.

SOCIAL DETERMINANTS OF HEALTH AND THE RESEARCH AGENDA

The goals of PHC direct our research attention to the SDH for both global and local research. The Commission on SDH, mentioned in previous chapters, conducted a three-year project into the SDH adopting a multidimensional research approach, using 'chains of reasoning' and social epidemiological approaches, to investigate the links between collective action and progress on the SDH (Marmot & Friel 2008). Their findings showed that collective action can lead to improved housing and employment conditions, which, in turn, can lead to health equity. Their program of research led the commissioners to argue that researching the SDH requires many types of evidence. This can be a combination of scientific evidence, such as demonstrating through a randomised controlled trial that nutritional supplements for young children can improve their cognitive and educational outcomes, and qualitative, descriptive evidence from case studies and action research, as to what structures and supports in the local community can help sustain these outcomes (Marmot & Friel 2008). Other researchers have recognised that the current research agendas that focus on population-level effects do not provide a realistic picture of the SDH, because they fail to analyse differential effects for various subgroups (Petticrew et al. 2009). Rather than confining studies to population-level causal factors as a basis for decisions about health care, they suggested the need for schematic descriptions of pathways between interventions and outcomes for different groups (Petticrew et al. 2009). The schematic representation of pathways to good health includes information from the policy agendas that help us progress towards equity and social justice at each stage of the life course. For example, when governments invest in healthy childhoods, adult skills development and workplace supports there is both an economic and social benefit. So generous social policies that support dual-earner families not only improve the family's economic and social condition, but that of the entire society, which contributes to social justice (Marmot & Friel 2008). These types of policies that support families and communities are a product of political and social trends, which influence what gets researched at the national, regional and local levels, and by whom.

In addition to the political and social agendas, research topics are also selected by researchers on the basis of their responsiveness to professional agendas. Trends within the fields of public and community health also affect topics for research. In the past, studies informing health-promotion strategies centred around strategies for influencing individual behaviour change. In the 21st century, health-promotion trends indicate a need for studies that include the ecological factors supporting behaviour changes, and how the environments of people's lives can support opportunities to make healthy choices. In addition, there has been a shift away from single-factor studies to comprehensive and multifactor studies that investigate the interactive and cumulative effect of proximal (under the control of the individual) and distal (features of the environments of people's lives) factors that contribute to health. To some extent, this multidimensional perspective has rescued the research agenda in community health from its insularity. Recognising the ecological relationships between human behaviour and environmental conditions, researchers today are more inclined to seek input from colleagues from diverse fields. They also tend to adopt varying combinations of approaches to study health-related questions from multiple perspectives.

The evolution of these research approaches and techniques have demonstrated societal benefit, whereas in the past there was an over-emphasis on 'methodological imperialism', which used to privilege scientific methods over a more eclectic approach that included social phenomena. For long-term community planning there is a need to adopt not only *multifactor* studies, but *multi-method* studies, which examine data from more than one perspective, and focus on the real-world context, inclusive of the conditions and outcomes that may not fall within the 'norm' or normal

pattern. As a result, research findings will be more dynamic and realistic, eminently better suited to influencing community health. Multi-method, multifactorial approaches provide opportunities to analyse new possibilities in the conception of each new study. Importantly, this allows researchers and those who use their research findings to maintain awareness of the dimensions of social relations that shape people's socio-ecological experience of health. This information provides a profusion of opportunities to inform change and to examine responses across time, developments, interventions and contexts.

CONDUCTING RESEARCH FOR POLICY AND PRACTICE

Research and policy development typically occur within a symbiotic relationship. As mentioned above, government policies can dictate research agendas. Reciprocally, research findings can lead to policies for better health. These policies tend to flow from strong coalitions of health planners, researchers and members of the community working toward the same goal. The combination of research evidence, the perspectives and preferences of health service users, and the experience of health practitioners can be invaluable in effecting change. When this type of information is available, research findings can be translated into practice; whether this is clinical or professional practice, education or management practice, or the practice of policy development.

Like New Zealand researchers, Professor Jeanine Young's research team from Queensland have also adopted this approach, focusing on the important role of nurses and other health professionals in promoting safe parenting. Using research data as a baseline, her team has developed an effective, accessible health promotion program for both parents and health professionals to promote safe sleeping. Based on epidemiological data showing that Queensland has one of the highest rates of SIDS/SUDI in Australia, the research team devised a set of studies to examine the extent to which Queensland nurses, midwives and parents were aware of the relevant policies and public health recommendations for safe sleeping. They found that many nurses had a lack of knowledge relating to SIDS/SUDI risk factors; some disagreed with current recommendations; and their knowledge deficits and attitudinal differences influenced nursing practice and information provided to parents. They also found that caregivers in Queensland were employing incorrect infant care practices, including sleep positioning, in greater numbers than their

EVIDENCE, TO EDUCATION, TO CHILD-HEALTH PRACTICE IN PREVENTING SIDS/SUDI

Australian and New Zealand child health professionals have spent the past decade researching sudden unexpected infant deaths. In partnership with public health policymakers, clinicians and community members, their work is directed towards ensuring translation of policy into the best possible practice. As the New Zealand group argues, preventative actions for better health need to be evidence-based; that is, coordinated, monitored and measured (Cowan & Bennett, Online. Available: www.changeforourchildren.co.nz 9 [accessed October 2013]). Significant work is being done to address the high rate of SIDS/SUDI among Māori and researchers are currently examining the efficacy of the *wahakura*. A wahakura is a hand-woven flax basket that the baby is put to sleep in (see Chapter 8). The wahakura with baby in it then stays in the bed so that baby is close to mum but has its own sleeping space. Researchers are undertaking a randomised controlled trial in which 240 mothers will be randomly allocated either a wahakura or portable cot. The sleep patterns of babies will be monitored at one and three months along with the safety and effects of the wahakura on breastfeeding rates, infant sleep duration, and bonding between mother and baby (Whakawhetu, Online. Available: www.whakawhetu.co.nz/ [accessed 3 April 2014])

EVIDENCE-BASED SAFE SLEEPING

- Baby on back
- Head and face uncovered
- Smoke-free environment
- Safe sleeping night and day
- Baby's own sleeping place in adult caregivers room for 6–12 months
- Breastfeed baby
- Keep immunisation up to date

(www.sidsandkids.org/safe-sleeping/, www.kidshealth.org.nz [accessed 8 October 2013])

non-Queensland counterparts, and these practices increased their infant's risk of SIDS/SUDI. The findings of these studies provided evidence that current advice relating to the Safe Sleeping messages may not be received, or may not be implemented, by a proportion of the population at risk. With her colleagues from Queensland Health and *SIDS and Kids Australia* Young designed an eLearning program that would be accessible to nurses and other child-health professionals irrespective of their location. The three-module program includes SUDI risk factors, evidence underpinning recommendations and parent advice, and an evaluation to measure learning outcomes. A pre-test/post-test design evaluated knowledge and knowledge application in those who completed the Safe Sleeping eLearning program, including allied health, medical, student, parent, Indigenous Health worker and SIDS and Kids employees. They found that the program increased knowledge, and self-reported and actual advice to parents. Follow-up has shown the program to be sustainable, effective and attractive. The program has now been developed in partnership with Aboriginal health professionals for health workers and parents, with culturally appropriate logos and information. As of 2013, nearly 2500 people have undertaken the program, which suggests an optimistic, healthy future for parents and infants (Young et al. 2013).

Why do you think nurses and other health professionals may not have been aware of current policies and guidelines related to safe sleeping? Do you think strategies other than the internet learning program would be as effective in promoting safe sleeping? **?**

Evidence-based practice

Since the 1970s the evidence-based practice (EBP) movement has worked towards involving health professionals throughout the world in evidence-based

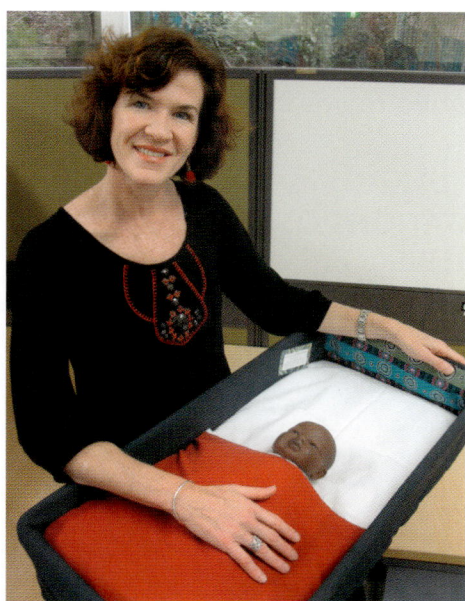

Professor Jeanine Young demonstrating safe sleeping pod (photo courtesy of Professor Jeanine Young)

EVIDENCE FOR PRACTICE

The best available research evidence, the clinician's knowledge and expertise, and the individual patient's views and preferences.

health planning and evidence-informed practice. The objective of EBP at the global level is to help societies achieve efficiency, effectiveness and equity (ICN 2012). At the local level many EBP initiatives are intended to achieve similar goals and, in the process, to advance knowledge that can be used to develop capacity for ongoing developments. EBP is often described in relation to evidence-based medicine (EBM), which was originally devised to inform a medical practitioner's intention to treat or intervene in a person's care. EBP is the integration of three things: the best available research evidence, the clinician's knowledge and expertise, and the individual patient's values. All of these inform decision-making regarding care and treatment (Sackett et al. 2000). Establishing a research culture of EBP in any health service or community promotes an attitude of inquiry among health professionals. A further benefit is that evidence can play a role in maintaining accountability for health resources by guiding decision-makers to plan appropriately (Hoffman et al. 2013). The process of EBP involves five steps. First, convert the need for information into an answerable research question. Some of the most important research questions for community health pose questions about how to promote health literacy or participation among certain groups, how outcomes may be moderated by various approaches to health promotion or the context of care, or the effectiveness of interventions across cultural groups or across the life course. The second step is to search for the best existing evidence to answer the research question, which involves searching databases or scholarly journals, or other sources of research such as local reports or reviews. The third step is to critically appraise existing evidence for its validity, impact and applicability. This step is made easier by the fact that in recent years helpful guidelines have been developed to help researchers appraise different types of studies. The EQUATOR network (Enhancing the Quality and Transparency of Health Research) is one of the most useful of these guidelines (www.equator-network.org). The fourth step in EBP is integration of the evidence with the researcher's existing knowledge, contextual information about the group or community circumstances and preferences, and any other situational information that may help

inform the research. The fifth step is concerned with quality in that it involves self-reflection on the thoroughness and accuracy of steps 1–4 (Hoffman et al. 2013).

STEPS IN EBP

- Researchable question
- Literature review
- Critical appraisal of studies
- Integrate knowledge with contextual information
- Re-check accuracy of steps above

In most cases, researchers begin by posing their question, then refining it to reduce ambiguity, to clarify what data they will collect, and to guide the literature search. It is helpful to collect and review the literature around the PICO mnemonic. That is, search for studies of the Population (children, adults etc.), the Intervention (smoking cessation), Comparisons (group versus individual health education and supports), and Outcomes (smoke-free days). In the process of searching the literature, researchers usually use synonyms and variant words and expressions, often in databases like CINAHL, MEDLINE, PUBMed or PROQUEST with which they are familiar, or in journals where similar studies have been published in the area of interest. In some cases, the research project *is* the literature review, either as a systematic review, integrative review or meta-analysis.

Systematic reviews, literature reviews, integrative reviews and meta-analyses

LIMITATIONS OF SYSTEMATIC REVIEWS

- Synthesising studies with different methods
- Disparate theoretical foundations
- Variable population groups
- Insufficient studies on a particular topic

A systematic review establishes the parameters for adequate or best available research evidence using preset criteria, derived primarily from randomised controlled clinical trials (RCTs) and other high-quality primary research studies. The original intention of systematic reviews for EBM was to provide the basis for treatment recommendations (Bero & Rennie 1995). In community health the 'best treatment' often means the best strategies for health promotion. The advantage of a systematic review is that it uses an explicit and auditable protocol, which is available from the resources of the Cochrane Collaboration (www.cochrane.org) or the Joanna Briggs Institute (www.joannabriggs.org). Another source of reviews is the *Guide to Community Preventive Services,* which analyses which interventions have been evaluated with what effects, and which aspects demonstrate proven effectiveness with what cost benefit (Brownson et al. 2009). Using a protocol ensures breadth and consistency in terms of appraising the participants, interventions and outcomes. The systematic review involves a clear definition of eligibility criteria for a study, a comprehensive search of all relevant studies available at the time of the review, explicit, reproducible and uniformly applied criteria in selecting studies for the review, rigorous appraisal of potential bias in the studies reviewed, and a synthesis of study results (Bennett et al. 2013). A *meta-analysis* takes the review to another level by combining and statistically analysing the evidence from a number of studies on a similar topic to enhance the validity of findings in relation to the outcomes of the study or the *effect size.* This statistical computation can provide a better estimate of a clinical effect than simply analysing the results from individual studies (Bennett et al. 2013). In cases where the studies selected cannot be combined statistically, the review can consist of a narrative analysis with other quasi-statistical methods (Whittemore & Knafl 2005).

SYSTEMATIC OR OTHER REVIEW?

Systematic review is the method of choice for EBP but it is important to evaluate the effectiveness and appropriateness of health care in differing contexts for different groups of people, which may require less structured reviews.

Diabetes is one area of community health that has attracted a proliferation of systematic reviews in recent times, which reflects its importance to clinicians and policymakers. Systematic reviews have been conducted on the links between exercise and glucose control (Avery et al. 2012), a diabetic person's ability to work (Breton et al. 2013), and numerous other aspects of living with diabetes. Other systematic reviews have been conducted on

THE PARACHUTE STUDY: A cautionary tale

Because of the myriad factors influencing community health, formulaic research strategies are not always appropriate. Community problems and issues require different paradigms that encourage researchers to articulate the range of problems and solutions in the context of the community or group. A persuasive argument for a multidimensional approach to research is cleverly presented in a study of parachute use to prevent death and major trauma related to gravitational challenge (Smith & Pell 2003). The authors' objective was to determine whether parachutes are effective in preventing major trauma. Predictably, they found no randomised controlled trials in their systematic review, and concluded that the effectiveness of parachutes has not been subjected to rigorous evaluation. They suggested that the most radical proponents of evidence-based practice, those who criticise observational studies, might want to conduct a double blind, randomized, placebo controlled, crossover trial of jumping out of a plane without a parachute!

different populations in relation to the uptake of programs and benefits of physical activity and/or good nutrition. For example, Purcher et al. (2013) conducted a systematic review of the link between physical activity, nutrition and academic performance in school children, whereas Pavey et al.'s (2012) systematic review was aimed at measuring adults' uptake and adherence when they were referred to exercise programs. Both of these studies could be used to help inform research into exercise, nutrition and academic performance, but for different population groups. By far, the greatest challenge in making sense of a wide range of studies lies in synthesising findings from research that may not have adopted a consistent approach. Each of these reviews conclude with statements about the limitations of the analysis in terms of disparate methods, the failure of some researchers to identify the theoretical foundations of their research, the difficulties in comparing different population groups and the need for more studies on a particular topic. These criticisms are typical of most systematic reviews, particularly where the reviewers try to draw definitive conclusions on appropriate intervention strategies or clinical guidelines from different research approaches. Researchers have come to realise that clinical guidelines are a crucial aspect of promoting knowledge transfer (KT). Techniques for developing clinical guidelines are rapidly evolving with the development of protocols for grading evidence and rating the strength of recommendations from research studies. The Cochrane Collaboration and other organisations maintain a repository of protocols or 'guidelines for developing guidelines' (www.cochrane.org). Some researchers argue that all research should be preceded by a systematic review; however, there are many aspects of community health for which systematic reviews are not available, so researchers setting out to conduct a study often review the literature available using alternative strategies such as *integrative reviews*. Integrative reviews also review the literature pertaining to a certain topic, but they are broader reviews than systematic reviews in that they include experimental and non-experimental studies (Whittemore & Knafl 2005). An integrative review can also be designed to define concepts, review theories, review evidence and analyse methodological issues (Whittemore & Knafl 2005). An excellent example of an integrative review is that conducted by Anthony and Jack (2009). Their review was intended to clarify case study methodology as it is being used in nursing research. Their work was extended by Freeman et al. (2012) in exploring how case study methodology could be used to study nurse migration, which is an issue of global interest. The main advantage of an integrative review is that combining and summarising several types of literature, including theoretical literature can provide a more complete picture of a phenomenon or health care problem (Whittemore & Knafl 2005). Others have used a *scoping review*, which is broader than a review of a single problem or issue in that it is intended to scope a broad topic. Bish et al.'s (2012) scoping review of issues in rural health leadership illustrates the use of this method in interpreting and reinterpreting the relevant literature to provide sufficient breadth for insightful analysis of the topic. Another useful type of review is the *concept analysis*, which can help build a common theoretical foundation for future studies from a consistent set of understandings. An example of this approach is the concept analysis of health assets (see Chapter 4) or Emmanuel and St John's (2010) concept analysis of maternal distress. The latter concept analysis was aimed at expanding our understandings of the transition to motherhood from a medicalised explanation of this phenomenon. Using Walker and Avant's (2005) guidelines for concept analysis these authors expanded the notion of maternal distress to include a woman's responses across the continuum from a normal postpartum stress response to the extent where a woman becomes mentally ill (Emmanuel & St John 2010). The research strategy involves analysis of how the concept is defined in the published literature, then analysis of antecedents, attributes, contributing factors and consequences of maternal distress. This provides a blueprint for theory development that helps subsequent researchers explore maternal distress from a consistent set of shared understandings that can help advance knowledge and practice.

CRITICAL INTERPRETIVE SYNTHESIS

Linking qualitative and quantitative data from studies addressing similar topics to study how the concepts and themes identified interact.

Systematic reviews can be useful in community health because they encourage researchers to develop a firm grounding before embarking on primary research, which also saves time and effort (Bambra 2011). However, to advance knowledge comprehensively, there is also a need to evaluate the effectiveness and appropriateness of health care or certain programs across specific contexts. For example, comparisons are difficult to reconcile when similar programs are conducted in general community settings for different population groups, such as Indigenous people, school health or occupational health (Aspin et al. 2012; Jolley et al. 2007; Young et al. 2012). Another issue concerns the 'disciplined subjectivity' required for analysing data, whether it is from a systematic review or another form of review (Sandelowski 2008:106). All reviews reflect the perspectives and preferences of reviewers, and the different way they conceive problems, pose research questions, and select and compare studies (Sandelowski 2008). Despite these differences the reviews identify gaps in knowledge to guide future research studies, particularly those that can establish the rationale for decision-making in practice. As professional knowledge evolves, new ways of combining data are being developed. One such approach is 'critical interpretive synthesis', which is a method for linking qualitative and quantitative data (Flemming 2010). The method is based on appraising quantitative and qualitative findings from studies addressing a similar topic (such as pain and pain management), translating the qualitative and quantitative findings into each other to study how the concepts and themes interface as a basis for comparison, and developing a synthesis of findings (Flemming 2010). This technique is promising for nursing research, and its use in community studies should prove to be informative in advancing the knowledge base.

Randomised controlled trials

Randomised controlled trials (RCTs) are described as the 'gold standard' in research, because they use an experimental study design, which allows the researcher the greatest control over the research (Goldenberg 2006). Some studies are 'quasi-experimental' in that the researcher may not have the degree of control expected of a scientific experiment, such as when they are unable to randomise subjects. Over the past two decades researchers have refined the techniques involved in conducting RCTs with a set of guidelines, the Consolidated Standards of Reporting Trials (CONSORT), which are widely used throughout the world to ensure consistency in reporting findings (Online. Available: www.bmj.com/content/328/7441/702 [accessed 15 November 2012]). At a basic level, the RCT uses a population sample, and randomly allocates approximately half to an experimental group and the other half to a control group. The experimental group receives an intervention, while the control group typically has 'usual care' or no intervention. The outcome of interest is measured in both groups before (pre-test) and after (post-test) the intervention. Changes that occur in the experimental group between the pre-test and the post-test are reasonably attributed to the intervention (Bennett & Hoffman 2013). This attribution relies on the condition that all other influences are controlled, which can be difficult for educational interventions. So, for example, if a researcher was introducing a program to teach parents about nutrition it would be necessary that the intervention group had no outside influences other than the education provided as part of the program. This would be a challenge as some parents may have pre-existing knowledge, others may have little access to the recommended foods, and others may have a child who was a fussy eater. In these cases, the challenge would be to eliminate extraneous influences by selecting participants with exactly the same knowledge level, similar access to the nutritious foods and infants with similar temperaments. Some researchers would find this level of control impossible, and they may revert to a more qualitative evaluation of their educational program.

Clearly, RCTs are important for developing well-verified, objective research studies, but in reducing the factors studied within tightly defined criteria they often fail to reveal the complexity within which people maintain health (Muncey 2009). Another criticism of RCTs is that the controlled conditions of a clinical trial are rarely available in communities. It would be unethical and not useful to allocate people to an RCT, giving one group the intervention, and withholding it from the other. On the other hand, a meta-analysis that combines the findings from a group of studies can be useful, especially if the findings and conclusions of the studies are synthesised into new ways of looking at the community or planning for community change. This information would then be combined with people's perspectives on how change can be implemented in their particular community or, where change has occurred, how they perceived the outcome (Morrison et al. 2008).

EVIDENCE FOR PRACTICE: Home visiting

We have noted throughout this book that home visiting is an important practice strategy for nurses. It is used as an intervention across the spectrum from prior to birth through to old age and palliative care. In particular, in Chapter 8 we outlined the important work of David Olds and colleagues who examined the positive outcomes among children and their mothers where the mothers had received intensive home visiting in the first two years of the child's life. Other research into home visiting programs in the early childhood period has, however, had more mixed results. In a local example, a nine-year follow-up study of children and families who had received intensive home visiting as part of the Early Start program in New Zealand, found that while some outcomes were encouraging others were less so. The positive outcomes included significantly reduced risk of hospital attendance for unintentional injury, lower risk of parent-reported harsh punishment, lower levels of physical punishment, higher parenting competence scores, and more positive child behavioural adjustment scores. However, there were no significant differences in a range of measures of parental behaviour and family outcomes such as maternal depression, parental substance use, intimate partner violence, adverse economic outcomes and life stress (Fergusson et al. 2013). Fergusson et al. (2013) conclude that while there were small to moderate benefits for children, these benefits did not extend to parents or the family overall.

A number of systematic reviews also suggest mixed outcomes from home visitation approaches. One review of home visitation schedules in the early postpartum period found there was no evidence of improvements in maternal and neonatal mortality, and no strong evidence that more postnatal home visits were associated with improvements in maternal health (Yonemoto et al. 2013). In two of the studies reviewed by Yonemoto et al. (2013), women receiving more home visits had higher mean depression scores. In both of these studies women already received four midwife home visits. One study then compared the addition of six versus one health visitor visits on top of the four midwife visits and the second added ten layperson visits in addition to the four midwife visits. Yonemoto et al. argue that the studies confirm an increased risk for depression due to more visits but attribute this to the possibility that more visits with health professionals meant women may have been more likely to disclose their feelings. The authors of one of the studies suggest that disruption of a woman's usual support systems may also contribute to the finding. It is important to note that in their study, Yonemoto et al. considered the number, rather than the frequency of visits, therefore it is not possible to determine if increased frequency of visits would have impacted on the depression scores. Similar to the Fergusson et al. (2013) findings, Yonemoto et al. did find there was some evidence of decreased hospital utilisation, at least among infants in the weeks following birth. There was also evidence that more home visits may encourage women to exclusively breastfeed and increase maternal satisfaction with postnatal care (Yonemoto et al. 2013). In a further review considering the needs of women with specific alcohol or drug problems in the pre or postpartum period, however, no significant differences were found in outcomes for women receiving home visits versus those who did not (Turnbull & Osborn 2012). Finally, a systematic review that looked at parenting programs found that parenting interventions most commonly provided in the home using multi-faceted interventions are effective in reducing child injury and may improve home safety (Kendrick et al. 2013).

? So how does the evidence guide our practice when there are such variable outcomes? While a systematic review gives us a useful overview of outcomes, it is also important to consider the context within which interventions are designed and implemented, and the research question that guides the review. The evidence suggests that home visitation programs are most effective when they focus on children through providing parents with new skills, knowledge and approaches to parenting, but less successful when targeted at changing long-standing parent or family issues and challenges. It is important that home visitation programs have clear goals and that nurses engaged in them are realistic about the outcomes that can be achieved. In translating research evidence into practice it is also important for researchers to adopt an incremental approach to research, whereby each research study adds a specific increment to our knowledge base in a defined area of practice. This would see researchers study home visiting across different contexts, as mentioned above, with consistent measurement of variables such as children's health status or developmental outcomes in relation to clearly specified visiting schedules and strategies.

Sources of evidence

The EBP movement is based on the notion that providing research evidence for all activities in the health professions ensures accountability to the population for clinical decision-making and interventions. Most nursing and health researchers today are aware of the importance of EBP through the work undertaken by the Cochrane Collaboration and the Joanna Briggs Institute, which maintain databases of systematic reviews of research on health care interventions in a wide range of clinical areas. Because not all community practitioners have the requisite high-level skills for literature retrieval and appraisal, or the time or management support to develop and use these skills in practice, many access 'predigested' sources of systematic reviews. These include the *Journal of Evidence-based Health Care*, and *Evidence Based Nursing*.

From the early days of EBP, 'evidence' was considered as quantifiable data situated within the paradigm of logical positivism. A paradigm is a set of beliefs or perspectives that creates a pattern for scholarly inquiry. Paradigms therefore encompass the philosophical assumptions that underpin the way we view natural phenomena (Polit & Beck 2012). Weaver and Olson's (2006) integrative review of nursing paradigms outlines those most often used in nursing research. The *positivist paradigm* is used in quantitative nursing studies, where the research is based on rigid rules of logic and measurement, truth, absolute principles and prediction (Weaver & Olson 2006). In contrast, the *interpretive paradigm* focuses on the meanings people ascribe to their actions and interactions. Another paradigm or philosophical perspective in nursing research is the *critical perspective,* sometimes called the *critical social theory* paradigm, which addresses social institutions, and issues of power and alienation as well as new opportunities (Weaver & Olson 2006). Interpretive research is undertaken on the assumption that reality is socially constructed through the use of language and shared meanings, so researchers seek to understand phenomena by listening to people or observing their actions (Pearson & Hannes 2013). Critical perspectives are based on the assumption that knowledge is value-laden, and shaped by historical, social, political, gender and economic conditions that, for some people, can be oppressive. Critical researchers therefore seek to answer *why* these conditions occur, and generate knowledge that can be used as a basis for change (Pearson & Hannes 2013).

> ### PARADIGMS
> - Positivist
> - Interpretive
> - Critical

Many researchers would argue that knowledge of communities must be contextualised and holistic, complete with cultural, spiritual and environmental dimensions. This type of knowing is multi-faceted, sometimes superseding that type of knowledge obtained from systematic assessments of prior research findings. It is often described as *naturalistic inquiry,* as information is gleaned from the natural setting, and interpreted using various *interpretive*, rather than *statistical* techniques. Naturalistic data can include informant interviews, focus groups (sometimes called 'yarning' groups), observational data and document analysis (Dimer et al. 2013). The knowledge gained from this type of research is an important element in informing policy and practice changes, especially when more than one type of inquiry is used in combination. Interpretive methods can be a useful approach to gathering and analysing data on the realities of community life for different groups of people. Three of the most common interpretive methods that are based on naturalistic inquiry are Phenomenology, Ethnography and Grounded Theory. Although there are variants of these methodological approaches, such as Phenomenography, Critical Ethnography, Cognitive Ethnography, and some differences in the way

Grounded Theory is constructed, we outline the three main methodological approaches below.

> ### NATURALISTIC INQUIRY
> Information gleaned from the natural setting of people's lives through interviews, observations and documents analysis.

Phenomenology is an interpretive approach that revolves around the essence of 'lived experience'; that is, primarily analysing what people say to try to reveal the essence of how they experience their lives. From a practical perspective, the research focus is on interpreting meanings from their experiences, presented usually as a set of themes, to make informed judgements about their needs as a basis for planning. *Ethnography* is another interpretive approach frequently used by researchers to study group cultural meanings. The conventions of ethnographic analysis are slightly different from analysing phenomenological data—in an ethnographic study, analysis adopts a structured approach to examining rich descriptions of shared cultural meanings as well as the artifacts and structures that maintain their culture. It is important to note that not all ethnographic studies are concerned with ethnic cultures. This methodological approach can be used to study the culture of a health care organisation, cultural commonalities among certain professional groups, the cultural features of a group of adolescents, young men, women or any other group with shared characteristics. *Grounded Theory* is basically a combination of an interpretive and deductive (positivist) approach that is aimed at developing a theory about the social psychological processes people use to create meaning and the actions they take in relation to a phenomenon of interest (studying, practising, organising, etc.) and contextual influences on the way they undertake these processes and activities. The theory is 'grounded' in the context from which data are collected on a specified phenomenon, so in this respect, the process begins in a similar way to a phenomenological study. The researcher analyses interviews, documents and/or observational data to generate explanatory codes and categories that will comprise elements and dimensions of the theory. The provisional categories are then analysed in conjunction with relevant theoretical concepts (called theoretical sampling). The process involves constant comparisons between sources, and multiple iterations through the data, to ultimately develop either a highly detailed set of propositions or a fully testable theory about the group or community. The grounded theory can then help guide identification of problems that need to be dealt with, or decisions that should be made to improve health.

Phenomenology

What is the lived experience?

Ethnography

What are the cultural meanings, structures and artifacts?

Grounded Theory

What social psychological processes explain how meanings are created, shared, negotiated?

BOX 15.1 **Adopt, adapt, act**

- Research—from carefully designed studies and comparative trials over time
- Knowledge and information—results of consultation, networking, internet information and analysis of documents
- Ideas and interests—expert knowledge shaped by personal and professional experience
- Politics—information relevant to government agendas, opportunities, crises or challenges
- Economics—cost-effectiveness or economic evaluation and opportunity cost data, for example, what opportunities are forgone when a program is developed

(Source: Bowen & Zwi 2005:166)

Decision-making for change requires not only research evidence, but a combination of content and procedural knowledge; what Benner (1984) calls 'knowing that' and 'knowing how'. This 'relational' knowledge (knowing what to do, and knowing how to do it) helps create an understanding of the community through critical reflection as well as data analysis, especially when evaluative data are gathered from members of the community. When this type of 'internal evidence' is used, any planned changes can be embedded in the local social structures, and based on community ownership of when and how change will occur (Abbott et al. 2008; Comino & Kemp 2008). Evidence-informed practice emanates from this type of community partnership approach. It represents a pathway to decision-making that involves generating the evidence, understanding how people make sense of their lives, and deciding how this knowledge can assist health promotion efforts (Nykiforuk et al. 2012). This is simplified in a three-step process of 'adopt, adapt, act' (see Box 15.1).

RESEARCH TO PRACTICE

Consider the current political environment, policy development arena, and your own clinical interests. Develop a research question that considers these varying contexts, that is applicable to your area of practice, and that meets the needs and priorities of the community in which you might practise.

The three-step approach described in Box 15.1 can be used as a guide to policy development. This requires the researcher working towards policy change to be engaged with at least the broad contours of government ideas, politics and economics (Labonte et al. 2005). One policy area common to the governments of Australia and New Zealand is the focus on PHC. Careful analysis of how PHC is understood in each country reveals some differences in relation to how various organisations at the national, state, territory or district level govern the practice of nurses and other health professionals. Understanding the policies and how they are applied in a practical sense is therefore important in terms of the constraints and facilitating factors that determine the extent to which changes can be made in a community. In some cases, local understandings provide the impetus for research that would inform policy, and in other cases, understanding government directions and priorities makes it easier to construct a rational argument for a research project that is responsive to the policy environment. So, for example, it might be easier for a nurse researcher to secure funding for a study that corresponds with or extends one of the areas that have been successful in recent research funding rounds, such as early childhood education, parental support, chronic illness prevention, or improving equity of access to care for older persons, helping to close the gap between Indigenous and non-Indigenous people in a specific way, or gathering data on migrant health needs. All of these topics resonate with the PHC agenda. They are also in synchrony with another trend, which is called translational research.

Translational research: knowledge translation and knowledge transfer (KT)

Translating research into policy and/or practice is a complex social process involving multiple interactions and linkages between producers and users of research (ICN 2012). Early researchers explained translational research in terms of two stages: from 'bench to bedside' (clinical laboratory to clinical application) and from clinical application in an ideal setting to real-world practice, also called the 'second translational gap' (Hay et al. 2012). KT in community health does not typically use the term 'bench to bedside'; instead the baseline data tend to be epidemiological data, which is then combined with input from members of the community and those involved in promoting their health to provide a comprehensive picture of assets and needs. The other difference between clinical and community translational research is the inclusion of life course epidemiological data, which gathers information on adverse life circumstances and the SDH (Hay et al. 2012). Together these sources of information comprise the best available evidence, professional knowledge and expertise, and people's preferences and expectations to improve outcomes (see Figure 15.1). The *transferability* of this type of evidence is dependent on whether or not there is the potential to extrapolate findings to other settings or other populations (Polit & Beck 2012).

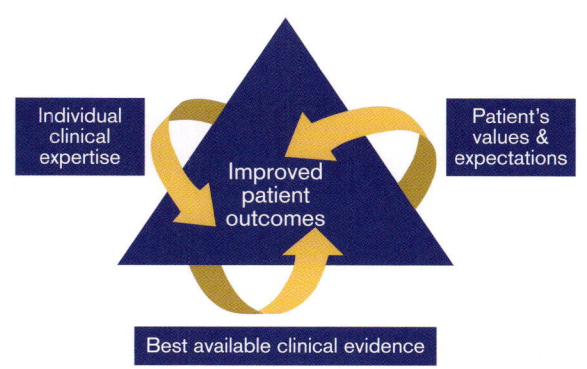

FIGURE 15.1
Translating evidence to practice

Contemporary researchers outline a multi-step process of translating knowledge to action or knowledge to practice within the context of theories or models. Although there is some debate about the use of terms, *theories* tend to be used when a set of relationships are explained and there is some predictive capability (Kitson et al. 2008). An example of this would be framing a research study within Rogers's (2003) Theory of the Diffusion of Innovations (see Chapter 6), which predicts that community members will be more likely to accept a change if they can see the relative advantage of the change, and its compatibility with their approach or goals. A *model*, on the other hand, is typically more diffuse, and usually refers to a specific way to implement research into practice. A good example of this would be the Stages of Change model (Prochaska & Velicer 1997), also described in Chapter 6. Models, like *conceptual frameworks*, can also be used as

translational devices. The Flinders program of chronic illness management (Flinders 2013) and the PRECEDE-PROCEED Model of Health Program Planning (Green & Kreuter 1991) are often used as conceptual frameworks for change. For example, Tramm et al. (2011) used the PRECEDE-PROCEED model to investigate whether it provided a robust framework for investigating health promotion in cancer survivors, and Lake et al. (2010) reported on the usefulness of the Flinders model in translating chronic disease self-management training into the practice of health professionals. Another example is DeGuzman and Kulbok's (2012) framework for researching the SDH with a focus on neighbourhoods and the built environment. Their framework is designed to gather data on inequalities, social and economic conditions and walkability of the built environment to analyse its potential for alleviating stress, encouraging healthy behaviours and providing supportive resources (DeGuzman & Kulbok 2012). This focus on 'place-based' research helps identify how a place is structured and perceived and impacts on people's place identity and engagement (Nykiforuk et al. 2012). As these and other studies show, although there has been a decline in theory development over the past decade (Yarcheski et al. 2012), community researchers continue to use and develop frameworks to guide health promotion practice. The use of a framework can help ensure some degree of consistency in the way researchers investigate the interaction between study variables.

Theoretical or conceptual frameworks tend to be used interchangeably, and these terms both present the bigger picture of translating knowledge into practice (Kitson et al. 2008). Frameworks add value to the rigour of research studies by providing a logical, empirical basis for the research, which guides the development of the study and the way findings are analysed, discussed and transferred into practice (Cane et al. 2012). By reporting the theoretical or conceptual framework along with study findings, other researchers can see where the findings fit with the body of knowledge, and how common understandings can help extend the knowledge base. In translating program knowledge to practice, partnerships with community members are integral to success, ensuring the acceptability of implementation strategies. Box 15.2 outlines one model for this type of knowledge translation.

Translational research is a burgeoning area of study in community and public health. As acknowledged in the model outlined in Box 15.2, successful translation of knowledge into practice is based on the principle of partnering with the community from the earliest stages of the research

(Miller et al. 2012). A number of other principles have emerged from researchers' experiences of translating programs across settings and populations. Australian rural health researchers have proposed a model to guide translation of evidence into practice with a focus on PHC. Their Health Services Research Impact Framework appraises the transferability of programs by integrating the strengths of several other models of research impact according to four broad areas (Buykx et al. 2012). These include research-related impact: *advancing knowledge*; policy impact: *informing decision-making*; service impact: *improving health and health systems*; and societal impact, which involves creating broad *social and economic benefit*. The model is promising in that it captures the major expectations of community health research. Once the framework is validated, the research team expects that it will prove useful in advancing KT for PHC research (Buykx et al. 2012).

BOX 15.2 Translating evidence to practice through community organisation partnerships

Steps	Evidence
Step 1 Needs assessment	Interpretive or mixed methods data collection, analysis and synthesis
Step 2 Adoption, adaptation	Review existing programs in relation to planned change
Step 3 Capacity development	Develop databases, systems for process and outcome data, staff training, outcome goals, sustainability
Step 4 EBP implementation, community engagement	Evaluation strategy, staff support
Step 5 Program evaluation	Data collection protocols, data collection, plan analysis, how to use data to inform practice
Step 6 Partnership development	Ongoing dialogue with partners on goals, priorities, challenges

(Source: Adapted from Miller et al. 2012)

Dose intervention
- Consistent protocol
- Similar group size
- Common incentives
- Participant training
- How changes contextualised

Dose response
- Population characteristics
- Environmental influences

Health promotion researchers have also developed implementation frameworks for KT. Cambon et al. (2012) developed a framework for appraising the merits of KT in promoting health across settings based on the notion of 'dose' and 'dose response'. In the context of health promotion initiatives, 'dose' refers to direct factors, and variable 'dose' response as indirect factors related to the intervention. Researchers have been using these terms to describe the outcomes of nursing interventions for several years, but most of the research has focused on clinical settings. In hospital studies, 'nurse dose' is used to explain how staffing variables (education, experience and skill mix) can impact on interventions (Manojlovich et al. 2011). Cambon et al.'s (2012) model represents another context for using these descriptors. In the health promotion example, 'dose intervention' is the degree to which those delivering the health promotion intervention followed the protocol, whether the group size was the same, which incentives were available to support participation, consistency of participant training and coaching in implementing the modifications, and how changes were contextualised. The level of direct influences ('dose response') depends on the population characteristics or environmental factors influencing the intervention (Cambon et al. 2012). Although this framework is not widely reported it does lend itself to health promotion studies in various settings.

This KT work by health promoters and community health professionals is on the cusp of providing researchers with valid frameworks to ensure rigour and efficiency in conducting research and using EBP to develop community capacity. As we have argued throughout this book, community capacity is developed from the grassroots level, with the researcher(s) adopting a guiding role in helping frame the way information is generated, shared and used. Where the objective is to study the outcome of nursing or health care interventions, the translational elements can include evaluation of the appropriateness, accessibility, acceptability, effectiveness, efficiency or equity of service improvements that have been implemented elsewhere (Maxwell 1984). Studies of appropriateness include such things as assets, preferences or satisfaction with services (Morgan & Ziglio 2007). Accessibility studies could address the services used by different population groups, such as young parents or older persons. Acceptability studies can address community perceptions of health interactions. Studies of effectiveness include evaluation of health promotion initiatives, such as antenatal care and its link with birth experiences. Efficiency is typically an examination of the cost-benefit of certain choices; for example, providing community support services for the homeless. Studies of equity generally have a broader reach, such as comparing the impact of affordable food or housing for different populations, including different cultural groups. Each of these questions is aligned with the KT approach in focusing on community partnerships.

APPRAISING EVIDENCE FOR CAPACITY DEVELOPMENT

- Appropriateness
- Accessibility
- Acceptability
- Effectiveness
- Efficiency
- Equity

COMMUNITY-BASED RESEARCH PARTNERSHIPS

One of the trends guiding research in nursing and other health disciplines is the move towards community-based research partnerships. Community-based research provides an ideal opportunity to inform policies from the ground up. It is also a way of providing feedback to policymakers of the applicability of policies on the ground, where people live, work, study or play. Funding bodies often support community partners such as government departments, hospitals or health districts, as collaborators in research studies, knowing that the information that will emerge will be more authentic than it would be if the researcher was working alone to investigate a community problem. Using qualitative research methods to interpret community members' perspectives can help explain the dimensions of health disparities and the role of social and culturally contextualised decision-making (Foster et al. 2012; Leeman & Sandelowski 2012). Local partnerships are also considered to have *ecological validity*; that is, real-world relevance (Polit & Beck 2012). Ecological validity is a construct that emerged from researchers' concerns with maintaining culturally relevant research strategies and findings (Johnson Crowder & Broome 2012). Bernal et al.'s (1995) framework for cultural evaluation in research is outlined below in Box 15.3.

PARTNERSHIP KNOWLEDGE

- Propositional
- Practical
- Experiential
- Presentational

Considering these aspects in planning and implementing research creates many kinds of knowledge. These include *propositional* knowledge gained from identifying the research question(s), *practical knowledge,* from developing the skills and competencies of research, *experiential knowledge* from participating in the research, and *presentational knowledge* from sharing information that will address the research question. Nykiforuk et al. (2012) explain that generating these types of knowledge through ongoing interaction between researchers and the many levels of stakeholders is crucial to translating evidence to practice for evidence-informed decision-making. The process also builds capacity, not only in knowledge development but in fostering skills and confidence among community

<table>
<tr><td colspan="2">

BOX 15.3 Framework for ecological validity

</td></tr>
<tr><td>

Dimension

</td><td>

Example

</td></tr>
<tr><td>Language</td><td>Age and culturally appropriate language</td></tr>
<tr><td>Persons</td><td>Ethnically inclusive strategies for team members</td></tr>
<tr><td>Metaphors</td><td>Symbols and metaphors that resonate with research partners</td></tr>
<tr><td>Content</td><td>Including unique social and economic factors, values</td></tr>
<tr><td>Concepts</td><td>Evaluations are consonant with culture</td></tr>
<tr><td>Goals</td><td>Congruent with values, customs, traditions</td></tr>
<tr><td>Methods</td><td>Cultural knowledge incorporated into methods, procedures</td></tr>
<tr><td>Context</td><td>Social, economic, political contexts are considered</td></tr>
</table>

(Source: Bernal et al. 1995)

BOX 15.4 Key principles of CBPR

1. Acknowledges community as the unit of identity
2. Builds on community strengths and resources
3. Facilitates collaborative, equitable involvement of all partners in all research phases
4. Integrates knowledge and action for mutual benefit
5. Promotes co-learning and empowerment to address social inequalities
6. Involves a cyclical and iterative process
7. Addresses health from both positive and ecological perspectives
8. Disseminates findings and knowledge to all partners
9. Involves a long-term commitment by all partners

(Source: Israel et al. 2001)

---

members for empowerment and long-term commitment (Masuda et al. 2011).

Community-based participatory research (CBPR)

Community-based participatory research has been described as systematic investigation with the participation of those affected by a certain issue with a view toward education, action or social change. It is used as a way of transforming societal power, so researchers use this approach in the context of addressing social disparities, democratising knowledge through multiple methods of discovery and dissemination, and promoting emancipatory actions for social justice (Masuda et al. 2011). Community members act as partners in the research process, and are valued for their unique strengths. CBPR is a culturally sensitive approach to community health research in that the researcher adopts an attitude of 'cultural humility', which is intended to redress power imbalances and maintain mutually respectful, dynamic community partnerships (Minkler 2005; Foster et al. 2012). CBPR is therefore appropriate for researching the SDH, especially the gender, culture and environmental aspects of disadvantage. Equity is therefore a central element of CBPR studies, many of which seek to foster organisational and social networks to help community members develop collective skills to address fundamental health inequities (Schulz et al. 2011). The key principles of CBPR are listed in Box 15.4, and Box 15.5 describes an example of CBPR in action.

CBPR

Research undertaken with the participation of community members affected by an issue with a view to education, action or social change.

ACTION RESEARCH

Action research revolves around flexible planning through iterative (repetitive) cycles, wherein the researchers and their partners in the community consider a research problem, then together engage in cycles of planning, proposed action, evaluation and further cycles of planning and action (Carr & Kemmis 1986). Action research studies are conducted within the interpretive paradigm and aimed at engaging with the people and/or issues under study, to understand the multiple dimensions of socially constructed behaviours and processes that affect their lives (Stringer 2004). Action research adopts a partnership approach similar to CBPR, in which all partners are considered co-researchers in exploring solutions to an issue of concern. As in CBPR, the researcher's role is to create a trusting environment, and to help keep the analysis on track with careful documentation, while helping others develop analytic skills and capacity. One of the most salient issues relevant to community health research is the capacity of action research studies to help people clarify their meanings, behaviours and

BOX 15.5 'Ngati and healthy' diabetes prevention program—CBPR in action

Just north of Gisborne on the rural East Coast of the North Island of New Zealand, about half the community have been identified as having diabetes or insulin resistance (IR) (Tipene-Leach et al. 2004). Implementation of a diabetes prevention program developed in collaboration with the local Māori tribe of Ngati Porou began in 2004. The intervention objectives are to:

1 increase the consumption of fruit and vegetables
2 increase the consumption of wholegrain foods
3 reduce the consumption of fat
4 increase exercise levels
5 reduce level of smoking
6 reduce alcohol intake.

Community members take an active part in the design and implementation of community initiatives (for example, walking groups and water-only schools). After two years, IR prevalence decreased from 35.5% to 25.4% ($p=0.003$) overall, most markedly among women aged 25 to 49 years (Coppell et al. 2009).

Further information on the project can be found at: www.otago.ac.nz/diabetes/research/ngati.html#pub1

interactions in the cultural contexts of their lives. When this type of research is planned and executed in partnership with community members, the researchers, and those using their research, are able to see how people make sense of their world, how they see one another, how they engage in resolving issues and problems and how they draw shared meanings from the processes (Stringer 2004). Understanding these dimensions of human behaviour can provide insights into how best to support community members through the changes they wish to make.

Participatory action research (PAR)

ACTION AND PAR RESEARCH

Researchers and their community partners work together through a cyclical process of planning, action, evaluation and reflection.

Participatory action research is an example of CBPR, wherein the focus is on collective, reflective inquiry aimed at understanding and change (Baum et al. 2006). The strength of PAR lies in it being a situational, collaborative approach (Carr & Kemmis 1986). PAR is similar to action research but sits in the critical paradigm rather than interpretive. Like other forms of CBPR, it is emancipatory, questioning the nature of knowledge, and how it represents and reinforces the interests of the more powerful people in society; drawing on experience as a basis for knowing; and using experiential knowledge to influence practice (Baum et al. 2006). As an action research approach, PAR is based on iterative cycles of collaborative decision-making, critical evaluation, action and reflection, which make it an ideal method to evaluate community changes. Two features of PAR that distinguish the method from other research are authentic participation and relevancy of actions, both controlled by the community, rather than external researchers (Burgess 2006). The process of PAR includes group reflections designed to identify mutual solutions which are *critical* or *emancipatory* (free from traditional restraints), because they emerge from the community (bottom-up) and not those who seek to study them (top-down). As the community members are engaged as partners in the research it is more likely than other methods to facilitate empowerment and sustainable change, especially as the community invests the project with energy and resources. PAR therefore embodies the values and purposes of CBPR. It is aimed at generating mindfulness: relational knowledge that captures the mutual understandings of human beings, connecting problems, critical analysis and values-based actions (Burgess 2006). When individual and collective perspectives are shared, there are often issues of inequities and power imbalances that become visible. Through mutual consciousness raising, the group can become empowered to speak freely and authentically, which ensures that appropriate information is being collected.

One innovative use of PAR is in working with children affected by illness or disability. Researchers in Tasmania and the UK have combined verbal and text-based approaches with drawing and photography as an arts-based approach to encourage children's engagement, communication, control and interpretation of their experiences (Carter & Ford 2013). These tools can help children identify concerns in an enjoyable environment where they feel sufficiently comfortable to express themselves in ways that can help health professionals understand their needs. Arts-based action research can also develop other capacities, as Nilson et al. (2013)

found, when they investigated young children's cognitive development in the process of preparing a work of art. Their findings revealed that the artistic endeavour ignited children's imagination and helped mobilise creativity and critical thinking, which had an important impact on their cognitive and social development (Nilson et al. 2013). Using participatory action research in the steps outlined in Box 15.6 can help bring to light issues that may be misunderstood in the context of promoting health.

Photovoice

Photovoice is a PAR method that has become popular with researchers throughout the past decade. It is based on the understanding that people are experts on their own lives and given the opportunity, they will be able to 'voice' their concerns and initiate grassroots change through photographs and stories (Wang et al. 2004). In this type of research, participants are provided with a camera, and take photographs that raise questions regarding how a certain situation exists, whether or not they wish to change it, and if so, how. Their photographs are intended to promote critical group discussion about personal and community issues and assets. This technique is based on the principle that images can

tell a story, and stories can influence policy. Photovoice researchers support the feminist notion that everyone has a particular story, a particular experience of class, race, gender, sexuality, family, country, displacement, alliances and other aspects of their lives (Wang et al. 2004). Wang, who is one of the pioneers of this method, and her colleagues explain how they used this technique originally in China, then in an American neighbourhood violence prevention collaborative, where people representing widely disparate ages, incomes, experiences, neighbourhoods and social power came together to develop photographs and narratives about their experiences. The images and multilayered stories they created were shared with policymakers, who, together with community leaders, were also asked to take photographs, which were then shared across groups during workshops. At the workshops conducted with both groups the researchers posed questions about what they each saw, what they believed was really happening, how this related to their lives, why the problem existed, and what could be done about it. The researchers acted as facilitators, bringing people together, providing them with the cameras, and collecting what the group believed were the most potent images. By sharing their perspectives and working together to choose the most significant images, there was a closer alignment among the groups in planning for change.

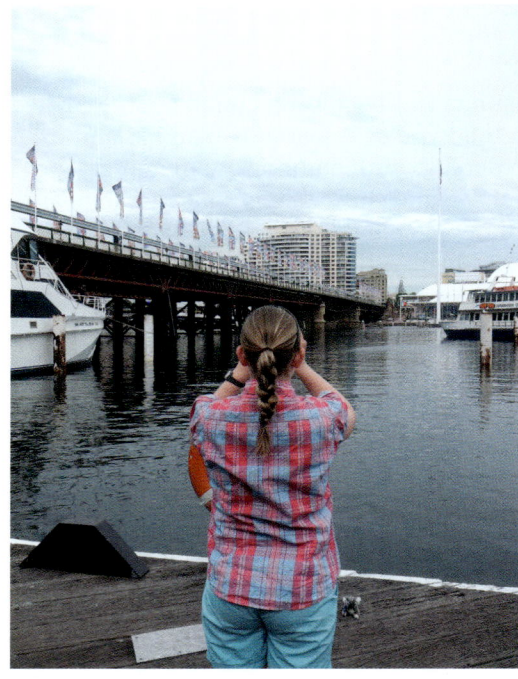

Photos capture many stories and perspectives that may differ from the written word (photo: Jill Clendon)

BOX 15.6 Steps in conducting PAR evaluations

1. Scoping—establishing what is to be accomplished, how change might occur, what resources are available, which principles underpin the project, and what people's accounts of what is occurring in the community can add to our understanding

2. Focusing—identifying what strategies are effective, what different people believe is working well

3. Gathering information—using different mechanisms to gather data: documents, verbal reports and interviews

4. Making meaning from information—engaging in reflection and group debriefing

5. Communication—drafting a report, discussing ideas with participants and others involved in the evaluation

6. Applying learning—fine tuning, making changes in the report, identifying key strategies and developing participants' skills in shaping the project, to begin the capacity development

(Source: Haviland 2004)

Since Wang et al.'s (2004) work was published other researchers have used photovoice to promote social action. Canadian researchers used the technique in Toronto to engage and empower immigrant residents to influence public policy and secure improved local services. Their research culminated in a display of photographs in a Community Forum and Exposition. Their 'expo' attracted the attention of policymakers, which brought about change in housing and economic conditions, two of the most profound SDH that were affecting their lives (Haque & Eng 2011). In Victoria, Australia, Adams et al. (2012) used PAR and photovoice to explore the meanings surrounding unhealthy eating and food insecurity in an Aboriginal Cooperative. The study showed that food selections were influenced by family harmony, collectivism and satiating hunger with fast foods. Subsequent action research cycles were used to depict healthy food portions, social cooking opportunities and a specialised cookbook. In all of these cases, photo-elicitation generated the type of dialogue that is so important in working closely with people to change their lives. Like other interpretive research strategies, these techniques lend themselves to mixed-methods approaches that combine both qualitative and quantitative data to capture this breadth of information. This has been called the 'primacy of the practical', where findings are seen to have applicability beyond those of a study that collects only quantitative data (Sandelowski 2004:1367). The research team is then able to interpret the social attributes and meanings held by the members of a group or a community, and examine the surrounding social conditions that shape their lives, all of which is research evidence for change. In some cases, the research question suggests a case study method.

CASE STUDY RESEARCH

Case study has rapidly become a mainstream method for nursing research. It is ideally suited to studies that seek to describe, explore and understand a phenomenon in its real-life context (Yin 2009). A case study is an intensive focus on one or more cases of the phenomenon, which the researcher constructs as a 'case' by defining its boundaries and units of analysis (Sandelowski 2011). Although case studies are not generalisable, they do provide important information on community health topics, by integrating multiple sources of evidence that have informational, rather than statistical, value (Anthony & Jack 2009; Luck et al. 2006). One impediment to case study research is a common misunderstanding of what can be analysed in this methodological

approach, particularly case studies that are exclusively interpretive. Although case studies are contextualised to a specific situation or cultural group, if data are carefully interpreted, both unique and common aspects of the case can be illuminated, providing a basis for comparison with other contexts or populations. This is accomplished by taking the analytic data that was used to profile the case and using techniques to 'decontextualise' the information. In interpretive case studies the researcher conducts a thematic analysis to identify themes, or units of meaning (Braun & Clarke 2006). Once these are identified, theoretical or process relationships can be explored among various clusters of meaning. These relationships are then studied to create new meanings, by reintegrating themes into larger clusters, across a larger number of cases. Reflecting on themes, and their relationships and implications in different settings, gives a depth of understanding that allows cross-case comparisons.

MIXED METHODS

The multifactor, social and cultural fabric of communities is well suited to mixed-method studies that can include the different world views of quantitative and qualitative methods either simultaneously or sequentially (Creswell & Plano Clark 2011). Incorporating contextual and cultural elements to the traditional designs of RCTs or quasi-experimental studies can help improve both theoretical and practical understandings that lie at the heart of community interventions. Similarly, discovering people's perspectives on health and wellbeing by listening to their stories or interview responses can lead to hypotheses that can be tested in the controlled conditions of quantitative research (Tashakkori & Teddlie 2003). Combining the findings of each type of study can include event analysis: measuring aspects of an event and interpreting interview accounts of an event; concurrent analysis of both types of data to ensure complementarity or completeness; or concurrent nested analysis to enrich descriptions with broader understandings. These techniques can provide a more complete picture of what is being researched through integration and interpretation (Happ et al. 2006).

EVENT ANALYSIS

- Measuring+interpreting
- Concurrent analysis
- Concurrent nested analysis

Questions that require a mixed-method design are those that cannot be explained by only one type of data; issues that require considerable breadth and depth; problems where there is a need to confirm or enhance findings with a second type of data; or studies where a research instrument is being developed from comprehensive information about the topic (Andrew & Halcomb 2009). In some cases, a qualitative element can be nested in a quantitative study, or a quantitative element nested in a qualitative study to provide important and unique insights (Happ et al. 2006). Using mixed methods is not a new technique, but it is growing in popularity for a number of reasons. These include increased reflexivity among nurses and other health professionals about the relationship between the researcher and the researched; heightened political awareness about the issues surrounding research, increased procedural knowledge about research governance and ethics, and a trend toward international collaboration (Brannen in Andrew & Halcomb 2009).

> ### MIXED METHODS
> Creating a broader 'picture' of community health.

Using a variety of research approaches to ascertain the merits of health promotion initiatives helps keep the focus on 'how' and 'why' questions. It also allows the researcher to evaluate many levels of outcomes, and to pose new questions for evaluation as the study progresses, especially if a PAR approach is being used. For example, as a program is being devised, evaluation might emphasise inter-organisational arrangements. The next phase might also include evaluating implementation of the program, and the skills required to deliver various components. A further iteration could add to these components a focus on maintenance and client outcomes (Goodman 2000). At any stage of this process, a comparative study of processes, or outcomes, or both, could be developed. Such a mixed-methods approach would allow the community to be considered a 'case' under study, with multiple dimensions of investigation, multiple methods, and in some cases multiple researchers, some focusing on ascertaining baseline information, some conducting comparative trials of interventions and some evaluating outcomes.

In an ecologically focused study, for example, the researcher would want to measure community or group change, and elements of the environment that either support or constrain the desired change, as

was used in the nutrition and exercise studies systematically reviewed by Avery et al. (2012) and Pavey et al. (2012). Using an additional method enhances the validity of studies by 'triangulation'. This involves interrogating the data from different perspectives, as a surveyor would triangulate a point of reference by viewing it from two different perspectives. For example, the study may ask:

- What conditions changed?
- To what extent?
- With what outcomes?

These questions could be answered using a quantitative survey, with responses analysed to judge whether and to what extent any responses were significant, or to provide a basis for predicting future initiatives (predictive validity). Following this phase, or simultaneously, an interpretive, qualitative element could be designed to address the questions:

- What factors support the change?
- Are there cultural barriers to change?
- What other influences affect the change?
- How do local residents believe the physical or social ecology of their community support or constrain the outcomes?
- Do they perceive any financial, policy or geographic barriers to gaining support for the changes?

The second group of questions requires an interpretive approach, and the methods used to gather data would typically include a combination of observations, interviews, document analysis, and knowledge of policy and social trends. The research team would seek to secure information that is comprehensive, and encompasses the reasons for change, or perceptions about the change. There would also be some detailed analysis of the social ecology or contextual factors involved in the change. To accomplish this, the researchers would likely plan a number of in-depth interviews and conduct a thematic analysis of people's responses to gain insight into the community and its particular areas of need or strength. These data would be analysed in a systematic way to produce new insights. Decisions on analysis of data would be made by the research team prior to data collection. In a *convergent* design quantitative and qualitative data would be collected concurrently, analysed separately, then merged to compare the findings. In an *explanatory* design data would be analysed sequentially, first quantitatively to decide what qualitative information would be required to produce the explanation sought by the research team. In an *embedded* design the primary data (either quantitative or qualitative) would be analysed, then a decision made as to how to connect the analysis of the other type of data. A transformative design could use either a convergent, explanatory or embedded design, and a *multiphase* design would connect data analysis for each phase or project of the study (Creswell & Plano Clark 2011). Any of these designs could be used to promote community health programs or interventions, depending on the research focus (see Figure 15.2).

MIXED METHODS DESIGNS

- Convergent
- Explanatory
- Embedded
- Multiphase

Researching culture

Over the past decades, research into cultural issues has grown steadily. As mentioned in previous chapters, this agenda should be extended to provide insights into the features of inclusive societies, intergenerational interactions in different cultures, and how expressions of culture affect health and wellbeing. Investigating cultural issues as a basis for practice is essential to successfully confront the needs of migrant groups during transitions to their new life, to anticipate influences on differing cultural groups' health and health service preferences throughout ageing, and to explore how families negotiate, change and work within the context of their cultural and social lives.

Naturalistic research, on its own, or in combination with other methods, is an ideal approach to begin a program of culturally oriented research, especially if the nascent ideas for the study arise from the cultural community itself. This often

occurs in a round table or discussion forum, where ideas can evolve into CBPR. One approach that has gained popularity with different cultural groups is *appreciative inquiry*, which is conducted within the interpretive or naturalistic paradigm. An appreciative inquiry is similar to PAR and participatory evaluation in that the objective is to ensure inclusive, empowering research processes that build hope, trust, respect and ultimately, capacity for change. The researcher attempts to bring people together to 'discover, dream, design and deliver' solutions to existing problems and innovations for change (Murphy et al. 2004:211). This can begin from a story-telling group, as is often the case in understanding cultural aspects of social life from individuals' oral histories. Research approaches such as photovoice could be considered as a form of appreciative inquiry, or an adjunct to ethnographic studies.

RESEARCHING TOGETHER

Naturalistic research is an ideal approach to researching culture, enabling the researcher to work alongside community members to explore their cultural needs and priorities.

Ethnography is traditionally seen as cultural research in that the focus is on the 'life world' as seen through cultural filters (Foster & Stanek 2007). This means that all data must be culturally contextualised. Where quantitative measures are taken, reliability and validity of instruments should be carefully tested with different groups, with special attention to cultural relevance of language and meaning at the individual, group and community level (Chesla & Rungreangkulkij 2001). Research studies that do not attend to these cultural aspects may be well intentioned, but they can potentially negate the socio-cultural reality of a vulnerable population (Wilson & Neville 2009). As mentioned above, ethnographers explore the artifacts, structures and dimensions of a culture that create people's life worlds, including their knowledge. Cognitive ethnography is another version of ethnographic research that examines how knowledge and resources are constructed and used in that culture (Ball & Ormerod 2000). This is interesting in light of today's communication technologies and the extent to which various cultural groups adopt technological innovations to help them maintain health, for example, using instant messaging systems converted to their language to become health literate.

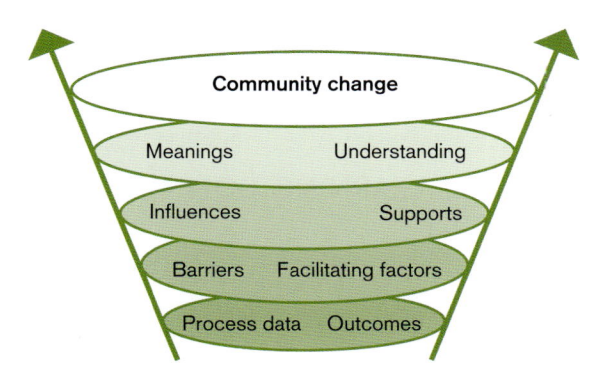

FIGURE 15.2
Using research information to understand community change

RESEARCHING WITH INDIGENOUS PEOPLE

Indigenous people have been the focus of many studies in Australia and New Zealand, and some of this research has not advanced the type of knowledge that contributes to their empowerment or self-determination. In some cases, researchers have forged relationships that have unearthed important features of Indigenous people's health, but in other cases, research reports have shown stereotypical perspectives of the researchers, rather than the researched. Some studies have actually damaged relationships, and violated the principles of cultural safety (Wilson & Neville 2009). This oversight has not been an intended goal of the research, but rather, a lack of understanding of the cultural and structural constraints on gathering meaningful data. Fredericks (2008) describes Australian Indigenous people as the most researched in the world, with many Indigenous students now studying research findings from studies that have yet to reflect Indigenous methodologies or knowledge.

CULTURALLY SAFE RESEARCH

Researchers involved in research with Indigenous people must approach any project from a position of humility and cultural safety. Research is never done *on* people but *with* people, acknowledging their rights, recognising their sovereignty and respecting their perspective.

In some cases, studies of Indigenous people have presented biased data because of the difficulty of accessing accurate statistics and participants (Priest et al. 2009). As mentioned in Chapter 13, some Indigenous people do not report their Indigenous status or do not wish to provide in-depth information to researchers for personal reasons (Kowanko et al. 2009). Many people, both Indigenous and non-Indigenous, prefer not to participate in research, some because they are transient residents of a community, and others because they do not see personal benefits in participating (Buckley 2008; Davies et al. 2008). A further issue for Indigenous researchers is the lack of a base of data from methodologically rigorous Indigenous intervention trials, despite a greater burden of disease among Indigenous people (Clifford et al. 2009). In some cases, studies have been structured according to Western scientific discourse with inconsistent terminology and culturally insensitive language (Cripps 2008; Priest et al. 2009). Dissemination

strategies have also been problematic, with passive distribution of clinical guidelines, or resources being used to communicate findings, instead of specific strategies that would help health care providers modify their practice (Clifford et al. 2009). Other problems in Indigenous research include the constraint of small sample sizes, a singular focus on descriptive studies, and a lack of infrastructure for research (Couzos et al. 2005). All of these problems indicate a need for researchers to educate themselves about the community and issues related to how members of the community will be affected by the research (Pyett et al. 2009).

Importantly, there is a need for external researchers to eliminate their propensity to draw comparisons between Indigenous and non-Indigenous populations, instead of studying phenomena or events in Indigenous groups over time (Cripps 2008; Couzos et al. 2005). In any context, researching people's experiences of health and wellbeing can be strengthened with a trajectory perspective, particularly over the life course. Trajectory research is a succinct and useful way to describe changes over time to identify assets and risks as a basis for planning how, when, and for whom nursing interventions and self-care are most effective (Henly et al. 2011). Longitudinal studies based on a synthesis of traditional and scientific approaches can provide meaningful information in terms of capturing the reality of Indigenous communities, and the issues that affect their health and wellbeing (Harvey 2009). Without meaningful and accurate data, it is difficult to monitor changes in health status, evaluate service access, or quantify and evaluate resources spent on Indigenous services (Draper et al. 2009). An important gap in the Indigenous research agenda is the social epidemiological approach to studying child health over time in urban environments (Priest et al. 2009). According to Priest et al. (2009) the focus on Indigenous rural and remote issues detracts from focusing on the needs of children living in cities, where they also experience disadvantage.

CULTURAL LEARNING COMMUNITIES

- Place-based
- Dialogue-focused
- Recognising Indigenous ways of knowing, being and valuing
- Accepting people's rights to think differently
- Co-production of knowledge

Canadian researchers have also drawn attention to the need for Aboriginal health research that encompasses the relationships between health and place (Anderson et al. 2011). They describe place-based communities as dialogue-based supportive networks that not only produce locally relevant knowledge, but that develop residents' research capacity. These networks offer the opportunity to focus on strengths with the premise of creating social change through empowerment, especially in reinforcing Aboriginal identity (Anderson et al. 2011). Academics can be part of these networks, framing cultural communities as learning communities where all members are co-producers of knowledge. Developing Indigenous research capacity can also help disseminate findings, which are not always published in the peer-reviewed literature (Clifford et al. 2009). One of the challenges involved in researching with Indigenous people is to develop ideas within an 'Indigenous minds' approach, valuing Aboriginal ways of knowing, being and valuing (Lindeman et al. 2011:275). This approach shifts the emphasis from trying to work out how Aboriginal people think, to accepting their right to think differently (Lindeman et al. 2011). Clearly, Indigenous community involvement in each phase of the research agenda is crucial, and is often overlooked by those who seek to address Indigenous health issues, but have not developed the cultural knowledge to do so (Couzos et al. 2005; Priest et al. 2009). According to Wilson and Neville (2009:72), studies with Indigenous groups should conform to the principles of the Treaty of Waitangi: 'partnership, participation, protection and power'. When these principles guide the research there is a greater likelihood of maintaining cultural safety. A major task for the researcher is to create safe spaces for dialogue and negotiation, so the group can determine the extent and nature of their involvement. Dimer et al.'s (2013) cardiac rehabilitation program for a group of Aboriginal people in Western Australia demonstrated the importance of engaging Aboriginal health professionals in program implementation and research. They adopted a partnership approach at each step of the way, using yarning groups to develop, implement and evaluate the program (Dimer et al. 2013). This approach is empowering, enabling mutual understanding and the type of cultural humility that characterises CBPR. Yarning is a culturally appropriate way of encouraging dialogue with Aboriginal and Torres Strait Islander people, wherein the researcher interacts with those in the group in a fluid, discursive way, entering a type of 'contact zone' for discussion (Power 2004:40). Power describes the researcher's role as turning down the volume of 'white noise' that represents preconceptions, values and conversational habits, in order to hear the Indigenous voices (Power 2004:40). This can help eliminate the structural disadvantage that often occurs with 'white standpoint', externally imposed research (Martin-McDonald & McCarthy 2007:129).

ACTION POINT

In order to fully hear Indigenous voices, turn down the 'white noise' that represents a researcher's preconceptions, values and conversational habits.

In New Zealand, concern and distrust over the way in which research on Māori has been practised and by whom has led to a growth in research using an approach called Kaupapa Māori research (Lawton et al. 2013). As described in Chapter 6 Kaupapa Māori is a term used by Māori to describe the practice and philosophy of living a life that is informed by Māori culture (Pihama et al. 2002). Kaupapa Māori research describes research that is conceived, developed and carried out by Māori with the end outcome of benefit to Māori (Walker et al. 2006). It is an approach that respects the belief that for indigenous research to be truly valid, it must include consultation with Māori and be both with and for Māori (Lawton et al. 2013). Although the approach developed firstly in education research, it has become a commonly used approach in health. Lawton et al. (2013) describe how a Kaupapa Māori approach to their research with young Māori mothers-to-be embeds the consultation process within the research from the outset. Three advisory groups have oversight of the research including one comprising Māori elders, one of young Māori mothers and a third of academic researchers. Ongoing consultation throughout the project ensures development, implementation and translation of findings into practice is done appropriately and in a manner that is acceptable to the community. This approach has many similarities to other participatory approaches in that it enables engagement and empowerment of participants and co-researchers. It is the embedding of cultural mores and values specific to Māori within Kaupapa Māori research that makes this approach unique. In addition, the approach contributes to tino rangatiratanga (self-determination) and mana motuhake (autonomy), specific rights that are guaranteed for Māori under the Treaty of Waitangi.

Confronting the researcher's cultural norms helps create an opportunity for Indigenous perspectives to take priority, helping people feel that the research is connected to the reality of their lives (Belfrage 2007; Couzos et al. 2005; Martin-McDonald & McCarthy 2007). Giving voice to Indigenous people is congruent with the critical social theory paradigm, where most research with culturally vulnerable groups is situated. In some cases, there is also a need to ensure the research is gender appropriate; such as in researching Indigenous women's issues. In this type of research it is necessary to plan the study in collaboration with the female custodians of Indigenous culture in the community, to ensure that all sensitivities are considered (Kildea et al. 2009).

ACTION POINT

The first step in ensuring cultural safety is to assume a reflexive attitude. Reflect on how your worldview might influence the research, the process of analysis and the dissemination of findings.

One of the most important elements of planning Indigenous research is for the researcher to assume a reflexive attitude as a first step in ensuring cultural safety. For a non-Indigenous researcher, this involves reflecting on how her/his worldview might influence the research, and the processes of analysis and dissemination of findings (Wilson & Neville 2009). Another important element is to actively pursue ethical approval for the research from Indigenous-controlled ethics committees, to ensure that Indigenous interests are represented in all processes (Dunbar & Scrimgeour 2006). These include committees such as the Māori Health Committee of the Health Research Council of New Zealand, the Queensland Aboriginal and Islander Health Forum, and the Western Australian Aboriginal Health Information and Ethics Committee. In other states of Australia besides Western Australia and Queensland, separate arrangements are made for ethical review through Aboriginal peak bodies at state and territory level (Couzos et al. 2005). What all have in common is adherence to the values and principles mandated by the National Health and Medical Research Councils of Australia and New Zealand, to ensure culturally appropriate research. These principles include *reciprocity* (including the community's perspectives), *respect* (transparent acknowledgement of Indigenous beliefs and practices), *equality* (through authentic research partnership strategies),

responsibility (developing cultural protocols for all stages of the research), *survival and protection* (promoting the crucial role of culture in the research), and *spirit and integrity* (demonstrating respect for the richness, diversity and integrity of the Indigenous community) (NHMRC 2003). Researchers in New Zealand are required to demonstrate clearly in applications for ethical approval how Māori have been consulted in relation to the research and what impact the research will have on Māori (National Ethics Advisory Committee 2012). There are a number of resources to assist with this including *Guidelines for Researchers on Health Research involving Māori* (NZ Health Research Council 2010). The values and principles for Indigenous research are embedded in the guidelines for researchers in Box 15.7.

RESEARCHING THE FUTURE

Although the research agenda for community health is growing, many areas remain inadequately researched, for a number of reasons. In most cases, the length of time required to investigate a web of factors or situations is prohibitive. Research may also be hampered by a lack of funding, due to the rigidity of many granting agencies to support broadly based studies. Dilution of interventions in large sites sometimes leads to a lack of clarity in the findings, which can be complicated by time trend effects. This occurs when the circumstances of the community change over time, or where the true costs of engaging with a community at each step of the process are underestimated.

ACTION POINT

Plan incremental, expanded programs of community health research to highlight aspects of community culture and social life in a way that will be useful to funders, providers, managers and community members.

Another difficulty is that there are varying cultural norms and expectations evident in community health research, which makes sharing the experience between different groups somewhat of a challenge. In action research studies, changes in health outcomes as a result of interventions are often not detectable for many years, which may create tensions on those waiting for results, including funding agencies. This is a particular problem if the effect of an intervention falls outside the political planning time frame. A

BOX 15.7 Characteristics of Indigenous-controlled health research

Setting the research agenda

- Community-driven research is strategic and based on priority needs.

- Power differentials between community representative bodies and external research bodies are balanced.

- Research focus is holistic, not just biomedical.

- Generalisability of research findings is considered.

- Capacity of community-controlled services is enhanced.

- Multi-centre research involves national community-based leadership.

Research project planning and approval

- Ethical clearance is granted by Indigenous human ethics committees.

- Benefits and risks of the research for individual and community are carefully examined.

- There is valid consent from community representative bodies.

- Support needed by community bodies for research to proceed is appraised.

- Any trial interventions are sustainable.

- Time required for planning and implementation are realistic.

(Source: Couzos et al. 2005:94 with permission)

- Cost required for planning and implementation is realistic.

Conduct of research

- There is no withholding of services while the research is being conducted.

- Research coordinators have skills in cross-cultural communication and are respectful of community structures.

- There is appropriate and informed client consent.

- Local community-based leadership and communication networks are harnessed.

- Approaches to data collection and management are flexible.

Analysis, dissemination and application of findings

- Ownership of intellectual property is vested in community-representative bodies.

- There is appropriate early community feedback.

- Communities are enabled to document their experiences.

- Research leads to actions promoting policy changes

further issue is related to the challenges of measuring place-based improvements at the neighbourhood or community level, especially if the research team has not enlisted team members who have cultural and statistical expertise. So, although the optimal approach is to investigate multidimensional studies of community health and wellness, the cautionary tale is that current funding agencies tend to seek out and fund research with short, sharp, measurable outcomes, within the parameters of their reporting requirements and political needs.

What remains for the future is to develop incremental, expanded programs of community health research that will highlight the aspects of community culture and social life, in a way that can be readily used for policymakers, health service managers and practitioners, and the community itself. This agenda includes the trajectory research mentioned earlier in the chapter, to assess change over time, including the effectiveness of interventions with individuals, families, groups or populations as they experience health and illness across settings and across the lifespan (Henly et al. 2011; Roberts & Ward 2011). The research to policy agenda will always have gaps to be filled with research into ways of shaping health care systems to provide appropriate, accessible, acceptable, effective, efficient and equitable care. It will also reflect trends and vested interests, particularly with budget constraints on health and research funding bodies. For those who are not working within large networks of researchers or organised programs of research, numerous research topics arise out of everyday practice with communities. Many practitioners at the cutting edge of practice have an ideal opportunity through research to make significant inroads into health care improvements or to manage care and interactions with greater efficiency and effectiveness.

> ## OPPORTUNISTIC RESEARCH
>
> Nurses at the cutting edge of practice often identify problems or issues that can be researched as part of their planning role.

As nurses or other health professionals it is important to include theory development in the research agenda (Diya et al. 2011), and professional issues that inform better health care for our communities. One of the most significant trends of the 21st century has seen the development of nurse and midwife entrepreneurs who practise as commercial health partners, and 'intrapreneurs' who undertake socially responsive entrepreneurial roles (Wilson et al. 2012). These models of community care are evolving in our area, especially in New Zealand, where 50% of midwives are engaged in independent practice, compared to the 1% worldwide (Wilson et al. 2012). Nurses have not yet reached visibility in this context, and in New Zealand, where 90% of health care interactions occur in PHC, 62% of nurses still practise in hospitals and rest homes (Betony & Yarwood 2013). This suggests a need to explore their knowledge base in relation to PHC and the SDH, and the extent to which their interactions with individuals and families in all care settings reflect an understanding of community needs. Similarly, community nurses, midwives and other health professionals need to ensure that their roles, and the barriers to their roles, are well researched and made visible, which can help reinforce their place in the health care system. In Australia the research agenda should extend to exploring the effectiveness of PHC nurses working to enhance (rather than substitute) GP practice in the GP superclinics as well as in regular GP practices.

Demographic changes are occurring in the community in tandem with the evolution of sophisticated research strategies that will enable greater clarity in investigating issues such as chronic conditions within a PHC, social justice ethos. It is crucial that Australian and New Zealand nurses add our voices to those of PHC nurses internationally to connect care, prevention and attention to the SDH at the grassroots level to global health policy (Betony & Yarwood 2013). Population ageing, exponential increase in chronic illness and lifestyle-related problems such as obesity, and mental health problems have heightened the need to research strategies for health literacy, empowerment and various versions of client-centred care (Kitson et al. 2010). Research studies need to include the rapidly growing cohort of baby boomers, who, as we have

mentioned previously, may want personalised accessible services with well-informed choices. Their needs and preferences may see the nursing role transformed into that of knowledge broker, culture broker and collaborative problem-solver partner. The Australian Institute for Family Studies (AIFS) indicates that we need further research on families. They have generated a list of studies for the future that includes: intergenerational issues, culture gaps in using technologies (especially with children staying in the family home longer), cohabitation relationships, diversity in family circumstances into which children are born, issues concerning successful settlement for migrant families, how key life stages are negotiated, influences of different types of care for different age groups when negotiating life stages, different care provided by different types of parents (same-sex, couple, grandparents), factors that prevent relationship breakdown, post-separation decision-making, time allocations, effects of the newly introduced National Disability Insurance Scheme, the influence of the built environment on family life across the life course, FIFO and defence force families, the role of isolation and vulnerability, child protection, bullying and peer victimisation, service provision for victims, service integration, collaboration, culturally sensitive services, stressors in parenting, social rejection, and dissemination of research findings (Australian Government 2012). Knowledge of family forms (cohabitation) and parenting research is also incomplete and this agenda needs to adopt the trajectory model if it is to help inform the way we help people resolve the stress of family transitions, including separation, widowhood, loneliness, fitness in ageing, and other gender issues. Studies need to take a transitions approach to research from risk/ assets to health or recovery, developing concepts, measures and models to link family roles and processes to outcomes using family-level analyses and behavioural genetics. This will help build a cumulative, cross-disciplinary body of knowledge, using multiple data sources and methods (Carr & Springer 2010).

Knowledge translation and knowledge exchange is the new focus for research that will help strengthen health systems (Bjork et al. 2013; Pentland et al. 2011). It is about creating, transferring and transforming knowledge from one social or organisational unit to another in a value-creating chain (Landry et al. 2006). Collaborative research formulation, production and dissemination provide local contextually and culturally appropriate knowledge, which should be theory based but locally translated to attract organisational support (Bjork et al. 2013; Pentland et al. 2011). An ideal research agenda could begin with the factors already known to promote healthy, safe and inclusive communities. For example, the Victorian Health Department's (VicHealth) framework for community wellbeing suggests a number of areas for research (Wiseman et al. 2007) (see Box 15.8).

The areas indicated above are simply suggestions for issues that are important to community health. Others include factors related to employment, work-life balance, housing, air and water quality and other aspects of the environments of people's lives that constitute the SDH. Although there are few audits of nursing research in Australia and New Zealand, a review of published studies in professional journals reveals some interesting trends. The *Journal of Community Health Nursing* publishes a wide range of community research, some of which is focused on behaviour change and chronic illness management, but research reports also include studies that advance knowledge, for example, by framing various interventions within a socio-ecological perspective of community life. The

journal *Family and Community Health* is another journal which reports studies on health promotion interventions for community residents, as well as social and environmental issues. These include studies of community environments that support injury prevention strategies, healthy adolescence and ageing, and reports of various specific nursing interventions. The journal *Health and Social Care in the Community* reports numerous studies of home care and other contexts for care giving. In the past few years, this journal has published widely on service organisation and the needs of carers. Studies also include those addressing the SDH: housing and homelessness, poverty, health inequalities and social inclusion. The *Australian Journal of Rural Health* contains reports of nursing research, but its major focus is on the rural community, so the reports are more interdisciplinary than some of the other nursing and midwifery journals. With workforce shortages, a large proportion of the research concerns recruitment and retention of health professionals, and professional issues related to attracting staff. The *Journal of Advanced Nursing* and the *Journal of Clinical Nursing* publish more frequently than some of the other nursing journals, and these have a strong mix of examples of evidence-based practice and topics addressing community health issues. Some of the more recent studies reported in these journals include research into psychosocial issues in health care, models of service delivery, and approaches for working with vulnerable groups.

BOX 15.8 Wellbeing indicators for healthy, safe and inclusive communities

Indicator	Potential research
Personal health and wellbeing	Health and quality of life Physical activity, weight Nutrition Alcohol, cigarette, drug use Mental health
Community connectedness	Community satisfaction Community caring, helping Volunteering Involvement in school activities Cultural inclusion
Early childhood development	Immunisation Breast feeding Child health monitoring
Personal and community safety	Public safety, transport Crime, violence Road trauma, injury Occupational health and safety
Lifelong learning	Literacy, numeracy School retention pathways to education Internet, library use
Service availability	Community perceptions of access, equity, appropriateness

RESEARCHING RESEARCH

Databases such as Proquest, Cinahl, Medline, PubMed, and Scopus provide extraordinary resources to support research

Australian journals such as *Contemporary Nurse*, *Collegian* and the *Australian Journal of Advanced Practice* also address a balanced mix of nursing and midwifery research that focuses on interventions, professional development, and the needs of communities. All publish international nursing studies. In some cases, the journals develop special issues dedicated to a certain topic, which can be particularly helpful to nurses and midwives working in the community. *Contemporary Nurse* publishes many special issues, with a strong emphasis on community and family topics, as well as culture and Indigenous health. *Nursing Praxis in New Zealand* publishes a range of nursing research specific to New Zealand and is an excellent source of New

Zealand specific studies. *Kai Tiaki Nursing Research* is a recently established New Zealand peer-reviewed nursing journal that publishes research on a range of topics specific to nursing and is another useful source of research specific to New Zealand.

There are many aspects of community life in Australia and New Zealand that have yet to be sufficiently researched. Our review of journals in which Australian and New Zealand nurses publish their research reveals a dearth of studies that respond to the SDH, although much of this work is published in a range of interdisciplinary journals, especially public health and health promotion journals. However, with the trend towards researching chronic conditions and ageing, numerous other journals publish studies relevant to all aspects of community practice. We have tried throughout this book to outline a wide range of resources from the most community-relevant journals. The best way to extend this work is by accessing further information through the large,

comprehensive databases that are available to most scholars and practitioners who have access to the internet. When all else fails, there is always Google! Some of the burning questions that remain are listed in Box 15.9.

The research questions found in Box 15.9 could be used to guide an entire program of research. However, the most important element in any investigation is the need to pose a manageable question; one that can be addressed in the timeframe allowed, using a defined pool of resources. Although other aspects of the research process are important, the method is ultimately driven by the research question. Box 15.10 outlines an approach to writing a study proposal, followed by some tips for arguing for the study to a granting body (Box 15.11). These tips are offered in the hope that we have persuaded all readers of this text to participate in generating and/or using the evidence base that will help communities become healthy, happy, vibrant and sustainable.

BOX 15.9 Community health study questions

- What community support mechanisms will create the best opportunities for empowerment and self-determinism among disadvantaged people? How can these be tailored to groups differentiated by race, ethnicity, gender, health status, age or geography?

- What policies and practices will create the best opportunities for enriched parenting? What are the barriers to good parenting for different age, stage and socio-economic groups? How can communities support parenting?

- What are the most helpful strategies in reducing alcohol and tobacco use/overuse for particular groups? How are these embedded in social and environmental factors?

- Which interventions have shown the most promise in fostering the combination of healthy nutrition and physical activity across the lifespan? What environmental influences facilitate healthy lifestyles for which groups?

- What are the moderators of workplace stress in promoting family health and happiness? Which occupational supports can help alleviate workplace stress for different types of workers?

- How can nurses enhance access to effective neighbourhood or community-based strategies for supporting families experiencing disruptions and transitions? Where and how are they most effective?

- What is good and best practice, or good and best process in maintaining mental health for different age groups? How are these practices implemented in rural and remote areas?

- How can schools support urban and rural adolescents through the crucial time of emerging identities?

- Which technologies are most helpful to develop health assets and meeting health needs for different age groups?

- How can health professionals participate in creating sustainable neighbourhoods to support healthy ageing?

- To what extent do emerging technologies, particularly telecommunications, provide health benefits for older rural residents?

- What are the barriers and facilitators involved in nurses becoming active advocates for social policies to protect human rights?

- In what ways can collaborative practice enhance health outcomes for communities?

- How do nurses understand the social determinants of health and how do they integrate this understanding into their practice?

- What are the most effective models of nursing care for chronic condition management, for health promotion, for community capacity building?

BOX 15.10 **Research proposal**

Getting started: from research question to solution

The basic ingredients for a successful research study are enthusiasm, perseverance and the art of argument. Developing a good research question can sometimes be extremely difficult. One of the best ways of identifying a good question to guide a research study is to contemplate what is already known in the area targeted for study, then to undertake a 'question framing' exercise. The research topic can be developed in consultation with community members, but then the researcher may want to do some further work on refining the topic into a specific question. Often, this can be done away from the research situation, when the researcher is able to think creatively. It also helps to talk to various people, as those with knowledge of the area of study can help to identify strengths and weaknesses in the question. A critical friend with little knowledge of the topic can also be helpful, as they may be able to interrogate ideas objectively and dispassionately in a way that helps the researcher clarify their thoughts.

Once a general topic has been decided, it is helpful to begin thinking of the research process as a strategic plan, as outlined below.

The question

The first step is to fill several pages with questions relating to the topic of study. Often, these questions are ones that a researcher has already thought about. Writing questions in a cohesive and simple manner is a very important step in the planning process. The questions will come from practice, reading, deliberate contemplation, discussion with community members and reflection on the intention of the study (the purpose). Once the questions have been written and considered, the second stage of the process begins.

The argument

A good argument is a well substantiated case for the following:

- what we do know about the topic
- what we do not know about it (the gap in knowledge)
- what we should know (how this piece of research can help to fill the knowledge gap)
- the implications of knowing this (so what?).

The argument has two major elements: the analysis of information, and the crafting of the idea (the proposal). Ultimately, a research study is aimed at generating and analysing data according to the conventions of rigorous research (the method), but all parts of the proposal must reflect precision and clarity, which are considered essential elements of research. The best way to learn to write in a scholarly style is to read widely from existing research. Although there is some variability in style in the published literature, there is a recognisable style of clear, concise writing. While reading research articles, researchers should attend to the features of style as well as to the mechanisms and findings of the research.

A good argument illustrates two major features: logical thinking and insight. Logical thinking is shown in the use of a disciplined presentation style (precise and clear), and the sequencing of thoughts about the topic from broad contextual issues, to more specific ones. Insight is the ability to clearly analyse the topic and synthesise ideas to create a new coalescence of knowledge.

Conceptual framework

A theoretical framework is a valid theory, used with reliability beyond its original setting. A conceptual framework or model may be a hybrid of one or more theories, or it may simply be an original framework devised from constructs (ideas) generated from the literature review (which should be ongoing throughout the process of writing the research proposal). The researcher's choice of whether to use a conceptual model or theoretical framework is argued briefly in the proposal. An introduction to the framework is given, followed by an explanation of the elements of the framework, and an indication of *how* the framework is to be used in the research. In quantitative studies, the framework is used to generate and guide the hypotheses, the strategies for testing these, and as a basis for reflecting on the findings. In qualitative (interpretive) studies, it is linked to the philosophical underpinnings of the method, and to the analysis of interpretations.

Steps in the Research Process

1. The question
2. The argument
3. The conceptual framework
4. The method
5. Research ethics
6. Findings/results
7. Discussion

BOX 15.10 **Research proposal—cont'd**

Method

The 'methods' argument should begin with an introduction to how the study is to be conducted, in what paradigm it is situated (for example, naturalistic or interpretive), and the philosophical foundation of the methodological approach. It should include any previous research in the area from which ideas are being extended or challenged. A researcher should then explain the design features of the research, including participants, data collection, and the analytic tests or techniques that will be used.

An explanation is provided of the actual method used, the sample, instruments, and reliability and validity data related to any instruments. If no instrumentation other than the researcher is used, the researcher must argue the data gathering as being justified in terms of the method. For example, in PAR, the process of working with the group is explained. In a case study, the way the case is bounded and what is to be included are explained. Other interpretive methods have their own conventions for design and analysis, and these should be described. Once the study is explained, the ethical considerations are outlined, including the source of ethical approval.

Research ethics

The major ethical considerations in conducting research studies are universally accepted, and these include ensuring confidentiality and anonymity of research participants, scientific validity and protection of vulnerable people, such as children, and those who become powerless by institutionalisation, or other factors. As mentioned above, where Indigenous people are part of the research, the proposal should be reviewed by the appropriate Indigenous research ethics committee in addition to institutional review by a university or health service sponsoring or hosting the study. Researchers' accountability to both those being researched and the scientific community holds them responsible to fully explain to research participants any known risks and benefits, regardless of how small, so that participants only consent to their involvement on the basis of being fully informed.

An explanation must be given to assure participants of the right to withdraw from the research at any time without recrimination, and where they will be able to access assistance if the need arises; that is, if they become distressed by the research process. The researcher must also explain how the data will be secured during the research process, and how and

when it will be destroyed at the end of the study. It is also helpful to assure participants of the purpose of the research; whether it is being conducted as part of a work/practice role, as a study for a higher degree, or as commissioned research. Participants should then be reassured that the findings will be published in aggregated form only, with all identifying data removed.

Researchers are also obliged to identify themselves and any others involved in the research (supervisors, co-researchers) and to provide feedback to those supplying information. This helps ensure that the participants are treated as partners, not simply as people supplying information to be taken away from the community. Participants should also be assured that data will be analysed in a culturally sensitive way, with cultural representation from someone who can guide the process if necessary, for cultural safety, and the benefit of the community. This also helps prevent researcher bias from compromising the research rigour and ethical standards. Involving the community should begin prior to the research, as it is helpful in framing the questions appropriately, in establishing the feasibility of the study, guiding the research process, and articulating the findings in language that is meaningful to the community. This creates a greater likelihood that community preferences will find their way into public policies.

Findings/results

Although different methods dictate different conventions for presenting results, it is often useful to organise the findings around the research questions or objectives. The object of presenting the results of research is to clearly demonstrate defensible findings from the evidence collected, and the appropriate use of analytic techniques.

Discussion

This section of the research is found after the presentation of findings, so it is not part of a research proposal. In presenting the findings, the discussion is often the most rewarding, as it revolves around that most important question: 'so what?'. This gives the researcher the opportunity to think creatively while maintaining an academic tone, especially in connecting the findings to the broader body of knowledge and the conceptual framework. A good research study typically moves from the discussion to implications for practice, education, management, system changes and/or policy recommendations and suggests further research, ending with a clear and concise summary of the study.

BOX 15.11 **Grant proposal**

Preliminary work

1 **Knowledge work**—are you sufficiently informed to write the proposal? Have you done or could you do some pilot work in the area?

- Write a current review of the topic.

- Imagine a conceptual framework for generating the question, establishing the method, analysing the data and discussing the findings.

- Compile a list of designs and methods previously used in studying the topic.

- Familiarise yourself with instruments or approaches to researching the variables of interest.

- Cite the right scholars in the field, including yourself.

2 **Funding/funders**—have you explored all options?

- Provide evidence of your expertise in conducting the type of study proposed.

- Outline the return on investment (ROI) for the funder.

- Establish the uniqueness of this study, conducted by your team.

- Explain how it fits with the priorities of the agency.

- Demonstrate knowledge of what that source has funded in the recent past (12 months?)—politics, priorities, possibilities.

- Consider the funding body's evaluation criteria, reviewers and processes.

- Contact people in the agency or those who have been successful in winning their grants.

- Cite the work of scholars funded by that agency.

- Provide evidence of cooperation at different sites, availability of facilities, project staff and consultants, sufficiency/feasibility of subject pool within timeframe of study, experience in managing complex projects.

- Find out if they accept resubmissions if you are rejected.

- Always value feedback from reviewers.

3 **Relationships**—collaborators, networking, critical friend

- Read successful proposals—study content, organisation, links between your goals and theirs, and between your aims, goals and plan for analysis, how proposal is marketed (tone, pitch, the art of argument), how much funding was awarded.

- Build the research team with complementary strengths and extra expertise (e.g. stats). It can be helpful to have someone on the team who has a track record of obtaining grants.

- Approach your own external reviewers—trade favours with people who know what to look for but don't seek admiration, rather someone who will be honest.

- Strategic plan for writing—allocate roles for each section, with specific deadlines, ensuring the strongest writer takes the lead.

- Meeting schedules are part of the plan; include brainstorming sessions.

4 **Budget**

- Be mindful of constraints—do not argue for more than what is available.

- Scale your study to available funds.

5 **The argument**

- Would it instruct a stranger but persuade an expert?

- Minimise jargon, write with logic, clarity and precision.

- Avoid grammatical errors.

- Use subheadings and a schedule of end points to help organise the proposal.

- Summarise key features in tables and figures.

- Argue from your pilot work—you are committed, you have a workable plan, you have already made an investment of time, money and knowledge.

- Write a balanced proposal in terms of the argument and the method.

6 **Time management**

- Consider timeline as another strategic planning exercise.

- Set timeline for developing drafts—thinking, editing, having drafts reviewed, rewriting.

- Plan backwards from due date—you need a draft ready at least a month before it's due.

- Consider permissions, approvals, feasibility of access to participants.

BOX 15.11 Grant proposal—cont'd

7   **Writing the proposal**

- Have a strategic plan: hypothesis, design including sampling strategy, analytic strategy and plan for dissemination.
- Ensure the argument is organised, logical—all aspects of proposal fit together, it is persuasive, authoritative and achievable, worthwhile and significant.
- Defend the methodology with strong rationale and congruence between background, rationale, hypotheses, framework, methods and budget.
- Rigor—utilise mechanisms for minimising, controlling, measuring or analysing bias.
- Ensure researchers have the skill needed to complete the study—right team to collect and analyse data.
- Take care with the writing style—aim for clarity, precision, artfulness—no sweeping indefensible statements or jargon.
- Discuss limitations and explain how they will not undermine the study or invalidate the evidence; justify limitations (e.g. cost) and remind reviewers how they were minimised.

Steps

1   Problem statement: what do we know, what don't we know, what should we know and so what? What is the consequence of not doing this study?

- Statement of unmet need
- Existing resources : availability, accessibility, acceptability
- Endorsement by partners

2   Goals, objectives, action steps, eloquently defended

- What specifically will be accomplished?
- Objectives are realistic, attainable, related to needs
- Articulate hypotheses and number these to add to flow of logic
- Action steps—outline what will be done or measured to reach each objective
- Literature critique provides justification of plan—it shouldn't be the main objective of the proposal
- Sampling strategy

3   Plan for evaluation/analysis

- Methodology—design features, interventions, data collection, analysis
- Formative evaluation of each stage and objectives, summative evaluation of effectiveness
- Plan for dissemination of findings—writing strategy, authorship, expectations of publications, elements of study to publish, sequencing preparation of publications

4   Budget

- Accurate spending plan, consistent with objectives
- Administrative tasks specified, link budget to timing of stages, equipment
- What is ROI for funders?

5   Abstract/summary

- A powerful first impression for reviewers—engage their interest, demonstrate research competence and sell the idea
- Summary will often determine who gets to review proposal

CASE STUDY: EBP to assist the Mason and Smith families

Nurses working in the mine site and in the home communities of both families are conscious of the need for evidence-based practice. A number of research findings have already affected the families, including global studies on sustainable environments and studies on family life and child health. For example, Huia has enrolled Jake in a research study to examine the effectiveness of nurse-led asthma clinics in managing childhood asthma. School health nurses in Perth are evaluating healthy school initiatives in relation to children's coping strategies. Public health researchers are working with nurses to identify the range of issues associated with FIFO family life to develop support programs.

REFLECTING ON THE BIG ISSUES

- Research is an important part of practice.
- Researching community health issues requires a broader approach than the traditional evidence-based practice methods.
- Mixed-method research can help provide the community perspective as well as specific investigation of designated variables.
- Research is time and resource intensive.
- Multidisciplinary studies can give a greater breadth to studies of community health.
- Special considerations must be given to researching with Indigenous people, to ensure their cultural safety.

- Community-based participatory research, especially participatory action research, is well suited to studies of the community.
- The research questions should dictate the research method, which then follows appropriate conventions for data collection, analysis and dissemination of findings.
- Translational studies are designed to transfer or translate knowledge into practice.
- The community research agenda has many gaps that indicate the need for ongoing research, particularly addressing the social determinants of health.
- Research is something that all nurses working in communities can and should be involved in.

REFLECTIVE QUESTIONS: How would I use this knowledge in practice?

1. Update the genogram you have been developing throughout the text and identify one research question for each family unit involved in the case study throughout the previous chapters.

2. Explain how you would investigate each of these questions.

3. How would the results of each study inform primary health care in your practice?

References

Abbott, S., Bickerton, J., Daly, M., et al., 2008. Evidence-based primary health care and local research: a necessary but problematic partnership. Prim. Health Care Res. Dev. 9, 191–198.

Adams, K., Burns, C., Liebzelt, A., et al., 2012. Use of participatory research and photo-voice to support urban Aboriginal healthy eating. Health Soc. Care Community 20 (5), 497–505.

Anderson, J., Pakula, B., Smye, V., et al., 2011. Strengthening Aboriginal health through a place-based learning community. Journal of Aboriginal Health (March), 42–53.

Andrew, S., Halcomb, E. (Eds.), 2009. Mixed methods research for nursing and health sciences. Wiley-Blackwell, Chichester.

Anthony, S., Jack, S., 2009. Qualitative case study methodology in nursing research: an integrative review. J. Adv. Nurs. 65 (6), 1171–1181.

Aspin, C., Brown, N., Jowsey, T., et al., 2012. Strategic approaches to health service delivery for Aboriginal and Torres Strait Islander people with chronic illness: a qualitative study. BMC Health Serv. Res. 12, 143–153.

Australian Government, 2012. AIFS research directions 2012–2015. AIFS, Melbourne.

Avery, L., Flynn, D., van Wersch, A., et al., 2012. Changing physical activity behavior in Type 2 Diabetes: A systematic review. Diabetes Care 35 (12), 2681–2690.

Ball, L., Ormerod, T., 2000. Putting ethnography to work: the case for a cognitive ethnography of design. Int. J. Hum. Comput. Stud. 53, 147–168.

Bambra, C., 2011. Real world reviews: a beginner's guide to undertaking systematic reviews of public health policy interventions. J. Epidemiol. Community Health 65, 14–19.

Baum, F., MacDougall, C., Smith, D., 2006. Participatory action research. J. Epidemiol. Community Health 60, 854–857.

Belfrage, M., 2007. Why 'culturally safe' health care? Med. J. Aust. 186 (10), 537–538.

Benner, P., 1984. From Novice to Expert: Power and Expertise in Nursing Practice. Aldine, Chicago.

Bennett, S., Hoffmann, T., 2013. Evidence about effects of interventions. In: Hoffmann, T., Bennett, S., Del Mar, C. (Eds.), Evidence Based Practice Across the Health Professions, second ed. Elsevier, Sydney, pp. 61–96.

Bennett, S., O'Connor, D., Hannes, K., et al., 2013. Appraising and understanding systematic reviews of quantitative and qualitative evidence. In: Hoffmann, T., Bennett, S., Del Mar, C. (Eds.), Evidence Based Practice Across the Health Professions, second ed. Elsevier, Sydney, pp. 283–312.

Bernal, G., Bonilla, J., Bellido, C., 1995. Ecological validity and cultural sensitivity for outcome research: Issues for the cultural adaptation and development of psychosocial treatments with Hispanics. J. Abnorm. Psychol. 23, 67–81.

Bero, L., Rennie, D., 1995. The Cochrane Collaboration: preparing, maintaining and disseminating systematic reviews of the effects of health care. J. Am. Med. Assoc. 274 (24), 1935–1938.

Betony, K., Yarwood, J., 2013. What exposure do student nurses have to primary health care and community nursing during the New Zealand undergraduate Bachelor of Nursing programme? Nurse Educ. Today 33, 1136–1142.

Bish, M., Kenny, A., Nay, R., 2012. A scoping review identifying contemporary issues in rural nursing leadership. J. Nurs. Scholarsh. 44 (4), 411–417.

Bjork, I., Lomborg, K., Much Nielsen, C., et al., 2013. From theoretical model to practical use: an example of knowledge translation. J. Adv. Nurs. 69 (10), 2336–2347.

Bowen, S., Zwi, A., 2005. Pathways to 'evidence-informed' policy and practice: a framework for action. PLoS Med. 2 (7), E166–E171.

Braun, V., Clarke, V., 2006. Using thematic analysis in psychology. Qualitative Research in Psychology 3 (77), 77–101.

Breton, M., Guenette, L., Amiche, M., 2013. Burden of diabetes on the ability to work: a systematic review. Diabetes Care 36 (3), 740–749.

Brownson, R., Fielding, J., Maylahn, C., 2009. Evidence-based public health: A fundamental concept for public health practice. Annu. Rev. Public Health 30, 175–201.

Buckley, B., 2008. The need for wider public understanding of health care research. Prim. Health Care Res. Dev. 9, 3–6.

Burgess, J., 2006. Participatory action research. First-person perspectives of a graduate student. Action Res. 4 (4), 419–437.

Buykx, P., Humphreys, J., Wakerman, J., et al., 2012. 'Making evidence count': a framework to monitor the impact of health services research. Aust. J. Rural Health 20, 51–58.

Cambon, L., Minary, L., Ridde, V., et al., 2012. Transferability of interventions in health education: a review. BMC Public Health 12, 497–510.

Cane, J., O'Connor, D., Michie, S., 2012. Validation of the theoretical domains framework for use in behaviour change and implementation research. Implement. Sci. 7, 37–54.

Carr, W., Kemmis, S., 1986. Becoming Critical: Education, Knowledge and Action Research. Falmer Press, London.

Carr, D., Springer, K., 2010. Advances in families and health research in the 21st century. J. Marriage Fam. 72, 743–761.

Carter, B., Ford, K., 2013. Researching children's health experiences: the place for participatory, child-centered, arts-based approaches. Res. Nurs. Health 36, 95–107.

Chesla, C., Rungreangkulkij, S., 2001. Nursing research on family processes in chronic illness in ethnically diverse families: a decade review. J. Fam. Nurs. 7 (3), 230–243.

Clifford, A., Jackson Pulver, L., Richmond, R., et al., 2009. Disseminating best-evidence health-care to Indigenous health-care settings and programs in Australia: identifying the gaps. Health Promot. Int. 24 (4), 404–415.

Comino, E., Kemp, L., 2008. Research-related activities in community-based child health services. J. Adv. Nurs. 63 (3), 266–275.

Coppell, K., Tipene-Leach, D., Pahau, H., et al., 2009. Two-year results from a community-wide diabetes prevention intervention in a high risk indigenous community: The Ngati and Healthy project. Diabetes Res. Clin. Pract. 85 (2), 220–227.

Couzos, S., Lea, T., Murray, R., et al., 2005. 'We are not just participants—we are in charge': the NACCHO ear trial and the process for Aboriginal community-controlled health research. Ethn. Health 10 (2), 91–111.

Creswell, J., Plano Clark, V., 2011. Designing and conducting mixed methods research, second ed. Sage, Los Angeles.

Cripps, K., 2008. Indigenous family violence: A statistical challenge. Injury, International Journal of Care of Injured 39 (S5), S25–S35.

Davies, G., Boothman, N., Duxbury, J., et al., 2008. An investigation of non-participation in health promotion interventions and its impact on population level outcomes. International Journal of Health Promotion and Education 45 (3), 107–112.

DeGuzman, P., Kulbok, P., 2012. Changing health outcomes of vulnerable populations through nursing's influence on neighbourhood built environment: A framework for nursing research. J. Nurs. Scholarsh. 44 (4), 341–348.

Dimer, L., Dowling, T., Jones, J., et al., 2013. Build it and they will come: outcomes from a successful cardiac rehabilitation program at an Aboriginal Medical Service. Aust. Health Rev. 37, 79–82.

Diya, L., Van den Heede, K., Sermeus, W., et al., 2011. The use of 'lives saved' measures in nurse staffing and patient safety research. Statistical considerations. Nurs. Res. 60 (2), 100–106.

Draper, G., Somerford, P., Pilkington, A., et al., 2009. What is the impact of missing Indigenous status on mortality estimates? An assessment using record linkage in Western Australia. Aust. N. Z. J. Public Health 33 (4), 325–331.

Dunbar, T., Scrimgeour, M., 2006. Ethics in Indigenous research—connecting with community. Bioeth. Inq. 3, 179–185.

Emmanuel, E., St John, W., 2010. Maternal distress: a concept analysis. J. Adv. Nurs. 66 (9), 2104–2115.

Fergusson, D., Boden, J., Horwood, L., 2013. Nine-year follow-up of a home-visitation program: A randomized trial. Pediatrics 131 (2), 297–303. <http://dx.doi.org/10.1542/peds.2012-1612>.

Flemming, K., 2010. Synthesis of quantitative and qualitative research: an example of Critical Interpretive Synthesis. J. Adv. Nurs. 66 (1), 201–217.

Flinders Program care planning process, 2013. Online. Available: <www.flinders.edu.au/medicine/sites/fhbhru/self-management.cfm> March 30, 2013.

Foster, J., Chiang, F., Burgos, R., et al., 2012. Community-based participatory research and the challenges of qualitative analysis enacted by lay, nurse, and academic researchers. Res. Nurs. Health 35, 550–559.

Foster, J., Stanek, K., 2007. Cross-cultural considerations in the conduct of community-based participatory research. Fam. Community Health 30 (1), 42–49.

Fredericks, B., 2008. Researching with Aboriginal women as an Aboriginal woman researcher. Aust. Fem. Stud. 23 (55), 113–129.

Freeman, M., Baumann, A., Fisher, A., et al., 2012. Case study methodology in nurse migration research: An integrative review. Appl. Nurs. Res. 25, 222–228.

Goldenberg, M., 2006. On evidence and evidence-based medicine. Lessons from the philosophy of science. Soc. Sci. Med. 62, 2621–2632.

Goodman, R., 2000. Evaluation of community-based health programs: An alternative perspective. In: Schneiderman, N., Speers, M., Silva, J., Tomes, H., Gentry, J., et al. (Eds.), Integrating Behavioral and Social Sciences with Public Health. American Psychological Association, Washington, pp. 293–304.

Green, L., Kreuter, M., 1991. Health Promotion Planning: An Educational and Environmental Approach. Mayfield Publishing Company, Mountain View.

Happ, M., DeVito Dabbs, A., Tate, J., et al., 2006. Exemplars of mixed methods data combination and analysis. Nurs. Res. 55 (2S), S43–S49.

Haque, N., Eng, B., 2011. Tackling inequity through a *Photovoice* project on the social determinants of health. Glob. Health Promot. 18 (1), 16–19.

Harvey, P., 2009. Indigenous health—evolving ways of knowing. Aust. Health Rev. 33 (4), 628–635.

Haviland, M., 2004. Doing participatory evaluation with community projects. AIFS Stronger Families Learning Exchange Bulletin 6 (Spring/Summer), 10–13.

Hay, A., Rortveit, G., Purdy, S., et al., 2012. Primary care research—an international responsibility. Fam. Pract. 29, 499–500.

Henly, S., Wyman, J., Findorff, M., 2011. Health and illness over time. The trajectory perspective in nursing science. Nurs. Res. 60 (3S), S5–S14.

Hoffmann, T., Bennett, S., Del Mar, C., 2013. Introduction to evidence-based practice. In: Hoffmann, T., Bennett, S., Del Mar, C. (Eds.), Evidence Based Practice Across the Health Professions, second ed. Elsevier, Sydney, pp. 1–15.

International Council of Nurses, 2012. Closing the gap: from evidence to action. ICN, Geneva.

Israel, B., Schulz, A., Parker, E., et al., 2001. Community based participatory research: Policy recommendations for promoting a partnership approach in health research. Educ. for Health 14 (2), 182–197.

Johnson Crowder, S., Broome, M., 2012. A framework to evaluate the cultural appropriateness of intervention research. West. J. Nurs. Res. 34 (8), 1002–1022.

Jolley, G., Lawless, A., Baum, F., et al., 2007. Building an evidence base for community health: a review of the quality of program evaluations. Aust. Health Rev. 31 (4), 603–610.

Kendrick, D., Mulvaney, C., Ye, L., et al., 2013. Parenting programs for the prevention of unintentional injuries in childhood. Cochrane Rev. Online. Available: <http://summaries.cochrane.org/CD006020/parenting-programmes-for-the-prevention-of-unintentional-injuries-in-childhood> 24 August 2013.

Kildea, S., Barclay, L., Wardaguga, M., et al., 2009. Participative research in a remote Australian Aboriginal setting. Action Res. 7 (2), 143–163.

Kitson, A., Conroy, T., Wengstrom, Y., et al., 2010. Defining the fundamentals of care. Int. J. Nurs. Pract. 16, 423–434.

Kitson, A., Rycroft-Malone, J., Harvey, G., et al., 2008. Evaluating the successful implementation of evidence into practice using the PARiHS framework: theoretical and practical challenges. Implement. Sci. 3 (1), doi:10.1186/1748-5908.

Kowanko, I., Stewart, T., Power, C., et al., 2009. An Aboriginal family and community healing program in metropolitan Adelaide: description and evaluation. Australian Indigenous Health Bulletin 9 (4), 1–12.

Labonte, R., Polanyi, M., Muhajarine, N., et al., 2005. Beyond the divides: Towards critical population health research. Crit. Public Health 15 (1), 5–17.

Lake, A., Staiger, P., 2010. Seeking the views of health professionals on translating chronic disease self-management models into practice. Patient Educ. Couns. 79 (1), 62–68.

Landry, R., Amara, N., Pablos-Mendes, A., et al., 2006. The knowledge-value chain: a conceptual framework for knowledge translation in health. Bull. World Health Organ. 84, 597–602.

Lawton, B., Cram, F., Makowharemahihi, C., et al., 2013. Developing a Kaupapa Māori research project to help reduce health disparities experienced by young Māori women and their babies [online]. Alternative: An International Journal of Indigenous Peoples 9 (3), 246–261.

Leeman, J., Sandelowski, M., 2012. Practice-based evidence and qualitative inquiry. J. Nurs. Scholarsh. 44 (2), 171–179.

Lindeman, M., Taylor, K., Binda Reid, J., 2011. Changing the thinking about priorities in Indigenous health research. Aust. J. Rural Health 19, 275.

Luck, L., Jackson, D., Usher, K., 2006. Case study: a bridge across paradigms. Nurs. Inq. 13, 103–109.

Manojlovich, M., Sidani, S., Covell, C., et al., 2011. Nurse dose. Linking staffing variables to adverse patient outcomes. Nurs. Res. 60 (4), 214–220.

Marmot, M., Friel, S., 2008. Global health equity: evidence for action on the social determinants of health. J. Epidemiol. Community Health 62, 1095–1097.

Martin-McDonald, K., McCarthy, A., 2007. 'Marking' the white terrain in indigenous health research: literature review. J. Adv. Nurs. 61 (2), 126–133.

Masuda, J., Creighton, G., Nixon, S., et al., 2011. Building capacity for community-based participatory research for health disparities in Canada: The case of 'partnerships in community health research'. Health Promot. Pract. 12 (2), 280–292.

Maxwell, R., 1984. Quality assessment in health. Br. Med. J. 288, 1470–1472.

Miller, A., Krusky, A., Franzen, S., et al., 2012. Partnering to translate evidence-based programs to community settings: Bridging the gap between research and practice. Health Promot. Pract. 13 (4), 559–566.

Minkler, M., 2005. Community-based research partnerships: challenges and opportunities. J. Urban Health 82 (2 Suppl. 2), doi:10.1093/urban/jti034.

Morgan, A., Ziglio, E., 2007. Revitalising the evidence-base for public health: an assets model. Promot. Educ. (Suppl. 2), 17–22.

Morrison, I., Stosz, L., Clift, S., 2008. An evidence base for mental health promotion through supported education: A practical application of Antonovsky's salutogenic model of health. International Journal of Health Promotion and Education 46 (1), 11–20.

Muncey, T., 2009. Does mixed methods constitute a change in paradigm? In: Andrew, S., Halcomb, E. (Eds.), Mixed methods research for nursing and the health sciences. Wiley-Blackwell, Chichester UK, pp. 13–30.

Murphy, L., Kordyl, P., Thorne, M., 2004. Appreciative inquiry: a method for measuring the impact of a project on the well being of an Indigenous community. Health Promot. J. Austr. 15 (30), 211–214.

National Ethics Advisory Committee, 2012. Ethical Guidelines for Observational Studies: Observational research, audits and related activities. Revised ed. Ministry of Health, Wellington.

National Health and Medical Research Council, 2003. Values and Ethics: Guidelines for ethical conduct in Aboriginal and Torres Strait Islander Health Research. Commonwealth of Australia, Canberra.

New Zealand Health Research Council, 2010. Guidelines for researchers on health research involving Māori. Health Research Council, Wellington.

Nilson, C., Fetherston, C., McMurray, A., 2013. Creative arts: An essential element in the teacher's toolkit when developing critical thinking in children. Australian Journal of Teacher Education 38 (7), 1–13.

Nykiforuk, C., Schopflocher, D., Vallianatos, H., et al., 2012. Community health and the built environment: examining place in a Canadian chronic disease prevention project. Health Promot. Int. doi:10.1093/heapro/dar093.

Pavey, T., Taylor, A., Hillsdon, M., et al., 2012. Levels and predictors of exercise referral scheme uptake and adherence: a systematic review. J. Epidemiol. Community Health 66, 737–744.

Pearson, A., Hannes, K., 2013. Evidence about patients' experiences and concerns. In: Hoffmann, T., Bennett, S., Del Mar, C. (Eds.), Evidence Based Practice Across the Health Professions, second ed. Elsevier, Sydney, pp. 221–239.

Pentland, D., Forsyth, K., Maciver, D., et al., 2011. Key characteristics of knowledge transfer and exchange in healthcare: integrative literature review. JAN 67 (7), 1408–1425.

Petticrew, M., Tugwell, P., Welch, V., et al., 2009. Better evidence about wicked issues in tackling health inequities. J. Public Health (Bangkok) 31 (3), 453–456.

Pihama, L., Cram, F., Walker, S., 2002. Creating methodological space: A literature review of Kaupapa Māori research Canadian Journal of Native Education 26 (1), 30–43.

Polit, C., Beck, C., 2012. Nursing research: generating and assessing evidence for nursing practice, ninth ed. Wolters Kluwer Health/Lippincott Williams & Wilkins, Storrs, Philadelphia.

Power, K., 2004. Yarning: A responsive research methodology. Journal of Australian Research in Early Childhood Education 11 (1), 37–46.

Priest, N., Mackean, T., Waters, E., et al., 2009. Indigenous child health research: a critical analysis of Australian studies. Aust. N. Z. J. Public Health 33 (1), 55–63.

Prochaska, J., Velicer, W., 1997. The transtheoretical model of health behavior change. Am. J. Health Promot. 12, 38–48.

Pucher, K., Boot, N., De Vries, N., 2013. Systematic review: School health promotion interventions targeting physical activity and nutrition can improve academic performance in primary and middle school children. Health Educ. 113 (5), 372–391.

Pyett, P., Waples-Crowe, P., van der Sterren, A., 2009. Engaging with Aboriginal communities in an urban context: some practical suggestions for public health researchers. Aust. N. Z. J. Public Health 33 (1), 51–54.

Roberts, T., Ward, S., 2011. Using latent transition analysis in nursing research to explore change over time. Nurs. Res. 60 (1), 73–79.

Rogers, E., 2003. Diffusion of innovations, fifth ed. The Free Press, New York.

Sackett, D., Straus, S., Richardson, W., et al., 2000. Evidence-based Medicine: How to Practice and Teach EBM. Churchill Livingstone, London.

Sandelowski, M., 2004. Using qualitative research. Qual. Health Res. 14 (10), 1366–1386.

Sandelowski, M., 2008. Reading, writing and systematic review. J. Adv. Nurs. 64 (1), 104–110.

Sandelowski, M., 2011. 'Casing' the research case study. Res. Nurs. Health 34, 153–159.

Schulz, A., Israel, B., Coombe, C., et al., 2011. A community-based participatory planning process and multilevel intervention design: Toward eliminating cardiovascular health inequities. Health Promot. Pract. 1296, 900–911.

Smith, C., Pell, J., 2003. Parachute use to prevent death and major trauma related to gravitational challenge:

systematic review of randomized controlled trials. Br. Med. J. 1459–1461.

Stringer, E., 2004. Action Research in Education. Pearson, Upper Saddle River, NJ.

Tashakkori, A., Teddlie, C., 2003. Handbook of mixed methods in social and behavioral research, second ed. Sage, Thousand Oaks, Ca.

Tipene-Leach, D., Pahau, H., Joseph, N., et al., 2004. Insulin resistance in a rural Māori community. N. Z. Med. J. 117, U1208.

Tramm, R., McCarthy, A., Yates, P., 2011. Using the Precede-Proceed Model of Health Program Planning in breast cancer nursing research. J. Adv. Nurs. 68 (8), 1870–1880.

Turnbull, C., Osborn, D., 2012. Home visits during pregnancy and after birth for women with an alcohol or drug problem. Cochrane Rev. Online. Available: <http://summaries.cochrane.org/CD004456/home-visits-during-pregnancy-and-after-birth-for-women-with-an-alcohol-or-drug-problem> 24 August 2013.

Venkatapuram, S., Marmot, M., 2009. Epidemiology and social justice in light of social determinants of health research. Bioethics 23 (2), 79–89.

Walker, L., Avant, K., 2005. Strategies for theory construction in nursing. Pearson Prentice Hall, Upper Saddle River, NJ.

Walker, S., Eketone, A., Gibbs, A., 2006. An exploration of Kaupapa Māori research, its principles, processes and applications. International Journal of Social Research Methodology 9 (4), 331–344.

Wallerstein, N., Yen, I., Syme, L., 2011. Integration of social epidemiology and community-engaged interventions to improve health equity. Am. J. Public Health 101 (5), 822–830.

Wang, C., Morrel-Samuels, S., Hutchison, P., et al., 2004. Flint photovoice: Community building among youths, adults, and policymakers. Am. J. Public Health 94 (6), 911–913.

Weaver, K., Olson, J., 2006. Understanding paradigms used for nursing research. J. Adv. Nurs. 53 (4), 459–469.

Whittemore, R., Knafl, K., 2005. The integrative review: updated methodology. J. Adv. Nurs. 52 (5), 546–553.

Wilson, D., Neville, S., 2009. Culturally safe research with vulnerable populations. Contemp. Nurse 33 (1), 69–79.

Wilson, A., Whitaker, N., Whitford, D., 2012. Rising to the challenge of health care reform with entrepreneurial and intrapreneurial nursing initiatives. Online J. Issues in Nurs. 17 (2), Manuscript 5:1–13.

Wiseman, J., McLeod, J., Zubrick, S., 2007. Promoting mental health and well-being: integrating individual, organizational and community-level indicators. Health Promot. J. Austr. 18 (3), 198–207.

World Health Organization (WHO), 2011. Hidden Cities: Unmasking and overcoming health inequities in urban settings. Online. Available: <http://hiddencities.org/downloads/WHO_UN-HABITAT_Hidden_Cities_Web.pdf> 21 January 2013.

Yarcheski, A., Mahon, N., Yarcheski, T., 2012. A descriptive study of research published in scientific nursing journals from 1985 to 2010. Int. J. Nurs. Stud. 49, 1112–1121.

Yin, R., 2009. Case Study Research: Design and Methods, fourth ed. Sage, Thousand Oaks.

Yonemoto, N., Dowswell, T., Nagai, S., et al., 2013. Schedules for home visits in the early post partum period. Cochrane Rev. Online. Available: <http://summaries.cochrane.org/CD009326/home-visits-in-the-early-period-after-the-birth-of-a-baby> 24 August 2013.

Young, M., Denny, G., Donnelly, J., 2012. Lessons from the trenches: Meeting evaluation challenges in school health education. J. Sch. Health 82 (11), 528–535.

Young, J., Higgins, N., Raven, L., 2013. Supporting child health professionals in health promotion roles: Efficacy, reach and sustainability of an eLearning group. Presentation, Research Seminar, University of the Sunshine Coast, 17 September.

Useful websites

http://joannabriggs.org/about.html—JBI and its networks

www.cochrane.org—Cochrane Collaboration

www.nhmrc.gov.au/about/organisation-overview/history-nhmrc/national-institute-clinical-studies—National Institute of Clinical Studies

www.phaa.net.au—Public Health Association of Australia

www.ruralhealth.org.au—Australian National Rural Health Alliance

www.who.int/mental_health/evidence/en/promoting_mhh.pdf—WHO Mental Health Evidence

www.who.int—World Health Organization

www.who.int/rpc/evipnet/en—WHO evidence-informed policy network

www.icn.ch—ICN

http://neac.health.govt.nz/home—National Ethics Advisory Committee of New Zealand

www.hrc.govt.nz—New Zealand Health Research Council

Appendices

Symbols Used in a Genogram

 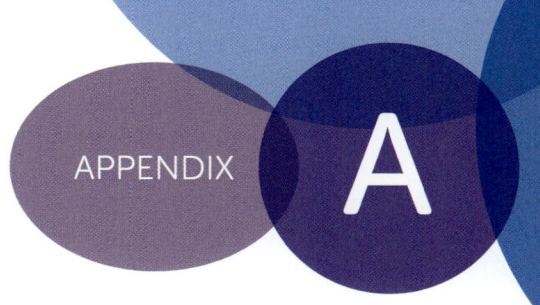

A genogram is a graphic representation of a family tree that displays the interaction of generations within a family. It goes beyond a traditional family tree by allowing the user to analyse family, emotional and social relationships within a group. It is used to identify repetitive patterns of behaviour and to recognise hereditary tendencies. Here are some of the basic components of a genogram.

Genogram symbols

In a genogram, males are represented by a square and females by a circle. If you are unsure of how to place individuals in complex family situations, such as reconstituted families, please visit the rules to build a genogram (www.genopro.com/genogram/rules/). GenoPro also has two other *gender symbols*, the diamond for a pet and the question mark for unknown gender.

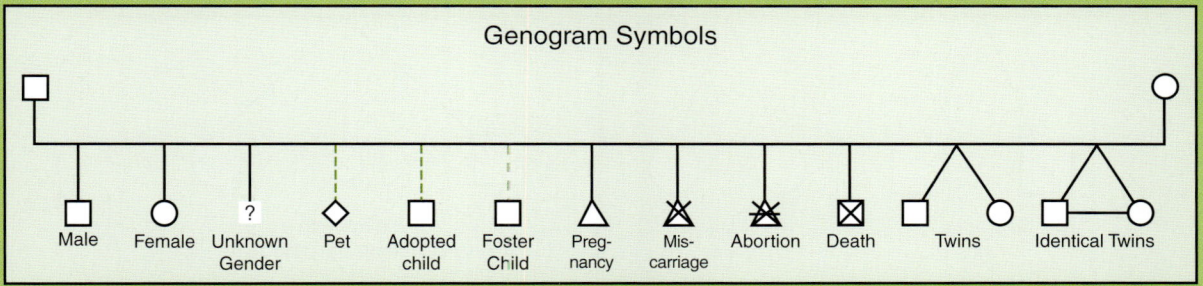

Standard gender symbols for a genogram

In a standard genogram, there are three different types of child: biological/natural child, adopted child and foster child. A triangle is used to represent a pregnancy, a miscarriage or an abortion. In the case of a miscarriage, there is a diagonal cross drawn on top of the triangle to indicate death. Abortions have a similar display to miscarriages, only they have an additional horizontal line. A still-birth is displayed by the gender symbol; the diagonal cross remains the same size, but the gender symbol is twice as small.

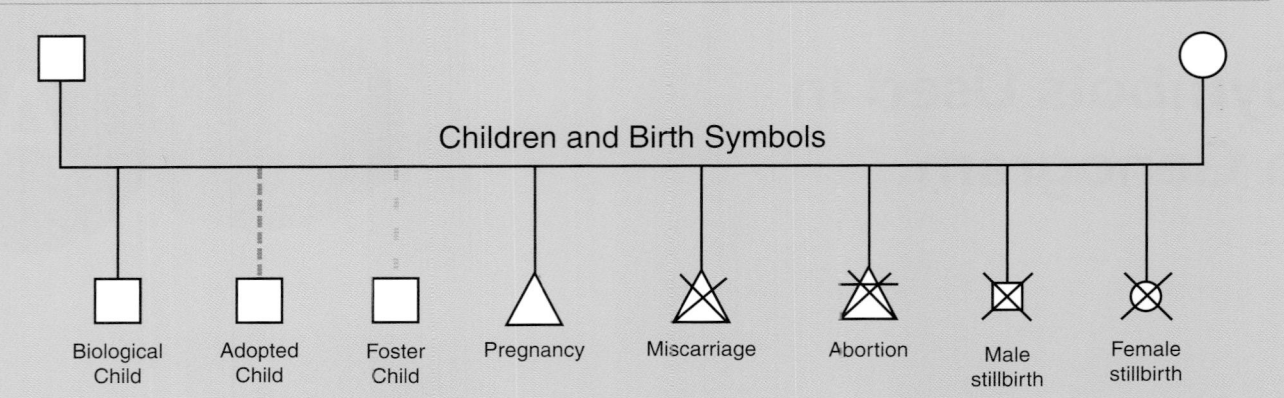

Genogram symbols for children's links and pregnancy terminations

In the case of multiple births such as twins, triplets, quadruplets, quintuplets, sextuplets, septuplets, octuplets, or more, the child links are joined together. GenoPro uses the term **twin** to describe any type of multiple birth. With GenoPro, creating twins is as simple as a single click on the toolbar button 'New Twins'. GenoPro take cares of all the drawing, including joining the lines together. Identical twins (or triplets ...) are displayed by a horizontal line between the siblings. In the example below, the mother gave birth to fraternal twin brothers, identical twin sisters and triplets, one of whom died at birth.

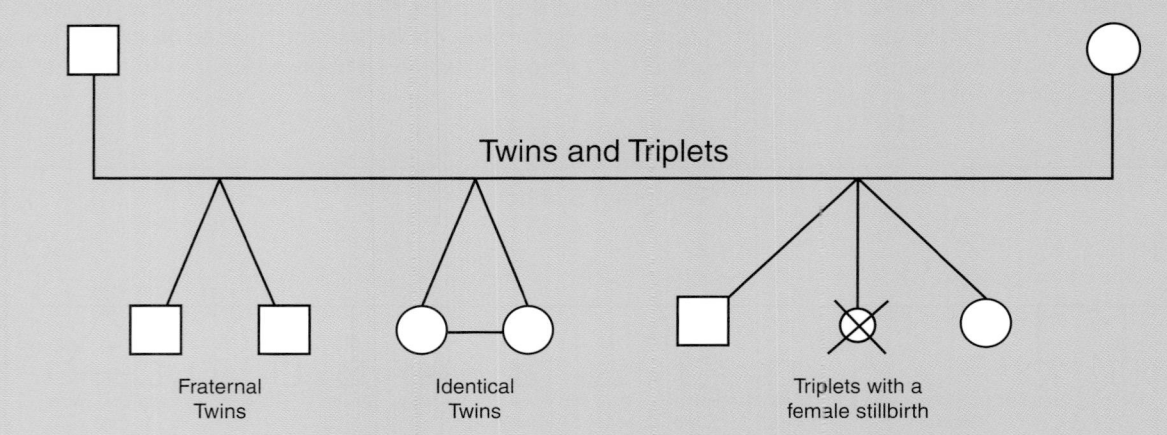

Child links are joined for multiple births such as twins and triplets

In addition to this, GenoPro supports medical genograms by using colour codes and special drawing in the gender symbol. To learn more, please visit medical genograms (www.genopro.com/genogram/symbols).

Genogram legend

At any time you can add a genogram legend by right-clicking on your mouse and selecting a new legend. The legend symbols have already been marked to be excluded from the report, so they will not appear when you generate a report.

(Source: Eenopro, with permission)

Jakarta Declaration on Leading Health Promotion into the 21st Century

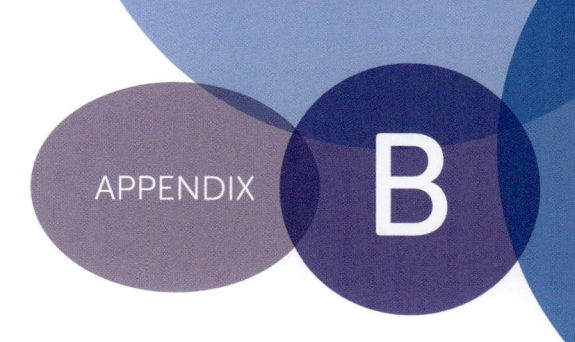

1   Promote social responsibility for health

Decision-makers must be firmly committed to social responsibility. Both the public and private sectors should promote health by pursuing policies and practices that:

- avoid harming the health of other individuals
- protect the environment and ensure sustainable use of resources
- restrict production and trade in inherently harmful goods and substances such as tobacco and armaments, as well as unhealthy marketing practices
- safeguard both the citizen in the marketplace and the individual in the workplace
- include equity-focused health impact assessments as an integral part of policy development.

2   Increase investments for health development

In many countries, current investment in health is inadequate and often ineffective. Increasing investment for health development requires a truly multisectoral approach, including additional resources to education, housing and the health sector. Greater investment for health, and reorientation of existing investments—both within and between countries—has the potential to significantly advance human development, health and quality of life.

Investments in health should reflect the needs of certain groups such as women, children, older people, indigenous, poor and marginalised populations.

3   Consolidate and expand partnerships for health

Health promotion requires partnerships for health and social development between the different sectors at all levels of governance and society. Existing partnerships need to be strengthened and the potential for new partnerships must be explored.

Partnerships offer mutual benefit for health through the sharing of expertise, skills and resources. Each partnership must be transparent and accountable and be based on agreed ethical principles, mutual understanding and respect. WHO guidelines should be adhered to.

4   Increase community capacity and empower the individual

Health promotion is carried out *by* and *with* people, not on or to people. It improves the ability of individuals to take action, and the capacity of groups, organisations or communities to influence the determinants of health.

Improving the capacity of communities for health promotion requires practical education, leadership training and access to resources. Empowering individuals demands more consistent, reliable access to the decision-making process and the skills and knowledge essential to effect change.

Both traditional communication and the new information media support this process. Social, cultural and spiritual resources need to be harnessed in innovative ways.

5   Secure an infrastructure for health promotion

To secure an infrastructure for health promotion, new mechanisms of funding it locally, nationally and globally must be found. Incentives should be developed to influence the actions of governments, non-government organisations (NGOs), educational institutions and the private sector to make sure that resource mobilisation for health promotion is maximised.

'Settings for health' represent the organisational base of the infrastructure required for health promotion. New health challenges mean that new and diverse networks need to be created to achieve intersectoral collaboration. Such networks should provide mutual assistance within and between countries and facilitate exchange of information on which strategies are effective in which settings.

Training and practice of local leadership skills should be encouraged to support health promotion activities. Documentation of experiences in health promotion through research and project reporting should be enhanced to improve planning, implementation and evaluation.

All countries should develop the appropriate political, legal, educational, social and economic environments required to support health promotion.

People's Health Charter

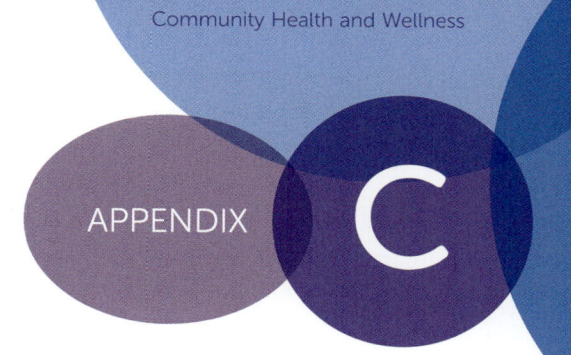

Introduction

In 1978, at the Alma-Ata Conference, ministers from 134 member countries in association with WHO and UNICEF declared 'Health for All by the Year 2000' selecting Primary Health Care as the best tool to achieve it.

Unfortunately, that dream never came true. The health status of third world populations has not improved. In many cases it has deteriorated further. Currently we are facing a global health crisis, characterised by growing inequalities within and between countries. New threats to health are continually emerging. This is compounded by negative forces of globalisation which prevent the equitable distribution of resources with regard to the health of people and especially that of the poor.

Within the health sector, failure to implement the principles of primary health care, as originally conceived in Alma-Ata has significantly aggravated the global health crisis.

Governments and the international bodies are fully responsible for this failure.

It has now become essential to build up a concerted international effort to put the goals of health for all to its rightful place on the development agenda. Genuine, people-centred initiatives must therefore be strengthened in order to increase pressure on decision-makers, governments and the private sector to ensure that the vision of Alma-Ata becomes a reality.

Several international organizations and civil society movements, NGOs and women's groups decided to work together towards this objective. This group together with others committed to the principles of primary health care and people's perspectives organised the 'People's Health Assembly' which took place from 4–8 December 2000 in Bangladesh, at Savar, on the campus of the Gonoshasthaya Kendra or GK (People's Health Centre).

1453 participants from 92 countries came to the Assembly which was the culmination of eighteen months of preparatory action around the globe. The preparatory process elicited unprecedented enthusiasm and participation of a broad cross section of people who have been involved in thousands of village meetings, district level workshops and national gatherings.

The plenary sessions at the Assembly covered five main themes: Health, Life and Well-Being; Inequality, Poverty and Health; Health Care and Health Services; Environment and Survival; and The Ways Forward. People from all over the world presented testimonies of deprivation and service failure as well as those of successful people's initiatives and organization. Over a hundred concurrent sessions made it possible for participants to share and discuss in greater detail different aspects of the major themes and give voice to their specific experiences and concerns. The five-day event gave participants the space to express themselves in their own idiom. They put forward the failures of their respective governments and international organizations and decided to fight together so that health and equitable development become top priorities in the policy-makers agendas at the local, national and international levels.

Having reviewed their problems and difficulties and shared their experiences, they have formulated and finally endorsed the People's Charter for Health. The charter from now on will be the common tool of a worldwide citizens' movement committed to make the Alma-Ata dream a reality.

We encourage and invite everyone who shares our concerns and aims to join us by endorsing the charter.

Preamble

Health is a social, economic and political issue and above all a fundamental human right. Inequality, poverty, exploitation, violence and injustice are at the root of ill-health and the deaths of poor and marginalised people. Health for all means that powerful interests have to be challenged, that globalisation has to be opposed, and that political and economic priorities have to be drastically changed. This Charter builds on perspectives of people whose voices have rarely been heard before, if at all. It encourages people to develop their own solutions and to hold accountable local authorities, national governments, international organisations and corporations.

Vision

Equity, ecologically-sustainable development and peace are at the heart of our vision of a better world—a world in which a healthy life for all is a reality; a world that respects, appreciates and celebrates all life and diversity; a world that enables the flowering of people's talents and abilities to enrich each other; a world in which people's voices guide the decisions that shape our lives. There are more than enough resources to achieve this vision.

The health crisis

'Illness and death every day anger us. Not because there are people who get sick or because there are people who die. We are angry because many illnesses and deaths have their roots in the economic and social policies that are imposed on us.'

(A voice from Central America)

In recent decades, economic changes world-wide have profoundly affected people's health and their access to health care and other social services.

Despite unprecedented levels of wealth in the world, poverty and hunger are increasing. The gap between rich and poor nations has widened, as have inequalities within countries, between social classes, between men and women and between young and old.

A large proportion of the world's population still lacks access to food, education, safe drinking water, sanitation, shelter, land and its resources, employment and health care services. Discrimination continues to prevail. It affects both the occurrence of disease and access to health care.

The planet's natural resources are being depleted at an alarming rate. The resulting degradation of the environment threatens everyone's health, especially the health of the poor. There has been an upsurge of new conflicts while weapons of mass destruction still pose a grave threat.

The world's resources are increasingly concentrated in the hands of a few who strive to maximise their private profit. Neoliberal political and economic policies are made by a small group of powerful governments, and by international institutions such as the World Bank, the International Monetary Fund and the World Trade Organization. These policies, together with the unregulated activities of transnational corporations, have had severe effects on the lives and livelihoods, health and well-being of people in both North and South.

Public services are not fulfilling people's needs, not least because they have deteriorated as a result of cuts in governments' social budgets. Health services have become less accessible, more unevenly distributed and more inappropriate.

Privatisation threatens to undermine access to health care still further and to compromise the essential principle of equity. The persistence of preventable ill-health, the resurgence of diseases such as tuberculosis and malaria, and the emergence and spread of new diseases such as HIV/AIDS are a stark reminder of our world's lack of commitment to principles of equity and justice.

Principles of the People's Charter for Health

- The attainment of the highest possible level of health and well-being is a fundamental human right, regardless of a person's colour, ethnic background, religion, gender, age, abilities, sexual orientation or class.

- The principles of universal, comprehensive Primary Health Care (PHC), envisioned in the 1978 Alma-Ata Declaration, should be the basis for formulating policies related to health. Now more than ever an equitable, participatory and intersectoral approach to health and health care is needed.

- Governments have a fundamental responsibility to ensure universal access to quality health care, education and other social services according to people's needs, not according to their ability to pay.

- The participation of people and people's organisations is essential to the formulation, implementation and evaluation of all health and social policies and programmes.

- Health is primarily determined by the political, economic, social and physical environment and should, along with equity and sustainable development, be a top priority in local, national and international policy-making.

A call for action

To combat the global health crisis, we need to take action at all levels—individual, community, national, regional and global—and in all sectors. The demands presented below provide a basis for action.

Health as a human right

Health is a reflection of a society's commitment to equity and justice. Health and human rights should prevail over economic and political concerns.

This Charter calls on people of the world to:

- Support all attempts to implement the right to health.

- Demand that governments and international organisations reformulate, implement and enforce policies and practices which respect the right to health.

- Build broad-based popular movements to pressure governments to incorporate health and human rights into national constitutions and legislation.

- Fight the exploitation of people's health needs for purposes of profit.

Tackling the broader determinants of health

Economic challenges

The economy has a profound influence on people's health. Economic policies that prioritise equity, health and social well-being can improve the health of the people as well as the economy.

Political, financial, agricultural and industrial policies which respond primarily to capitalist needs, imposed by national governments and international organisations, alienate people from their lives and livelihoods. The processes of economic globalisation and liberalisation have increased inequalities between and within nations. Many countries of the world and especially the most powerful ones are using their resources, including economic sanctions and military interventions, to consolidate and expand their positions, with devastating effects on people's lives.

This Charter calls on people of the world to:

- Demand transformation of the World Trade Organization and the global trading system so that it ceases to violate social, environmental, economic and health rights of people and begins to discriminate positively in favour of countries of the South. In order to protect public health, such transformation must include intellectual property regimes such as patents and the Trade Related aspects of Intellectual Property Rights (TRIPS) agreement.

- Demand the cancellation of Third World debt.

- Demand radical transformation of the World Bank and International Monetary Fund so that

these institutions reflect and actively promote the rights and interests of developing countries.

- Demand effective regulation to ensure that TNCs do not have negative effects on people's health, exploit their workforce, degrade the environment or impinge on national sovereignty.

- Ensure that governments implement agricultural policies attuned to people's needs and not to the demands of the market, thereby guaranteeing food security and equitable access to food.

- Demand that national governments act to protect public health rights in intellectual property laws.

- Demand the control and taxation of speculative international capital flows.

- Insist that all economic policies be subject to health, equity, gender and environmental impact assessments and include enforceable regulatory measures to ensure compliance.

- Challenge growth-centred economic theories and replace them with alternatives that create humane and sustainable societies. Economic theories should recognise environmental constraints, the fundamental importance of equity and health, and the contribution of unpaid labour, especially the unrecognised work of women.

Social and political challenges

Comprehensive social policies have positive effects on people's lives and livelihoods. Economic globalisation and privatisation have profoundly disrupted communities, families and cultures. Women are essential to sustaining the social fabric of societies everywhere, yet their basic needs are often ignored or denied, and their rights and persons violated.

Public institutions have been undermined and weakened. Many of their responsibilities have been transferred to the private sector, particularly corporations, or to other national and international institutions, which are rarely accountable to the people. Furthermore, the power of political parties and trade unions has been severely curtailed, while conservative and fundamentalist forces are on the rise. Participatory democracy in political organisations and civic structures should thrive. There is an urgent need to foster and ensure transparency and accountability.

This Charter calls on people of the world to:

- Demand and support the development and implementation of comprehensive social policies with full participation of people.

- Ensure that all women and all men have equal rights to work, livelihoods, to freedom of expression, to political participation, to exercise religious choice, to education and to freedom from violence.

- Pressure governments to introduce and enforce legislation to protect and promote the physical, mental and spiritual health and human rights of marginalised groups.

- Demand that education and health are placed at the top of the political agenda. This calls for free and compulsory quality education for all children and adults, particularly girl children and women, and for quality early childhood education and care.

- Demand that the activities of public institutions, such as child care services, food distribution systems, and housing provisions, benefit the health of individuals and communities.

- Condemn and seek the reversal of any policies, which result in the forced displacement of people from their lands, homes or jobs.

- Oppose fundamentalist forces that threaten the rights and liberties of individuals, particularly the lives of women, children and minorities.

- Oppose sex tourism and the global traffic of women and children.

Environmental challenges

Water and air pollution, rapid climate change, ozone layer depletion, nuclear energy and waste, toxic chemicals and pesticides, loss of biodiversity, deforestation and soil erosion have far-reaching effects on people's health. The root causes of this destruction include the unsustainable exploitation of natural resources, the absence of a long-term holistic vision, the spread of individualistic and profit-maximising behaviours, and over-consumption by the rich. This destruction must be confronted and reversed immediately and effectively.

This Charter calls on people of the world to:

- Hold transnational and national corporations, public institutions and the military accountable for their destructive and hazardous activities that impact on the environment and people's health.

- Demand that all development projects be evaluated against health and environmental criteria and that caution and restraint be applied whenever technologies or policies pose potential threats to health and the environment (the precautionary principle).

- Demand that governments rapidly commit themselves to reductions of greenhouse gases from their own territories far stricter than those set out in the international climate change agreement, without resorting to hazardous or inappropriate technologies and practices.

- Oppose the shifting of hazardous industries and toxic and radioactive waste to poorer countries and marginalised communities and encourage solutions that minimise waste production.

- Reduce over-consumption and non-sustainable lifestyles—both in the North and the South. Pressure wealthy industrialised countries to reduce their consumption and pollution by 90 per cent.

- Demand measures to ensure occupational health and safety, including worker-centred monitoring of working conditions.

- Demand measures to prevent accidents and injuries in the workplace, the community and in homes.

- Reject patents on life and oppose bio-piracy of traditional and indigenous knowledge and resources.

- Develop people-centred, community-based indicators of environmental and social progress, and press for the development and adoption of regular audits that measure environmental degradation and the health status of the population.

War, violence, conflict and natural disasters

War, violence, conflict and natural disasters devastate communities and destroy human dignity. They have a severe impact on the physical and mental health of their members, especially women and children. Increased arms procurement and an aggressive and corrupt international arms trade undermine social, political and economic stability and the allocation of resources to the social sector.

This Charter calls on people of the world to:

- Support campaigns and movements for peace and disarmament.

- Support campaigns against aggression, and the research, production, testing and use of weapons of mass destruction and other arms, including all types of landmines.

- Support people's initiatives to achieve a just and lasting peace, especially in countries with experiences of civil war and genocide.

- Condemn the use of child soldiers, and the abuse and rape, torture and killing of women and children.

- Demand the end of occupation as one of the most destructive tools to human dignity.

- Oppose the militarisation of humanitarian relief interventions.

- Demand the radical transformation of the UN Security Council so that it functions democratically.

- Demand that the United Nations and individual states end all kinds of sanctions used as an instrument of aggression which can damage the health of civilian populations.

- Encourage independent, people-based initiatives to declare neighbourhoods, communities and cities areas of peace and zones free of weapons.

- Support actions and campaigns for the prevention and reduction of aggressive and violent behaviour, especially in men, and the fostering of peaceful coexistence.

- Support actions and campaigns for the prevention of natural disasters and the reduction of subsequent human suffering.

A people-centred health sector

This Charter calls for the provision of universal and comprehensive Primary Health Care, irrespective of people's ability to pay. Health services must be democratic and accountable with sufficient resources to achieve this.

This Charter calls on people of the world to:

- Oppose international and national policies that privatise health care and turn it into a commodity.

- Demand that governments promote, finance and provide comprehensive Primary Health Care as the most effective way of addressing health problems and organising public health services so as to ensure free and universal access.

- Pressure governments to adopt, implement and enforce national health and drugs policies.

- Demand that governments oppose the privatisation of public health services and ensure effective regulation of the private medical sector, including charitable and NGO medical services.

- Demand a radical transformation of the World Health Organization (WHO) so that it responds to health challenges in a manner which benefits the poor, avoids vertical approaches, ensures intersectoral work, involves people's organisations in the World Health Assembly, and ensures independence from corporate interests.

- Promote, support and engage in actions that encourage people's power and control in decision-making in health at all levels, including patient and consumer rights.

- Support, recognise and promote traditional and holistic healing systems and practitioners and their integration into Primary Health Care.

- Demand changes in the training of health personnel so that they become more

problem-oriented and practice based, understand better the impact of global issues in their communities, and are encouraged to work with and respect the community and its diversities.

- Demystify medical and health technologies (including medicines) and demand that they be subordinated to the health needs of the people.

- Demand that research in health, including genetic research and the development of medicines and reproductive technologies, is carried out in a participatory, needs-based manner by accountable institutions. It should be people- and public health-oriented, respecting universal ethical principles.

- Support people's rights to reproductive and sexual self-determination and oppose all coercive measures in population and family planning policies. This support includes the right to the full range of safe and effective methods of fertility regulation.

People's participation for a healthy world

Strong people's organisations and movements are fundamental to more democratic, transparent and accountable decision-making processes. It is essential that people's civil, political, economic, social and cultural rights are ensured. While governments have the primary responsibility for promoting a more equitable approach to health and human rights, a wide range of civil society groups and movements, and the media have an important role to play in ensuring people's power and control in policy development and in the monitoring of its implementation.

This Charter calls on people of the world to:

- Build and strengthen people's organisations to create a basis for analysis and action.

- Promote, support and engage in actions that encourage people's involvement in decision-making in public services at all levels.

- Demand that people's organisations be represented in local, national and international fora that are relevant to health.

- Support local initiatives towards participatory democracy through the establishment of people-centred solidarity networks across the world.

Amendment

After the endorsement of the PCH on December 8, 2000, it was called to the attention of the drafting group that action points number 1 and 2 under Economic Challenges could be interpreted as supporting the social clause proposed by the WTO, which actually serves to strengthen the WTO and its neoliberal agenda. Given that this countervails the PHA demands for change of the WTO and the global trading system, the two paragraphs were merged and amended.

The section of War, Violence and Conflict has been amended to include natural disasters. A new action point, number 5 in this version, was added to demand the end of occupation. Furthermore, action point number 7, now number 8, was amended to read to end all kinds of sanctions. An additional action point number 11 was added concerning natural disasters.

The People's Health Assembly and the Charter

The idea of a People's Health Assembly (PHA) has been discussed for more than a decade. In 1998 a number of organisations launched the PHA process and started to plan a large international Assembly meeting, held in Bangladesh at the end of 2000. A range of pre- and post-Assembly activities were initiated including regional workshops, the collection of people's health-related stories and the drafting of a People's Charter for Health. The present Charter builds upon the views of citizens and people's organisations from around the world, and was first approved and opened for endorsement at the Assembly meeting in Savar, Bangladesh, in December 2000. The Charter is an expression of our common concerns, our vision of a better and healthier world, and of our calls for radical action. It is a tool for advocacy and a rallying point around which a global health movement can gather and other networks and coalitions can be formed.

Join us—endorse the Charter

We call upon all individuals and organisations to join this global movement and invite you to endorse and help implement the People's Charter for Health.

PHM Global Secretariat

Email: secretariat@phmovement.org

Web: www.phmovement.org

Endorse the People's Charter for Health

Personal information

Name

First: _____.

Last: _____.

Mailing address

Street and no.: _____

City: _____.

State: _____

Zip code: _____

Country: _____.

Email: _____

Organisation

Name: _____

Website: _____

Comments on the Charter

_____
_____
_____
_____
_____
_____
_____
_____
_____
_____

Ary suggestions for the PHM?

_____
_____
_____
_____
_____
_____
_____
_____
_____
_____
_____
_____
_____
_____
_____
_____

Don't be hesitant to add any further suggestions in separate papers.

Please fill in and send to: secretariat@phmovement.org

The People's Health Charter was produced by the People's Health Movement and endorsed at the first People's Health Assembly held in Savar Bangladesh in December 2000. It resulted from a consultation process with grassroots communities across the globe about the health issues that most concerned them.

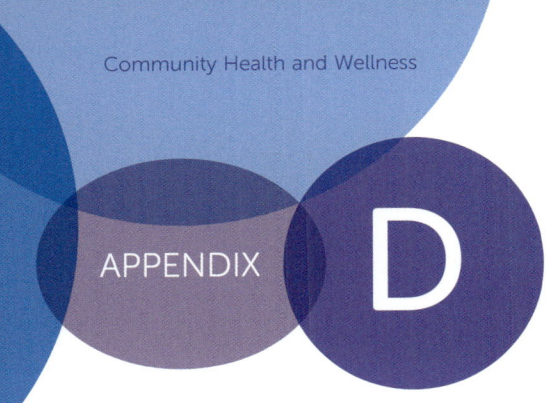

D The Bangkok Charter for Health Promotion in a Globalized World

Introduction

Scope

The Bangkok Charter identifies actions, commitments and pledges required to address the determinants of health in a globalized world through health promotion.

Purpose

The Bangkok Charter affirms that policies and partnerships to empower communities, and to improve health and health equality, should be at the centre of global and national development.

The Bangkok Charter complements and builds upon the values, principles and action strategies of health promotion established by the *Ottawa Charter for Health Promotion* and the recommendations of the subsequent global health promotion conferences which have been confirmed by Member States through the World Health Assembly.

Audience

The Bangkok Charter reaches out to people, groups and organizations that are critical to the achievement of health, including:

- governments and politicians at all levels
- civil society
- the private sector
- international organizations, and
- the public health community.

Health promotion

The United Nations recognizes that the enjoyment of the highest attainable standard of health is one of the fundamental rights of every human being without discrimination.

Health promotion is based on this critical human right and offers a positive and inclusive concept of health as a determinant of the quality of life and encompassing mental and spiritual wellbeing.

Health promotion is the process of enabling people to increase control over their health and its determinants, and thereby improve their health. It is a core function of public health and contributes to the work of tackling communicable and non-communicable diseases and other threats to health.

Addressing the determinants of health

Changing context

The global context for health promotion has changed markedly since the development of the *Ottawa Charter*.

Critical factors

Some of the critical factors that now influence health include:

- increasing inequalities within and between countries
- new patterns of consumption and communication
- commercialization
- global environmental change, and
- urbanization.

Further challenges

Other factors that influence health include rapid and often adverse social, economic and demographic changes that affect working conditions, learning environments, family patterns, and the culture and social fabric of communities.

Women and men are affected differently and the vulnerability of children and exclusion of marginalized, disabled and indigenous peoples have increased.

New opportunities

Globalization opens up new opportunities for cooperation to improve health and reduce transnational health risks; these opportunities include:

- enhanced information and communications technology, and

- improved mechanisms for global governance and the sharing of experiences.

Policy coherence

To manage the challenges of globalization, policy must be coherent across all:

- levels of governments
- United Nations bodies, and
- other organizations, including the private sector.

This coherence will strengthen compliance, transparency and accountability with international agreements and treaties that affect health.

Progress made

Progress has been made in placing health at the centre of development, for example through the Millennium Development Goals, but much more remains to be achieved; the active participation of civil society is crucial in this process.

Strategies for health promotion in a globalized world

Effective interventions

Progress towards a healthier world requires strong political action, broad participation and sustained advocacy.

Health promotion has an established repertoire of proven effective strategies which need to be fully utilized.

Required actions

To make further advances in implementing these strategies, all sectors and settings must act to:

- **advocate** for health based on human rights and solidarity
- **invest** in sustainable policies, actions and infrastructure to address the determinants of health
- **build capacity** for policy development, leadership, health promotion practice, knowledge transfer and research, and health literacy
- **regulate and legislate** to ensure a high level of protection from harm and enable equal opportunity for health and wellbeing for all people
- **partner and build alliances** with public, private, non-governmental and international organizations and civil society to create sustainable actions.

Commitments to health for all

Rationale

The health sector has a key role to provide leadership in building policies and partnerships for health promotion.

An integrated policy approach within government and international organizations, and a commitment to working with civil society and the private sector and across settings, are essential to make progress in addressing the determinants of health.

Key commitments

The four key commitments are to make the promotion of health:

1   central to the global development agenda
2   a core responsibility for all of government
3   a key focus of communities and civil society
4   a requirement for good corporate practice.

1   Make the promotion of health central to the global development agenda

Strong intergovernmental agreements that increase health and collective health security are needed. Government and international bodies must act to close the health gap between rich and poor. Effective mechanisms for global governance for health are required to address all the harmful effects of:

- trade
- products
- services, and
- marketing strategies.

Health promotion must become an integral part of domestic and foreign policy and international relations, including in situations of war and conflict.

This requires actions to promote dialogue and cooperation among nation states, civil society, and the private sector. These efforts can build on the example of existing treaties such as the World Health Organization Framework Convention for Tobacco Control.

2   Make the promotion of health a core responsibility for all of government

All governments at all levels must tackle poor health and inequalities as a matter of urgency because health determines socio-economic and political development.

Local, regional and national governments must:

- give priority to investments in health, within and outside the health sector
- provide sustainable financing for health promotion.

To ensure this, all levels of government should make the health consequences of policies and legislation explicit, using tools such as equity-focused health impact assessment.

3 Make the promotion of health a key focus of communities and civil society

Communities and civil society often lead in initiating, shaping and undertaking health promotion. They need to have the rights, resources and opportunities so that their contributions are amplified and sustained. In less developed communities, support for capacity building is particularly important.

Well organized and empowered communities are highly effective in determining their own health, and are capable of making governments and the private sector accountable for the health consequences of their policies and practices.

Civil society needs to exercise its power in the marketplace by giving preference to the goods, services and shares of companies that exemplify corporate social responsibility.

Grass-roots community projects, civil society groups, and women's organizations have demonstrated their effectiveness in health promotion, and provide models of practice for others to follow.

Health professional associations have a special contribution to make.

4 Make the promotion of health a requirement for good corporate practice

The corporate sector has a direct impact on the health of people and on the determinants of health through its influence on:

- local settings
- national cultures
- environments, and
- wealth distribution.

The private sector, like other employers and the informal sector, has a responsibility to ensure health and safety in the workplace, and to promote the health and wellbeing of their employees, their families and communities.

The private sector can also contribute to lessening wider global health impacts, such as those associated with global environmental change by complying with local, national and international regulations and agreements that promote and protect health. Ethical and responsible business practices and fair trade exemplify the type of business practice that should be supported by consumers and civil society, and by government incentives and regulations.

A global pledge to make it happen

All for health

Meeting these commitments requires better application of proven strategies, as well as the use of new entry points and innovative responses.

Partnerships, alliances, networks and collaborations provide exciting and rewarding ways of bringing people and organizations together around common goals and joint actions to improve the health of populations.

Each sector—intergovernmental, government, civil society and private—has a unique role and responsibility.

Closing the implementation gap

Since the adoption of the *Ottawa Charter*, a significant number of resolutions at national and global level have been signed in support of health promotion, but these have not always been followed by action. The participants of this Bangkok Conference forcefully call on Member States of the World Health Organization to close this implementation gap and move to policies and partnerships for action.

Call for action

Conference participants request the World Health Organization, in collaboration with others, and its Member States, to allocate resources for health promotion, initiate plans of action and monitor performance through appropriate indicators and targets, and to report on progress at regular intervals. United Nations organizations are asked to explore the benefits of developing a Global Treaty for Health.

Worldwide partnership

This Bangkok Charter urges all stakeholders to join in a worldwide partnership to promote health, with both global and local engagement and action.

Commitment to improve health

We, the participants of the 6th Global Conference on Health Promotion in Bangkok, Thailand, pledge to advance these actions and commitments to improve health.

11 August 2005

Note: This charter contains the collective views of an international group of experts, participants to the 6th Global Conference on Health Promotion, Bangkok, Thailand, August 2005, and does not necessarily represent the decisions or the stated policy of the World Health Organization.

Nairobi Call to Action

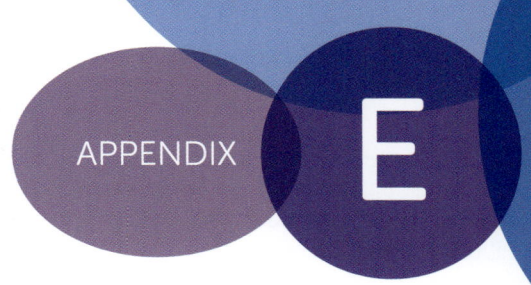

THE NAIROBI CALL TO ACTION FOR CLOSING THE IMPLEMENTATION GAP IN HEALTH PROMOTION

1. INTRODUCTION

PURPOSE

The Nairobi Call to Action identifies key strategies and commitments urgently required for closing the implementation gap in health and development through health promotion.

Health promotion is a core and the most cost-effective strategy to improve health and quality of life, and reduces health inequities and poverty. In so doing, it helps achieve national and international health and development goals such as the Millennium Development Goals. Implementing health promotion creates fairer societies that enable people to lead lives that they value by increasing their control over their health and the necessary resources for wellbeing.

AUDIENCE

The Nairobi Call to Action reaches out to:

- WHO and other UN partners;
- International development organisations;
- Governments, politicians and policy makers at all levels;
- Public, civil society, non-governmental and private organizations, and practitioners;
- Individuals, families, communities, community-based organizations and social networks.

Urgent responsibilities:

- **Strengthen leadership and workforces**
- **Mainstream health promotion**
- **Empower communities and individuals**
- **Enhance participatory processes**
- **Build and apply knowledge**

PROCESS

The Nairobi Call to Action was developed by participants at the 7th Global Conference on Health Promotion, Nairobi, Kenya, in October 2009, hosted by the World Health Organization and the Republic of Kenya.

Over 600 experts from more than 100 countries participated including Ministers of Health, politicians, senior public servants, health practitioners, policy makers, researchers, teachers, and community representatives. They were complemented by an equal number of virtual participants who registered on a new social networking site (www.connect2change.org). Utilising multiple participatory processes, the Call to Action was developed during the five day meeting and is complemented by a full Conference Report and a series of technical papers.

BACKGROUND

The Call to Action aligns with the aspirations of Member States, reflects the vision of the Alma Ata Declaration and supports the recommendations of the WHO Commission on the Social Determinants of Health.

The Call reaffirms the values, principles and action strategies of health promotion codified in the Ottawa Charter for Health Promotion 1986 and in subsequent global health promotion conferences[1] including The Bangkok Charter for Health Promotion in a Globalized World 2005, which has been confirmed by Member States through the World Health Assembly.

Health promotion has demonstrated its effectiveness and return on investment at local, regional, national and international levels. Although many of the challenges that drove the development of health promotion remain the same, new threats continue to emerge or escalate rapidly.

Health promotion can greatly contribute to tackling development and equity challenges and to the realisation of human rights. However, implementation gaps exist, in evidence, policy, practice, governance and political will, resulting in a failure to realise this potential. This represents a lost opportunity, measured in avoidable illness and suffering as well as the broader social and economic impacts.

2. GLOBAL COMMITMENT

We, the participants of the 7th Global Conference on Health Promotion, recognising the changing context and acute challenges, call on all governments and stakeholders to respond urgently to this Call to Action and the strategies and actions that follow.

TO USE THE UNTAPPED POTENTIAL OF HEALTH PROMOTION

We pledge, as champions, to:

- Use the existing evidence to prove to policy-makers that health promotion is fundamental to managing national and global challenges such as population ageing, climate change, global pandemic threats, maternal mortality, migration, conflict and economic crises;

- Revitalise primary health care by fostering community participation, healthy public policy and putting people at the centre of care;

- Build on the resilience of communities by harnessing their resources to address the double burden of non-communicable and communicable diseases.

---

[1] Adelaide Australia 1988, Sundsvall Sweden 1991, Jakarta Indonesia 1997, Mexico City Mexico 2000, Bangkok 2005

TO MAKE HEALTH PROMOTION PRINCIPLES INTEGRAL TO THE POLICY AND DEVELOPMENT AGENDA

We call on governments to exercise their responsibility for public health, including working across sectors and in partnership with citizens, in particular to:

- Promote social justice and equity in health by implementing the recommendations of the WHO Commission on the Social Determinants of Health;

- Accelerate the attainment of national and international development goals by building and redistributing resources to strengthen capacity and leadership for health promotion;

- Be accountable for improving people's quality of life and well being.

TO DEVELOP EFFECTIVE AND SUSTAINABLE DELIVERY MECHANISMS

We request Member States to mandate WHO to:

- Develop a Global Health Promotion Strategy and action plans, with regional follow-up that respond to the major health needs and incorporate cost-effective and equitable interventions;

- Strengthen its internal capacity for health promotion, and assist Member States to develop sustainably funded structures and set up accountable reporting mechanisms for investment in the promotion of health;

- Disseminate compelling evidence on the social, economic, health and other benefits of health promotion to key sectors.

3. STRATEGIES AND ACTIONS

The following strategies and actions are presented under the five sub-themes of the Conference: building capacity for health promotion, strengthening health systems, partnerships and intersectoral action, community empowerment, and health literacy and health behaviours. Actions across the sub-themes complement each other.

BUILDING CAPACITY FOR HEALTH PROMOTION

Building sustainable health promotion infrastructure and capacity at all levels is fundamental to closing the implementation gap.

ACTIONS THAT MAKE A DIFFERENCE:

Strengthen leadership

... by establishing good governance with respect to integrity, transparency, and accountability;

... by developing individuals and institutions to create a sustainable health promotion infrastructure;

... by building skills in advocacy and stewardship to address determinants of health.

Secure adequate financing

... by establishing stable and sustainable financing at all levels, for example health promotion foundations, and by levering financing from sectoral, bi-lateral and multi-lateral donor programs.

Grow practitioner skill-base

... by reorienting the understanding and skills of health promotion in current health workers;

... by providing structures and incentives to train, maintain and retain health promotion capacity across the health system, and other sectors that impact on health;

... by setting accreditation competencies and standards for health promotion, and revising the curricula of health and health-related professionals in training to include health promotion;

... by establishing and strengthening national, regional and institutional capacity to implement systematic training to develop a critical mass of health promotion practitioners able to perform to specified competencies;

... by promoting teaching of core values underlying basic human rights and equity;

... by ensuring timely and accurate dissemination of information and resources for the preparedness and response to emergencies and epidemics;

... by expanding and strengthening WHO Collaborating Centers for Health Promotion in all regions to reflect emerging and unmet needs.

Enhance system-wide approaches

... by assessing the national capacity for health promotion using validated tools and methods as a routine process for quality improvement;

... by developing, adapting and applying quality improvement tools and methods to ensure intervention effectiveness and sustainability at all levels.

Improve performance management

... by strengthening information systems to benchmark and monitor health promotion implementation, regarding policies, processes and outcomes;

... by embedding determinants of health and equity and risk factors in current surveillance, monitoring and evaluation systems.

STRENGTHENING HEALTH SYSTEMS

To be sustainable, health promotion interventions must be embedded in health systems that support equity in health and meet high performance standards. Integrating health promotion in all health systems functions and at all levels improves the overall performance of health systems.

ACTIONS THAT MAKE A DIFFERENCE:

Strengthen leadership

... by governments advocating for the promotion of health in all sectors and settings, supporting inter-sectoral and inter-disciplinary action, including the opportunities through regulation and legislation;.

... by ensuring community participation in governance of health systems at all levels;

... by ensuring effective stewardship and oversight.

Enhance policy

... by systematically integrating health promotion across the continuum of health care and other social and community services, throughout the lifecourse;

... by ensuring that health promotion is mainstreamed into priority programmes such as HIV/AIDS, malaria, tuberculosis, mental health, maternal and child health, violence and injury, neglected tropical diseases, and noncommunicable diseases such as diabetes;

... by using targets, quality measures and incentives for systematic and sustainable health promotion;

... by developing specific approaches to reach women, in light of their unique role in ensuring the success of health promotion programmes, as both beneficiaries and primary care givers in most societies;

... by implementing health promotion strategies with people with disabilities, to improve quality of life , wellbeing and promote development.

Assure universal access

... by guaranteeing that health systems provide accessible, appropriate and comprehensive health services for all, including measuring performance for marginalized groups;

... by insisting that health systems provide accessible and comprehensive information and resources for health promotion that are culturally, linguistically, age, gender and ability appropriate;

... by addressing financial and other resource barriers with innovative approaches.

Build and apply the evidence base

... by investing in research and evaluation, and its dissemination, to increase the adoption of better practices in health promotion;

... by setting up databases including clearing-houses on research evidence and rapid response mechanisms to meet policymakers and practitioners' needs for evidence-informed policy formulation and decision making.

PARTNERSHIPS AND INTERSECTORAL ACTION

Effectively addressing the determinants of health and achieving health equity requires actions and partnerships that extend beyond the health sector to implement forms of collaboration, cooperation and integration between sectors.

ACTIONS THAT MAKE A DIFFERENCE:

Strengthen leadership

... by negotiating and adopting shared goals and objectives and working towards common results across sectors and institutions, at all levels of governance;

... by ensuring that the private sector and other players accept their responsibilities to safeguard and promote the health of their clients, workers, customers and communities.

Enhance policy

... by developing political momentum and leadership for health in all policies and settings;

... by mainstreaming health promotion and social determinants of health approaches across all policies, programs, and research agendas with a focus on health equity, ensuring integrated planning, capacity-building and resource allocation;

... by establishing health equity as a key social indicator to measure the performance of intersectoral initiatives;

... by creating functional inter-governmental regional bodies, such as an African Health Promotion Partnership, to set a vision and agenda for health promotion, and advocate and mobilize resources in the region to achieve these.

Enhance implementation

... by developing and adapting to country context, tools, mechanisms and capacities to create opportunities at local, regional and national levels for intersectoral action on health equity;

... by encouraging credible role modeling for healthy living;

... by strengthening and supporting civil society to develop common and effective approaches;

... by utilising the opportunities of 'mass events' for health promotion such as international sports tournaments;

... by being proactive and partnering with the media in an informed and mutually supportive way.

Build and apply the evidence base

... by developing and incorporating indicators of equity and intersectoral action, focusing both on health outcomes and determinants;

... by evaluating initiatives to determine critical success factors for scaling up.

COMMUNITY EMPOWERMENT

Communities must share the power, resources and decision-making to assure and sustain conditions for health equity.

ACTIONS THAT MAKE A DIFFERENCE:

Enable community ownership

... by listening to and starting with the voices and aspirations of the community in planning and action;

... by recognizing and appreciating indigenous culture, traditional ways, and the contribution of migrant groups;

... by assuring meaningful and equitable participation and control in decision making among all groups including those experiencing social, economic or political exclusion;

... by involving people with passion, people with power and people with influence in partnerships for change and improvement;

... by building community capacity during planning, implementation, monitoring and evaluation.

Develop sustainable resources

... by establishing financing mechanisms that assure coordinated, integrated and holistic responses to community-determined goals over an extended time frame.

Build and apply the evidence base

... by including narratives and empirical evidence of success and lessons learned;

... by incorporating indigenous knowledge systems into planned curriculum and mainstreaming its application across key sectors.

HEALTH LITERACY AND HEALTH BEHAVIOURS

Basic literacy is an essential building block for development and health promotion. Health literacy interventions need to be designed based on health, social and cultural needs.

ACTIONS THAT MAKE A DIFFERENCE:

Support empowerment

... by ensuring basic education for all citizens;

... by building on existing community resources and networks to ensure sustainability and enhance community participation;

... by designing health literacy interventions based on community needs and priorities in their political, social and cultural context, with particular consideration for the needs of people with disability;

... by ensuring that communities are able to access and act on knowledge and overcome any barriers.

Embrace information and communication technologies (ICT)

... by formulating a strategic framework on ICT to equitably improve health literacy;

... by ensuring that public policies increase affordable access to ICT through wider coverage of remote and underserved areas;

... by building the ICT capacity of health professionals and communities, and maximize the use of available ICT tools.

Build and apply the evidence base

... by developing a core set of evidence-based health literacy indicators and tools based on constructs and concepts relevant to health using quantitative and qualitative methods;

... by surveying and monitoring health literacy levels of individuals and communities;

... by setting up a system to monitor, evaluate, document and disseminate health literacy interventions.

Acting together

Developing and developed countries are facing a surge of preventable disease that threatens to undermine their future economic development.

Five urgent responsibilities for governments and stakeholders:

- ○ Strengthen leadership and workforces
- ○ Mainstream health promotion
- ○ Empower communities and individuals
- ○ Enhance participatory processes
- ○ Build and apply knowledge

The Nairobi Call to Action for Closing the Implementation Gap in Health Promotion has strong global support, is urgently needed and will make a profound difference to people's lives.

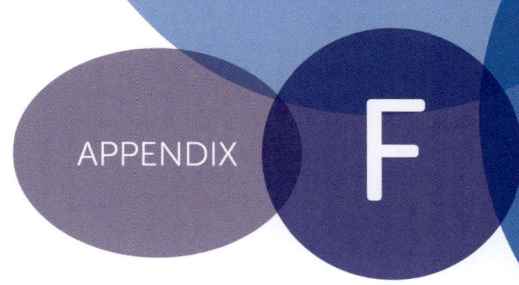

Helsinki Statement on Health in All Policies

The 8th Global Conference on Health Promotion, Helsinki, Finland, 10-14 June 2013

The Helsinki Statement on Health in All Policies

Building on our heritage, looking to our future

The 8th Global Conference on Health Promotion was held in Helsinki, Finland from 10-14 June 2013. The meeting builds upon a rich heritage of ideas, actions and evidence originally inspired by the *Alma Ata Declaration on Primary Health Care* (1978) and the *Ottawa Charter for Health Promotion* (1986). These identified intersectoral action and healthy public policy as central elements for the promotion of health, the achievement of health equity, and the realization of health as a human right. Subsequent WHO global health promotion conferences[1] cemented key principles for health promotion action. These principles have been reinforced in the 2011 *Rio Political Declaration on Social Determinants of Health*, the 2011 *Political Declaration of the UN High-level Meeting of the General Assembly on the Prevention and Control of Non-communicable Diseases*, and the 2012 Rio+20 Outcome Document (*the Future We Want*). They are also reflected in many other WHO frameworks, strategies and resolutions, and contribute to the formulation of the post-2015 development goals.

Health for All is a major societal goal of governments, and the cornerstone of sustainable development

We, the participants of this conference

Affirm our commitment to equity in health and recognize that the enjoyment of the highest attainable standard of health is one of the fundamental rights of every human being without distinction of race, religion, political belief, economic or social condition. We recognize that governments have a responsibility for the health of their people and that equity in health is an expression of social justice. We know that good health enhances quality of life, increases capacity for learning, strengthens families and communities and improves workforce productivity. Likewise, action aimed at promoting equity significantly contributes to health, poverty reduction, social inclusion and security.

Health inequities between and within countries are politically, socially and economically unacceptable, as well as unfair and avoidable. Policies made in all sectors can have a profound effect on population health and health equity. In our interconnected world, health is shaped by many powerful forces, especially demographic change, rapid urbanization, climate change and globalization. While some diseases are disappearing as living conditions improve, many diseases of poverty still persist in developing countries. In many countries lifestyles and living and working environments are influenced by unrestrained marketing and subject to unsustainable production and consumption patterns. The health of the people is not only a health sector responsibility, it also embraces wider political issues such as trade and foreign policy. Tackling this requires political will to engage the whole of government in health.

[1] Subsequent conferences were held in Adelaide (1988); Sundsvall (1991); Jakarta (1997); Mexico City (2000); Bangkok (2005); Nairobi (2009).

Health in All Policies is an approach to public policies across sectors that systematically takes into account the health implications of decisions, seeks synergies, and avoids harmful health impacts in order to improve population health and health equity. It improves accountability of policymakers for health impacts at all levels of policy-making. It includes an emphasis on the consequences of public policies on health systems, determinants of health and well-being.

We recognize that governments have a range of priorities in which health and equity do not automatically gain precedence over other policy objectives. We call on them to ensure that health considerations are transparently taken into account in policy-making, and to open up opportunities for co-benefits across sectors and society at large.

Policies designed to enable people to lead healthy lives face opposition from many sides. Often they are challenged by the interests of powerful economic forces that resist regulation. Business interests and market power can affect the ability of governments and health systems to promote and protect health and respond to health needs. *Health in All Policies* is a practical response to these challenges. It can provide a framework for regulation and practical tools that combine health, social and equity goals with economic development, and manage conflicts of interest transparently. These can support relationships with all sectors, including the private sector, to contribute positively to public health outcomes.

We see *Health in All Policies* as a constituent part of countries' contribution to achieving the United Nations *Millennium Development Goals* and it must remain a key consideration in the drafting of the post-2015 Development Agenda.

We, the participants of this conference

- Prioritize health and equity as a core responsibility of governments to its peoples.
- Affirm the compelling and urgent need for effective policy coherence for health and well-being.
- Recognize that this will require political will, courage and strategic foresight.

We call on governments

to fulfil their obligations to their peoples' health and well-being by taking the following actions:

- **Commit to health and health equity as a political priority** by adopting the principles of Health in All Policies and taking action on the social determinants of health.
- **Ensure effective structures, processes and resources** that enable implementation of the Health in All Policies approach across governments at all levels and between governments.
- **Strengthen the capacity of Ministries of Health to engage other sectors of government** through leadership, partnership, advocacy and mediation to achieve improved health outcomes.
- **Build institutional capacity and skills** that enable the implementation of Health in All Policies and provide evidence on the determinants of health and inequity and on effective responses.
- **Adopt transparent audit and accountability mechanisms** for health and equity impacts that build trust across government and between governments and their people.
- **Establish conflict of interest measures** that include effective safeguards to protect policies from distortion by commercial and vested interests and influence.
- **Include communities, social movements and civil society** in the development, implementation and monitoring of Health in All Policies, building health literacy in the population.

We call on WHO to

- Support Member States to put Health in All Policies into practice
- Strengthen its own capacity in Health in All Policies
- Use the Health in All Policies approach in working with United Nations agencies and other partners on the unfinished Millennium Development Goals agenda and the post-2015 Development Agenda
- Urge the United Nations family, other international organizations, multilateral development banks and development agencies to achieve coherence and synergy in their work with Member States to enable implementation of Health in All Policies

We, the participants of this conference

- Commit ourselves to communicate the key messages of this Helsinki Statement to our governments, institutions and communities.

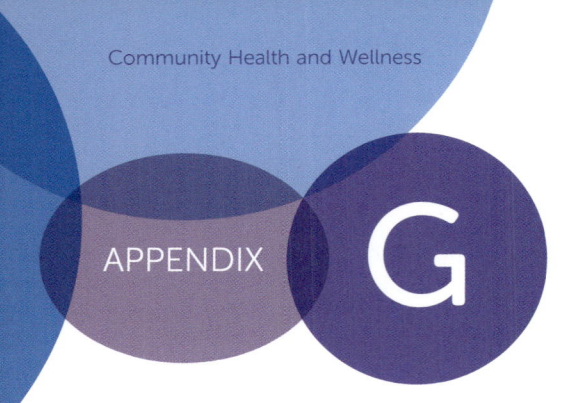

National School Nursing Professional Practice Standards

The following summary is an excerpt from *National School Nursing Professional Practice Standards*, 2nd edition, Maureen Ward, 2012 (copyright Victorian School Nurses, Australian Nursing Federation [Victorian Branch] Special Interest Group, and Australian Nursing Federation, Federal Office, 2012).

The full document, published by the Australian Nursing Federation, is available at http://anmf.org.au/pages/school-nursing-standards

Summary of professional practice domains

Domain: professional practice

Standard one

Demonstrates a comprehensive knowledge of school nursing incorporating child and adolescent health and development.

Standard two

Practises within a professional and ethical nursing framework.

Standard three

Practises in accordance with legislation related to school nursing practice and child and adolescent healthcare.

Standard four

Advocates for and protects the rights of children and young people.

Standard five

Effectively manages human and material resources.

Domain: provision and coordination of care

Standard six

Effectively addresses the healthcare needs of students and groups considering a whole of school community approach.

Standard seven

Coordinates, organises and provides health promotion considering a whole of school community approach.

Standard eight

Contributes to the maintenance of a healthy work and learning environment that is respectful, safe and supportive of students and the school community.

Domain: collaborative and therapeutic practice

Standard nine

Uses a range of effective communication skills.

Standard ten

Engages in collaborative practice to provide comprehensive school nursing care.

Domain: critical thinking and analysis

Standard eleven

Participates in ongoing professional development of self and others.

Standard twelve

Identifies the relevance of research in improving individual student and whole of school community health outcomes.

Australian Family Strengths Nursing Assessment Guide

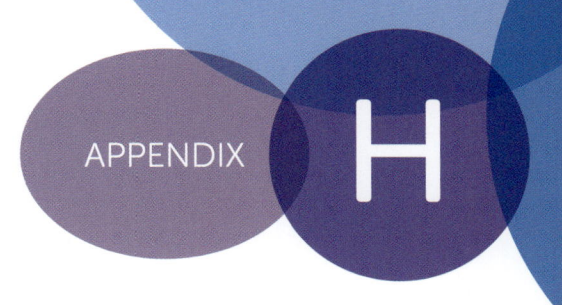

APPENDIX H

Family strength	Strength (S) or growth (G) area and comments

Togetherness
- In your family, what shared beliefs really matter to you?
- Do you share beliefs that really matter that you would like to follow during this admission/time of health care?
- What are some of the things that cause you to celebrate together?
- Can you tell me about some of your family's shared memories?

Sharing activities
- When does the family spend time together?
- How often would you play together as a family?
- Can you tell me about when you have good times together in your family?

Affection
- How do you show your love for each other?
- How would others know you care about each other?
- If I were to ask your best friend about how you care about each other, what would they say?
- What sorts of things do you do for each other?

Support
- Can you tell me of times when you as a family 'share the load' and help each other?
- What does it mean in your family to be 'there for each other'?
- What new things have others in your family been encouraged to try?

Communication
- What helps your family to listen to each other?
- Tell me about when you talk openly with each other.
- Can you tell me about some of the times when you laugh together?

Family strength	Strength (S) or growth (G) area and comments

Acceptance

- In what ways does your family accept your individual differences?
- When are you most likely to give each other space?
- How do you show the members of your family that you respect each other's point of view?
- What does 'forgiveness of each other' look like in your family?
- What different responsibilities do each of you have?

Commitment

- What helps you feel safe and secure with each other?
- Can you list some of the things your family does for your community?
- What rules do you have in your family and how should these be followed during this admission?

Resilience

- In what ways has this admission changed your plans?
- What helps keep each other hopeful?
- Can you tell me about when your family pulled together in a crisis?
- When you have a problem, what helps you discuss your problems?
- What do other people say they admire in your family?

Spiritual wellbeing

It is recommended that, with families who share beliefs that really matter to them, these further question/s are asked:

- Is spiritual wellbeing an important strength for your family?
- What do you do as a family to maintain your spiritual wellbeing?
- Would you like help to maintain any of your spiritual activities during this admission/time of health care?

The AFS Nursing Assessment Guide was developed by L Smith (2008) with permission from *Our scrapbook of strengths* (Family Action Centre and St Luke's Innovative Resources, 2003), using the language that Australian families use when talking about their own family and updated in 2013. The spiritual wellbeing section was added following evaluation of v1 and recent research evidence highlighting the positive impact of spiritual wellbeing on healthy outcomes.

ARACY Call to Action: Transforming Australia for Our Children's Future

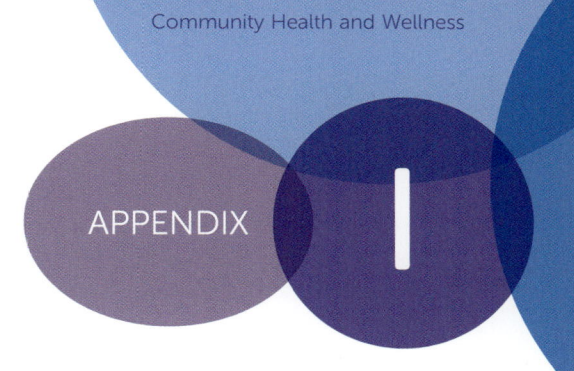

APPENDIX I

ARACY 2009 Conference declaration and call to action

From 2 to 4 September 2009 more than 560 delegates joined the Australian Research Alliance for Children and Youth in Melbourne to examine the theme 'Transforming Australia for our children's future: making prevention work'.

Eminent speakers at the ARACY conference discussed the urgent need to transform Australia into a society that truly nurtures and respects children and young people, to improve their wellbeing and prevent the problems that are increasingly affecting them.

The conference concluded with delegates showing overwhelming support for the following Declaration and call to action to the entire Australian community—to the Australian Government; to state, territory and local governments; and to community and business leaders.

ARACY is taking the Declaration to federal, state and territory governments, local governments and community leaders and organisations around the country. We welcome the use of the Declaration by community organisations, governments and business committed to improve the wellbeing of children and young people. If you are using the Declaration or would like more information, please contact ARACY.

We, the delegates to the national conference of the Australian Research Alliance for Children and Youth held in Melbourne from 2 to 4 September 2009,

- representing a wide range of research, policy and community interests and perspectives
- believing that Australia must raise its international standing on child and youth wellbeing to match the best of the Organisation for Economic Co-operation and Development (OECD) countries
- confident that by working together to transform Australia into a society that truly values, nurtures and respects children and young people, we can create a community with a greater sense of

wellbeing where all children and young people can thrive and achieve their potential

have agreed on the following Declaration as a call to the entire Australian community and to all levels of government, to take action to change Australia to improve the wellbeing of our children and young people.

Principles for action

Action to improve the wellbeing of Australia's children and young people must be firmly guided by the following principles:

1. All Australian children and young people have a right to the care, conditions and opportunities they need for their wellbeing and to achieve their potential.

2. Nurturing and trusting relationships with parents and carers are essential for the long-term wellbeing of children and young people.

3. The physical, social, cultural and economic environments in which children and young people live play a key role in their wellbeing.

4. Australia must urgently lower the levels of poverty and inequality to improve the wellbeing of all children and young people.

5. Children and young people have the right to be respected and heard in matters affecting their wellbeing.

6. All Australians share responsibility for the wellbeing of children and young people, and need to value the role of parents, carers, families and people who work with them.

7. Empowered, active communities working in partnership with active governments play a critical part in enhancing the wellbeing of children and young people.

8. What is good for children and young people is good for all of us. The entire Australian community bears the social and economic cost caused by preventable problems.

9 Australia must learn from cultures with a positive attitude to children and young people. We must also learn from public policies that achieve high levels of child wellbeing; adequate support for parents, carers and families; and low levels of child poverty (for example, policies in the Nordic countries).

10 Effective prevention requires a strong theoretical framework; a sound evidence base; and effective design, implementation and evaluation.

Critical issues and challenges facing Australia today

1 Relative to Organisation for Economic Co-operation and Development (OECD) standards, Australian children and young people are not faring well. This is particularly so for Indigenous children.

2 The link between poverty, inequality and poor outcomes for children is clear. One in seven Australian children live in poverty, including 50 percent of all Indigenous children.

3 Problems that are mostly preventable compromise the wellbeing of many young Australians.

4 Preventing problems is more ethical than a focus on treatment. Prevention delivers improved health and wellbeing to individuals, and social and economic benefits to the community. However funding for prevention remains only a fraction of recurrent funding for treatment.

5 A strong and effective preventive approach requires a major change in the way we operate. Practice, policy and research, and also governments and non-government funders, need to adopt preventive approaches and longer timeframes to achieve sustainable outcomes.

6 Many initiatives by the Australian Government, states and territories and not-for-profits are building blocks contributing to the wellbeing of children and young people. We will be successful if we sustain the current momentum towards change over the long term, with better integration of initiatives and effective collaboration across sectors and disciplines.

Four key strategies for action

Four key strategies will address these challenges and improve the wellbeing of Australia's children and young people.

Strategy 1: Make the wellbeing of children and young people a national priority.

• Critical elements—whole-of-nation social change is the key to advancing the prevention agenda to reduce the level of problems affecting children and young people.

The critical elements of a social change strategy are:

(a) achieving widespread public agreement that the entire community shares responsibility for the wellbeing of children and young people

(b) increasing the value Australians place on children, young people and those who care for them

(c) empowering and supporting parents and carers, increasing their confidence and competence

(d) empowering communities to form local partnerships to improve the wellbeing of children and young people

(e) ensuring that every government department, every organisation, every profession, every business, and every local community group thinks about and acts with the wellbeing of children in mind, and

(f) listening to the voices of children and young people.

• Who should take action?—The Australian community, in partnership with business, non-government organisations and all levels of government. ARACY is asking the Australian Government to take leadership by supporting ARACY's national strategy for social change. This comprehensive strategy involves all sections of the community. It promotes a long-term, integrated program of public information; coordination of existing and new initiatives; and partnerships (national and local) between communities, non-government organisations, business and government to increase the wellbeing of children and young people.

• Timeframe—Action must start immediately and will need to be sustained over at least 10 to 15 years to achieve lasting social change.

Strategy 2: Set internationally comparable health and wellbeing targets for children and young people for the next 20 years.

Critical elements of this strategy are:

(a) adopting international indicators and gathering the data required to ensure Australia can fully participate in international comparisons of child wellbeing

(b) raising Australia's international standing to high levels of child and youth wellbeing, to match the levels achieved by the Nordic countries (as determined by the OECD report Doing better for children or similar indicators), and

(c) listening to the voices of children and young people.

- Who should take action?—The Australian Government and its statutory agencies such as the Australian Institute for Health and Welfare and the Australian Bureau of Statistics, in consultation with relevant non-government organisations.
- Timeframe—From September 2009.

Strategy 3: Agree on a national child and youth development agenda integrating existing early years, middle years and youth agendas.

Critical elements of this strategy are:

(a) ensuring a whole-of-government approach to children and young people

(b) integrating child-focused programs

(c) supporting parents, carers and families, and promoting their key role for the wellbeing of children and young people

(d) achieving an effective balance between targeted prevention (focused on single issues or risk groups) and holistic (primary prevention) approaches

(e) developing, supporting and retaining workers to enable them to deliver the national agenda

(f) assessing all government policies for 'child and youth impact' before implementing, and

(g) listening to the voices of children and young people.

- Who should take action?—Collaboration between the Australian and state/territory governments, Council of Australian Governments (COAG), and non-government organisations, building on and integrating existing government initiatives such as COAG's National Early Childhood Development Strategy—Investing in the Early Years, the Office for Youth's Work and the Social Inclusion Agenda.
- Timeframe—A meeting should be convened in March 2010 to discuss broad parameters with government, non-government and business; and the aim should be to finalise the national agenda by the end of 2010.

Strategy 4: Develop a collaborative research plan on the prevention of problems affecting children and young people, linked with the child and youth development agenda.

Critical elements of this strategy are:

(a) achieving a better understanding of causal pathways to problem outcomes and developing effective preventive interventions to tackle them

(b) increasing our knowledge on dissemination, implementation and evaluation of preventive strategies in 'real world' situations

(c) building the evidence base on what works for priority areas (e.g. Aboriginal populations), and

(d) listening to the voices of children and young people.

- Who should take action?—Collaborations of researchers, practitioners and policy-makers; for example, ARACY's Prevention Science Network.
- Timeframes—The research plan should be finalised by the end of 2010.

For more information, contact ARACY:

Email: enquiries@aracy.org.au

Phone:

Canberra	Melbourne	Sydney	Perth
02 6232 4503	03 9345 5145	02 9085 7247	08 9476 7800

September 2009

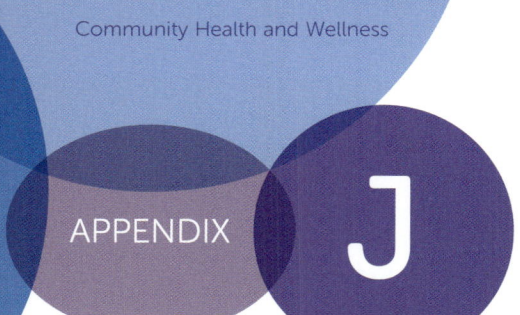

HEEADSSS Assessment Tool for Use with Adolescents

A psychosocial assessment of young people is equally as important as a physical assessment. The following tool is based on Goldenring & Cohen's (1988), Goldenring's (2004), and the Ministry of Health New Zealand (2002) HEEADSSS method of interviewing. HEEADSSS stands for **H**ome, **E**ducation/ employment, **E**ating, peer group **A**ctivities, **D**rugs, **S**exuality, **S**uicide/depression, and **S**afety. We suggest that you also consider exploring the adolescent's level of community involvement as this may be an area of strength for the individual or an area where support can be found.

We recommend you undertake formal training in the use of the HEEADSSS assessment tool prior to use.

Goldenring J 2004 Getting inside adolescents heads: an essential update. Contemporary Pediatrics

Goldenring J, Cohen E 1988 Getting into adolescents' heads. Contemporary Paediatrics: 75–90

Ministry of Health New Zealand 2002 Family Violence Intervention Guidelines: Child and Partner Abuse. Ministry of Health, Wellington

Home

In home we cover family, culture and connections, looking for both resiliency and risk issues.

- Where do you live? Who do you live with?
- Ask about extended family links and culture—iwi, hapu, whanau, tribe.
- Where were you born? How long have you been here?
- Do you belong to a church? What activities and length of time have you been involved with the church?
- Do you have jobs or responsibilities at your place?
- Who makes the rules? What happens if rules are broken?
- What happens when you fight at your house?
- Is there any violence occurring at your house?

- Who in your family do you get along well with? Not so well?
- Who is the person who you talk to most?

Education

- Do you go to school/training course/work?
- If no—how long have you been out of school/ work? Why? Plans? What do you do with your time now?
- If yes—which school? What is good about school? Not so good?
- Do you have friends at school? Is there a teacher you get along well with?
- How do you do in your school work and classes?
- Do you have ideas about what you might like to do when you leave school?
- Do you miss much school? Why?
- Are you bullied at school?

Eating

- What do you like and not like about your body?
- Have there been any recent changes in your diet?
- Have you dieted in the last year? How? How often?
- Have you done anything else to try to manage your weight?
- How much exercise do you get in an average day? Week?
- What do you think would be a healthy diet? How does that compare to your current eating patterns?

Activities

Here we cover what you do; for example, with your friends, with your family and in your community.

- What do you and your friends do for fun? (With whom, where and when?)

- What do you and your family do for fun? (With whom, where and when?)
- Do you participate in any sports or other activities?
- Do you regularly attend a church group, club or other organised activity?
- Are you involved in any community activities?
- How do you get money?
- How do you get around? Do you drive sometimes?
- What about sleeping? Do you sleep well?

Drugs/Alcohol

Introduce, for example, 'We know that many young people try alcohol and drugs; is it all right if I ask you some questions about that now?'

- Do young people at your school smoke? Do your friends smoke? Do you smoke?
- Do your friends/parents ever drink alcohol? Do you?
- Have you ever used marijuana? What other drugs/solvents are young people using these days?
- What do you think about that? What have you tried?
- If the young person is using:
    ○ How much are you using? In what circumstances? What do you like and not like about using?
    ○ What risks do you take when using? Have you ever considered using less?

Sexuality

Introduce, for example, 'We ask everyone about sexuality because that is a very important aspect of young people's lives and can affect their health so much. Is that OK with you? You can "pass" on questions if you want to.'

- Have you had any sexuality education at school? What was that like?
- Do your friends have sexual relationships? Do you?
- Are any of them wondering about sexual orientation—liking girls or boys? Are you?
- What do you know about safe sex?
- What do you do (in terms of keeping sexually safe)? Do you use condoms? How much of the time (every time, just when you can get them, sometimes)?
- What could you do if you thought you might be pregnant?

- Has anybody ever touched you in a way that you don't like?
- If you ever felt uncomfortable or something unpleasant happened to you, is there anyone that you could tell?
- Are there adults you can go to for advice/help about sex and relationships?
- Do you want to talk about anything else about relationships or sex?

Suicide and Depression

In this we cover issues of mental health and self-harm.

- How would you describe your mood/feelings most of the time? (Scale 1–10)
- Do you have really good/bad times?

If low mood is an issue, review sleeping, eating, energy, concentration, feelings of guilt/worthlessness and safety.

- Do you ever have worries or hassles that bother you?

If yes:

- Do they keep you awake at night?
- Do you have to do anything to keep them under control?
- Do you sometimes feel that life is not worth it?
- Have you ever harmed yourself deliberately?

If no, you may not need to continue this line of questioning.

- Have you ever thought of ending your pain once and for all?
- Do you know anyone who has died from suicide? Who? When?
- How often do you think about doing it? How did you think you would do it?
- How strong are these feelings for you at the moment?
- Do you think you might try?
- What if something went wrong for you? (Relationship break-up, etc.)
- Who could you tell about feeling suicidal?

Regarding previous suicidal behaviour:

- What did they do? How many times? How long ago? What happened?
- How do they feel about the fact that they did not die?
- Do they wish they had died?
- Have things changed since then? What?
- Do they think that they might try again?

Safety

- Have you ever been seriously injured? How? How about anyone else you know?
- Do you always wear a seatbelt in the car?
- Have you ever ridden with a driver who was drunk or high? When? How often?
- Do you use safety equipment for sports and/or other physical activities (e.g. helmets for biking or skateboarding)?
- Is there any violence in your home?
- Does the violence ever get physical?
- Is there a lot of violence at your school? In your neighbourhood? Among your friends?
- Have you ever been physically or sexually abused? Have you ever been raped on a date or at any other time?
- Have you ever been in a car or motorbike accident? (What happened?)
- Have you ever been picked on or bullied? Is that still a problem?
- Have you gotten into any physical fights in school or in your neighbourhood? Do you still feel that way?
- Have you ever felt like you needed to carry a knife, gun or other weapon to protect yourself? Do you still feel that way?

Ecomap

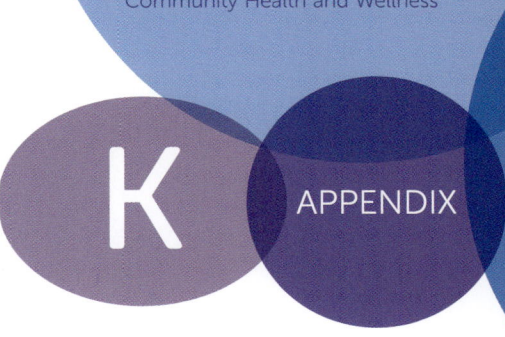

School

Work

Church

FAMILY

Friends

Extended
family

Key

══════	Strong
- - - -	Tenuous
+++++	Stressful
⟶	Energy flow

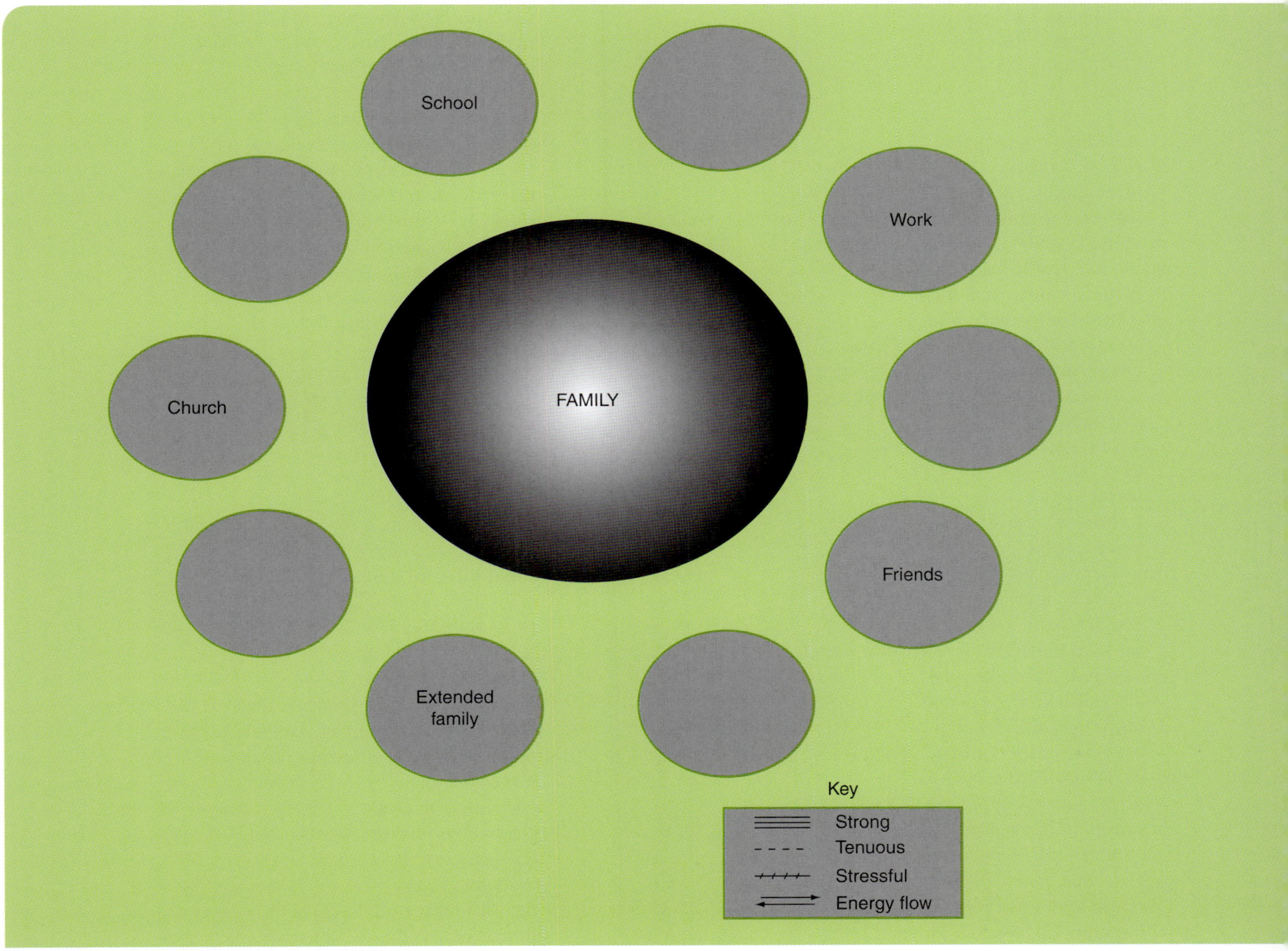

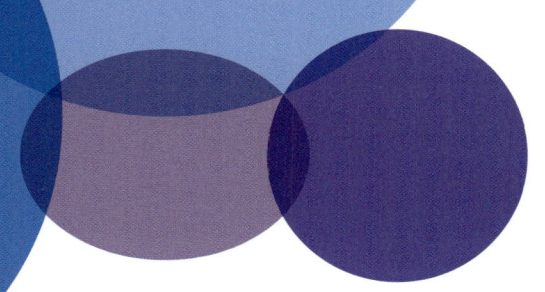

Index

Page numbers followed by "f" indicate figures, "t" indicate tables, and "b" indicate boxes.

548